Handbook of Neurologic Rating Scales

Second Edition

Handbook of Neurologic Rating Scales

Second Edition

Edited by

Robert M. Herndon, M.D.

Demos

Demos Medical Publishing, LLC, 386 Park Avenue South, New York, New York 10016

Visit our Web site at http://www.demosmedpub.com

Library of Congress Cataloging-in-Publication Data

Handbook of neurologic rating scales / edited by Robert M. Herndon.—2nd ed.
      p. ; cm.
  Includes bibliographical references and index.
  ISBN 1-888799-92-7
  1. Neurologic examination—Handbooks, manuals, etc. 2. Psychiatric rating scales —
Handbooks, manuals, etc.
  [DNLM: 1. Nervous System Diseases—diagnosis. 2. Neurologic Examination—methods. 3. Psychological Tests. WL 141 H23648 2006] I. Herndon, Robert M.
  RC348.H296 2006
  616.8'0475—dc22
               2005028798

Made in the United States of America

To access the downloadable PDFs that come with your purchase of this title, please go to:

www.demosmedpub.com/neuroscales.html

and use the word "scales" when prompted for a password.

Contents

To access the downloadable PDFs that come with your purchase of this title, please go to:

www.demosmedpub.com/neuroscales.html

and use the word "scales" when prompted for a password.

Foreword

In an earlier era, clinicians in neurology had their own personal approach for measuring the changes in the patients before them. These were not only personal approaches, but also the clinicians were very proud of their innovative ways to elucidate the nature and course of neurologic disease. Their students would learn their methods and apply these in their practice and teaching. There was no consistency across neurology, even though some of these personal methods, often named after the clinician, became widely known.

In the post–World War II era, large case series and early clinical trials became more frequent and increasingly structured. Slowly, the need for consistency in the use of the measurement tools became recognized. If a group of clinicians in North America were studying progression in multiple sclerosis or amyotrophic lateral sclerosis or dementia, they needed to recognize the similarities and the differences in their results when compared to the studies being done in Sweden or Australia using other methods of measurement for the same condition. Different scales for measuring the progress of dementia, for example, may measure different things and have varying results depending on at what stage and in what circumstances they are used. It does not mean that there could not be many scales, but it was necessary to know what each assesses best, their advantages and disadvantages, and whether they had been validated in various situations.

The first edition of Robert M. Herndon's *Handbook of Neurologic Rating Scales* quickly became an invaluable reference work on the increasing array of scales for measuring neurologic disease. Since the first edition, the importance of this book has only increased. When Herndon and his coauthors brought together under one cover a collection of the most used and validated scales, clinicians had a convenient reference source for the design of clinical trials and also an aid to understanding the increasing literature of clinical trials in neurology.

Having completed the initial ground-breaking work, they recognized the need for a new edition to add the increased experience and understanding of current scales, the adaptations and variations on older scales, and to incorporate the new scales since the first edition appeared in 1997.

Dr. Herndon has a long experience caring for neurologic patients and in the design, organization, and management of clinical trials in neurology. He has brought together other experts on aspects of pediatric and adult neurology, symptom management, and rehabilitation to provide clinicians with a timely and expanded reference source on the many rating scales used in neurology.

The publication of the initial edition of this work was a major contribution to the neurologic literature, and this edition is even more useful and helpful to clinicians and researchers in the efforts to advance knowledge of neurologic disease and bring advances in treatment and care to those who suffer from neurologic disease. It is in the interest of these patients and their families that this difficult and exacting work is being done.

Jock Murray, M.D.
Professor of Medicine (Neurology)
Professor of Medical Humanities
Dalhousie University
Halifax, Nova Scotia
Canada

Preface

Advances in the treatment of diseases of the nervous system continue to depend on careful measurement of the results of treatment. The number of clinical trials has been steadily increasing for at least a half century. The number and quality of measurement tools needed to conduct clinical trials continues to develop at a rapid pace. In the 8 years since the first edition of this book, numerous new scales have appeared. To accommodate these developments, we have added new chapters, including chapters on general use scales, ataxia scales, and peripheral nerve scales and have updated and expanded most of the chapters.

Most drugs used to treat neurologic disease are, at best, partially effective. Advances are made incrementally, and, as treatment improves, new drugs and combinations need to be compared to older therapies. This requires even more precise and accurate measurement than that required for placebo-controlled trials, because differences between groups are likely to be much smaller. This volume provides a review of some of the tools used to compare different therapies for a variety of neurologic diseases in formal trials and for outcomes research.

The prevalence and economic consequences of neurologic disease continue to increase steadily. One unfortunate economic consequence of the partially effective therapies common in neurologic diseases is that treatment goes on for longer periods of time—many years or even decades. In addition, the prevalence of chronic neurologic disease increases with age, and our population is aging. Thus, the expense of neurologic care can be expected to continue to increase. On the positive side, many of those with chronic neurologic disease are able to continue productive work much longer than they could previously.

Understanding the qualities of a scale is important not only for those planning clinical trials but also for clinicians who wish to interpret trials reported in the literature and who want to compare treatments reported using different scales. Scales vary enormously in complexity, precision, and reliability. Precision and reliability, in large part, determine the number of patients needed in a clinical trial and are important for interpreting results of a trial. Too much precision may detect statistical differences between treatments that are clinically insignificant, whereas too little precision may result in failure to detect clinically important differences.

Clinical trials are the basis for evidence-based medicine. Medical care is becoming increasingly evidence-based, although much of medicine remains empiric. With the development of new, better, and more precisely targeted medications, the quality of evidence needed to obtain approval by the U.S. Food and Drug Administration and other similar organizations has also increased. Bringing a new medication to market requires much more study, more extensive trials, and better documentation of results than ever before. The cost of developing a new medication is now approaching $1 billion. On the other hand, we know much more about the new medications and their side effects and risks, as well as their benefits, but, also, we see a corresponding increase in cost.

One factor that helps to control the cost of new medications is development of better, more precise scales. In pilot trials, scales can often demonstrate sufficient benefit to warrant further development or, alternatively, insufficient promise to warrant further expenditure. As a result, we see continuing development of better and more efficient scales in neurology.

Inevitably, in a volume such as this, some important developments are left out. There are far too many scales to include them all. We have had to be selective but have endeavored to include the most important, widely used, and validated scales. We trust that this text proves valuable to those planning clinical trials and those who wish to have a better understanding of the meaning of trials.

Robert M. Herndon, M.D.
Jackson, MS
August 2005

Contributors

Benjamin Rix Brooks, M.D.
Department of Neurology
William S. Middleton Memorial VA Hospital
Madison, Wisconsin

Roger A. Brumback, M.D.
Departments of Pathology and Psychiatry
Creighton University Medical Center
Omaha, Nebraska

Richard Camicioli, M.D.
Department of Medicine
Division of Neurology
University of Alberta
Alberta, Edmonton
Canada

James J. Cereghino, M.D.
Department of Neurology
Oregon Health and Science University
Portland, Oregon

Wayne M. Clark, M.D.
Department of Neurology
Oregon Health Science and University
Portland, Oregon

Gary Cutter, Ph.D.
Department of Biostatistics
University of Alabama
School of Public Health
Birmingham, Alabama

Domenic Esposito, M.D.
Department of Neurosurgery
The University of Mississippi
  Medical Center
Jackson, Mississippi

Stephen T. Gancher, M.D.
Department of Neurology
Kaiser Permanente
Portland, Oregon

Michelle D. Gaugh, M.A.
Department of Neurology
University of Rochester Medical Center
Rochester, New York

Samuel T. Gontkovsky, Psy.D.
Center for Neuroscience and
  Neurological Recovery
Methodist Rehabilitation Center
Jackson, Mississippi

Jeffrey I. Greenstein, M.D.
Multiple Sclerosis Research Institute
Philadelphia, Pennsylvania

Cathy F. Hansen, M.S., P.T.
Department of Rehabilitation Services
The University of Mississippi
  Medical Center
Jackson, Mississippi

Robert M. Herndon, M.D.
Department of Neurology
G.V.(Sonny) Montgomery VAMC
Jackson, Mississippi

J. Maurice Hourihane, M.B., M.R.C.P.I.
Dent Neurologic Institute
Amherst, New York

Edward L. Manning, Ph.D.
Department of Neurology
The University of Mississippi Medical Center
Jackson, Mississippi

Risa Nakase-Richardson, Ph.D.
Neuropsychology Department
Brain Injury Program
Methodist Rehabilitation Center
Jackson, Mississippi

Elcio J. Piovesan, M.D
Department of Internal Medicine
Division of Neurology
Hospital de Clinicas
  da Universidade Federal do Parana
Curitiba, Brazil

Giovanni Schifitto, M.D.
Department of Neurology
University of Rochester Medical Center
Rochester, New York

Stephen D. Silberstein, M.D.
Department of Neurology
  and Jefferson Headache Center
Thomas Jefferson University
Philadelphia, Pennsylvania

Raphael Corcoran Sneed, M.D.
Children's Rehabilitation Service
Department of Pediatrics
The University of Mississippi Medical Center
Jackson, Mississippi

Frances Spinosa, R.N.
Department of Neurosurgery
The University of Mississippi Medical Center
Jackson, Mississippi

Charles F. Swearingen, B.S.
Brain Injury Program
Methodist Rehabilitation Center
Jackson, Mississippi

Katherine Wild, Ph.D.
Department of Neurology
  and Layton Aging and Alzheimer's Disease Center
Oregon Health and Science University
Portland, Oregon

1

Introduction to Clinical Neurologic Scales

Robert M. Herndon, M.D., and Gary Cutter, Ph.D.

"One's knowledge of science begins when he can measure what he is speaking about and express it in numbers." *Lord Nelson*

Clinical trials invariably require measurement of the effect of a medication or procedure on a disease process. Measurement of the effects of neurologic disease and of the effect of treatment on the disease requires appropriate tools. In general, these tools are scales in one form or another. Scales to measure neurologic disease began to appear around 1950, but the number and variety of neurologic scales have increased dramatically since the early 1980s. Medicine is progressively changing from the empirical art it was at the beginning of the twentieth century to an information-based, more scientific enterprise.

A surprising amount of medical therapy remains empirical, but the change to evidence-based medicine is accelerating. Much of the change is due to U.S. Food and Drug Administration (FDA) requirements, which require quantifiable evidence of efficacy and/or effectiveness, and some is related to the continu-ing increase in medical costs and the pressures to establish the effectiveness and the cost effectiveness of medications and procedures. It is also driven by the desire of physicians and others to improve care. Controlled clinical trials and outcomes research are at the heart of information-based medicine. Unlike treatments for blood pressure or survival times for cancers, which are easily defined and measurable, neurology is often focused on the constellation of effects produced. Thus, neurologic scales are essential tools in clinical trials designed to provide the information for improved care. As much as clinicians may dislike the idea, if it cannot be demonstrated objectively that treatment is effective, it will not be reimbursed. Even effective therapies are likely to fall by the wayside if studies to prove their effectiveness are not done.

The earliest reported controlled trial appears to be that of Dr. James Lind (Bollet, 1987). In 1747, he assessed the value of various popular remedies for scurvy aboard a Royal Navy ship. He took 12 scorbutic sailors and put them all on the same diet with the exception of the experimental treatment. He put two each on the following remedies:

1. A quart of cider a day
2. Twenty-five drops of vitriol three times a day
3. Two spoonfuls of vinegar three times a day on an empty stomach
4. Two spoonfuls of vinegar three times a day with vinegar used to spice their food
5. A half pint of sea water a day
6. Two oranges and one lemon a day

The result was that, after 6 days, one of those who had received the oranges and lemon was back at work and the other much improved. Those who received the cider were a little better, and the others were not improved. Given the dramatic response, one wonders if a controlled trial was really necessary, but despite the obvious effectiveness of the therapy, it was decades before it was widely used even in the Royal Navy. Of interest is the fact that prevention of scurvy in the Royal Navy had a major impact on the Battle of Trafalgar. The British fleet had been at sea long enough that the opposing forces expected the British sailors to have diminished effectiveness because of the well-known extremely high frequency of scurvy after long periods at sea and its profound effect on the crews.

In the trial by Lind, the outcome was really return to work and improvement in the condition of the sailor. The outcome was judged solely by the author. Today, clinicians and the FDA require defined criteria to judge improvement and objective criteria defining return to work.

Many principles of clinical trials were being formulated in the medical literature, changing from the dogma of the authoritarian approaches of Galen to a more outcome-oriented profession. By the early 1900s, a more formal approach to outcomes was evolving. In 1910, the Flexner report (Flexner, 1910) cited the need for outcomes to be measured. Codman, a surgeon, in 1914 wrote that treatments should be analyzed systematically, followed long enough to determine success, and if not, why not (Codman, 1914). Controlled trials remained rare and did not become common until after World War II. At that time, with the expansion of the National Institutes of Health and its training and research grant programs, controlled trials became more common. Three seminal trials, the sulfa drug trials in 1948 in Britain, the streptomycin trial (*BMJ* 1998), and in 1956 one of the largest trials ever undertaken in the United States, the Salk polio vaccine trials (Francis et al., 1955), were initiated. This trial used the incidence of polio to confirm the benefits of vaccination and involved large numbers of children randomized to pla-

cebo or the Salk vaccine. The success in demonstrating conclusively the benefits of vaccination had a great impact on medical practice as well as the approach to establishing effectiveness. Clinical trials received added impetus in the late 1960s after the Kefauver committee report with changes in the FDA, which included the requirement that efficacy as well as safety be established before a new drug could be approved for marketing. Before this time, only safety had to be determined, as established by changes in the agency in the 1930s.

The number of controlled trials of new therapies for agents affecting neurologic function has expanded exponentially since 1970, with the explosion of new information in immunology and transmitter/receptor physiology, chemistry, and now the information from the Human Genome Project. New medications are now usually rationally designed for a specific mode of action rather than developed empirically. With this enormous expansion, a plethora of new scales to measure neurologic function have been and continue to be developed. These range from very simple and straightforward scales that directly measure the function of interest, such as the ambulation index, to scales quite remote from the pathology such as quality-of-life scales. Some are well-designed and carefully validated, whereas others are used without much thought as to what is actually being measured, the efficiency or reliability of the measurement, or the validity of the scale being used.

The purpose of this book is to provide a resource for clinicians and clinical investigators in the broad field of neurology and neurologic rehabilitation to help them (1) evaluate the clinical trials literature by providing information on the scales being used, (2) evaluate and select appropriate and efficient scales for clinical trials and outcomes research and to monitor their patients, and (3) provide information that helps them to develop new scales or measures or to improve existing ones.

This is not a clinical trials book, and the reader is referred to some of the excellent books on trial design and methodology such as Meinert's (1986) *Clinical Trials, Design, Conduct and Analysis*; Friedman and colleague's (1996) *Fundamentals of Clinical Trials*; Stuart Pocock's (1984) *Clinical Trials*; or Meier's (1975) Statistics and Medical Experimentation for further information regarding trial design and planning. Nevertheless, to understand the purposes and uses of neurologic scales, it is necessary to understand some of the basics of clinical trials.

Outcomes research involves the systematic comparison of pre-existing risk factors, treatment, and outcome. This has been done very effectively with some surgical procedures, such as coronary artery bypass grafts and balloon angioplasty, for which programs have been developed that assess risk factors and predict outcome. With these programs, because of the large number of patients undergoing these procedures, it is possible to put in such factors as age, weight, cardiac ejection fraction, diabetes, smoking, and so forth and derive an overall risk of various surgical complications. Although generally more difficult to do in neurologic disease, it is being done in a variety of illnesses and injuries, particularly head and spine trauma and stroke. Outcomes research is also very important in establishing the effectiveness and cost-effectiveness of various approaches to rehabilitation in neurologic disease. The difficulty here is the fact that comparing processes of treatment such as rehabilitation becomes complex when trying to decide the value of any particular part of the process.

There are many types of clinical trials. The most common are (1) open trials, in which both the patient and investigator know what each patient is receiving, (2) single-blind trials, in which the investigator knows what treatment the patient is receiving but the patient does not know, (3) double-blind trials, in which neither the patient nor the investigator knows who is receiving which treatment, and (4) modified double-blind trials, in which the patient and an examining physician do not know what the patient is receiving but there is a monitor or treating physician who either knows from the outset what the patient is receiving or who, because of the drug side effects or laboratory abnormalities, is in a position to make an educated guess as to who is receiving which therapy. Although many trials are placebo-controlled, when an effective treatment already exists, comparison trials are more usual, and these also can be open or blinded.

Open trials are often used early in the investigation of a new drug in what are commonly known as *phase I trials* or *early phase II*. Here the investigator is trying to determine dose and safety, whether or not there is enough indication of efficacy to warrant further trial, and what dosage might be both safe and effective. Open trials may also be used after definitive trials to continue to assess safety and toxicity in a larger population than that in the initial trial to detect rare side effects and/or complications before or, more commonly, after marketing, known as *postmarket surveillance*. Sometimes, single-blind trials are used in phase I, often with a crossover design. This can help to adjust for placebo effects and suggestibility and may give a clearer picture of the nature of the drug effects and nature and severity of side effects. Furthermore, it

enables the investigator to explain that each patient will receive active drug for some period of time. Although, when one is dealing with a drug that is clearly rapidly curative, as with penicillin for lobar pneumonia, one may not need a controlled trial to establish effectiveness, but it is likely that the FDA will require a clinical trial to demonstrate the claim. However, when dealing with therapies that have a palliative or a limited effect in a chronic disease or when comparing two treatments of somewhat similar effectiveness, controlled trials become essential.

Phase II trials are designed to demonstrate safety and show at least a hint of efficacy and are typically *double-blind* or *double masked*. These are typically larger than phase I trials and may provide clear evidence of efficacy; however, they generally lack the power to provide definitive evidence of efficacy. Their main purpose is to demonstrate relative safety and to provide information for the design of definitive trials. Blinding, or masking, is a key element to obtaining objective results. Although it is antithetical for medicine to deliver therapies unknown to the provider, observing responses and evaluating safety void of preconceived biases is essential. Blinding patients and clinicians to which treatment a patient is receiving can be an important part of assessing results. To do this in an ethical manner, all treatments must be clearly defined and identified to both the clinicians and the patients. Both must be assured that adequate monitoring will occur so that if efficacy is clearly demonstrated, the study will be terminated and the patients on the inferior treatment offered effective therapy. Similarly if a therapy is harmful, the study will be terminated and both the provider and patients notified and more effective or less harmful therapy offered. These assurances are no longer merely implicit in clinical trials, but structurally and legally mandated.

Phase III trials, often referred to as *pivotal trials*, are larger trials designed to establish both safety and efficacy and are generally required for FDA approval. These trials are almost invariably double-blind or modified double-blind, placebo-controlled trials. From a statistical perspective, it is easier to show efficacy against no treatment or a treatment using a placebo (mimicking all components of the therapy without using the active agents). This presents an ethical problem in many instances in which there are already partially effective therapies. Is it ethical to fail to treat a multiple sclerosis patient with the best current therapy or to use placebo in a seriously ill schizophrenic so the clinician can compare no treatment with a new drug? Is it ethical to do a placebo-controlled trial in the case of malignancies for which there are treatments that are known to prolong survival? In many cases, the authors believe a comparison trial with best current therapy would be both more ethical and provide as good or better evidence of the drugs effectiveness, but these studies require larger sample sizes and/or longer duration to establish the results.

Irrespective of the nature of the trial, the outcome must be defined before commencing the trial. Objective end points, such as death, reduction in blood pressure, and so forth, are much easier to define in this manner. Scales are often used when such outcomes are not available or pertinent. The World Health Organization has developed a system of classification of diseases that is extensive and detailed, International Classification of Functioning, Disability and Health 2. Although it has its uses, it also has serious limitations. Its main applicability is in the area of rehabilitation, and clinical research in the area of rehabilitation usually should take account of the classification. Nevertheless, in the opinion of the authors, *the most important question in designing or choosing a scale is how well it is suited to the task at hand in terms of validity, efficiency, sensitivity, and specificity*, not how well it agrees with this or some other theoretical construct.

World Health Organization Classification: "International Classification of Functioning, Disability and Health"

The International Classification of Functioning, Disability and Health 2 is a detailed numerical classification system that resembles the International Classification of Diseases Revision 10 and is intended to be complementary to it. It is far too extensive and complex to be adequately covered in this volume. It is an attempt to combine the medical model of disability with the social model. It is likely that it will have increasing application and relevance to the classification of disability and handicap and has limited relevance to clinical trials outside the area of rehabilitation where ability to function in the community and limitations imposed by the community come into play. For clinical trials in neurology and for outcomes research, it makes sense to use the simplest and most efficient measure that accomplishes the task.

In some situations, it may be desirable to use a direct measure of physical impairment, but it is often far more efficient to use surrogate measures in the form of a few simple, timed functional tests. The Multiple Sclerosis

Functional Composite scale was developed as a more quantitative scale than the Kurtzke Expanded Disability Status Scale (EDSS) (Kurtzke, 1983). It consists of timed 25-foot walk, the Nine Hole Peg Test, and the Paced Auditory Serial Addition Test. It is much more precise and reliable than the EDSS and at the same time is more sensitive to change. It is, however, subject to controversy in that proving it is a valid surrogate requires years of experience. Furthermore, in multiple sclerosis, the outcome that the surrogate must reflect has not been sufficiently defined. Although the EDSS has become sort of a gold standard, clearly patients in the upper ranges have problems not addressed by the EDSS. Thus, defining a surrogate without a gold standard creates enormous problems in establishing a surrogate. Blood pressure has become a well-accepted surrogate for cardiovascular disease. A single elevated blood pressure is, of course, not a death sentence, but, on average, people with higher blood pressure do experience substantial increases in cardiovascular mortality. Intervening on blood pressure has been shown to lower cardiovascular mortality, and thus, it satisfies some important necessary conditions for a surrogate. The surrogate predicts the outcome usually sooner, and changing the value of the surrogate by intervening produces a consistent change in the outcome.

In multiple sclerosis, magnetic resonance imaging has been used as a more or less direct measure of pathology, but it correlates rather poorly with impairment and disability and thus is not a very satisfactory surrogate for either disability or pathology.

Characteristics of Useful Scales

A useful measure or scale should have the following characteristics:

1. It should be appropriate to the task.
2. It should be valid—that is, it should measure what it purports to measure.
3. It must be accurate. It should accurately measure what it purports to measure.
4. It must be reliably reproducible (precise).
5. It should be efficient and easy to use, with little special training.
6. It should be sensitive to change in the underlying condition yet relatively insensitive to symptom fluctuation.
7. It should be consistent over time—that is, not subject to so-called frame-of-reference shifts.

Scale Should Be Appropriate to the Task

Many scales are used for tasks other than the one for which they were designed. It would generally not be appropriate to use a handicap scale to assess pathology or to use an impairment scale to assess rehabilitation. Some scales, such as quality-of-life scales, are intended to cover a broad range of diseases or conditions. Sometimes, global measures comparing across diseases can be important such as those used to ascertain allocation of resources. Others are appropriate only for a very limited range of problems. A scale used for a purpose other than the one for which it was designed usually requires validation for the new use.

Scale Must Have Demonstrated Validity

A valid scale, or measure, is one that measures what it purports to measure. These concepts are analogous to laboratory accuracy and precision. With a laboratory test, accuracy can be measured using spiked or created samples to ensure accuracy. Precision is discussed in Scale Results Should Be Reproducible (Precise) as reliability, or the ability of the test to consistently read the same sample. Several terms are used to describe various types and aspects of validity.

Face validity is the apparent congruence between what is to be measured and the measurement. Wade (1992) has described this as the "apparent sensibility of the measure and its components." Face validity is only rarely adequate. Hauser and colleague's (1983) ambulation index has obvious face validity for the assessment of mobility. It is, in fact, a simple direct assessment of the person's mobility and requirement for mobility aids. On the other hand, the ambulation index would not have face validity as a measure of urinary function, although it might be shown to have some predictive value.

Construct validity is the extent to which results from the measure concur with results predicted from the theoretical model of how things should behave. If it is assumed that weakness and spasticity in the legs impair gait, then independent measures of strength and spasticity should correlate with gait impairment. If there is no correlation, the measure is probably not valid for the purpose intended. If the correlation is perfect, the measure is redundant. A good surrogate measure has high correlation with the expected outcome.

Criterion-related validity is the extent to which a measure agrees with some external criterion. This may be another widely accepted measure or the opinion of experts. A "gold standard" is not always available, however. For example, although the Kurtzke EDSS is widely regarded as inadequate and outdated, it remains the standard for clinical research in multiple sclerosis, and until a better measure is devised and accepted, any new proposed scale will be measured against this standard. The Multiple Sclerosis Functional Composite scale, as it goes through further development, may become the standard, but at this time still lacks wide acceptance. One problem with a faulty criterion variable is how to know if the new measure is better. If it does not agree substantially, it is likely faulty, but if it agrees too much, it cannot offer new information to displace the old "tarnished" gold standard.

Content validity is the extent to which a measure with multiple items covers all aspects of the model and avoids irrelevancies. For example, the Hauser ambulation index is a valid measure of mobility in multiple sclerosis but would not be valid as an overall measure of disability in multiple sclerosis because it ignores upper extremity function, vision, and other systems frequently affected by the disease.

Ecological validity is the validity of the measure in the context in which it is to be used. For example, the ability of a wheelchair-bound woman with multiple sclerosis to prepare a meal in a kitchen designed for the handicapped may have little validity if she has access to only a kitchen designed for the physically able that has not been modified.

Predictive validity is how well the scale measure at a prior point in time can predict future change. For example, the Multiple Sclerosis Functional Composite scale can predict the future EDSS as well or better than the EDSS itself.

Scale Results Should Be Reliable (Accurate)

Scale results should accurately measure what they purport to measure. Results should correlate with other measures of the same impairment or disability. Laboratory tests are often compared to standards and calibration samples to ensure accuracy. Scales must attempt this same targeting of results. With scales, however, clear exact values are rarely known, and validity is established comparing well-characterized groups of patients with very different stages of disease or disabilities.

Scale Results Should Be Reproducible (Precise)

The same patient, in the absence of change in the disease, should receive the same score from either the same or a different examiner. Because borders between levels on a given scale are rarely sharp, this is a difficult but important standard. Some measures such as timed gait, walking distance, requirement for walking aids, and timed upper extremity functions such as the Nine Hole Peg Test and Box and Blocks test can have clear, fairly well-defined and consistent boundaries. On the other hand, with items such as weakness or coordination scored as mild, moderate, or severe, different observers have different boundaries, and the same observer may define the boundaries differently on different days. Thus, measures that use only categories such as mild, moderate, and severe often have lower reliability than more continuous variables. Reproducibility or precision is often called *reliability*. With a laboratory test, the coefficient of variance or percent variation is often used to characterize the reliability. Tests with more than 10–15% variance are often considered poor tests or having poorer reliability.

Scale Should Be Efficient

Many measures fall by the wayside because they require too much time to administer or score. Often, a busy clinician tries to take a shortcut. For example, in the middle range of the Kurtzke EDSS, a great deal depends on how far the patient can walk without a rest. Accurate determination requires walking the patient, but it is quite common for the examiner to simply ask the patient how far he or she can walk. This is simply not adequate for a reliable determination. Even if the measure is self-administered or administered by a technician, efficiency is important. Patients do not want to spend long periods filling out questionnaires, technicians must be paid, clinical studies usually require a substantial number of patients, and time savings from using efficient measures mean that more individuals can be studied in the same time or with the same amount of money. In addition, for outcomes research for which the assessment is commonly made during a routine office visit, efficiency is imperative. Patient burden, staff burden, and documentation and process requirements should always be kept in mind when considering scales or measurements. This does not always mean that a shorter scale is better; it is merely one of the criteria that must be weighed in the selection process.

Scale Should Be Sensitive to Change in the Underlying Condition, Yet Relatively Insensitive to Day-to-Day Symptom Fluctuation

For clinical trials in chronic diseases in which change in clinical condition may occur very slowly,

sensitivity is very important. A number of studies in multiple sclerosis have failed to show an effect on disease progression despite effects on number of attacks. This is almost certainly not because there is no effect on the course of disease, but because the effect was too small to show on the Kurtzke scale which, in some parts of its range, is insensitive to small changes. This problem is also seen in other degenerative diseases such as parkinsonism, where marked fluctuation in patient performance occurs even minute to minute. In this case, the frequency and severity of the fluctuations themselves may be represented on a scale. Care must be taken to avoid identifying spurious improvement or worsening that results from fluctuation in symptoms or mere measurement rather than change in the underlying disease.

Types of Scales

The type of the scale used sets some limits on the appropriate uses of the scale. Scales may be classed as *nominal*, *ordinal*, *interval*, or *ratio*. Nominal measures are not really measures at all but represent classification. The terms *diseased* or *not diseased* are commonly used. Gender is a nominal variable. Nominal scales are useful for determining the frequency or prevalence of a particular item in a population but are not really scales in the usual sense and are not dealt with further here.

Ordinal scales are scales that produce a rank order, but the intervals on the scale may be nonuniform. Education is often recorded as an ordinal variable: less than high school, high school graduate, some college, college graduate, or higher. Most neurologic scales are ordinal scales and use relatively crude classifications without sharp borders such as absent, mild, moderate, or severe.

Likert scales are a subgroup of ordinal scales. Most readers are familiar with Likert scales from continuing education questionnaires. They consist of a series of statements, and the test taker has a series of choices expressing opinion regarding the statement. Most commonly, five levels are used—strongly agree, agree, undecided, somewhat disagree, and strongly disagree. They are usually scored numerically from 5 for strongly agree to 1 for strongly disagree. The sum of the individual scores is interpreted in terms of empiric norms. Pain scales or comfort scales are also of this type, although they are sometimes scored on a

100-point scale. Nevertheless, the meaning of 1 point on the scale may not be the same at all levels of the scale. Many laboratory scales, if put on an ordinal scale, might be normal, borderline, or abnormal. For example, diastolic blood pressure might be classified as normal (less than 90 mm Hg), mild (90–105 mm Hg), and high (more than 105 mm Hg).

Use of parametric statistics such as the t-test is often inappropriate with ordinal scales, although a perusal of the literature indicates that the Student's t-test has often been used with such scales. Generally, statistical analysis should involve nonparametric tests such as the Wilcoxon Rank Sum Test, the Mann-Whitney test, or categorical analyses using chi-square tests.

Interval scales are similar to ordinal scales but are continuous (are similar to a number line or length of a line segment), and there is a uniform distance between points (the difference between two points is essentially the same regardless of what part of the scale one is in). The difference between a 1 and a 2 on the scale should be the same as the difference between 4 and 5 or 99 and 100. A thermometer is an interval scale, as is a timed 10-meter walk or a measure of height or weight. There are few interval scales in use in neurology. Those that are used are generally timed tasks, including such items as timed gait, the Perdue Pegboard, and the Nine Hole Peg Test. Laboratory tests are often considered on an interval scale. Interval scales can also be discrete or count data. Such is the case with gadolinium-enhanced lesions on magnetic resonance imaging or the Paced Auditory Serial Addition Test, in which the score is the number of additions correctly done by the patient.

Scale Selection

Selection of a scale or scales is one of the most important steps in planning a clinical research project. The scales and the related statistical methods determine, to a very large extent, how many patients are needed to achieve a specified statistical power—that is, how likely one is to see a difference if it exists. They also determine what kind of statistics that can be used, how much time and effort will be required to gather the essential data, and how many personnel will be needed to help with the study.

In some instances, measures other than the main scale on which a trial depends are needed. For example, in the interferon beta-1a (Avonex) trial,

attack frequency was used even though the investigators considered it a poor measure. It was included because it had been used in other phase III trials and there was a need to be able to compare this trial with the interferon beta-1b (Betaseron) and copolymer-1 (Copaxone) trials. Similarly, despite the fact that there are better measures, it is still almost imperative that the Kurtzke EDSS be included in any multiple sclerosis trial so that results can be compared with previous trials.

Whatever scales are chosen, it is important that they have demonstrated validity for the purpose for which they are being used. It would not be appropriate, for example, to use a Parkinson's disease scale in a stroke trial, or even in another movement disorder trial, without first demonstrating that it has some validity for that purpose.

The efficiency of the scale(s) selected for a trial is also important. When possible, the most efficient scale(s) that do the job should be selected. Efficiency is important whether the examiner is a physician, a psychologist, a medical assistant, or the patient filling out extensive questionnaires. Patients become impatient with extended testing and may drop out rather than put up with testing that fatigues them or takes too much of their time. Even if they persevere, the fatigue of the assessment may cause unreliable answers to be obtained. Thus, pilot testing of whatever is selected should be done to ensure the set of measures is appropriate. The need for comparison with earlier trials and to use well-validated scales often limits ones ability to use only the more efficient measures, however.

References

Bollet AJ. The purpura nautica, or low C on the high seas. In: *Plagues and poxes*. New York: Demos Publications, 1987:1–8.

Codman EA. The product of a hospital. *J Surg Gynecol Obstet* 1914;18:491–96.

Flexner A. *Medical education in the United States and Canada*. Boston: Merrymount Press, 1910.

Francis T, Korns RF, Voight RB, et al. An evaluation of the 1954 poliomyelitis vaccine trials. *Am J Pub Health* 1955; 45(Suppl):1–63.

Friedman LM, Furberg CD, DeMets DL. *Fundamentals of clinical trials*. St. Louis: Mosby-Year Book, 1996.

Hauser SL, Dawson DM, Lehrich JR, et al. Intensive immunosuppression in progressive multiple sclerosis: a randomized three-arm study of high dose intravenous cyclophosphamide, plasma exchange and ACTH. *N Engl J Med* 1983;308:173–80.

Kurtzke JF. Rating neurologic impairment in multiple sclerosis: an expanded disability status scale (EDSS). *Neurology* 1983;33:1444–52.

Meinert CL. *Clinical trials, design, conduct and analysis.* New York: Oxford University Press, 1986.

Meier P. Statistics and medical experimentation. *Biometrics* 1975;31:511–29.

Pocock SJ. *Clinical trials: a practical approach.* Chichester: Wiley, 1984.

Streptomycin in pulmonary tuberculosis (reprinted from *BMJ* 1948:ii:790–1) *BMJ* 1998;317:1248.

Wade DT. *Measurement in neurological rehabilitation.* New York: Oxford University Press, 1992:38.

2 Generic and General Use Scales

Robert M. Herndon, M.D.

Several neurologic scales do not fit neatly into a specific disease or subspecialty category but are used across a variety of diseases. Some of these are used widely, well beyond the field of neurology, such as the generic quality-of-life scales, depression scales, and pain scales, whereas others, such as the Ashworth scale, are used almost exclusively in neurology but are useful in many different neurologic disorders. The purpose of this chapter is to describe some of the scales that do not fit easily into other chapters but nevertheless are sufficiently widely used to be important to neurologists and scales for areas that are not sufficiently developed to warrant a full chapter at this time.

Quality-of-Life Scales

There are many general scales for comparing health status in different diseases. These *quality-of-life* scales include the Sickness Impact Profile, the Short Form 20, and the Quality of Life Index, among others. The Short Form 36 is widely used and is used as a base for extended disease-specific scales (Ware & Sherbourne, 1992). It forms the basis for some extended scales in neurologic disease, such as the Multiple Sclerosis Quality of Life-54 and the Multiple Sclerosis Quality of Life Inventory, which are discussed in Chapter 7, and the Epilepsy Surgery Inventory-55, discussed in Chapter 14. Use of the Short Form 36 requires permission/license from the Rand Corporation for use. Short Form 36 forms are available from the Medical Outcomes Trust, 235 Wyman Street, Suite 130, Waltham, MA 02541, http://www.outcomes-trust.org. Presentation and review of general quality-of-life scales are beyond the scope of this volume. A thorough discussion of these scales can be found in *Measuring Health,* 2nd edition, by McDowell and Newell (1996).

Ashworth and Modified Ashworth Scales for Spasticity

Description

Ashworth and Modified Ashworth Scales for Spasticity (Table 2-1) are simple scales done for

Table 2-1. Ashworth Scale and Modified Ashworth Scale

Ashworth Scale	
0	No increase in tone
1	Slight increase in tone giving a catch when the limb moved in flexion or extension
2	More marked increase in tone but limb easily flexed
3	Considerable increase in tone, passive movement difficult
4	Limb rigid in flexion or extension
Modified Ashworth Scale	
0	No increase in tone
1	Slight increase in muscle tone, manifested by a catch and release or by minimal resistance at the end of the range of motion when the affected part(s) is moved in flexion or extension
1+	Slight increase in muscle tone, manifested by a catch, followed by minimal resistance throughout the remainder (less than one-half) of the range of movement
2	More marked increase in muscle tone through most of the range of motion but affected part(s) easily moved
3	Considerable increase in muscle tone, passive movement difficult
4	Affected part(s) rigid in flexion or extension

assessment of spasticity. They can be done in considerable detail, assessing each individual muscle group, as is typically done in assessing patients being considered for intrathecal baclofen treatment, or may be assessed on only a few larger muscle groups.

Administration

The scales are most commonly done by physical therapists, although they are also done by neurologists and physiatrists.

Time to Administer

Time to administer varies from a few minutes to 10–15 minutes depending on the number of muscle groups tested.

Validation

The scales have good face validity, but reliability has been limited (Pandyan et al., 2003; Haas et al., 1996). Intra-observer reliability appears to be considerably better than inter-observer reliability (Blackburn et al., 2002).

Disadvantages

Inter-observer reliability has been poor, although intra-observer reliability is fairly good.

Advantages

These are the only widely used scales for spasticity, and their overall meaning is widely understood even though reliability is somewhat limited.

Walking while Talking

Description

Walking while talking is a divided-attention walking task used to estimate risk of falling in the elderly.

Validation

The test was validated in a community-based cohort of 60 nondemented elderly aged 65–98 years. The test included a simple and complex version. The simple version had a sensitivity of 46% and specificity of 89%. For the complex version, the sensitivity was 39% and specificity 96%. Thus, it appears to have only fair sensitivity but good specificity as a test for prediction of falls in the elderly.

Time to Administer

Time to administer varies from a few minutes up to perhaps 10–15 minutes depending on the individual tested and his or her walking speed and endurance.

Administration

The time to walk 20 feet and return (40 feet in all) is timed. This is repeated with the patient reciting the alphabet aloud (walking while talking—simple) and again with the patient reciting alternate letters of the alphabet (walking while talking—complex). Cutoff scores are set at 1 standard deviation from the norm. A time of 18 seconds or longer for the timed gait, 18 seconds or longer for walking while talking—simple, and 33 seconds or longer for walking while talking—complex are considered abnormal.

Advantages

Walking while talking is a simple test that has fair sensitivity and good specificity for prediction of falls in the elderly.

Disadvantages

Walking while talking is a bit time-consuming for a predictive test for use in the general population of elderly. Thus, it is most likely to be used in defined populations in whom some indication of a risk of falling is already present. It appears to have much less sensitivity than the "timed up and go," with slightly better specificity. Further validation in a larger population is desirable.

Timed Up and Go

Description

Timed up and go is a simple timed test of mobility designed for use with the frail elderly.

Validation

As a simple, straightforward timed test of functional mobility, up and go has excellent face validity. It has good predictive validity, with 87% sensitivity and 87% specificity for predicting falls in the elderly (Shumway Cook et al., 2000). The authors also looked at the timed up and go with a concurrent task of counting backwards by 3s from a random number between 20 and 100 and while carrying a full glass of water, but the additional conditions added little. Pandyan et al. (1999, 2003) showed that a time of more than 17 seconds in the simple up and go was predictive of a decline in basic activities of daily living.

Time to Administer

Time to administer is 1–3 minutes.

Administration

The timed up and go is the time required to get up from a straight-backed arm chair, walk to a line 3 m from the front legs of the chair, and return and sit down (Podsiadlo & Richardson, 1991).

Advantages

Timed up and go is a simple, highly efficient test of mobility for frail elderly. It appears useful in assessing mobility, safety, and particularly risk of falls in the frail elderly. Specificity is a little less than walking while talking, but sensitivity is much better.

Disadvantages

The test may not pick up intermittent difficulty in gait such as might be seen in Parkinson's disease, in which the on or off state may be important, and will likely not pick up falls related to postural hypotension.

Affective Lability

A large number of terms have been used for the lability of affective expression related to pseudobulbar palsy. These include *pathologic laughing and weeping, affective lability, emotional lability, emotional incontinence, lability of affective expression,* and *pathologic emotionality.* The terms are used to describe the markedly exaggerated laughing and/or crying typically seen in those with pseudobulbar palsy. It occurs in a large variety of diseases, including amyotrophic lateral sclerosis, stroke, Alzheimer's disease, and multiple sclerosis. The most widely used term currently is *pseudobulbar affect.* The affective expression is typically either dissociated from or greatly exaggerated relative to the stimulus. Thus, a slightly sad event may lead to uncontrollable laughter or uncontrolled weeping. There are two published scales for the assessment of this condition: the Center for Neurological Study Lability Scale and the Pathological Laughter and Crying Scale.

Center for Neurological Study Lability Scale

Description

The Center for Neurological Study Lability Scale is a self-report measure of affective lability, also variously called *pathologic laughing and weeping, pseudobulbar emotionality, emotional lability,* and *lability of emotional expression,* among others (Table 2-2). Perhaps the best term is *affective dysregulation syndrome* because it is a

Table 2-2. Center for Neurological Study Lability Scale

Applies Never	Applies Rarely	Applies Occasionally	Applies Frequently	Applies Most of the Time
1	2	3	4	5

1. There are times when I feel fine one minute, and then I'll become tearful the next over something small or for no reason at all.

| 1 | 2 | 3 | 4 | 5 |

2. Others have told me that I seem to become amused very easily or that I seem to become amused about things that really aren't funny.

| 1 | 2 | 3 | 4 | 5 |

3. I find myself crying very easily.

| 1 | 2 | 3 | 4 | 5 |

4. I find that even when I try to control my laughter I am often unable to do so.

| 1 | 2 | 3 | 4 | 5 |

5. There are times when I won't be thinking of anything happy or funny at all, but then I'll suddenly be overcome by funny or happy thoughts.

| 1 | 2 | 3 | 4 | 5 |

6. I find that even when I try to control my crying I am often unable to do so.

| 1 | 2 | 3 | 4 | 5 |

7. I find that I am easily overcome by laughter.

| 1 | 2 | 3 | 4 | 5 |

From Moore SR, Gresham, LS, Bromberg MB, et al. A self report measure of affective lability. *J Neurol Neurosurg Psychiatry* 1997;63:89–93, with permission.

problem of regulation of affect (expressed emotion) and not of emotion (internal state).

Validation

This is a well-validated scale; it has excellent face validity, test/retest reliability, construct validity, convergent validity, and predictive validity. Validation has been done only for amyotrophic lateral sclerosis, but it should be applicable in any disease state in which this syndrome occurs (Brooks et al., 2004; Moore et al., 1997; Smith et al., 2004).

Administration

This is a self-administered Likert scale that requires only a few minutes for the patient to complete. Scoring is simple and can be done by anyone, requiring only a few minutes.

Time to Administer

Time to administer is 1–5 minutes.

Advantages

The Center for Neurological Study Lability Scale is a simple, well-validated, and efficient measure of lability of affective expression. It can be used to detect or assess emotional lability.

Disadvantages

The scale does not clearly distinguish between weeping related to depression and that due to affective dysregulation. Therefore, separate assessment of depression must be done in anyone with pseudobulbar affect because the affective expression may or may not relate to internal emotional state, and severe depression can coexist with and is difficult to recognize in the presence of pathologic laughter.

Summary

This is a relatively new, well-validated scale for assessing affective dysregulation. It is a simple scale, easy to administer, and applicable to any disease state in which the syndrome of affective dysregulation occurs.

Pathological Laughter and Crying Scale

Description

The Pathological Laughter and Crying Scale is an 18-item Likert scale that was used to examine the effect of nortriptyline on pseudobulbar affective state after stroke (Table 2-3) (Robinson et al., 1993).

Time to Administer

Time to administer is 2–5 minutes.

Validation

The original report includes validation on a group of 54 stroke patients. Its sensitivity for lability clinically diagnosed by a psychiatrist blind to the diagnosis using a cutoff of 13 was 0.88, with a specificity of 0.94. Further validation was done by interviewing relatives, and the Pearson's correlation coefficient was 0.86. There was no correlation with the Hamilton depression scale or Mini-Mental State Examination.

Advantages

The scale is a little longer and more detailed than the Center for Neurological Study Lability Scale. It appears to separate affective expression from internal emotional state a bit better than the Center for Neurological Study Lability Scale. Despite being a bit longer, it is still brief and efficient and has good sensitivity and specificity.

Disadvantages

There are no substantial disadvantages. Separate assessment of depression may still be required.

Table 2-3. Pathological Laughter and Crying Scale (Patient Interview)

Ratings are based on clinical assessment. Initial probe questions are given for each item. However, further questions may be used for clarification. Write the number in the spaces provided that most accurately reflects clinical symptoms.

1. Have you recently experienced sudden episodes of laughter?

    ___Rate the frequency of the episodes during the past 2 wk.

    0. Rarely or not at all

    1. Occasionally

    2. Quite often

    3. Frequently

2. Have you recently experienced sudden episodes of crying?

    ___Rate the frequency of the episodes during the past 2 wk.

    0. Rarely or not at all

    1. Occasionally

    2. Quite often

    3. Frequently

If you have experienced sudden episodes of laughter, please answer the following (questions 3–10), otherwise skip to question 11.

3. Have these episodes occurred without any cause in your surroundings?

    ___Rate the frequency with which the episodes have occurred without external stimuli in the past 2 wk.

    0. Rarely or not at all

    1. Occasionally

    2. Quite often

    3. Frequently

(continued)

Table 2-3. *(continued)*

4. Have these episodes lasted for a long period of time?

___Rate the average duration of the episodes during the past 2 wk.

0. Very brief

1. A few seconds

2. Moderate (<30 sec)

3. Prolonged (>30 sec)

5. Have these episodes been uncontrollable by you?

___Rate the ability to control the episodes during the past 2 wk.

0. Rarely or not at all

1. Occasionally

2. Quite often

3. Frequently

6. Have these episodes occurred as a result of feelings of happiness?

___Rate the frequency with which the episodes have occurred as a result of happiness in the past 2 wk.

0. Rarely or not at all

1. Occasionally

2. Quite often

3. Frequently

7. Have these episodes occurred in excess of feelings of happiness?

___Rate the frequency with which the episodes have been disproportionate to the emotional state in the past 2 wk.

0. Rarely or not at all

1. Occasionally

2. Quite often

3. Frequently

8. Have these episodes of laughter occurred with feelings of sadness?

___Rate the frequency of association between the episode and the paradoxical emotion in the past 2 wk. The sadness must precede or accompany the episode and not be a reaction to it.

0. Rarely or not at all

1. Occasionally

2. Quite often

3. Frequently

9. Have these episodes occurred with any emotions other than happiness or sadness, such as nervousness, anger, fear, etc.?

___Rate the frequency of association between the episodes and emotions in the past 2 wk. The emotions must precede or accompany the episode and not be a reaction to it.

0. Rarely or not at all

1. Occasionally

2. Quite often

3. Frequently

Table 2-3. *(continued)*

10. Have these episodes caused you any distress or social embarrassment?

___Rate the degree of distress or embarrassment caused by the episodes in the past 2 wk.

0. Rarely or not at all

1. Occasionally

2. Quite often

3. Frequently

If you have experienced sudden episodes of crying, please answer the following (questions 11–18).

11. Have these episodes occurred without any cause in your surroundings?

___Rate the frequency with which the episodes have occurred without external stimuli in the past 2 wk.

0. Rarely or not at all

1. Occasionally

2. Quite often

3. Frequently

12. Have these episodes lasted for a long period of time?

___Rate the average duration of the episodes during the past 2 wk.

0. Very brief

1. Short (a few seconds)

2. Moderate (<30 sec)

3. Prolonged (>30 sec)

13. Have these episodes been uncontrollable by you?

___Rate the ability to control the episodes during the past 2 wk.

0. Rarely or not at all

1. Occasionally

2. Quite often

3. Frequently

14. Have these episodes occurred as a result of feelings of sadness?

___Rate the frequency with which the episodes have occurred as a result of sadness in the past 2 wk. The sadness must precede or accompany the crying and not be a reaction to it.

0. Rarely or not at all

1. Occasionally

2. Quite often

3. Frequently

15. Have these episodes occurred in excess of feelings of sadness?

___Rate the frequency with which the episodes have been disproportionate to the emotional state in the past 2 wk.

0. Rarely or not at all

1. Occasionally

2. Quite often

3. Frequently

(continued)

Table 2-3. *(continued)*

16. Have these episodes of crying occurred with feelings of happiness?

___Rate the frequency of association between the episode and the paradoxical emotion in the past 2 wk. The happiness must precede or accompany the crying.

0. Rarely or not at all

1. Occasionally

2. Quite often

3. Frequently

17. Have these episodes occurred with any emotions other than sadness or happiness, such as nervousness, anger, fear, etc.?

___Rate the frequency of association between the episodes and emotions in the past 2 wk. The emotions must precede or accompany the episode and not be a reaction to it.

0. Rarely or not at all

1. Occasionally

2. Quite often

3. Frequently

18. Have these episodes caused you any distress or social embarrassment?

___Rate the degree of distress or embarrassment caused by the episodes in the past 2 wk.

0. Rarely or not at all

1. Occasionally

2. Quite often

3. Frequently

References

Blackburn M, van Vliet P, Mockett SP. Reliability of measurements obtained with the modified Ashworth scale in the lower extremities of people with stroke. *Phys Ther* 2002;82:25–34.

Brooks BR, Thisted RA, Appel SH, et al. Treatment of pseudobulbar affect in ALS with dextromethorphan/quinidine: randomized trial. *Neurology* 2004;63:1364–70.

Haas BM, Bergström E, Jamous A, et al. The inter rater reliability of the original and of the modified Ashworth scare for the assessment of spasticity in patients with spinal cord injury. *Spinal Cord* 1996;34:560–64.

McDowell I, Newell, C. *Measuring health* (2nd ed.). New York: Oxford University Press, 1996.

Moore SR, Gresham LS, Bromberg MB, et al. A self report measure of affective lability. *J Neurol Neurosurg Psychiatry* 1997;63:89–93.

Okumiya K, Matsubayashi K, Nakamura T, et al. The "timed up and go" test and manual bottom score are useful predictors of functional decline in basic and instrumental ADL in community-dwelling older people. *J Am Geriatr Soc* 1999;46:677–82.

Pandyan AD, Johnson GR, Price CIM, et al. A review of the properties and limitations of the Ashworth and modified Ashworth Scales as measures of spasticity. *Clin Rehab* 1999;13:373–83.

Pandyan AD, Price CI, Barnes MP, et al. A biomechanical investigation into the validity of the modified Ashworth Scale as a measure of elbow spasticity. *Clin Rehabil* 2003;17:290–93.

Podsiadlo D, Richardson S. The timed "Up and Go": a test of functional mobility for frail elderly persons. *J Am Geriatr Soc* 1991;39:142–48.

Robinson RG, Parikj RM, Lipsey JR, et al. Pathological laughing and crying following stroke: validation of a measurement scale and a double blind treatment study. *Am J Psychiatry* 1993;150:286–93.

Shumway Cook A, Brauer S, Woollacott M. Predicting the probability of falls in community-dwelling older adults using the Timed Up and Go Test. *Phys Ther* 2000; 81:1060–61.

Smith RA, Berg JE, Pope LE, et al. Validation of the CNS emotional lability scale for pseudobulbar affect (pathological laughing and crying) in multiple sclerosis patients. *Mult Scler* 2004;10:679–85.

Ware JE, Sherbourne CD. The MOS 36-item short form health survey (SF-36). I. Conceptual framework and item selection. *Med Care* 1992;30:473–83.

3 Pediatric Developmental Scales

Roger A. Brumback, M.D.

M any of the scales that have been developed in clinical neuroscience for evaluation of adults can be adapted for use in children [an example is the Mini-Mental State Examination (Folstein et al., 1975; Ouvrier et al., 1993), which has been in its pediatric version renamed School-Years Screening Test for the Evaluation of Mental Status (Ouvrier et al., 1999)]. However, the unique aspect of pediatric neurology is the developmental changes that occur in children. Many scales have been developed to assess the development for a variety of functions. Many of these are used routinely by pediatricians as well as pediatric neurologists. One of the most important scales is the simple measurement of the fronto-occipital head circumference. Growth charts for plotting head circumference (as well as height and weight) are widely available in all hospitals with pediatric services and in pediatrician offices. Many of the scales for evaluating children are proprietary, and copies must be purchased or permission obtained from various companies or individuals for their use (see also Hammill et al., 1992; Raskin, 1985; Spreen & Strauss, 1991; Wodrich, 1997).

American Association on Mental Retardation Adaptive Behavior Scale

Adaptive behavior assessment is an important part of diagnosing mental retardation (Grossman, 1983), as the diagnosis of mental retardation requires subnormal functioning in both intelligence and in adaptive behavior. Thus, the American Association on Mental Retardation has published scales for use in the assessment of adaptive behavior (Fogelman, 1974; Nihira et al., 1969; Schalock & Braddock, 1999).

Description

The Adaptive Behavior Scale has two versions: Adaptive Behavior Scale—School for children aged 3–21 years and the Adaptive Behavior Scale—Residential and Community for residentially confined individuals and adults with disabilities. This scale consists of two parts. The part I behavioral domains are developmentally organized and measure basic survival skills and behaviors important for independent living; the part II domains assess maladaptive behaviors (Table 3-1).

Table 3-1. American Association on Mental Retardation Adaptive Behavior Scale

Part I Behavioral domains
Independent functioning
Physical development
Economic activity
Language development
Number and time concepts
Domestic activity (in Adaptive Behavior Scale—Residential and Community version)
Prevocational/vocational activity
Self-direction
Responsibility
Socialization
Part II Behavioral domains
Violent and destructive behavior
Antisocial behavior
Rebellious behavior
Untrustworthy behavior
Withdrawal
Stereotyped behavioral and odd mannerisms
Inappropriate interpersonal manners
Unacceptable or eccentric habits
Unacceptable vocal habits
Self-abusive behavior
Hyperactive tendencies
Sexually aberrant behavior
Psychological disturbances

Administration requires approximately 15–30 minutes. Scores on individual domains can be grouped together into three broad factors (each reported as a standard score): personal self-sufficiency, community self-sufficiency, and social responsibility. Norms are available down to age 3 years.

Bayley Scales of Infant Development II

The Bayley Scales of Infant Development II, designed for the age range of 1 month to 3.5 years, is now one of the most widely used measures for infant development (Bayley, 1970, 1993; Damarin, 1978; Lehr et al., 1987).

Description

This test measures mental and motor development. It consists of three parts: mental scale (measures sensory-perceptual acuity, discrimination, object constancy, memory, learning, problem solving, vocalization, early verbalization, and early abstract thinking), motor scale (body control, coordination, and finger manipulation), and behavior rating scale (affective behavior, motivation, and interest). Items are numbered according to difficulty (age level), and all items are tested between a basal level, at which all items are passed, and a ceiling level, at which no items are passed. The Bayley Scales of Infant Development II has 178 items in the mental scale, 97 items in the motor scale, and 30 items in the behavior rating scale. Items at many levels use similar test situations—for example, item 3 is response to the sound of a rattle, item 36 is the child playing with the rattle, item 48 is turning the head to the sound of the rattle, and item 59 is the child finding the rattle after it has been taken away. Scoring results in a mental development index and psychomotor development index. These scores can also be converted to age-equivalents. Administration time is approximately 30–40 minutes.

The Bayley Scales of Infant Development II has been standardized on a large sample (more than 1,000) of normal children. Studies suggest a considerable variability in scores from repeat testing at close intervals (Horner, 1988), indicating that any score from a single session needs to be correlated with other observations of the child or that multiple repeat tests should be averaged to correct information about the child's functioning. This is also why the predictive value of this test for later intelligence scores is not completely settled (Ramey et al., 1973).

Bellevue Index of Depression

In 1973, Weinberg and colleagues published criteria for establishing the diagnosis of depression in children (Weinberg et al., 1973). Subsequently, Petti (1978) used these criteria to develop a semistructured interview questionnaire termed the Bellevue Index of Depression administered separately to the child and the parent or caretaker.

Description

The Bellevue Index of Depression consists of 40 items in 10 categories (Table 3-2). Each item is rated on a four-part scale of "not at all," "a little," "quite a bit," or "very much" and for duration of less than 1 month, 1–6 months, 6 months to 2 years, or always. The items

Table 3-2. Bellevue Index of Depression

I. Dysphoric mood
1. Statements or appearance of sadness, loneliness, unhappiness, hopelessness, and/or pessimism
2. Mood swings, moodiness
3. Irritable, easily annoyed
4. Hypersensitive, cries easily
5. Negative, difficult to please

II. Self-deprecatory ideation
6. Feelings of being worthless, useless, dumb, stupid, ugly, guilty
7. Beliefs of persecution
8. Death wishes
9. Suicidal thoughts
10. Suicidal attempts

III. Aggressive behavior (agitation)
11. Difficult to get along with
12. Quarrelsome
13. Disrespectful of authority
14. Belligerent, hostile, agitated
15. Excessive fighting or sudden anger

IV. Sleep disturbance
16. Initial insomnia
17. Restless sleep
18. Terminal insomnia
19. Difficulty awakening in the morning

V. Change in school performance
20. Frequent complaints from teachers ("daydreaming," "poor concentration," "poor memory")

21. Loss of usual work effort in school subjects
22. Loss of usual interest in nonacademic school activities
23. Much incomplete school work
24. Much incomplete homework
25. A drop in usual grades
26. Finds homework difficult

VI. Diminished socialization
27. Less group participation
28. Less friendly, less outgoing
29. Socially withdrawing
30. Loss of usual social interests

VII. Change in attitude toward school
31. Does not enjoy school activities
32. Does not want or refuses to attend school

VIII. Somatic complaints
33. Non-migraine headaches
34. Abdominal pain
35. Muscle aches or pains
36. Other somatic complaints or concerns (specify)

IX. Loss of usual energy
37. Loss of usual personal interests or pursuits (other than school; e.g., hobbies, playing)
38. Decreased activity level; mental and/or physical fatigue

X. Unusual change in appetite and/or of weight
39. Anorexia or polyphagia
40. Unusual weight change in past 4 mo

are administered on a written form for parents and in a semistructured interview format with the child.

A summary score is obtained from both the child's answers and the parent's form, with the higher of the summary scores considered the total score for the test purposes. The total score above a cutoff value is considered evidence of depression, with greater severity of depression relating to higher scores. Age range is from 6 to 12 years. Completion requires approximately 15–30 minutes.

Inter-rater reliability is good, it is relatively easy to administer, and it can be used to identify changes with therapy (Petti & Conners, 1983; Petti & Law, 1982).

Brazelton Neonatal Behavioral Assessment Scale

The Brazelton Scale was originally introduced in 1973 as a means of evaluating the behavior of infants, particularly the ability of infants to interact with the environment (Brazelton, 1973; Brazelton, 1984; Brazelton & Nugent, 1995).

Description

The Brazelton Scale includes 28 behavioral items (scored on a 9-point scale), 18 reflex items (scored on

Table 3-3.   Brazelton Neonatal Behavioral Assessment Scale

Behavioral items	Reflex items
Response decrement to light	Plantar grasp
Response decrement to rattle	Babinski's
Response decrement to bell	Ankle clonus
Response decrement to tactile stimulation of foot	Rooting
Orientation—inanimate visual	Sucking
Orientation—inanimate auditory	Glabella
Orientation—inanimate visual and auditory	Passive movements—arms
Orientation—animate visual	Passive movements—legs
Orientation—animate auditory	Palmar grasp
Orientation—animate visual and auditory	Placing
Alertness	Standing
General tonus	Walking
Motor maturity	Crawling
Pull-to-sit	Incurvation (Gallant response)
Defensive movements	Tonic deviation of head and eyes
Activity level	Nystagmus
Peak of excitement	Tonic neck reflex
Rapidity of buildup	Moro
Irritability	Supplementary items
Lability of states	Quality of alertness
Cuddliness	Cost of attention
Consolability	Examiner facilitation
Self-quieting	General irritability
Hand-to-mouth	Robustness and endurance
Tremulousness	State regulation
Startles	Examiner's emotional response
Lability of skin color	
Smiles	

a 4-point scale), and seven supplementary items (scored on a 9-point scale) of particular value in assessing frail premature infants (Table 3-3).

This scale has been used in a variety of obstetrical and neonatal research studies to ascertain effects on the newborns (Dixon et al., 1984; Field et al., 1986; Fowles, 1999; Stjernqvist & Svenningsen, 1990).

Children's Depression Inventory

The popular 21-item Beck Depression Inventory (Beck, 1967) was modified for use in children as the Children's Depression Inventory (Kovacs, 1980–1981).

Description

The Children's Depression Inventory is a 27-item self-report scale that evaluates a range of depressive symptoms. Each item is rated with three choices of severity (scored from 0 to 2). The total score correlates with severity of depressive symptomatology and can be used to follow changes in severity. Age range is 6–16 years. The test requires a first grade reading level (Kazden & Petti, 1982). Completion requires approximately 15 minutes.

Children's Depression Rating Scale—Revised

The Children's Depression Rating Scale can be used as a clinical screening device for depression and as a measure of change with treatment (Poznanski et al., 1979, 1984, 1985).

Description

The Children's Depression Rating Scale—Revised consists of 17 items administered in a semi-structured interview. Fourteen of the items are rated on the basis of the answers by the child during the interview, and three are rated by the examiner on the basis of observation of the child's nonverbal behavior. Severity ratings for each item reflect both intensity and frequency of the symptom. The total score above a cutoff value is considered evidence of depression, with greater severity relating to higher scores. Age range is 6–12 years. Testing requires approximately 20–30 minutes.

Conners' Parent Rating Scale

The Conners' Parent Rating Scale is one of the most widely used scales for assessment of childhood behavioral disturbances in psychopharmacologic studies (Conners, 1985). Two versions exist, the original version introduced by Conners (1970) and a shorter revised version by Goyette et al. (1978).

Description

The original version has 93 questions (the revised version only 48 questions) (Table 3-4). The test is completed by the parent or caretaker of the child for the symptoms that are currently evident (previous symptoms—i.e., not present during the past month—are not to be rated). Areas assessed by the questionnaire include conduct problems, hyperactivity, inattention, aggression, anxiety, somatic complaints, fears, obsessive-compulsive behavior, and school adjustment problems. Each item is to be rated by the parent on a four-part scale of "not at all," "just a little," "pretty much," or "very much," with scores of 0, 1, 2, and 3 for these respective responses.

Summary scores and factor scores can be obtained. Age range is 6–14 years. Completion requires approximately 10–15 minutes.

This test has been shown to have a relatively consistent practice effect on successive administrations resulting in lower scores (Werry & Sprague, 1974); thus, several baseline administrations are necessary before beginning any therapeutic trials.

Conners' Teacher Rating Scale

The Conners' Teacher Rating Scale is the most widely used scale in assessing stimulant drug effects in hyperactive children (Conners, 1969). There are the original version introduced, in 1969, and a shortened revised version, but the original version has been more extensively used (Trites et al., 1982a, 1982b).

Description

The original version has 39 items (the revised version has 28) (Table 3-5). The test is completed by the homeroom teacher. Items are divided into three groups—classroom behavior, group participation, and attitude toward authority. Each item is rated on a four-part scale of "not at all," "just a little," "pretty much," or "very much," with scores of 0, 1, 2, and 3 for these respective responses.

Summary scores and factor scores can be obtained. Age range is 6–17 years. Completion requires approximately 5–10 minutes.

Denver II (Denver Developmental Screening Test)

The Denver Developmental Screening Test was first introduced in 1969 by Frankenburg and Dodds and almost immediately became a favorite technique for pediatricians to quickly assess the developmental level of infants and young children (Frankenburg et al., 1988a, 1988b; Frankenburg & Camp, 1975). The current revision of the test underwent extensive restandardization and is now known as the Denver II (Frankenburg et al., 1992).

Description

The Denver II measures four domains of behavior: personal-social, fine motor-adaptive, language, and gross motor (Figure 3-1). The test consists of 125 items arranged in order of difficulty. Test forms give the ages at which 25%, 50%, 75%, and 90% of children correctly pass each item. The age-equivalent developmental level for each of the domains is determined by the last item the child successfully completes. Some test items can be passed by report of a caretaker. Age range is birth to 6 years (the age scale conforms to the schedule of the American Academy of Pediatrics Health Supervision Visit Schedule). Administration requires approximately 20 minutes.

Table 3-4. Conners' Parent Rating Scale

Problems of eating
    1. Picky and finicky
    2. Will not eat enough
    3. Overweight
Problems of sleep
    4. Restless
    5. Nightmares
    6. Awakens at night
    7. Cannot fall asleep
Fear and worries
    8. Afraid of new situations
    9. Afraid of people
    10. Afraid of being alone
    11. Worries about illness and death
Muscular tension
    12. Gets stiff and rigid
    13. Twitches, jerks, etc.
    14. Shakes
Speech problems
    15. Stuttering
    16. Hard to understand
Wetting
    17. Bed wetting
    18. Runs to bathroom constantly
Bowel problems
    19. Soiling self
    20. Holds back bowel movements
Complains of following symptoms even though doctor
    can find nothing wrong
    21. Headaches
    22. Stomachaches
    23. Vomiting
    24. Aches and pains
    25. Loose bowels
Problems of sucking, chewing, or picking
    26. Sucks thumb
    27. Bites or picks nails
    28. Chews on clothes, blankets, or other items
    29. Picks at things such as hair, clothing, etc.

Childish or immature
    30. Does not act his age
    31. Cries easily
    32. Wants help doing things he should do alone
    33. Clings to parents or other adults
    34. Baby talk
Trouble with feelings
    35. Keeps anger to himself
    36. Lets himself get pushed around by other children
    34. Unhappy
    38. Carries a chip on his shoulder
Overasserts himself
    39. Bullying
    40. Bragging and boasting
    41. Sassy to grown-ups
Problems making friends
    42. Shy
    43. Afraid they do not like him
    44. Feelings easily hurt
    45. Has no friends
Problems with brothers and sisters
    46. Feels cheated
    47. Mean
    48. Fights constantly
Problems keeping friends
    49. Disturbs other children
    50. Wants to run things
    51. Picks on other children
Restless
    52. Restless or overactive
    53. Excitable, impulsive
    54. Fails to finish things he starts—short attention
       span
Temper
    55. Temper outbursts, explosive and unpredictable
       behavior
    56. Throws himself around
    57. Throws and breaks things
    58. Pouts and sulks

Table 3-4. *(continued)*

Sex

    59. Plays with own sex organs

    60. Involved in sex play with others

    61. Modest about his body

Problems in school

    62. Is not learning

    63. Does not like to go to school

    64. Is afraid to go to school

    65. Daydreams

    66. Truancy

    67. Will not obey school rules

Lying

    68. Denies having done wrong

    69. Blames others for his mistakes

    70. Tells stories that did not happen

Stealing

    71. From parents

    72. At school

    73. From stores and other places

Fire setting

    74. Sets fires

Trouble with police

    75. Gets into trouble with police

Perfectionism

    76. Everything must be just so

    77. Things must be done same way every time

    78. Sets goals too high

Additional problems

    79. Inattentive, easily distracted

    80. Constantly fidgeting

    81. Cannot be left alone

    82. Always climbing

    83. A very early riser

    84. Will run around between mouthfuls at meals

    85. Demands must be met immediately—easily frustrated

    86. Cannot stand too much excitement

    87. Laces and zippers always open

    88. Cries often and easily

    89. Unable to stop a repetitive activity

    90. Acts as if driven by a motor

    91. Mood changes quickly and drastically

    92. Poorly aware of surroundings or time of day

    93. Still cannot tie shoelaces

Developmental Test of Visual-Motor Integration

The Beery Developmental Test of Visual-Motor Integration is a copying test modeled after the visual perception test of Frostig (Frostig et al., 1966) and is similar to the Bender-Gestalt Test (Armstrong & Knopf, 1982). The test was originally introduced in 1967 (Beery & Buktenica, 1967) but has since been revised (Beery, 1982, 1989).

Description

This test consists of 24 designs of progressive difficulty, from a vertical line to three-dimensional cube that the child is told to copy into a blank space directly below the stimulus figure. The test is in two forms—the short form, with only the first 15 designs for use in ages 2–8 years, and the long form, with all designs for use up to age $14^{11}/12$ years. Scoring results in a standard score and an age-equivalent. Completion requires approximately 20 minutes.

Although the original normative data were criticized on ethnic and socioeconomic grounds (Martin et al., 1977), the restandardization in more than 3,000 children for the revision has overcome this problem (Beery, 1989).

Dubowitz Scale

The Dubowitz scale uses a series of 10 neuromuscular criteria to assess gestational age of a newborn infant (Dubowitz et al., 1970). These neuromuscular criteria in combination with 12 physical criteria can be used to determine gestational age from 26 to 44 weeks (Dubowitz & Dubowitz, 1981). Ballard and colleagues (1991) reduced the neuromuscular items to six and the

Table 3-5. Conners' Teacher Rating Scale

Classroom behavior

1. Constantly fidgeting
2. Hums and makes other odd noises
3. Demands must be met immediately—easily frustrated
4. Coordination poor
5. Restless or overactive
6. Excitable, impulsive
7. Inattentive, easily distracted
8. Fails to finish things he starts—short attention span
9. Overly sensitive
10. Overly serious or sad
11. Daydreams
12. Sullen or sulky
13. Cries often and easily
14. Disturbs other children
15. Quarrelsome
16. Mood changes quickly and drastically
17. Acts "smart"
18. Destructive
19. Steals
20. Lies
21. Temper outbursts, explosive and unpredictable behavior

Group participation

22. Isolates himself from other children
23. Appears to be unaccepted by group
24. Appears to be easily led
25. No sense of fair play
26. Appears to lack leadership
27. Does not get along with opposite sex
28. Does not get along with same sex
29. Teases other children or interferes with their activities

Attitude toward authority

30. Submissive
31. Defiant
32. Impudent
33. Shy
34. Fearful
35. Excessive demands for teacher's attention
36. Stubborn
37. Overly anxious to please
38. Uncooperative
39. Attendance problem

physical maturity items to six to define a scale that accurately assesses infants from 20 to 44 weeks' gestational age (Ballard et al., 1991).

Description

The original Dubowitz scale has 10 neuromuscular items, but the new Ballard Score adaptation includes only the six most reproducible neuromuscular items (Figure 3-2). The evaluation must be performed within the first 12 hours of life.

Posture: Posture is observed with infant quiet and in supine position (score 0: arms and legs extended; 1: beginning of flexion of hips and knees, arms extended; 2: stronger flexion of legs, arms extended; 3: arms slightly flexed, legs flexed and abducted; 4: full flexion of arms and legs).

Square Window: The hand is flexed on the forearm between the thumb and index finger of the examiner. Enough pressure is applied to get as full a flexion as possible, and the angle between the hypothenar eminence and the ventral aspect of the forearm is measured and graded according to diagram. (Care is taken not to rotate the infant's wrist while doing this maneuver.)

Arm Recoil: With the infant in the supine position, the forearms are first flexed for 5 seconds, then fully extended by pulling on the hands, and then released. The sign is fully positive if the arms return briskly to full flexion (score 2). If the arms return to incomplete flexion or the response is sluggish, it is graded as score 1. If they remain extended or

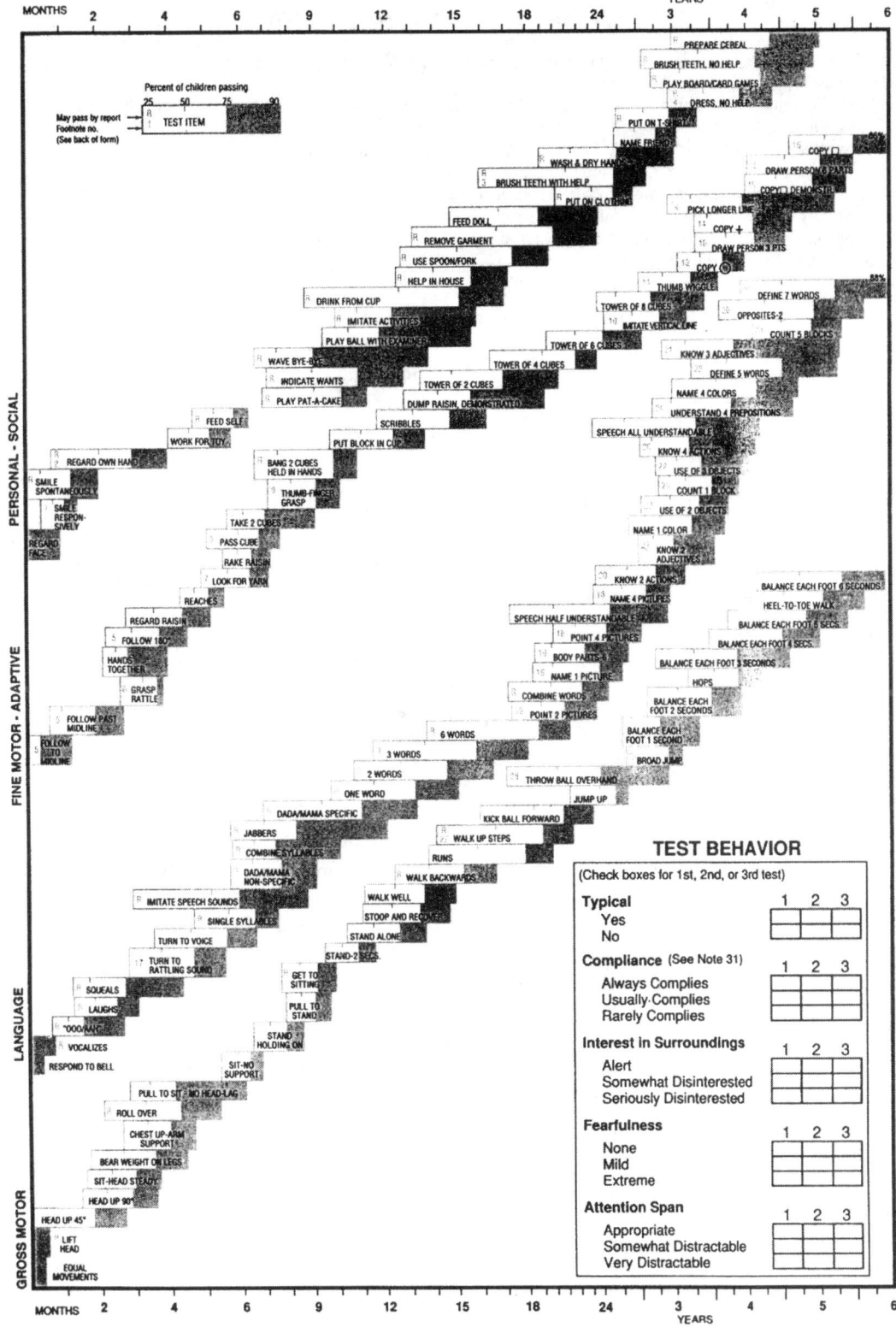

Figure 3-1. (continued)

DIRECTIONS FOR ADMINISTRATION

1. Try to get child to smile by smiling, talking or waving. Do not touch him/her.
2. Child must stare at hand several seconds.
3. Parent may help guide toothbrush and put toothpaste on brush.
4. Child does not have to be able to tie shoes or button/zip in the back.
5. Move yarn slowly in an arc from one side to the other, about 8" above child's face.
6. Pass if child grasps rattle when it is touched to the backs or tips of fingers.
7. Pass if child tries to see where yarn went. Yarn should be dropped quickly from sight from tester's hand without arm movement.
8. Child must transfer cube from hand to hand without help of body, mouth, or table.
9. Pass if child picks up raisin with any part of thumb and finger.
10. Line can vary only 30 degrees or less from tester's line. |/
11. Make a fist with thumb pointing upward and wiggle only the thumb. Pass if child imitates and does not move any fingers other than the thumb.

12. Pass any enclosed form. Fail continuous round motions.
13. Which line is longer? (Not bigger.) Turn paper upside down and repeat. (pass 3 of 3 or 5 of 6)
14. Pass any lines crossing near midpoint.
15. Have child copy first. If failed, demonstrate.

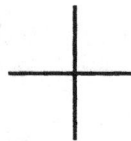

When giving items 12, 14, and 15, do not name the forms. Do not demonstrate 12 and 14.

16. When scoring, each pair (2 arms, 2 legs, etc.) counts as one part.
17. Place one cube in cup and shake gently near child's ear, but out of sight. Repeat for other ear.
18. Point to picture and have child name it. (No credit is given for sounds only.)
    If less than 4 pictures are named correctly, have child point to picture as each is named by tester.

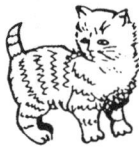

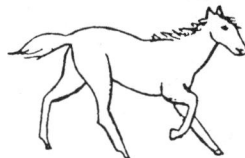

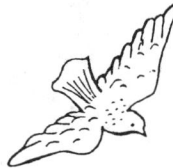

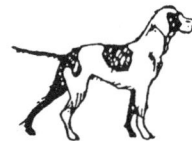

19. Using doll, tell child: Show me the nose, eyes, ears, mouth, hands, feet, tummy, hair. Pass 6 of 8.
20. Using pictures, ask child: Which one flies?... says meow?... talks?... barks?... gallops? Pass 2 of 5, 4 of 5.
21. Ask child: What do you do when you are cold?... tired?... hungry? Pass 2 of 3, 3 of 3.
22. Ask child: What do you do with a cup? What is a chair used for? What is a pencil used for?
    Action words must be included in answers.
23. Pass if child correctly places and says how many blocks are on paper. (1, 5).
24. Tell child: Put block on table; under table; in front of me, behind me. Pass 4 of 4.
    (Do not help child by pointing, moving head or eyes.)
25. Ask child: What is a ball?... lake?... desk?... house?... banana?... curtain?... fence?... ceiling? Pass if defined in terms of use, shape, what it is made of, or general category (such as banana is fruit, not just yellow). Pass 5 of 8, 7 of 8.
26. Ask child: If a horse is big, a mouse is __? If fire is hot, ice is __? If the sun shines during the day, the moon shines during the __? Pass 2 of 3.
27. Child may use wall or rail only, not person. May not crawl.
28. Child must throw ball overhand 3 feet to within arm's reach of tester.
29. Child must perform standing broad jump over width of test sheet (8 1/2 inches).
30. Tell child to walk forward, ⟳⟳⟳⟳➤ heel within 1 inch of toe. Tester may demonstrate.
    Child must walk 4 consecutive steps.
31. In the second year, half of normal children are non-compliant.

OBSERVATIONS:

Figure 3-1. *continued*

Neuromuscular Maturity

	-1	0	1	2	3	4	5
Posture							
Square Window (wrist)	>90°	90°	60°	45°	30°	0°	
Arm Recoil		180°	140°-180°	110°-140°	90-110°	<90°	
Popliteal Angle	180°	160°	140°	120°	100°	90°	<90°
Scarf Sign							
Heel to Ear							

Physical Maturity

Skin	sticky friable transparent	gelatinous red, translucent	smooth pink, visible veins	superficial peeling &/or rash. few veins	cracking pale areas rare veins	parchment deep cracking no vessels	leathery cracked wrinkled
Lanugo	none	sparse	abundant	thinning	bald areas	mostly bald	
Plantar Surface	heel-toe 40-50 mm: -1 <40 mm: -2	>50mm no crease	faint red marks	anterior transverse crease only	creases ant. 2/3	creases over entire sole	
Breast	imperceptible	barely perceptible	flat areola no bud	stippled areola 1-2mm bud	raised areola 3-4mm bud	full areola 5-10mm bud	
Eye/Ear	lids fused loosely: -1 tightly: -2	lids open pinna flat stays folded	sl. curved pinna; soft; slow recoil	well-curved pinna; soft but ready recoil	formed & firm instant recoil	thick cartilage ear stiff	
Genitals male	scrotum flat, smooth	scrotum empty faint rugae	testes in upper canal rare rugae	testes descending few rugae	testes down good rugae	testes pendulous deep rugae	
Genitals female	clitoris prominent labia flat	prominent clitoris small labia minora	prominent clitoris enlarging minora	majora & minora equally prominent	majora large minora small	majora cover clitoris & minora	

Maturity Rating

score	weeks
-10	20
-5	22
0	24
5	26
10	28
15	30
20	32
25	34
30	36
35	38
40	40
45	42
50	44

Figure 3-2.

are only followed by random movements, the score is 0.

Popliteal Angle: With the infant supine and his pelvis flat on the examining couch, the thigh is held in the knee–chest position by the examiner's left index finger and thumb supporting the knee. The leg is then extended by gentle pressure from the examiner's right index finger behind the ankle, and the popliteal angle is measured.

Heel-to-Ear Maneuver: With the baby supine, draw the baby's foot as near to the head as it will go without forcing it. Observe the distance between the foot and the head as well as the degree of extension at the knee. Note that the knee is left free and may draw down alongside the abdomen.

Scarf Sign: With the baby supine, take the infant's hand, and try to put it around the neck and as far posteriorly as possible around the opposite shoulder. Assist this maneuver by lifting the elbow across the body. See how far the elbow goes across (score 0: elbow reaches opposite axillary line; 1: elbow between midline and opposite axillary line; 2: elbow reaches midline; 3: elbow does not reach midline).

Kaufman Assessment Battery for Children

The Kaufman Assessment Battery for Children (K-ABC) is the newest of the intelligence tests and uses a different theoretical model than the two standard tests—the Stanford-Binet and the Wechsler scales. The theoretical model is of sequential and simultaneous processing of information, which is presumably based on the theories of Luria (Das et al., 1979; Luria, 1980). It incorporates six achievement tests and 10 mental process subtests (seven of which are *simultaneous* and three *sequential*). Six subtests are considered nonverbal and suitable for children with language problems (Kaufman et al., 1987).

Description

The K-ABC consists of 16 subtests (Table 3-6). Although the test is designed for ages $2^6/_{12}$–$12^6/_{12}$ years, not all subtests are administered to all ages.

Testing involves sequential administration of each item from a basal level to a ceiling level (last item

correctly answered), with raw score consisting of the ceiling item minus errors. This score can be translated into a scaled score and age-appropriate standard scores. In addition to a mental processing composite score, scores for four scales are available (sequential processing scale, simultaneous processing scale, achievement scale, and nonverbal scale). Average administration time ranges from 30 minutes for 3-year-olds to 75 minutes for 12-year-olds.

The K-ABC has been well-standardized (Kaufman & Kaufman, 1983). Disadvantages are that it does not identify mental retardation in young children (Sattler, 1988), and it is not equivalent to the Wechsler scales or the Stanford-Binet test (the K-ABC overestimates intelligence quotient [IQ] by up to 8 points), but it does offer some additional information supplementary to these tests (Naglieri, 1985).

Kaufman Adolescent and Adult Intelligence Test

For individuals aged 11 years and older, the Kaufman Adolescent and Adult Intelligence Test is a novel intelligence test that incorporates concepts of neuropsychology and cognitive psychology (Kaufman & Kaufman, 1993).

Description

The Kaufman Adolescent and Adult Intelligence Test incorporates both standard intelligence test materials in several subtests (definitions, double meaning, famous faces, and auditory comprehension) and novel neuropsychology-based test materials in additional subtests (rebus learning, logical steps, mystery code, and memory for block designs).

The Kaufman Adolescent and Adult Intelligence Test appears to be particularly useful in assessing children who seem brighter than their standard intelligence test scores (Wodrich, 1997) and in children and adolescents with traumatic brain injury (Dumond & Hagberg, 1994).

KeyMath—Revised Test

The KeyMath—Revised Test is a revision of the earlier diagnostic arithmetic test that assesses mathematical skills (Connolly, 1988; Connolly et al., 1976).

Table 3-6.   Kaufman Assessment Battery for Children

1. Magic window (15 items; simultaneous; age range $2^{6}/_{12}$–$4^{11}/_{12}$ yr)—child must name an object (e.g., a car) rotated behind a narrow slit that allows only part of the object to be seen at any one time

2. Face recognition (15 items; simultaneous; age range $2^{6}/_{12}$–$4^{11}/_{12}$ yr)—child briefly views picture of face and must pick same face with different pose out of a group photograph

3. Hand movements (21 items; sequential; all ages)—child must copy exact sequence of taps on table with fist, palm, or side of hand

4. Gestalt closure (25 items; simultaneous; all ages)—child must name or describe an incomplete ink drawing

5. Number recall (19 items; sequential; all ages)—a digit repetition task

6. Triangles (18 items; simultaneous; age range $4^{0}/_{12}$–$12^{6}/_{12}$ yr)—child assembles identical rubber triangles (blue on one side, yellow on other side) to match an abstract design

7. Word order (20 items; sequential; age range $4^{0}/_{12}$–$12^{6}/_{12}$ yr)—child points to outlines of common objects in same order as named by examiner

8. Matrix analogies (20 items; simultaneous; age range $5^{0}/_{12}$–$12^{6}/_{12}$ yr)—child selects from an array the design that matches the test design

9. Spatial memory (21 items; simultaneous; age range $5^{0}/_{12}$–$12^{6}/_{12}$ yr)—child has to recall location of pictures arranged randomly on page

10. Photo series (17 items; simultaneous; age range $6^{0}/_{12}$–$12^{6}/_{12}$ yr)—child arranges photographs in proper time sequence

11. Expressive vocabulary (24 items; achievement; age range $2^{6}/_{12}$–$4^{11}/_{12}$ yr)—child names photographed objects

12. Faces and places (35 items; achievement; all ages)—child identifies fictional characters and famous persons and places (e.g., Santa Claus)

13. Arithmetic (38 items; achievement; age range $3^{0}/_{12}$–$12^{6}/_{12}$ yr)—various tasks such as counting, recognizing shapes, identifying numbers, and solving verbal arithmetic problems

14. Riddles (32 items; achievement; age range $3^{0}/_{12}$–$12^{6}/_{12}$ yr)—child must infer name from characteristics (e.g., "What has fur, wags its tail, and barks?")

15. Reading/decoding (38 items; achievement; age range $5^{0}/_{12}$–$12^{6}/_{12}$ yr)—child identifies letters and reads words

16. Reading/understanding (24 items; achievement; age range $7^{0}/_{12}$–$12^{6}/_{12}$ yr)—child must act out printed commands

Description

The test consists of subtests divided into three areas. The basic concepts area subtests—numeration, fractions, and geometry and symbols—evaluate the understanding of basic arithmetic operations. The operations area subtests—addition, subtraction, multiplication, division, mental computation, and numerical reasoning—evaluate computational abilities. The applications area subtests—word problems, missing elements, money, measurements, and time—evaluate the ability to use arithmetic in everyday life. The test items of increasing difficulty are presented orally as open-ended questions by the examiner. For most items, the child must respond orally, although for a few of the more difficult items, written computation may be necessary. Results are expressed as subtest scores, areas scores, and a composite grade-equivalent score. Age range is pre-school through grade 6. Administration requires 30–40 minutes.

The KeyMath Test is a grade-equivalency test and does not allow for age comparisons (Price, 1984). It is a particularly useful test for evaluating individuals with poor reading and writing skills because these are not required.

Neurological Examination for Subtle Signs

Subtle neurologic signs ("soft signs") are frequently evident in children with a variety of neurologic, learning, and behavior problems. The Physical and Neurological Examination for Soft Signs was developed to quantitate these findings (Camp et al., 1978; Holden et al., 1982). It was subsequently revised and renamed the Neurological Examination for Subtle Signs (Denckla, 1985).

Description

The Neurological Examination for Subtle Signs consists of 21 items that test lateral preferences, gait and station, and coordination (10 of the items are timed). Items include various walking (on the heels, on the toes, and on the sides of the feet), rapid alternating movement, and balancing tasks. Age range is approximately 4–15 years. Administration requires approximately 15–20 minutes.

Although norms have been published from the National Institutes of Health sample for some of the timed tasks, this examination is observer-dependent, and thus norms need to be established for each investigator on his or her own population. However, the test does provide a systematic method for reproducibly examining and detecting subtle neurologic signs in children.

Peabody Picture Vocabulary Test—Revised

Peabody Picture Vocabulary Test—Revised is a multiple choice test designed to evaluate receptive vocabulary, originally introduced in 1965 and revised in 1981 (Dunn & Dunn, 1981). The test requires no reading ability. Two equivalent alternate forms are available.

Description

The child is asked to pick one of four pictured items that depict the word spoken by the examiner. There are five training questions and 175 test questions of increasing difficulty. The test is stopped after failures on six out of eight consecutive questions. The score is the total number of items passed, which can be translated into a standard score or age-equivalent (note that in the original test, these translations of the score were termed *IQ* and *mental age,* implying that the Peabody Picture Vocabulary Test was a test of verbal intelligence). Average administration time is 10 minutes. Age range is 2 years to adulthood.

The Peabody Picture Vocabulary Test was standardized on a sample ranging in age from 2.5 years to 40 years. Retest reliability is very high with readministration within 2 weeks using the alternate form or with the same form after several months (Tillinghas et al., 1983).

Stanford-Binet Intelligence Scale—Revised

In 1905 in France, Binet introduced an intelligence test that was subsequently introduced in North America by Terman in 1916. Later revisions were introduced in 1937, 1960, and 1986. The current form is the fourth edition (Thorndike et al., 1986a, 1986b).

Description

The Stanford-Binet Intelligence Scale consists of 15 subtests (Table 3-7). The vocabulary subtest is administered first to obtain a basal level for beginning items in all the other subtests. The basal level for each test is established when two consecutive items are passed; the ceiling level is established by four consecutive failures. The only timed subtest is pattern analysis (subtest 5).

The subtests are grouped into four broad areas—verbal reasoning, abstract/visual reasoning, quantitative reasoning, and short-term memory—and a composite score is derived from the area scores. These standard age scores (equivalent to IQ scores) have a mean of 100 and standard deviation of 16. The test is designed for ages 2–23 years. Administration requires an average of 60–90 minutes.

Vineland Adaptive Behavior Scales

The purpose of the Vineland Adaptive Behavior Scales is to evaluate the various social adaptive behaviors normally important in daily living (Evans & Bradley-Johnson, 1988). This test is an extensive revision of the original Vineland Social Maturity Scales (Doll, 1935).

Description

The test is not administered to the subject but to the caretaker or person most familiar with the subject. The test items are administered in a semistructured interview. For example, for the item "speaks in full sentences," the examiner must ask the caretaker about this with probing questions in such a way as to be certain of the correct understanding and response by the caretaker. Thus, considerable training and skill on the part of the examiner is necessary to accurately administer this test. The survey form consists of 297 items, and the expanded form has an additional 280 items. There are four domains (and multiple subdomains) of behavior assessed with this test: communication (receptive, expressive, and written), daily living skills (personal, domestic, and community), socialization (interpersonal relationships, play and leisure time, and coping skills), and motor skills (gross motor and fine motor). Scoring of each item is as follows: 2 points for activity satisfactorily performed often, 1 point for new or sometimes correctly performed activities, and 0 for

Table 3-7. Stanford-Binet Intelligence Scale—Revised

1. Vocabulary (46 items)—child names pictures (to item 14) and gives word definitions

2. Comprehension (42 items)—child answers questions (e.g., "Give two reasons why there are commercials on television.")

3. Absurdities (32 items)—child must point out incongruities in pictures (e.g., girl writing on a piece of paper with a fork)

4. Verbal relations (18 items)—child is shown cards, each containing four words, and is instructed to describe how the fourth word differs from the other three words (e.g., boy, girl, man, dog)

5. Pattern analysis (42 items)—child must properly place blocks in holes (to item 10) and arrange up to nine blocks in a design

6. Copying (28 items)—child must copy the arrangement of four blocks shown by the examiner (to item 12) and copy geometric shapes shown on cards

7. Matrices (26 items)—child must choose correct geometric design or letter pattern to fill empty box in 2 × 2 and 3 × 3 matrices

8. Paper folding and cutting—child is asked to pick which pattern of folded paper would produce the paper form shown as the test item

9. Quantitative (40 items)—child must correctly arrange blocks with varying numbers of dots, count, and perform simple arithmetic

10. Number series (26 items)—child determines the next two numbers in various number series

11. Equation building (18 items)—child must arrange numbers and arithmetic symbols to produce equations

12. Bead memory (42 items)—child must pick the correct bead or arrange beads on a stick after being shown a card for 5 sec

13. Memory for sentences (42 items)—child repeats sentences ranging in length from 2 to 22 words

14. Memory for digits (26 items)—child must repeat in correct order and in reverse order three to nine digits

15. Memory for objects—child must find two to eight objects in correct sequence as shown previously on cards

no performance of the activity. Scoring yields an adaptive behavior composite score, individual domain and subdomain scores, and age-equivalents. An optional set of questions covers maladaptive behaviors such as bedwetting, impulsiveness, and so forth. Age range is birth to 19 years (which is presumable an adult ceiling for adaptive behavior). Administration time is approximately 20–40 minutes for the survey form and 60–90 minutes for the expanded form.

Standardization of the test involved administration to 3,000 normals (Sparrow et al., 1984). This is an advantage because correlations have been made with other tests. The disadvantage of the test is that it requires extensive training of examiners. In addition, administration time can be greatly increased with poorly informed or uneducated caretakers.

Wechsler Intelligence Tests

The Wechsler intelligence tests have three forms for different age ranges—the Wechsler Preschool and Primary Scale of Intelligence—Revised (WPPSI-R), for age 3–7³/₁₂ years; the Wechsler Intelligence Scale for Children—Third Edition (WISC-III), for ages 6–16¹¹/₁₂ years; and the Wechsler Adult Intelligence Scale—Revised (WAIS-R), for ages 16–74 years. There are individually administered tests that provide a measure of general intelligence and are the most popular tests used for such evaluation (Kaufman, 1979, 1994; Kaufman et al., 1986; Wechsler, 1989, 1991).

Description

The test consists of a series of subtests dichotomized as to verbal or performance subtests. The WISC-III consists of five verbal subtests and five performance subtests (plus 1 optional subtest in the verbal and two optional subtest in the performance categories), as described in Table 3-8.

The WPPSI-R is similar to the WISC-III, with five performance subtests and five verbal subtests (plus 1 optional subtest in both verbal and performance categories). Nine subtests (information, similarities, arithmetic, vocabulary, comprehension, picture completion,

Table 3-8. Wechsler Intelligence Tests

1. Information (verbal)—child is asked questions such as "How many days are there in a week?" or "Who discovered America?" that assess the basic fund of knowledge

2. Similarities (verbal)—child is told to describe how two objects go together or are alike (e.g., "cat" and "mouse"), which assesses higher order conceptual abilities and language facility

3. Arithmetic (verbal)—child is asked to count objects or compute simple word problems without assistance of paper and pencil (e.g., "If I cut an apple in half, how many pieces will I have left?")

4. Vocabulary (verbal)—child is asked to define words (e.g., "bicycle," "nail," "affliction"), which assesses receptive vocabulary

5. Comprehension (verbal)—child is asked questions that require practical reasoning (e.g., "What is the thing to do when you cut your finger?" or "Why should a promise be kept?")

6. Digit span (verbal; optional test)—child repeats series of from three to nine numbers forward and series of two to eight numbers backward, which assesses attention and short-term memory (although anxiety and difficulties with sequential organization can impair performance)

7. Picture completion (performance)—child is asked to identify what parts are missing in a series of pictures (e.g., "leg of an elephant," "slot in a screw"), which assesses part–whole relationships

8. Picture arrangement (performance; timed)—child is asked to arrange a set of jumbled pictures to tell a story, which assesses visual sequencing, social awareness, planning, and appreciation of the relationships of events

9. Block design (performance; timed)—child must recreate designs using blocks with sides that are all red, all white, or half red/half white, which assesses visual-motor coordination

10. Object assembly (performance; timed)—child must assemble puzzle pieces to produce five objects (e.g., child, horse, car, human face, ball), which assesses visual-motor coordination

11. Coding (performance; timed)—this is a substitution task in which the child must fill a blank row of squares above a row of shapes (coding A) or numbers (coding B) with the appropriate symbol keyed to the same number or shape, which assesses visual-motor coordination and motor efficiency

12. Symbol search (performance; optional; timed)—child must determine whether the example shapes are included among a group of test shapes, which assesses visual-motor coordination

13. Mazes (performance; optional; timed)—child must draw a line from the middle of the maze to the exit without entering any "blind alleys," which assesses visual-motor skills and planning

block design, object assembly, and mazes) are the same in both the WPPSI-R and the WISC-III, but the versions are simpler in the WPPSI-R. The sentences subtest is an optional subtest that substitutes for digit span in the verbal category. The animal pegs subtest is an optional subtest in the performance category that substitutes for the coding subtest. The geometric design subtest in the performance category has no counterpart in the WISC-III (Table 3-9).

Scoring produces subtest scaled scores, composite scores for the verbal and performance sections (verbal IQ and performance IQ), and an overall score (full scale IQ). Administration requires an average of 90 minutes.

The Wechsler scales are probably the most widely used intelligence tests in the United States and have been extensively studied, and the previous version, the WISC-R, was the most extensively cited test in the psy-

Table 3-9. Wechsler Preschool and Primary Scale of Intelligence—Revised

1. Sentences (verbal; optional)—child must repeat verbatim a sentence read aloud by the examiner (e.g., "Fish swim."), which assesses short-term memory and attention

2. Animal pegs (performance; optional)—child must place a colored peg next to a picture of an animal according to a key

3. Geometric design (performance)—consists of two parts: in the visual recognition/discrimination items, child must identify an example shape among a group of test shapes; in the drawing items, child must copy a series of figures, which assesses visual-motor coordination

chology literature (Kaufman, 1979, 1990). In addition to correlations with the verbal, performance, and full scale IQ scores, many factor analyses have been performed on the various subtests (Wechsler, 1991).

Weinberg Screening Affective Scale

In 1973, Weinberg and colleagues published criteria for establishing the diagnosis of depression in children. Weinberg subsequently developed a question-naire that can be used to screen for depression in individual settings or with group administration (Weinberg & Emslie, 1988).

Description

The test is used as a screening measure for evidence of depression in children and adolescents (Table 3-10). The test consists of 56 "yes-no" items.

The WSAS has been used in one study to survey a school population for evidence of depression (Emslie et al. 1990).

Table 3-10. Weinberg Screening Affective Scale

Instructions: We would like to ask you some very serious and very important questions. We want to know how you feel about yourself. If you agree with the statement, circle Yes. If you do not agree with the statement, circle No. We consider these questions and your answers very important.		
1. I will try to give my honest feelings on these questions.	Yes	No
2. I feel dumb and stupid too much of the time.	Yes	No
3. I can't do my homework anymore.	Yes	No
4. I wish that I could stay in bed all day.	Yes	No
5. I can't do anything right.	Yes	No
6. Sometimes I wish I were dead.	Yes	No
7. I don't like other people.	Yes	No
8. I don't like school anymore.	Yes	No
9. I feel sad too much of the time.	Yes	No
10. I can't do my school work anymore; it's too hard.	Yes	No
11. It's hard to have any fun anymore.	Yes	No
12. School makes me feel sick.	Yes	No
13. I have too many bad moods.	Yes	No
14. This is not a good world.	Yes	No
15. I don't like to eat anymore.	Yes	No
16. I feel lonely too much of the time.	Yes	No
17. I have too much trouble remembering things.	Yes	No
18. Nothing is ever done the way I like it.	Yes	No
19. I eat too much.	Yes	No
20. I am not as good as other people.	Yes	No
21. It seems like I'm always in trouble for fighting, and that is not fair.	Yes	No
22. I have gained too much weight.	Yes	No
23. I have too many headaches.	Yes	No
24. I don't want to go to school anymore.	Yes	No
25. I don't have fun playing with my friends anymore.	Yes	No
26. I feel too tired to play.	Yes	No
27. It seems like some part of my body always hurts me.	Yes	No
28. It makes me feel good to tease other people.	Yes	No

(continued)

Table 3-10. *(continued)*

29. People are always talking about me when I'm not there.	Yes	No
30. I can't sit still, and that is a problem for me.	Yes	No
31. My friends don't want to be with me anymore.	Yes	No
32. I'm too hard to get along with.	Yes	No
33. I can't concentrate on my work.	Yes	No
34. I daydream too much in school.	Yes	No
35. I never seem to be able to finish my work in school.	Yes	No
36. I have too many stomachaches.	Yes	No
37. I have too many aches and pains in my muscles.	Yes	No
38. I don't want to get out of bed in the morning.	Yes	No
39. I talk too much, and that causes a problem for me.	Yes	No
40. I'm always grouchy, and that's bad.	Yes	No
41. It's hard to fall asleep, and that bothers me.	Yes	No
42. My friends don't like me anymore.	Yes	No
43. When I wake up at night, it is hard to go back to sleep.	Yes	No
44. I am losing too much weight.	Yes	No
45. I cause trouble for everybody.	Yes	No
46. I don't want to be with my friends anymore.	Yes	No
47. Everybody picks on me.	Yes	No
48. I get angry easily.	Yes	No
49. School makes me feel nervous.	Yes	No
50. I cry a lot.	Yes	No
51. I talk back to grown-ups.	Yes	No
52. I wake up too early in the morning, and it is hard to go back to sleep.	Yes	No
53. I can't have any fun anymore.	Yes	No
54. I think a lot about killing myself.	Yes	No
55. My answers are how I have been feeling most of the time.	Yes	No
56. These answers represent my honest feelings.	Yes	No

Score sheet

Criteria for depression by self-report

A. I and II plus four (4) or more of III–X

B. Two or more positive items per major symptom category: I–X

C. "Yes" response on question 55

	Number of positive items	Criteria	
I: 9,13,14,16,18,40,48,50	_____	Yes	No
II: 2,5,6,20,21,29,31,42,47,54	_____	Yes	No
III: 28,32,45,51	_____	Yes	No
IV: 38,41,43,52	_____	Yes	No
V: 3,10,17,33,34,35	_____	Yes	No
VI: 7,25,46	_____	Yes	No
VII: 8,12,24,49	_____	Yes	No

Table 3-10. *(continued)*

VIII: 23,27,36,37		_____	Yes	No
IX: 4,11,26,53		_____	Yes	No
X: 15,19,22,44		_____	Yes	No
	Total: _____			
Total number of positive categories				
I II III IV V VI VII VIII IX X:		_____		
Response to question 55:			Yes	No
Depression by self-report:			Yes	No
Death wish—positive on item 6:			Yes	No
Suicidal ideation—positive on item 54:			Yes	No

References

Armstrong BB, Knopf KF. Comparison of the Bender-Gestalt and Revised Developmental Test of Visual-Motor Integration. *Percept Mot Skills* 1982;55:164–66.

Ballard J, Khoury JC, Wedig K, et al. New Ballard Score, expanded to include extremely premature infants. *J Pediatr* 1991;119:417–23.

Bayley N. *Bayley Scales of Infant Development* (2nd ed.). San Antonio: The Psychological Corporation, 1993.

Bayley N. Development of mental abilities. In: Mussen PH (ed.). *Carmichael's manual of child psychology* (3rd ed.). New York: Wiley, 1970.

Beck AT. *Depression: clinical, experimental, and theoretical aspects.* New York: Harper & Row, 1967.

Beery KE. *Developmental Test of Visual-Motor Integration.* Austin, TX: PRO-ED, 1989.

Beery KE. *Revised administration, scoring, and teaching manual for the Developmental Test of Visual-Motor Integration.* Cleveland: Modern Curriculum Press, 1982.

Beery KE, Buktenica NA. *Developmental Test of Visual-Motor Integration.* Chicago: Follett Publishing, 1967.

Brazelton TB. *Neonatal Behavioral Assessment Scale.* London: Spastics International Medical Publications, 1973.

Brazelton TB. *Neonatal Behavioral Assessment Scale* (2nd ed.). London: Spastics International Medical Publications, 1984.

Brazelton TB, Nugent JK. *Neonatal Behavioral Assessment Scale* (3rd ed.). London: Mac Keith Press, 1995.

Camp JA, Bialer I, Sverd J, et al. Clinical usefulness of the NIMH Physical and Neurological Examination for Soft Signs. *Am J Psychiatry* 1978;135:362–64.

Conners CK. A teacher rating scale for use in drug studies with children. *Am J Psychiatry* 1969;126:884–88.

Conners CK. Symptom patterns in hyperkinetic, neurotic, and normal children. *Child Dev* 1970;41:667–82.

Conners CK. *The Conners' rating scales.* Austin, TX: PRO-ED, 1985.

Connolly AJ. *KeyMath—Revised: manual.* Circle Pines, MN: American Guidance Service, 1988.

Connolly AJ, Nachtman W, Pritchett EM. *The KeyMath Diagnostic Arithmetic Test.* Circle Pines, MN: American Guidance Service, 1976.

Damarin F. Bayley Scales of Infant Development. In: Buros OK (ed.). *The eighth mental measurement yearbook.* Vol. 1. Highland Park, NJ: Gryphon, 1978:290–93.

Das JP, Kirby JR, Jarman RF. *Simultaneous and successive cognitive processes.* New York: Academic Press: 1979.

Denckla MB. Revised Neurological Examination for Subtle Signs. *Psychopharmacol Bull* 1985;21:773–800.

Dixon SD, Synder J, Holve R, et al. Behavioral effects of circumcision with and without anesthesia. *J Dev Behav Pediatr* 1984;3:246–50.

Doll EA. A genetic scale of social maturity. *Am J Orthopsychiatry* 1935;5:180–88.

Dubowitz L, Dubowitz V. *The neurological assessment of the preterm and fullterm newborn infant.* London: Spastics International Medical Publications, 1981.

Dubowitz LMS, Dubowitz V, Goldberg C. Clinical assessment of gestational age in the newborn infant. *J Pediatr* 1970;77:1–10.

Dumond R, Hagberg C. Review of the Kaufman Adolescent and Adult Intelligence Test. *J Psychoed Assess* 1994; 12:190–96.

Dunn LM, Dunn LM. *Peabody Picture Vocabulary Test—Revised.* Circle Pines, MN: American Guidance Service, 1981.

Emslie GJ, Weinberg WA, Rush AJ, et al. Depressive symptoms by self-report in adolescence: phase I of the development of a questionnaire for depression by self-report. *J Child Neurol* 1990;3:114–21.

Evans LD, Bradley-Johnson S. A review of recently developed measures of adaptive behavior. *J Clinl Psychol* 1988;44:276–87.

Field T, Schanberg SM, Scafidi F, et al. Tactile/kinesthetic stimulation effects on preterm neonates. *Pediatrics* 1986;77:654–58.

Fogelman C (ed.). *Manual for the AAMD Adaptive Behavior Scales: 1974 revision.* Washington, DC: American Association on Mental Deficiency, 1974.

Folstein MF, Folstein SE, McHugh PR. "Mini-Mental State." A practical method for grading the cognitive state of patients for the clinician. *J Psychiatric Res* 1975;12:189–98.

Fowles ER. The Brazelton Neonatal Behavioral Assessment Scale and Maternal Identity. *Am J Matern Child Nurs* 1999;24:287–93.

Frankenburg WK, Camp BW (eds.). *Pediatric screening tests.* Springfield, IL: Charles C. Thomas, 1975.

Frankenburg WK, Chen J, Thornton SM. Common pitfalls in the evaluation of developmental screening tests. *J Pediatr* 1988a;113:1110–13.

Frankenburg WK, Dodds J, Archer P, et al. The Denver II: a major revision and standardization of the Denver Developmental Screening Test. *Pediatrics* 1992;89:91–97.

Frankenburg WK, Ker CY, Engelke S, et al. Validation of key Denver Developmental Screening Test items: a preliminary study. *J Pediatr* 1988b;112:560–66.

Frostig M, Lefever DW, Whittlesey JRB. *Administration and scoring manual for the Frostig Developmental Test of Visual Perception.* Palo Alto, CA: Consulting Psychologists Press, 1966.

Goyette C, Conner CK, Ulrich R. Normative data on revised Conners parent and teacher rating scales. *J Abnorm Child Psychol* 1978;6:221–36.

Grossman HJ. *Manual on terminology and classification in mental retardation* (revised ed.). Washington, DC: American Association on Mental Deficiency, 1983.

Hammill DD, Brown L, Bryant BR. *A consumer's guide to tests in print* (2nd ed.). Austin, TX: PRO-ED, 1992.

Holden EW, Tranowski KJ, Prinz RJ. Reliability of neurological soft sign in children: reevaluation of the PANESS. *J Abnorm Child Psychol* 1982;10:163–72.

Horner TM. Single versus repeated assessments of infant abilities using the Bayley Scales of Infant Development. *Infant Mental Health Journal* 1988;9:209–17.

Kaufman AS. *Intelligent testing with the WISC-R.* New York: Wiley, 1979.

Kaufman AS. *Assessing adolescent and adult intelligence.* Boston: Allyn and Bacon, 1990.

Kaufman AS. *Intelligent testing with the WISC-III.* New York: Wiley, 1994.

Kaufman AS, Kaufman NL. *K-ABC: Kaufman Assessment Battery for Children.* Circle Pines, MN: American Guidance Service, 1983.

Kaufman AS, Kaufman NL. *Manual for the Kaufman Adolescent and Adult Intelligence Test.* Circle Pines, MN: American Guidance Service, 1993.

Kaufman AS, Long SW, O'Neal MR. Topical review of the WISC-R for pediatric neuroclinicians. *J Child Neurol* 1986;1:89–98.

Kaufman AS, O'Neal MR, Avant AH, et al. Introduction to the Kaufman Assessment Battery for Children (K-ABC) for pediatric neuroclinicians. *J Child Neurol* 1987;2:3–16.

Kazdin AE, Petti TA. Self-report and interview measures of childhood and adolescent depression. *J Child Psychol Psychiatry* 1982;23:437–57.

Kovacs M. Rating scales to assess depression in school-aged children. *Acta Paedopsychiatrica* 1980–1981;46:305–15.

Lehr CA, Ysseldyke JE, Thurlow ML. Assessment practices in model early childhood special education programs. *Psychology in the Schools* 1987;24:390–99.

Luria A. *Higher cortical function in man* (2nd ed.). New York: Basic Books, 1980.

Martin R, Sewell T, Manni J. Effects of race and social class on pre-school performance of the Developmental Test of Visual-Motor Integration. *Psychology in the Schools* 1977;14:466–70.

Naglieri JA. Use of the WISC-R and the K-ABC with learning disabled, borderline mentally retarded, and normal children. *Psychology in the Schools* 1985;22:133–41.

Nihira K, Foster R, Shelihaas M, et al. *Adaptive Behavior Scales.* Washington, DC: American Association on Mental Deficiency, 1969.

Ouvrier R, Hendy J, Bornholt L, et al. SYSTEMS: School-Years Screening Test for the Evaluation of Mental Status. *J Child Neurol* 1999;14:772–80.

Ouvrier RA, Goldsmith RF, Ouvrier S, et al. The value of the Mini-Mental State Examination in childhood: a preliminary study. *J Child Neurol* 1993;8:145–48.

Petti TA. Depression in hospitalized child psychiatry patients: approaches to measuring depression. *J Am Acad Child Psychiatry* 1978;17:49–59.

Petti TA, Conners CK. Changes in behavioral ratings of depressed children treated with imipramine. *J Am Acad Child Psychiatry* 1983;22:355–60.

Petti TA, Law W. Imipramine treatment of depressed children: a double-blind study. *J Clin Psychopharmacol* 1982;2:107–10.

Poznanski EO, Cook SC, Carroll BJ. A depression rating scale for children. *Pediatrics* 1979;64:442–50.

Poznanski EO, Freeman LN, Mokros HB. Children's Depression Rating Scale—Revised. *Psychopharmacol Bull* 1985;21:979–89.

Poznanski EO, Grossman JA, Buchsbaum Y. Preliminary studies of the reliability and validity of the Children's Depression Rating Scale. *J Am Academy Child Psychiatry* 1984;23:191–97.

Price PA. A comparative study of the California Achievement Test (forms C and D) and the KeyMath Diagnostic Arithmetic Test with secondary LH students. *J Learn Disabil* 1984;17:392–96.

Ramey CT, Campbell FA, Nicholson JE. The predictive power of the Bayley Scales of Infant Development and the Stanford-Binet Intelligence Test in a relatively constant environment. *Child Dev* 1973;44:790–95.

Raskin A (ed.). *Psychopharmacol Bull* 1985;21:713–1124.

Sattler JM. *Assessment of children.* San Diego: Jerome M. Sattler Publisher, 1988.

Schalock RL, Braddock DL (eds.). *Adaptive behavior and its measurement: Implications for the field of mental retardation.* Washington, DC: American Association on Mental Retardation, 1999.

Sparrow SS, Balla DA, Cicchetti DV. *Vineland Adaptive Behavior Scales.* Circle Pines, MN: American Guidance Service, 1984.

Spreen O, Strauss E. *A compendium of neuropsychological tests: administration, norms, and commentary.* New York: Oxford, 1991.

Stjernqvist K, Svenningsen NW. Neurobehavioural development at term of extremely low-birthweight infants (less than 901g). *Dev Med Child Neurol* 1990;32:679–88.

Thorndike RL, Hagen EP, Sattler JM. *Stanford-Binet Intelligence Scale* (4th ed.). Chicago: Riverside Publishing, 1986a.

Thorndike RL, Hagen EP, Sattler JM. *Technical manual: Stanford-Binet Intelligence Scale* (4th ed.). Chicago: Riverside Publishing, 1986b.

Tillinghas BS, Morrow JE, Uhlig GE. Retest and alternate form reliability of the PPVT-R with fourth, fifth, and sixth grade pupils. *J Education Res* 1983;76:243–44.

Trites RL, Blouin AG, Ferguson HB, et al. The Conners Teacher Rating Scale: an epidemiological inter-rater reliability and follow-up investigation. In: Gadow K, Loney J (eds.). *Psychosocial aspects of drug treatment for hyperactivity.* Boulder, CO: Westview Press, 1982a.

Trites RL, Blouin AGA, Laprade K. Factor analysis of the Conners Teacher Rating Scale based on a large normative sample. *J Consult Clin Psychol* 1982b;50:615–23.

Wechsler D. *Manual for the Wechsler Preschool and Primary Scale of Intelligence—Revised.* San Antonio: The Psychological Corporation, 1989.

Wechsler D. *Manual for the Wechsler Intelligence Scale for Children Third Edition.* San Antonio: The Psychological Corporation, 1991.

Weinberg WA, Emslie GJ. Weinberg screening affective scales (WSAS and WSAS-SF). *J Child Neurol* 1988; 3:294–96.

Weinberg WA, Rutman J, Sullivan L, et al. Depression in children referred to an educational diagnostic center: Diagnosis and treatment. *J Pediatr* 1973;83:1065–72.

Werry JS, Sprague RL. Methylphenidate in children—effect of dosage. *Aust N Z J Psychiatry* 1974;8:9–19.

Wodrich DL. *Children's psychological testing: a guide for non-psychologists* (3rd ed.). Baltimore: Paul H. Brookes Publishing, 1997.

4 Pediatric Neurologic and Rehabilitation Rating Scales

Raphael Corcoran Sneed, M.D., Edward L. Manning, Ph.D., and Cathy F. Hansen, M.S., P.T.

"Children Are Not Small Adults"

The simple and important mantra in pediatrics, "children are not small adults," is often forgotten or ignored by adult-orientated physicians, especially when considering pediatric neurologic and rehabilitation rating scales. Such rating scales are not new. As far back as 1935 physical and functional scales were attempted for "crippled children" (Sheldon, 1935). However, neurologic and functional rating scales did not come to the forefront until the last quarter of the twentieth century. Physicians face unique challenges in formulating measurement outcomes for children, perhaps even more so than for adults (Bax, 1993). This coincides with an increasing emphasis in medicine, including pediatrics, for more scientific confirmation of treatments and interventions for which appropriate rating scales in research, prognostication, and benchmarking of management are critical (Bax, 1986, 1988, 1993, 1999; Butler, 1995; Majnemer & Limperopoulos, 2002; O'Donnell & Roxborough, 2002; Sussman, 2001).

The principal features of pediatrics and children are (1) growth and development and the corollary of (2) the effect of age on human pathological conditions. These features raise several issues in applying rating and outcome scales. First, children are constantly changing, which makes a single rating or outcome scale extremely difficult to develop. This is especially true in regard to "What is normal?" when the correct question should be "What is normal *for what age*?" A newborn is *normally* dependent in almost all activities, whereas older children are partially dependent and adolescents mostly independent for the same evaluated function. An acutely injured child at 9 months of age may normally be nonambulatory but when reexamined 6 months later be walking independently. Although the same rating scale done at each of these times shows change, was the improvement in mobility due to normal maturation or to some intervention during this period, or both? Thus normalized scales become extremely difficult and complex if they are to be thorough and accurate. Yet there is a recognition that the more complex the scale, the less likely it will be used and the greater the concerns about interrelater reliability.

Second, incidences and etiologies for specific disorders (e.g., stroke, spinal cord injury [SCI], multiple sclerosis) are often quite different in children than adults. For example, cerebral vascular accidents are much less frequent in childhood but have a much greater range of etiologies than for adults. Multiple sclerosis is very uncommon in childhood; but one finds much more literature regarding cerebral palsy. Furthermore, most adult inpatient rehabilitation centers and outpatient clinics group patients by diagnosis in *dedicated* or *program-specific* units (e.g., stroke, brain injury, SCI, geriatric). Whereas a pediatric unit usually has a plethora of mixed diagnoses. Age is the divider traditionally used for children, etiology for adults.

A third issue for rating and outcome scales is the same problem physicians often face when prescribing medications for pediatric patients. In 1968, Dr. Harry Shirkey coined the term *therapeutic orphans* (therapeutic orphan syndrome or TOS) for the lack of studies about the safety, proper dosage, and efficacy for drugs for children that have been approved for adults (Shirkey, 1968). The same holds true for most major neurologic rating scales, as there are few or no studies that validate results for children of all ages. Most of the scales were developed for adult use only, just as most drugs developed for adults lack research for their use in children. The scales' validity for children of varying ages may be open to question. Results must be viewed with caution unless specific literature exists to validate the scales' pediatric application to all ages tested. On further inspection, age may also affect assessments in adults, especially as scales are increasingly undergoing subset revisions for elderly populations.

A problem for any rating scale is pushing it beyond the original limits of its development and, even more so, applying it to groups for which it has not been *normed*. Thus, investigators may apply adult-derived scales without taking into account that the developing child is undergoing continued neuromuscular and cognitive changes, especially in the first 5–7 years of life, or that *abnormal* reflexes (*primitive reflexes*) may be normal at certain ages. Nor are children able to cognitively cooperate before reaching certain developmental stages. For example, it is generally accepted that most children cannot sufficiently cooperate to perform a manual muscle test of strength until a chronological and mental age of approximately 5 years is reached. In doing sensation testing of dermatomes scoring, a younger child may be able by "blinding" to tell if pain is felt or not felt, but unable to quantify whether pain is present but has decreased. Furthermore, if the young child is not "blinded," he or she age-appropriately cries emotionally even at the sight of the approaching pin, negating any accurate testing of true sensation. Additionally, whereas adults of all ages (excluding perhaps for the very elderly) are assumed to perform all motor and cognitive normed tasks equally well, "norms" for children are changing with age and development. A child given a score at age 1 who then achieves a higher score at a later age for the same areas rated may appear on paper to have improved; in reality the child may still be well below the norms appropriate for the later age.

Problems with Pediatric Scales

Many of the pediatric scales were developed and tested for specific diagnostic categories such as cerebral palsy, traumatic brain injury (TBI) or Down syndrome. Therefore, caution is urged with their use in a new group of subjects because they may lack validation for these children. Although both have SCI, children with spina bifida (S/B) may behave and respond quite differently from those with acquired traumatic SCI or have many associated problems that affect test results.

One must also take care in blind acceptance of numbers in rating scales, especially when gleaned from a review of clinical charts. Inter-rater reliability may be poor. In a controlled environment study with ongoing training and recredentialing of the staff, scoring may be fairly accurate. However, in noncontrolled settings, knowledge and definition of the ratings by the observers may be quite variable. For example, studies have previously shown that pediatric residents have little training in physical medicine and rehabilitation (Coury, 1990; Paul & Kathirithamby, 1991; Sneed et al., 2000). Thus, their knowledge of American Spinal Injury Association (ASIA) scoring, manual muscle strength testing, Glasgow Coma Scale, Rancho Los Amigos Cognitive Scale, and other testing may be less than ideal.

Physical Rehabilitation Medicine involves the focused monitoring and measuring of a person's current physical and cognitive functional status, along with a prediction of later physical, cognitive, and social outcomes in a community environment. One should take care not to look only at composite scores. A child with good motor scores but cognitive impairment may have the same total score as a child with poor motor scores but intact cognition. But cognition may be the key in the long-term outcome of rehabilitation. "Carry over" must also be considered. Certain therapeutic regimens have been known to show improvements in a child in a controlled environment or with a therapist but not in a community environment or with other caregivers. Thus ratings in controlled settings may not be the same as outside in daily life.

Existing Pediatric Neurologic Rating Scales

As many of the scales are reviewed in depth elsewhere in this book, we will not repeat the evaluations but comment on those areas that have additional pediatric modifications. Given the voluminous reports published almost monthly on new rating scales, another question arises. At what point should a newly developed scale be accepted for general and valid use?

A multitude of rating scales for children exist that the neurologist should be familiar with, although many of these focus on growth and development and on behavior rather than on motor or functional status. Several excellent reviews of such scales already exist (Gormley & Krach, 1997; Lollar et al., 2000; Molnar & Sobus, 1999; Robbins & Crowley, 1999; Taggart & Aguilar, 2000). Previously well covered materials in the above references will not be repeated here, except for commentary on a few of the major and commonly used scales. Instead, areas not reviewed previously will be the focus. Table 4-1 is provided with a summation of some of the existing scales for quick review along with references or resource location for further inquiry. A detailed discussion of the more commonly used scales follows.

The Apgar score (Apgar, 1953) is perhaps the most venerable and widely used (almost everyone born in a United States hospital has one) pediatric-specific rating scale and a good example of the phenomena of attempting to stretch a rating scale beyond its original intent. The Apgar score is not a neurologic rating scale, although both parents and physicians, including neurologists, have attempted to use it as such. It is an objective method to guide physicians for resuscitative efforts needed in infants after delivery and nothing more (Shevell, 1999). It may not even correlate well with the presence of "birth asphyxia" (Marrin & Paes, 1988). This is not surprising, as it is now recognized that most causes of cerebral palsy occur prebirth, rather than from "lack of oxygen at birth." Studies performed to try to correlate Apgar with later neurologic outcome continue but so far have shown a lack of sensitivity and specificity for hypoxia at birth or for later neurologic outcome (Jepson et al., 1991). Also the shorter the gestational age of premature infants, the greater the question of its acceptability as compared with mature infants (Juretschke, 2000).

Growth and Development

Growth charts to monitor length/height, weight, and head circumference are a mainstay of pediatrics for monitoring developmental and neurologic disorders. Growth charts adapted from the National Center for Health Statistics data and copied by Ross Laboratories have been among the most widely used. In 2000 the U.S. Centers for Disease Control and Prevention (CDC) released newly revised growth charts for children (available for downloading and printing at http://www.cdc.gov/growthcharts). The older charts had a narrower range of geographic, ethnic, and socioeconomic status whereas the CDC charts are more nationally diverse. Neurologists should note that there are definite differences in head circumference measures in the CDC charts compared with the older charts. Additional curves for body mass index have been added (A body mass index calculator is available for downloading at http://www.cdc.gov/nccdphp/dnpa/bmi/calc-bmi.htm). Further software (Epi Info 2000) is also available from the CDC (http://www.cdc.gov/epiinfo).

Although not a neurologic rating scale, sequence of growth and sexual development does have potential profound effect on the motor and cognitive/social functions of the developing child. Therefore, clinicians and researchers should be aware of the markers of sexual maturation, particularly the five stages of genital and breast development of both sexes as proposed by Tanner (Tanner scale) (Tanner, 1966).

Infantile reflex development is important to the motor development of the maturing child, both in the disappearance of the "primitive", intrauterine, and birth reflexes at the appropriate ages (or their inappropriate persistence due to neurologic insult) and the age appropriate obtainment of the protective and postural reflexes (or the failure to do so, which may lead to mobility dysfunction) (Milani-Comparetti & Gidoni, 1967a, 1967b; Capute, 1986; Molnar & Sobus, 1999). When performing rating scale assessments, especially with more adult-orientated scales, one must recognize that certain primitive reflexes, such as the Babinski up to a year or so, may normally be present and others may normally not appear until after certain ages.

Table 4-1. Neurologic Rating Scales Applicable to Pediatrics

Name and Reference	Age Range	Purpose	How Long	Advantages
ABILITIES Index (Bailey et al., 1993)		Document the nature and extent of childhood disability		
Activities Scale for Kids (Pencharz et al., 2001)		Musculoskeletal disorders		
Alberta Infant Motor Scales (Long & Tieman, 1998; Piper & Dorrah, 1993; Piper et al.)	0–18 mo	Motor	Quick, 15 min	Emphasis on motor milestones; quick; minimal equipment; only observation involved
Assessment for Gestational Age (Amiel-Tison & Grenier, 1968)	Neonates	Neurologic, gestational age		
Amount of Assistance Questionnaire		Amount of assistance to complete standard daily tasks	15 min	
Apgar (Apgar, 1953)	Neonates (newborn 1, 5, 10, 15 min)	Resuscitative intervention	Quick	
Ashworth Score (Ashworth, 1964)		Spasticity/tone		
American Spinal Injury Association (American Spinal Injury Association, 2002)				
Assessment of Movement Activities in Infants (Haley et al., 1989)	Infants	Motor		
Assessment of Preterm Infant Behavior (Als et al., 1982)	Preterm Infants	Neurologic		
Assessment, Evaluation and Programming System for Children (Bricker, 1993)	1 mo–3 yr	Behavioral		
Battelle Developmental Inventory (Newborg et al., 1984; Filiatrault et al., 1991)	0–8 yr, 1 mo–9 yr	Development		
Bayley Infant Neurodevelopmental Screener (Aylward, 1992)	3–24 mo	Brain and behavioral relationship with maturation	15 min	
Bayley Scales of Infant Development-II (Bayley, 1969; The Psychological Corporation, 1993)	2–30 mo, 0–42 mo, 1–42 mo	Developmental delay, cognitive, motor, behavior	45 min for mental, 45 min for motor, some children may require 75 min	One of best standardized techniques for determining developmental status (one of the most widely used in infant research)
Beery-Buktenica Developmental Test of Visual Motor Integration (Beery, 1989)				

Disadvantages	Summary	GM	FM	ADL	AB	LC	RD	S/M	HS/QL	C/B
									Yes	
		Yes								
							Yes			
		Yes		Yes	Yes	Yes				
		Yes								
										Yes
		Yes	Yes							
										Yes
										Yes
Must undergo special training.		Yes	Yes		Yes	Yes	Yes			Yes

(continued)

Table 4-1. *(continued)*

Name and Reference	Age Range	Purpose	How Long	Advantages
Behavior Assessment System for Children (Reynolds & Kamphaus, 1992)	4–18 yr	To aid in the identification and differential diagnosis of emotional and behavioral disorders in children	10–20 min	Allows for comparison of the typography and intensity of problematic behavior (as well as the identification of positive aspects of behavior) across home and school settings
Behavior Rating Inventory of Executive Function (Gioia et al., 2001)	5–18 yr	Designed to assess the presence of executive function deficits based on informant observation; an 86-item scale (each descriptor is rated none, sometimes, often) yielding composite measures for behavioral regulation, metacognition, and a global executive function		A useful observation-based method for identification of executive function deficits
Bleck (Bleck, 1975)				
Bobath (motor treatment technique rather than rating scale) (Bobath, 1967)				
Bobath Test Chart of Motor Ability (Bobath, 1980)	Childhood	Motor		
Boston Naming Test (Kaplan et al., 1983)	>5.5 yr	To assess confrontational naming skills		A sensitive measure of confrontational naming
Brigance Inventory of Early Development (Brigance, 1978)	0–7 yr	Developmental		
Bruininks-Oseretsky Test of Motor Proficiency (Bruininks, 1978)	4.5–14.5 yr	Motor	45–60 min, 15–20 min short form	Has short form
Brunnstrom (motor treatment technique rather than rating scale)				
California Verbal Learning Test Children's Version (Delis et al., 1994)	5–16 yr	Designed to assess verbal learning and memory	55 min	A sensitive measure for the identification of components of verbal learning and memory
Canadian Occupational Performance Measure (Law et al., 1994)	Variable, 7 yr–adult	Variable	45 min	
Carolina Curriculum for Infants and Toddlers with Special Needs, 2nd ed. (Johnson-Martin et al., 1991)	0–36 mo	Behavioral		
Cerebral Palsy Assessment Chart (Semans, 1965)	Childhood	Motor; cerebral palsy		
Chandler Movement Assessment of Infants: Screening Test (Chandler et al., 1980)	0–<12 mo	Neurologic		

Disadvantages	Summary	GM	FM	ADL	AB	LC	RD	S/M	HS/QL	C/B
Measures for preschoolers are not as psychometrically sound and should be interpreted with caution.	A well-designed and developed series of measures for the identification of emotional and behavioral disorders in children									Yes
Further research is needed demonstrating correlations between the rating and objective measures of executive dysfunction.	An informant-based method for identification of executive function deficits									
		Yes								
	A 60-item measure of confrontational naming	Yes	Yes	Yes	Yes	Yes				
May have too lengthy and complex instructions for young children		Yes	Yes							
Hand scoring is tedious.	A well-designed and sensitive measure of components of verbal learning and memory									Yes
		Yes	Yes		Yes	Yes				
		Yes					Yes			
		Yes					Yes			

(continued)

Table 4-1.   *(continued)*

Name and Reference	Age Range	Purpose	How Long	Advantages
Child Behavior Checklist (Achenbach, 1994)	2–18 yr	To assess the competencies and problems of children and adolescents using ratings from different formats	15 min	Developed for the collection of information across informants, facilitating identification and differential diagnosis of behavioral and emotional problems
Child Health and Illness Profile-Adolescent Edition (Starfield et al., 1993)	11–17 yr	Health assessment specifically for adolescents	30 min	Measures differences among age, gender, and socioeconomic status; may evaluate impact on health care interventions
Child Health Questionnaire (Landgraf et al., 1996)	One version for 5–15 yr, one for 2 mo–5 yr, and one for parents	Compares health of general and specific groups		Eliminates the benefits of alternative treatments; has been translated and used in several non-English–speaking countries
Child Health Questionnaire Parent Form (Landgraf et al., 1996)		Musculoskeletal disorders		
Children's Auditory Verbal Learning Test-2 (Talley, 1993)	6 yr 6 mo–17 yr 11 mo	Assess the presence and severity of learning and memory impairment in children		
Children's Depression Inventory (Kovacs, 1982)	7–17 yr	Self-rating index of depressive symptoms	10–15 min	Clinical and research utility for assessing self-report of depressive symptoms
Children's Memory Scale (Cohen, 1998)	5–16 yr	To evaluate learning and memory functions in children and adolescents; the complete scale consists of nine subtests that assess functions in three domains—auditory/verbal, visual/nonverbal, and attention/concentration	20–50 min	A subgroup of the examinees was also administered the Wechsler Intelligence Scale for Children-Third Edition or the Wechsler Preschool and Primary Scale of Intelligence-Revised, allowing for the evaluation of relationships and discrepancies between IQ and memory.
Children's Orientation and Amnesia Test (Msall, 1996)	3–15 yr	Cognition	10 min	
Coma/Near-Coma Scale	>1 yr		20 min	
Comprehensive Developmental Scales				
Conners' Continuous Performance Tests	6 yr–adult	To assess attention problems	14 min	A sensitive measure of attention/vigilance
DeGangi-Berk Test of Sensory Integration (Berk & DeGangi, 1983)	3–5 yr	Sensory motor, postural control; bilateral motor integration, reflex integration	30 min	Diagnostic tool
Denver II (Frankenburg et al., 1967, 1970; Glascoe et al., 1992)	1 mo–6 yr, 2 wk–6 yr	Developmental	25 min	
Developmental Hand Dysfunction: Theory, Assessment and Treatment (Erhardt, 1994)	15 mo–adult	Evaluation of hand dysfunction in neurologic conditions		

Disadvantages	Summary	GM	FM	ADL	AB	LC	RD	S/M	HS/QL	C/B
Some scales do have low levels of reliability, suggesting caution with interpretation.	A series of self-report, parent and/or teacher report measures that allow for a broad-based screening of behavioral and emotional disorders									Yes
									Yes	
									Yes	
										Yes
	A 27-item self-report measure of depressive symptoms in children									Yes
One reviewer's experience is that administration of the scale was longer than another memory battery for children (Wide Range Assessment of Memory and Learning). Administration time can also vary considerably with neurologically impaired children.	A psychometrically sound measure of learning/memory functions for children 5–16 yr									Yes
									Yes	
										Yes
	A computer-administered measure of attention problems									Yes
Requires 2 hr of training to administer		Yes	Yes				Yes			
		Yes	Yes		Yes	Yes	Yes			
			Yes							

(continued)

Table 4-1. *(continued)*

Name and Reference	Age Range	Purpose	How Long	Advantages
Developmental Test of Visual Perception (Hammill et al., 1993a)				
Developmental Test of Visual-Motor Integration (Beery, 1989)	2–15 yr	Developmental		
Developmental Visual Dysfunction Assessment (Erhardt, 1993)	6 mo–adult	Measures visual-motor development		
Dubowitz (Neurologic Assessment of the Preterm and Full-term Newborn Infant) (Dubowitz & Dubowitz, 1981; Dubowitz et al., 1998)	Preterm and term infants	Neurologic	Quick	
Early Intervention Developmental Profile (Brown et al., 1997; Rogers & D'Eugenio, 1977)	0–36 mo	Developmental delay		Comprehensive record of skills
Early Learning Accomplishment Profile (Glover et al., 1978)	0–36 mo	Developmental		
Erhardt Developmental Prehension Test	Neonatal–6 yr, 0–15 mo	Hand function, developmental		
Erhardt Developmental Visual Assessment (Erhardt, 1993)				
First Step (screening test for evaluating preschoolers) (Miller, 1993)	2 yr 9 mo–6 yr 2 mo	Developmental	15 min	
Fugl-Meyer Scale of Functional Return after Hemiplegia (Berglund & Fugl-Meyer, 1986; Duncan et al., 1983; Filiatrault et al., 1991; Fugl-Meyer et al., 1975;)				
Functional Activities Score (Msall et al., 1993)	All ages	Spina bifida		
Functional Independence Measure (Granger et al.,1998)				
Functional Rehabilitation Evaluation of Sensori-Neurologic Outcomes (Roberts et al., 1999)		Global, functional	45 min	
Functional Status II-R (Stein & Jessop, 1990)	0–16 yr	Evaluates parent's perceptions of impact of illness on child's physical, social, and psychological functions	30 min	Has good psychometric properties

Disadvantages	Summary	GM	FM	ADL	AB	LC	RD	S/M	HS/QL	C/B
		Yes	Yes							
								Yes		
		Yes					Yes			
Small sample sizes for reliability/ validity testing; not used for diagnosis or prediction of future capabilities		Yes	Yes		Yes					
		Yes	Yes	Yes		Yes				
			Yes							
		Yes			Yes	Yes				
		Yes								
		Yes			Yes		Yes			
Limited in health status measures, mental health assessments, and the interdependence among items									Yes	

(continued)

Table 4-1. *(continued)*

Name and Reference	Age Range	Purpose	How Long	Advantages
Gesell Revised Developmental Diagnosis (Gesell & Amatruda, 1974; Knoblock et al., 1987)	1–36 mo	Developmental delay	45 min	
Glasgow Coma Scale (Raimondi & Hirschauer, 1984)				
Glasgow Outcome Scale (Raimondi & Hirschauer, 1984)				
Gross Motor Function Measure (Gross Motor Measures Group, 1993)	>6 mo, childhood, 5 mo–16 yr	Motor	60 min, 45–60 min	
Gross Motor Function Measure-66 (Russell et al., 2000)				
Gross Motor Function Measure-88				
Gross Motor Functional Classification System (Palisano et al., 1997)	Childhood	Motor		
Halstead-Reitan Neuropsychological Test Battery for Children (Reitan, 1993a)	5–8 yr	Developed to assess a variety of cognitive or neuropsychological functions in children; 14 subtests assessing factors including attention and concentration, language, sensorimotor and motor functions, visuospatial and visuomotor functions, and concept formation		Developed essentially as a downward extension of the adult version of this battery; sensitive to brain–behavior relationships. Individual subtests can be selected to address specific questions.
Halstead-Reitan Neuropsychological Test Battery for Older Children (Reitan, 1993b)	9–14 yr	To assess a range of neuropsychological functions in older children; 12 subtests assessing areas including attention and concentration; sensory, sensorimotor, visuospatial, visuomotor, and motor functions; language; concept formation; and memory		Basically designed as a downward extension of the adult version of this battery, individual tests have demonstrated sensitivity to brain–behavior relationships. Individual tests can be selectively administered to address specific questions.
Harris Infant Neuromotor Test (Harris & Daniels, 1996)	3–12 mo	Detects early signs of cognitive and motor delays	30 min	
Hawaii Early Learning Profile (Furuno et al., 1988; Parks et al., 1988)	3–6 yr, 0–36 mo	Development, global		
Home Observation for Measure of the Environment (Cauldwell, 1984)	Birth–36 mo	Adaptive		
Infant Monitoring Questionnaires (Squires & Bricker, 1989)	4–36 mo	Developmental		

Disadvantages	Summary	GM	FM	ADL	AB	LC	RD	S/M	HS/QL	C/B
		Yes	Yes		Yes	Yes				
		Yes								
		Yes								
Formal training is recommended/ required for administration, scoring, and interpretation; lengthy evaluation if all subtests are performed	A fairly comprehensive battery of tests for a range of neuro-psychological functions for young children									Yes
Formal training is recommended for administration, scoring, and interpretation. Testing using the entire battery can be a lengthy process.	A battery of tests designed to assess a variety of neuropsy-chological functions in older children									Yes
										Yes
		Yes	Yes	Yes	Yes	Yes				
					Yes					

(continued)

Table 4-1. *(continued)*

Name and Reference	Age Range	Purpose	How Long	Advantages
Infant Motor Screen (Nickel et al., 1989)	Preterm for corrected ages of 4–16 mo	Neurologic		
Infant Neurological International Battery (Ellison et al., 1994)	0–9 mo	Neurologic		
Infant Toddler Scale for Every Baby (Miller, 1992)	3–42 mo	Developmental		
Jebsen Test of Hand Function (Jebsen et al., 1969; Taylor et al., 1973)	6 yr and older	Hand function		
Kaufman Assessment Battery for Children (Kaufman & Kaufman, 1983)	2.5–12.5 yr	Designed as a test of intelligence and achievement. The 15 subtests produce four scales—sequential and simultaneous processing, achievement, and nonverbal.	35–75 min, depending on age	The test may prove useful when information is needed about nonverbal abilities.
Kaufman Brief Intelligence Test (Kaufman & Kaufman, 1990)	4–90 yr	To provide a brief measure of verbal and nonverbal intelligence	15–30 min	Useful as a screening measure of verbal and nonverbal abilities
Manual Muscle Testing (Kendall, 1993)				
Milani-Comparetti Motor Development Screening Test (Milani-Comparetti & Gidoni, 1967a, 1967b; Stuberg et al., 1989)	2–24 mo, 1–16 mo	Cerebral palsy, motor		
Miller Assessment for Preschoolers (Miller, 1982)	2 yr 9 mo–5 yr 8 mo	Developmental, sensorimotor, cognitive	Lengthy	
Modified Ashworth (Bohannon & Smith, 1987a)				
Molnar (Molnar & Gordon, 1976)				
Motor Control Assessment (Steel et al., 1991)	2–17 yr	Motor	30–60 min	
Motor Free Visual Perceptual Test (Colarusso & Hammill, 1996)				
Movement Assessment Battery for Children (Henderson & Sugden, 1992)	4–12 yr	Developmental		
Movement Assessment of Infants (Brander et al., 1993)	0–12 mo	Motor	90 min, lengthy	
Movement Assessment of Infants-Revised	0–12 mo	Motor		

Disadvantages	Summary	GM	FM	ADL	AB	LC	RD	S/M	HS/QL	C/B
							Yes			
							Yes			
				Yes	Yes					
			Yes							
Norms for this test are >20 yr old and possibly out of date. As noted earlier, factor analytic studies may not support the designation of sequential processing, simultaneous processing, and achievement designations.	A measure designed to assess general intelligence and achievement in children									Yes
Should not be used as a substitute for more thorough measures of intelligence										Yes
Questionable under 5 yr										
		Yes					Yes			
		Yes	Yes	Yes						Yes
		Yes					Yes			
			Yes							
		Yes					Yes			

(continued)

Table 4-1. (continued)

Name and Reference	Age Range	Purpose	How Long	Advantages
Mullen Scales of Early Learning (Mullen, 1995)	Birth–68 mo	A comprehensive measure of cognitive functions for infants and preschool children. The Mullen is comprised of a gross motor scale (administered to children from birth to 33 mo) and four cognitive scales (visual receptive, fine motor, receptive language).	15–60 min	A useful measure for the assessment of cognitive abilities and gross motor skills for young children
Multilingual Aphasia Examination, Third Edition (Benton et al., 1994)	6–69 yr	To evaluate the presence, severity, and qualitative aspects of aphasia	Not reported	A relatively brief test sensitive to various aspects of receptive and expressive language dysfunction
Naturalistic Observation of Newborn Behavior (Als, 1981)	0–4 wk	Behavioral		
Neurodevelopmental Treatment (motor treatment technique rather than rating scale) (Bobath, 1967)				
Neonatal Behavioral Assessment Scale (Brazelton, 1973)	0–4 wk			
Neonatal Neurobehavioral Exam (Morgan et al., 1988)	<32-wk gestation to 40-wk gestation	Developmental		
Neonatal Oral-Motor Assessment Scale (Braun & Palmer, 1985)	Neonate	Oral motor		
NEPSY: a developmental neuropsychological assessment (Korkman et al., 1998)	3–12 yr	Designed to assess neuropsychological development for children ages 3–12 yr, with separate forms for ages 3–4 yr and 5–12 yr. The NEPSY is designed to measure functions in five domains: attention/executive functions, language, sensorimotor, visuospatial processing.	45–120 min	Considered by one reviewer to be a strong developmental neuropsychological instrument based on sound theory and research. Selected subtests can be administered to address specific questions in place of administration of the entire battery.
Neurobehavioral Assessment of Preterm Infant (Korner & Thom, 1990)	32–42 wk gestation	Neurologic	Long	
Neurologic Exam of the Full-Term Infant (Prechtl, 1977)	Newborn 38–42 wk gestation	Neurologic	Long	

Disadvantages	Summary	GM	FM	ADL	AB	LC	RD	S/M	HS/QL	C/B
None reported. The Mullen is a revised version of the Mullen Scales of Early Learning, and the authors appear to have addressed some of the concerns identified with the original measure.	A comprehensive measure for gross motor skills for children from birth to 33 mo and for general cognitive abilities for children from birth to 68 mo									Yes
The manual does not describe reliability data.	A measure of receptive and expressive language skills comprised of nine subtests and two rating scales that yield findings in five domains—oral expression, spelling, oral verbal understanding, reading, and ratings for articulation and praxic features of writing									Yes
		Yes					Yes			
							Yes			
		Yes								
Some training and practice are required to facilitate administration, scoring, and interpretation of what can be a lengthy battery with older children. Formal training is recommended.	A well-developed measure of developmental neuropsychological functions for children ages 3–12 yr									Yes
		Yes					Yes			
		Yes					Yes			

(continued)

Table 4-1. *(continued)*

Name and Reference	Age Range	Purpose	How Long	Advantages
Nursing Child Assessment Satellite Training and Feeding Scales (Barnerd, 1979)	Teaching, 0–3 yr; feeding, 0–1 yr	Adaptive		
Peabody Developmental Motor Scales (Folio & Fewell, 1983)	0–83 mo	Motor	45–60 min	Can be used to quantify gains in severely handicapped
Peabody Individual Achievement Test-Revised (Markwardt, 1989)	5–22 yr	Designed to measure academic achievement. The test is comprised of six subtests, including general information, reading recognition, reading comprehension, mathematics, spelling, and written expression.	60 min	Several subtests do not require expressive language and, as such, can be useful for assessing subjects with adequate receptive but poor expressive language skills.
Peabody Picture Vocabulary Test-III (Markwardt, 1989)	2.5–90 yr	To measure receptive vocabulary skills and as a screening test of verbal ability	11–12 min	A relatively easy-to-administer measure
Pediatric Assessment of Self-Activities (Coley, 1978)	Childhood	Motor		
Pediatric Evaluation of Disability (Nichols & Case-Smith, 1996)	6 mo–7 yr, 6 mo–7.5 yr	Global, motor	90 min, 20–30 min	
Pediatric Glasgow Coma Scale (Hahn, 1988)	0–3 yr	Consciousness	10 min	
Pediatric Levels of Consciousness (Brink & Imbus, 1982)				
Pediatric Orthopaedic Society of North America Pediatric Musculoskeletal Functional Health Questionnaire				
Pediatric Outcomes Data Collection Instrument (Pencharz et al., 2001)		Musculoskeletal disorders		
Personality Inventory for Children-Second Edition (Seat & Broen, 1977)	5–19 yr	A survey of children's behavior covering behavioral, emotional, cognitive, and interpersonal adjustment		The inventory covers a wide range of psychological and adjustment problems, provides useful validity scales (which reflect reporting tendencies of the informant), and provides useful interpretation guidelines.
Posture and Fine Motor Assessment of Infants (Case-Smith & Bigsby, 2000)	2–12 mo	Motor delays	25–30 min	Better correlations for posture than fine motor
Preschool Test of Visual Motor Integration				

Disadvantages	Summary	GM	FM	ADL	AB	LC	RD	S/M	HS/QL	C/B
					Yes					
Activity cards available, but of little use		Yes	Yes		Yes		Yes			
The reading comprehension measure may be confounded by memory; the spelling measure requires the subject to point to the correct spelling (out of four choices) and, as such, may not provide an accurate index of spelling ability.	An acceptable comprehensive test of academic achievement for areas other than written expression									Yes
None reported	A relatively brief and easy-to-administer measure of receptive language									Yes
		Yes		Yes	Yes					
		Yes		Yes	Yes					
									Yes	
Low reliability is reported for some subscales, suggesting the need for additional research.	An informant-based assessment of psychological, emotional, and cognitive adjustment									
Low reliability scores; use as an adjunct to other tests to determine motor age		Yes	Yes							
New scale: limited data on validity/reliability										

(continued)

Table 4-1. *(continued)*

Name and Reference	Age Range	Purpose	How Long	Advantages
Proprioceptive Neuromuscular Facilitation (motor treatment technique rather than rating scale) (Knott & Voss, 1968)				
Purdue Pegboard Test (Tiffin & Asher, 1948)	2.5 yr–adult	To evaluate gross movement and dexterity of upper extremities. The test consists of two rows of 25 holes into which pins are inserted (fewer holes are used for younger children). Scores are reported for trials for dominant, nondominant, and both hands.	3–9 min	A brief measure of upper extremity dexterity
Quality of Life				
Quality of Well-Being Scale	14 yr and older and adults		20 min to administer and 6-day follow-back format	
Questionnaire for Identifying Children with Chronic Conditions				
Quick Neurological Screen Test-II (Matti et al., 1989)	6–17 yr			
Ranchos Los Amigos Cognitive Scale (Hagen et al.,1974)	0–7 yr	Cognition	10 min	
Rand Health Status Measure for Children	Version for 0–4 yr and version for 5–13 yr	Assesses child's health-related outcomes		Also a scale for adults to compare with
Reflex Testing Methods for Evaluation of Central Nervous System Development (Fiorentino, 1963)	Infancy–6 yr	Motor		
Revised Gesell and Amatruda Developmental Neurological Exam (Knoblock et al., 1987)	4 wk–5 yr	Developmental		
Rey Auditory Verbal Learning Test (Schmidt, 1996)	7–89 yr	Designed to measure verbal learning and memory	15 min	An easily administered measure of verbal learning. Alternate versions of the list are available, enabling the possibility of serial administrations with limited practice effect.
Scales of Independent Behavior (Bruininks et al., 1984)	0–adult	Developmental		

Disadvantages	Summary	GM	FM	ADL	AB	LC	RD	S/M	HS/QL	C/B
	A measure of upper extremity dexterity for children and adults									
Lengthy, complex to administer, only developed on adults									Yes	
									Yes	
		Yes	Yes				Yes			
										Yes
									Yes	
		Yes					Yes			
		Yes	Yes		Yes	Yes				
Care should be taken to locate norms appropriate for the population being evaluated.	An easily administered and sensitive measure of verbal learning for ages 7–89 yr									Yes

(continued)

Table 4-1. *(continued)*

Name and Reference	Age Range	Purpose	How Long	Advantages
Scales of Independent Behavior-Revised (Bruininks et al., 1996)	Infants to adults, with or without developmental disabilities	To assess functional independence and adaptive functioning across settings—school, home, employment, and community	60 min	A useful instrument for professionals determining the eligibility of individuals for educational and/or support services. It allows the examiner to identify skills an individual can or could perform and provides information about the presence of problems.
School Function Assessment Test (Coster et al., 1998)	Elementary school age children with disabilities	Functional activities; evaluation of school performance	1.5–2.0 hr	No special training required to administer
Sensory Integration and Praxis Test (Ayres, 1989)	4 yr–8 yr 11 mo	Sensory integration; vestibular, proprioception, kinesthesia, tactile, visual	1.5–2.0 hr	
Sensory Integration and Praxis Test (Southern California Integration Test) (Ayres, 1989)	4–9 yr, 2 yr 9 mo–5 yr 8 mo	Learning impairment; assessment of developmental status	25–35 min	Statistically sound, identifies strengths and weaknesses
Sensory Profile (Dunn, 1999)	5–10 yr	Assess sensory processing abilities	30 min for caregiver, 10 min for sensory profile, 20–30 min for examiner to complete score sheet	Measures response during course of daily life
Spina Bifida Neurological Scale (Oi & Matsumoto, 1992)	2 yr–adult	Spina bifida		
Standard Recording of Central Motor Deficit (Evans & Alberman, 1985; Evans et al., 1986, 1989)	Childhood	Central nervous system deficit, global		
Tardieu Scale (Tardieu et al., 1954)		Tone		
Test for Gross Motor and Reflex Development (Hoskins & Squires, 1973)	2–24 mo	Motor		
Test of Infant Motor Performance (Campbell, 1993)	32-wk gestation to 3.5 mo after term delivery	Motor	25–40 min	

Disadvantages	Summary	GM	FM	ADL	AB	LC	RD	S/M	HS/QL	C/B
Hand scoring can be tedious. The Problem Behavior Scale, although useful, is a limited sample of items. No validity measures are reported comparing adaptive behaviors reported by informants and adaptive behaviors demonstrated by an individual and/or observed by the examiner.	The scales are a useful measure for rating the functional behavior of a wide age range of individuals and provides for the preliminary indication of the presence of a problem or maladaptive behavior.									
Lengthy to administer		Yes	Yes	Yes	Yes	Yes				
Not to be used with children with severe neuromotor dysfunction								Yes		
		Yes	Yes	Yes	Yes					
					Yes		Yes			
		Yes			Yes		Yes			
		Yes	Yes		Yes	Yes				
		Yes								
		Yes					Yes			
		Yes					Yes			

(continued)

Table 4-1. *(continued)*

Name and Reference	Age Range	Purpose	How Long	Advantages
Test of Memory and Learning (Reynolds & Bigler, 1994)	5–19 yr	Developed to evaluate children and adolescents for a range of learning and memory skills	40–45 min	Described by one reviewer as a highly reliable and well-normed measure for the assessment of learning and memory
Test of Nonverbal Intelligence, Third Edition (Brown et al., 1977)	6–89 yr 11 mo	Designed to assess problem solving and abstract reasoning abilities in a language-free format	15–20 min	A useful screening measure of nonverbal reasoning ability in a language-free format
Test of Sensory Functions in Infants (DeGangi & Greenspan, 1989)	4–18 mo, best suited for 7–18 mo	Measure of sensory processing and reactivity: pressure; adaptive motor function; visual-tactile integration; ocular-motor control; reactivity to vestibular stimulation	20–30 min	Diagnostic tool to be used in conjunction with Bayley Scales of Infant Development
Test of Visual Motor Integration (Hammill et al., 1993b)				
Test of Visual Motor Skills-Revised (Gardner, 1995)				
Test of Visual Perceptual Skills (non-motor) (Gardner, 1988)	4–12 yr 11 mo	Determination of visual-perceptual strengths and weaknesses based (non-motor)	7–15 min	Measures seven subsets of visual perception; does not require verbal response
The Gordon Diagnostic System (Gordon, 1996)	Children to adults	To assess attention/vigilance	9 min per task	A series of measures of simple and complex attention processes
The Token Test for Children (DiSimoni, 1978)	3–12 yr	To assess receptive language dysfunction	8 min	A brief screening measure of receptive language
Toddler and Infant Motor Evaluation (Long & Tieman, 1998; Miller & Roid, 1994)	0–42 mo, 4.0 mo–3.5 yr	Motor	10–20 min for younger children; 20–40 min for older children	Diagnostic tool, development of remediation, treatment research
Transdisciplinary Play Based Assessment (Linder, 1990)	6 mo–6 yr	Adaptive, developmental		
TUFTS Assessment of Motor Performance (Haley et al., 1991)	3 yr and older	Global, motor		
Vienna Vigilance Score (Berger et al., 2001)				

Disadvantages	Summary	GM	FM	ADL	AB	LC	RD	S/M	HS/QL	C/B
One reviewer has indicated that children find the test long and tedious. Another reviewer expressed concerns about methods used to identify and eliminate item and test bias for groups and, as such, expressed concerns about interpretations of test scores with minority groups.	A reliable and sensitive measure of learning and memory for ages 5–19 yr									Yes
Should not be used in the place of more thorough measures of intelligence	A language-free format for assessing problem-solving skills									Yes
Should not be used on infants with delays until 10 mo old								Yes		
							(Visual perception)			
A stand-alone unit that is somewhat expensive. Continuous performance tests have not demonstrated effectiveness with regard to differential diagnosis of attention-related disorders as of yet.	A computer-administered measure of attention/vigilance									Yes
Lack of reliability and validity limits the level of interpretation available with this test.	A brief measure of a child's receptive language skills									
Complex scoring		Yes	Yes	Yes						
						Yes				
		Yes	Yes	Yes	Yes					
										Yes

(continued)

Table 4-1. *(continued)*

Name and Reference	Age Range	Purpose	How Long	Advantages
Vineland Adaptive Behavior Scales (Sparrow et al., 1984)	0–19 yr	Cognitive		
Wechsler Abbreviated Scale of Intelligence (WASI) (The Psychological Corporation, 1999)	6–89 yr	Designed as a brief, reliable measure of general intelligence. One review suggests that this test may be thought of as a combination of the Wechsler Intelligence Scale for Children-Third Edition and the WASI-III. This measure consists of four subtests, two verbal measures (vocabulary and similarities) and two performances measures (block design and matrices).	15–30 min	A brief, yet psychometrically sound measure reflecting general intellectual functions
Wechsler Intelligence Scale for Children-Third Edition (The Psychological Corporation, 1992)	6–16 yr 11 mo	A measure of a child's general intelligence. A collection of 13 subtests. The six verbal subtests use language-based items, and the seven performance subtests use visual-motor items that are less dependent on language.	50–75 min	This test and its predecessor, the Wechsler Intelligence Scale For Children-Revised, are probably the most popular, widely researched, and widely used measures of general intellectual functions for this age range. This measure provides a thorough evaluation of a number of verbal and performance constructs of general intelligence.
Wechsler Preschool and Primary Scale of Intelligence-Revised (Wechsler, 1989)	3.0–7.3 yr	Developed to assess constructs of general intelligence in children	75 min	Excellent standardization; provides useful diagnostic information with regard to constructs of general intelligence
Wechsler Individual Achievement Test-II (The Psychological Corporation, 2001)	4 yr to adult	To assess achievement. The full version provides information on language skills, reading, spelling and written expression, and math skills.	Varies with age	Co-normed with Wechsler intelligence tests to facilitate examination of intelligence–achievement relationships
Wee-Functional Independence Measure (Granger et al., 1998)	6 mo–7 yr, 0–18 yr	Global, motor	30 min	
Westmead Post-Traumatic Amnesia (Marosszeky et al.,1993)				
Wide Range Achievement Test-3 (Wilkinson, 1993)	5–75 yr	Assessment of basic achievement skills for reading, spelling, and arithmetic	15–30 min	A brief but accurate measure of reading recognition, spelling accuracy, and mathematical skills

Disadvantages	Summary	GM	FM	ADL	AB	LC	RD	S/M	HS/QL	C/B
				Yes	Yes					
Limited with regard to some of the concepts typically assessed by measures of general intelligence because of its brevity	A brief (two to four subtests) measure of general intelligence									Yes
Administration of the entire battery, including supplemental subtests, can be time-consuming. Formal training is necessary for accurate administration, scoring, and interpretation.										Yes
Long administration time; low reliability of individual subtests; limited floor for certain subtests; possible difficulties in scoring for some responses. Those issues and others highlight the need for extensive training for administration, scoring, and interpretation.	A well-developed measure of constructs of general intelligence for this age range									Yes
Requires formal training for appropriate administration, scoring, and interpretation	A measure of a comprehensive range of general educational achievement skills									Yes
		Yes		Yes	Yes					
										Yes
	A brief but accurate measure of basic achievement skills for reading, spelling, and math									Yes

(continued)

Table 4-1. *(continued)*

Name and Reference	Age Range	Purpose	How Long	Advantages
Wide Range Assessment of Memory and Learning (Adams & Sheslow, 1990)	5–17 yr	Designed to evaluate a child's learning and memory ability across a variety of verbally and visually presented tasks. The battery has nine subtests, each of which yields a norm-referenced score. These subtests are combined to yield composite scores including verbal memory, visual memory, and learning indices.	45–60 min	Relatively easy to administer and score. Test reviews in Buros Mental Measurements Yearbook suggest it is an effective measure of short-term concentration and attention.
Wisconsin Card Sorting Test (Heaton et al., 1993)	6.5–89.0 yr	Developed initially as a measure of abstract reasoning among adult populations, this measure is used with children and adults as a clinical neuropsychological measure of complex problem solving.	20–30 min	Designed as a measure of executive functions, scoring is available for not only overall level of performance (number of correct category sorts), but also for a typography of performance (number of errors, perseverative responses and errors, etc.), which allows for additional research and clinical applications.
Youth Quality of Life Instrument-Research Version (Patrick et al., 1998)	12–18 yr			Allows cross-cultural comparisons

AB = adaptive behavior; ADL = activities of daily living; C/B = cognitive and/or behavioral; FM = fine motor; GM = gross motor; HS/QL = health status/quality of life; LC = language/communication; RD = reflex development; SM = sensory motor.
Note: Many of the referenced reports do not provide sufficient information to complete the category columns. Only selected scales considered to be most widely used or of significant historical content are reviewed in the text. Scales are referenced so that the reader may review in more detail.
Modified and expanded from Haley et al. (1992), Long (1995), Gormley Jr. & Krach (1997), Molnar & Sobus (1999), Robbins & Crowley (1999), and Taggart & Aquilar (2000).

Motor

Across all rating scales for motor function measures is the long standing observed phenomena of normal neurologic motor changes, which with normal maturation appear to complete and plateau between the ages of 5 and 7 years. This appears to coincide with completion of myelination of the nervous system of the child. This "plateau" accounts for the necessity of caution in attributing improvement on a rating scale observed during a treatment to the treatment itself. The improvement may be attributable to normal maturation or a combination of both.

Manual Muscle Testing

The development of testing for muscle strength is attributed to a number of investigators. Dr. Robert W. Lovett published in 1916 a description of manual muscle testing (MMT) in his book on the treatment of infantile paralysis (Lovett, 1916). In 1927, Charles L. Lowman, M.D. described a numerical system for muscle grades (Lowman, 1927). Henry O. and Florence P. Kendall originated a percentage system of muscle grades in 1936 and published their work as a text in 1949 with the latest revision in 1993 (Kendall et al., 1993). Daniels and Worthingham published a second major text on MMT in the 1940's with the most recent

Disadvantages	Summary	GM	FM	ADL	AB	LC	RD	S/M	HS/QL	C/B
										Yes
Although designed to assist clinicians working with developmentally disabled children, those children were not part of the standardization sample.	A relatively easy to administer measure of learning and memory for children ages 5–17 yr									
Somewhat complex with regard to hand scoring; often referred to as an index of frontal lobe functions, although data do not support this level of specificity	A sensitive measure of executive functions, available in hand- and computer-scored versions, for ages 6.5 yr and older									Yes
									Yes	

edition appearing in a modified version by Hislop and Montgomery (1995). Nancy B. Reese has published the more recent text incorporating muscle testing and sensory functions with an extensive section devoted to pediatrics by Venita Lovelace-Chandler (Reese, 1999).

The need for accurate and reliable measurement of strength is important in the field of rehabilitation. Strength testing is performed to determine the capability of muscle groups or individual muscles to function in movement and their ability to provide stability and support (Kendall et al., 1993). Assessment of muscle function can be used as an indicator of improvement, decline, or prognostication for function based on the results of interventions. MMT is designed to measure the ability of muscle to develop tension against resistance (Sepega, 1990). Many factors must be considered to achieve accurate and reproducible measures to optimize validity and reliability of MMT. Patient positioning, stabilization, muscle palpation, application of resistance, and choice of grading scale should be as uniform as possible.

Although MMT is widely used due to its versatility and common acceptance, there have been problems in terms of inter-tester and intra-tester reliability. Early studies reported complete agreement between examiners of 60–66% and agreement within plus or minus one full grade in 91–95% of the manual muscle tests given (Blair, 1957; Lilienfield et al., 1954).

A lower level of reliability was reported by Iddings et al. (1961) with complete inter-rater agreement of 41–51% and agreement within plus or minus one full grade in 96–98% of the tests. Later studies suggest that MMT has limited inter-rater and test-retest reliability (Beasley, 1961; Bohannon, 1986b; Hinderer & Hinderer, 1993). Even though there is controversy in the literature regarding intra-rater and inter-rater reliability for MMT, Reese (1999) has observed that studies reporting lower inter-rater reliabilities used a research protocol that allowed examiners to use their own method of MMT. Studies that used a uniform method of MMT demonstrated higher inter-rater reliability.

MMT is designed to measure the entire range of muscle strength from no evidence of muscle contraction to movement through the complete range of motion against gravity and maximum resistance (Reese, 1999). The validity of MMT has been well documented by many researchers (Aitkens et al., 1989; Beasley, 1956; Bohannon, 1986b). Evidence demonstrates that MMT possesses predictive validity following SCI (Brown et al., 1991; Lazar et al., 1989). Disagreement exists over the validity of MMT in the strength discernment of muscle grades above 3 (fair) (Scull & Arthreya, 1995). MMT loses ability to discriminate between gradations of strength above the grade of 3 where whole gradations of strength are difficult to discriminate. Much subjectivity exists with terms, such as "maximum," "moderate," or "minimal," when describing force for resistance. The use of isokinetic dynamometry and hand-held dynamometers has been demonstrated as a more valid alternative for gradations of strength above 4 (Aitkens et al., 1989; Bohannon, 1986b; Schwartz et al., 1992).

Numerous methods exist for MMT grading. Multiple grading scale systems can lead to confusion in interpretation or discussion of muscle grades. The chart depicted in Table 4-2 from Kendall (1993) depicts numbers, words, and letter grades. Not indicated on this chart is the system of pluses that correspond to normal (four pluses), good (three pluses), fair (two pluses), poor (one plus), and zero. The form more commonly used is similar to one used in the ASIA

Table 4-2. Key to Muscle Grading

	Function of the Muscle	*Grade Symbols*		
No movement	No contraction felt in the muscle	Zero	0	0
	Tendon becomes prominent or feeble contraction felt in the muscle, but no visible movement of the part	Trace	T	T
Test movement	Movement in horizontal plane			
	Moves through partial range of motion	Poor–	P–	1
	Moves through complete range of motion	Poor	P	2
	Moves to completion of range against resistance or moves to completion of range and holds against pressure	Poor+	P+	3
	Antigravity position	Poor+	P+	3
	Moves through partial range of motion	Poor+	P+	3
Test position	Gradual release from test position	Fair–	F–	4
	Holds test position (no added pressure)	Fair	F	5
	Holds test position against slight pressure	Fair+	F+	6
	Holds test position against slight to moderate pressure	Good–	G–	7
	Holds test position against moderate pressure	Good	G	8
	Holds test position against moderate to strong pressure	Good+	G+	9
	Holds test position against strong pressure	Normal	N	10

From Kendall FP, McCreary EK, Provance PG. *Muscles: testing and function* (4th ed). Baltimore: Williams & Wilkins, 1993, with permission.

Table 4-3. Motor Examination

0 = Total paralysis

1 = Palpable or visible contraction

2 = Active movement, full ROM with gravity eliminated

3 = Active movement, full ROM against gravity

4 = Active movement, full ROM against moderate resistance

5 = (Normal) active movement, full ROM against full resistance

5* = (Normal) active movement, full ROM against sufficient resistance to be considered normal if identified inhibiting factors were not present

ROM = range of motion.
From American Spinal Injury Association: *International standards for neurological classification of spinal cord injury, revised 2002*. Chicago: American Spinal Injury Association, 2002, with permission.

Standards (Table 4-3). Several authors call for standardization of the description of tests and symbols used for recording MMT results to avoid confusion and aid in research (Kendall et al., 1993; Reese, 1999).

MMT is the most inexpensive and convenient method for assessing muscle strength. It may be the most accurate method of assessing strength in very weak muscles (Reese, 1999). For more accurate assessment of strength when muscle strength approaches normal, other methods of testing with dynamometers may be more appropriate (Soderberg, 1999). The mastery of MMT skills requires repeated practice on normal and impaired persons. There are concerns of reliability and validity as previously discussed.

The pediatric population poses special problems for MMT. Much depends on the age and ability of the child to follow directions. Kendall states that "young children seldom cooperate in strong test movements. Very often tests must be recorded as 'apparently normal' which indicates that strength may be normal, although one cannot be sure" (Kendall et al., 1993). Assessment of muscle strength in infants and children below the age of five is more often performed through observation of movement and function. Pediatric assessment procedures do not rely on MMT alone for information on motor activity. Reflex responses, movement against gravity, movement patterns, and functional performance are part of a comprehensive evaluation to assess motor function (Connolly, 1995; Donohoe & Bleakney, 1994). Muscle testing below the age of 5 years may not offer a reliable muscle test (Gajdosik & Gajdosik, 1994). However, Lovelace-Chandler (1999) presents an eloquent description of gravity-resisted techniques for birth through 12 months along with a discussion regarding the difficulties encountered with pediatric populations.

Isolation of specific muscle groups, prevention of substitutions, stabilization, and observation of joint motion in relation to gravity is at the heart of MMT. Upper motor neuron dysfunctions with abnormalities of tone cloud the use of MMT. Isolated muscle function is a task that is limited when spasticity is present. Those difficulties have been well documented by many authors describing motor function in cerebral palsy and adult hemiplegia (Bobath, 1967, 1980; Reynolds et al., 1958). Patterns of movement in association with spasticity for adults and children have been thoroughly described by Bobath (1967), Brunnstrom (1970), and Knott and Voss (1968). Disputes exist over the validity of strength assessments when spasticity is present. Past practices have advocated against MMT as a measure of strength due to the limitations of muscle isolation when patterns of movement are present (Gajdosik & Gajdosik, 1994). However, more recent evidence suggests that hand-held dynamometer measures may be a reliable indicator of strength gains for populations with spasticity (Bohannon, 1986a; Bohannon & Smith, 1987b). Strength assessment in children with specific pathologic conditions, such as Duchenne's muscular dystrophy and myelodysplasia, are described by Agre et al. (1987), Florence et al. (1992), and Stuberg and Metcalf (1988).

MMT remains the most convenient and inexpensive method of examining muscle strength despite the problems that have been documented. It has been shown to be reliable in accurately describing strength in very weak muscles. Examiners are urged to be consistent with grading scales, terminology, and techniques so that reliability of MMT will not suffer.

Brunnstrom Recovery Stages (for Hemiplegia)

Physical therapist Signe Brunnstrom observed large numbers of hemiplegic patients and noted similar sequences of events during recovery. Those stages are described in detail in the text, *Movement Therapy in Hemiplegia: A Neurophysiological Approach* (Brunnstrom, 1970). A brief synopsis of recovery stages follows:

Stage 1: Flaccidity and no movements of the limb can be initiated.

Stage 2: Associated reaction or minimal voluntary movement may be present; beginning of spasticity development.

Stage 3: Voluntary control of movement synergies (flexor synergy and extensor synergy); spasticity increases and may become severe.

Stage 4: Movement combinations that do not follow synergistic movements are mastered with initial difficulty progressing to ease; spasticity begins to diminish.

Stage 5: If progress continues, basic limb synergies decline with more difficult motor combinations evident.

Stage 6: Spasticity disappears and individual joint movements are demonstrated and coordination approaches normal.

Brunnstrom recovery stages have historically been utilized in adult populations. Hemiplegia due to stroke in children is a relatively rare occurrence, so there is little if any documentation in the literature of the staging utilized with children.

Bayley Scales of Infant Development-II

The Bayley Scales of Infant Development-II (BSID-II; The Psychological Corporation, 1993) is a revision of the 1969 BSID. The Bayley Scales, originally developed by Nancy Bayley, are a comprehensive assessment of developmental status for children from 1 to 30 months. The original version was intended to assess normal development of young children. It is one of the most widely used assessment tools in infant research. Norm-referenced motor and mental scales include memory, object permanence, manipulation, problem solving, verbal communication, and gross and fine motor function. Revisions reflect current norms, a broader age range (1–42 months), additional skill range, new scoring procedures, updated stimulus material, and improved psychometric properties.

The revised version remains a three-part evaluation of developmental status of children. The three parts are the Mental Scale, Motor Scale, and Behavior Rating Scale. A test kit with all materials is included except for stairs and a balance board. The manual is extensive in its discussion of procedures and test progression.

Numerous studies have established the validity of the original BSID and the BSID-II in terms of con-

struct, predictive, and discriminate validity (DiLalla et al., 1990; Field et al., 1979; Matheny, 1980). The predictive value is moderate in cognitive areas with lower scores more predictive. The Bayley mental score is correlated at 0.57 with the Stanford-Binet Intelligence scale for children above age 2 and has approximately 90% agreement on items noted on inter-rater reliability assessments.

Health care professionals administer the test. Administration times vary depending on the child's age. The approximate time is 45 minutes for the Mental Scale and 45 minutes for the Motor Scale. The Mental Scale is administered first followed by the Motor Scale.

Individual record forms are used to record responses. Grading is as follows: pass (P), fail (F), omit (O), refuse (R), or reported by mother (RPT). Raw scores are converted to the Mental Development Index and the Psycho-Motor Development Index by referencing norms for the child's age as computed by Bayley.

The BSID and BSID-II represent the best-standardized techniques for assessing development in infants. They are widely used in research and assist in identifying the developmental status for a particular age. Examiners must undergo extensive training to become validated as a tester. The scales are limited in their ability to provide in-depth motor assessment and delineation of gross and fine motor development (Palisano, 1986). Examiners are advised to be conservative with regard to assuming normality from old BSID scores. The norms represented in the older version were done prior to 1969. The revised version scores have not been demonstrated to be stable based on scores of infants tested longitudinally in the first year (Coryell et al., 1989).

Bruininks-Oseretsky Test of Motor Proficiency

Dr. Robert H. Bruininks developed the Bruininks-Oseretsky Test of Motor Proficiency (BOT) in 1972. It is based on the adaptation of the Oseretsky Tests of Motor Proficiency. Similarities exist between the two tests, but the revised test reflects important advances in content, structure, and technical qualities (Bruininks, 1978). The test is designed to assess important aspects of motor development using eight subtests. Gross motor and fine motor components are assessed: coordination of upper limbs, speed of response, visuo-motor control, speed and dexterity of upper limbs, speed and agility while turning, balance, bilateral coordination, and strength. It is appropriate for children from 4.5 to 14.5 years of age. It can be used with normal and developmentally disabled children. The test is standardized and norm referenced.

The average test–retest reliability for the complete battery is 0.87. Reliability of 0.98 and 0.90 for interobserver reliability is reported by Bruininks (1978). According to Bruininks (1978) the validity of the BOT "is based on its ability to assess the construct of motor development or proficiency." The test is usually administered by a variety of professionals. No special training is required. The testing procedure is standardized and scores are normed. All supplies needed are included in the test kit. A large area with little distraction is recommended. Administration time varies for the short form at 15–20 minutes to 45–60 minutes for the long form. Younger children may require two short sessions for completion. Raw scores are converted to point scores, then to standardized scores for age equivalents. Interpretation of performance is done by comparing derived scores with the scores of subjects tested in the standardized program in relation to a national reference group.

The BOT is an excellent instrument for evaluation of school-age children demonstrating motor problems but who do not have obvious physical handicaps. Its ability to discriminate between populations makes it a valuable research tool. Only the potential for space requirements in its administration limits its usefulness. The BOT is a valid and reliable test for assessing gross and fine motor functioning in children so that appropriate education and therapeutic interventions can be made.

School Function Assessment

School function refers to a student's ability to perform important functional activities that enable participation in educational programs. The need for a standardized instrument to guide assessment and program planning was underscored by the influx of students with disabilities in regular education settings (Coster et al., 1998). The School Function Assessment (SFA) is a three-part, judgment-based (questionnaire) assessment used to measure a student's performance of functional tasks that support participation in the academic and social aspects of an elementary school program (grades K–6). It is designed to assist with collaborative program planning for students with a variety of disabling conditions. The three parts consist of participation, task supports, and activity performance.

Participation is one scale evaluating the student's participation in six major school-related activ-

ity settings. The *Task Supports* consists of four scales; Physical Tasks Assistance, Physical Tasks Adaptation, Cognitive/Behavioral Tasks Assistance, and Cognitive/Behavioral Tasks Adaptations. The *Activity Performance* consists of 21 separate scales for a comprehensive set of activities such as travel, maintaining and changing positions, eating and drinking, hygiene, memory and understanding, and safety, to mention a few. A raw score total is developed for each of the scales.

Test developers report reliability coefficients between 0.82 and 0.98 for test-retest reliability. Two test–retest studies were conducted during development of the SFA. Reliability estimates using Pearson *r* and intra-class correlation was reported as similar. Internal consistency using the coefficient alpha method ranged from 0.92 to 0.98. Validity measures were conducted for content and construct validity. The results indicated that the instrument was perceived to be both comprehensive and relevant for the population of students with disabilities in elementary schools (Coster et al., 1998). The authors cite the need for additional research to establish the relationship between scores from the SFA and existing tests with similar content.

No special training is required for administration. A variety of school professionals, such as educators, physical and occupational therapists, speech language pathologists, and psychologists, may administer the instrument. Administration time ranges from 1.5 to 2.0 hours. Scores are recorded on the Record Form. Several methods may be used to gather the information either by one individual or through a collaborative team. Ratings are based on the student's typical or most consistent level in each of the three parts. Raw scores are converted using the *Rating Scale Guide*.

The SFA is a multi-level model of functional performance that reflects the focus of legislation on achieving full participation of students with disabilities. Items are applicable to students with a wide variety of special needs. It is transdisciplinary in focus and language. A disadvantage of the instrument is the length of time it takes to administer. Further research is needed to validate the instrument. The SFA is best used when a team perspective is needed on school functional performance.

Beals, Bleck, and Molnar/Gordon Ratings

To assess motor function, Beals (1966) developed a Severity Index for children with cerebral palsy either "spastic paraplegia or diplegia" for prognosis for ambulation. He used select standardized items of motor development expected to be accomplished by the chronological age of 3 years, the child's highest actual performance of motor age development. Chronological age is divided by motor age to obtain a motor quotient. Two separate motor quotients could be determined before age 3 years to project the 3-year-old quotient. A Severity Index of 12 or more predicted free ambulation by 7 years. An index of 10 was the lowest with free ambulation. Nine or more could achieve crutch walking. An index of 4 was the lowest for crutch-walking. Bleck (1975) used clinical scoring of persistence of five primitive reflexes beyond time of suppression or lack of development of two postural protective reflexes by 12 months or older to predict locomotion progress. Molnar and Gordon (1976) used clinical evaluations of the persistence of six selected primitive reflexes after 18–24 months age for ambulation potential. Inability to sit by 2 years old and intellectual impairments correlated negatively. Correlations were also made with types of cerebral palsy regarding most, least, and indefinite for ambulation.

Gross Motor Function Measures

Gross Motor Function Measure (GMFM) is a widely used and accepted scale. It has been primarily developed for children with cerebral palsy. Adversely there is less validation for other diagnoses, such as acquired brain injury or developmental disabilities, although there are some studies in children with Down syndrome (Russell et al., 1989, 1994). GMFM and its derivatives are proprietary through the Centre for Childhood Disability Research (CanChild) at http://www.fhs.mcmaster.ca/canchild. GMFM-88 is the older version with 88 items. It has been modified to a newer, updated, and shorter version GMFM-66 which consists of 66 items (Russell et al., 2000). Pros for the scale include the following: a shorter time for administration, ordering of items evaluated by difficulty, improved interpretation of magnitude of changes for each item as well as for the total score due to the interval scale, and direct comparison of changes with different functional abilities for clinical research and program evaluations. It classifies by age specific gross motor activities: <2 years old, 2–4 years old, 4–6 years old, and 6–12 years old. A con is that a computer program is needed to score. Recently the use of the GMFM-66 and its derivative the Gross Motor Function Classification System (GMFCS) (Palisano et al., 1997) has been found to provide evidence-based prognostication for gross motor progress in children with cerebral palsy (Kinsman, 2002; Rosenbaum et al., 2002).

Sensory Integration

Sensory Integration is an assessment and treatment approach that focuses on sensory aspects of the child and their effect on motivation, movement, attention, and socioemotional well-being (Blanche et al., 1995). Sensory integrative dysfunction can lead to deficits in motor planning and execution (Fisher & Bundy, 1992). Ayres (1964, 1979) and Gilfoyle et al. (1981) described the normalization of tactile and vestibular functions as essential for refinements in fine and gross motor skills and in motor planning abilities. Several Sensory Integration assessment instruments are noted in the accompanying Table 4-1. Children with developmental delays, learning disorders, attention deficits, autism, and motor coordination deficits can benefit from the use of sensory integrative assessment and treatment.

Cognition

The Glasgow Coma Scale and its later expansion to the separate Glasgow Outcome Scale again share the TOS, having been developed on adult patients and recognized to be increasingly problematic, especially in a "gray zone" of 4–5 years of age and especially in children 3 years of age and under. Several modifications have been attempted including a Coma Scoring and Outcome Scale (also since known as the *Children's Coma Score*) by Raimondi and Hirschauer (1984) and modifications of the Glasgow Coma Scale (Adelaide Paediatric Scale) by Reilly et al. (1988) and Hahn et al. (1988), especially for use in children under 4 years of age (Table 4-4). A later variation, the Vienna Vigilance Score (Berger et al., 2001) has been attempted to avoid painful stimuli to elicit a reaction, but it requires a rehabilitation team to observe activities. It is much more complex in items, training of examiners, and difficulty to learn as well as requiring a complex process of team scoring. The collective process of all members of a multidisciplinary team in a consensus conference to derive a score of the child's past 7 days' activities suggests a strong element of subjectivity. It also raises the possibility of more assertive members influencing less sure members as well as the question of correlation of results between multiple teams and institutions. We feel that widespread use is yet to be determined.

Rancho Los Amigos Levels of Cognitive Function and its revised version in 1974 (Hagen et al.,

Table 4-4. Pediatric Modifications of Glasgow Coma Scale

Children's Coma Scale[a,b]	Adelaide Pediatric Scale[c,d]	Children's Coma Scale[e] (Modified Glasgow Coma Scale)	Modified Glasgow Coma Scale[f] (Modified by Pediatric Department of Donau Hospital, Vienna)
Ocular response	*Eye opening*	*Eye opening*	*Eye opening*
4 Pursuit	Same as Adult Glasgow Coma Scale	4 Spontaneous	4 Spontaneous
3 EOM intact, reactive pupils		3 Reaction to speech	3 Reaction to speech
2 Fixed pupils or EOM impaired		2 Reaction to pain	2 Reaction to pain
1 Fixed pupils and EOM paralyzed	*Best verbal response*	1 No response	1 No response
	5 Oriented		
	4 Words	*Best verbal response*	*Best verbal response*
Verbal response	3 Vocal sounds	(GCS subscore) (CCS subscore)	>5 yr 2–5 yr 0–23 mo
3 Cries	2 Cries	5 Oriented 5 Smiles, oriented to sound, follows objects, interacts	5 Oriented and speaking 5 Adequate words 5 Adequate smile or babbling
2 Spontaneous respirations	1 None	Crying Interacts	4 Disoriented & speaking 4 Inadequate words 4 Cries but consolable
1 Apneic		4 Confused/ disoriented 4 Consolable Inappropriate	3 Inadequate words 3 Continual crying 3 Continual crying
	Best motor response	3 Inappropriate words 3 Inconsistently consolable Moaning	2 Incomprehensible sounds 2 Moaning or babbling 2 Moaning, restlessness
Motor response	Same as Adult GCS	2 Incomprehensible 2 Inconsolable Irritable, restless	1 No response 1 No response 1 No response
4 Flexes and extends		1 No response 1 No response No response	
3 Withdraws from painful stimuli			*Best motor response*
2 Hypertonic			>1 yr <1 yr
1 Flaccid		*Best motor response*	6 Obeys commands 6 Spontaneous movements
		6 Spontaneous (obeys verbal commands)	5 Local protective reaction against pain 5 Local protective reaction against pain
		5 Localizes pain	4 Withdraws to pain 4 Withdraws to pain
		4 Withdraws in response to pain	3 Flexion to pain 3 Flexion to pain
		3 Abnormal flexion to pain (decorticate posture)	2 Extension to pain 2 Extension to pain
		2 Abnormal extension to pain (decerebrate posture)	1 No response 1 No response
		1 No response	

CCS, Children's Coma Scale; EOM, extraocular muscles; GCS, Glasgow Coma Scale.
[a]Raimondi and Hirschauer (1984).
[b]The maximum score assignable is 11, and the minimal 3.
[c]Reilly et al. (1988).
[d]Normal aggregate score: birth to 6 months, 9; <6–12 mo, 11; <1–2 yr, 13; <5 yr, 14.
[e]Hahn et al. (1988).
[f]Berger et al. (2001).

1974) has been long and widely used as an evaluation scale for monitoring stages of recovery after acquired brain injury. However, it was principally designed for adults (TOS). Recognizing the problems of application to those of decreasing age, researchers developed a subsequent Pediatric Levels of Consciousness for acquired brain injury in children (Brink & Imbus, 1982). It is subdivided into three age groups: (1) infants, 6 months to 2 years old, (2) preschool, 2–5 years old, and (3) school age, 5 years and older. There are five, compared to ten in the adult Rancho Levels of Cognitive Function, scoring classes applied to each group for items or actions appropriate to each age group: (1) orientation to time and place, (2) responsiveness to environment, (3) localized response to sensory stimuli, (4) generalized response to sensory stimuli, and (5) no response to stimuli. Although more age appropriate, the pediatric form does not yet enjoy the familiarity or widespread use of its adult version counterpart.

Higher Cognitive/Behavioral

When discussing functional outcomes and quality-of-life (QOL) rating scales, one area that is often overlooked is higher neurocognitive and behavioral issues. Patients may have good physical outcomes and fair-to-complete preservation of basic cognitive skills in memory and routine reasoning. Yet, in certain types of injuries, such as from TBI with countercoup phenomena involving the frontal and/or temporal lobes or hypoxic encephalopathies with cerebral cortex injury, one may have subtle impairments such as higher judgment reasoning, decreased safety awareness, emotional lability or aggression, or inappropriate sexual activity. For example, in the past, guidelines for returning to sports or recreational activities were based strictly on physically orientated scales, with such sports as riflery and archery being allowed. Yet, who would want to be in front of a rifle-carrying person on a dove hunt with poor safety awareness or impulse control? A person with complete quadriplegia at C-5 spinal cord level could still write this book chapter, but even a mild stroke leading to disinhibition and judgment may completely negate this activity. Thus by most rating scales the person may show excellent recovery, unless thought is given to incorporating these areas.

Investigation of the cognitive or neuropsychological sequelae of acquired and congenital disorders facilitates the identification of objective findings for any cognitive deficits associated with a particular dis-order. Those findings in turn facilitate both research and clinical endeavors.

With regard to research, for example, the possibility exists to identify the heterogeneity or homogeneity of strengths and deficits for various populations (e.g., TBI, stroke), which facilitates a greater understanding of brain–behavior relationships. The availability of objective measures also permits comparison with patient (and family) subjective complaints. For example, pediatric (and adult) patients with mild TBI often have a higher rate of subjective complaints than patients who have sustained moderate or severe TBI. Repeat administration of various tests and measures allows for an increased understanding of the time course of sequelae and, from a clinical perspective, can serve as an aid in treatment planning.

From a clinical perspective, identification of cognitive deficits associated with a particular disorder facilitates the development of habilitation and rehabilitation efforts, both in an acute care setting and in transition to community (e.g., school) settings. These findings also provide the opportunity for patient and family training, an issue that addresses not only the need for cognitive rehabilitation efforts but also facilitates the patient's (and family's) psychological adaptation to their condition.

The cognitive or neurobehavioral parameters assessed may vary with regard to patient status, the nature of referral questions, etc. But typically they include the following: measures of arousal (including agitation), attention and vigilance, receptive and expressive language, paralinguistic features of speech, general intelligence, measures of traditional academic achievement, reasoning and problem-solving, learning and memory, visual, visuospatial, and visuomotor functions, sensory and sensorimotor functions, motor functions, and personality and/or behavioral/affect ratings (Yeates, 2000).

As with any evaluation process in an acute care setting, the level of complexity of the evaluation is dependent on patient status and will be driven by the changing typography of patient cognition and behavior in evolving conditions. For example, early assessments of TBI patients focus more on general level of arousal, consistency of response to external stimuli, the presence or absence of agitation, and command following. As noted earlier, scales initially developed for the assessment of those issues with adults (coma recovery scales) are generally used for that purpose, although it remains an empirical question as to the appropriateness of any particular item from those scales in its application to children. After the child has demonstrated improvement to a consistently wakeful state, the next issue of importance is residual post-traumatic amnesia and confusion. At this stage, application of complicated and lengthy assessment batteries would be frustrating for the child and would yield little information other than an index of that confusion. Accordingly, a number of scales (Children's Orientation & Amnesia Test [Ewing-Cobbs et al., 1990], Westmead Post-Traumatic Amnesia [Marosszeky et al., 1993; Shores et al., 1986]) are typically used to assess, by way of serial assessments, the resolution of post-traumatic amnesia and confusion before more complex measures are used.

A review of the literature, unfortunately, does not indicate the availability of reliable, valid, and useful (e.g., brief, not subject to significant practice effects) bedside measures for assessing various cognitive functions in children. As such, clinicians are usually left with choices including downward extension of adult measures, development of informal measures, and the use of selected measures from existing tests. Each of these choices has its potential pitfalls. Downward extension of existing adult tests makes numerous assumptions about the appropriateness of individual items for children. Along with the choice of development of informal measures, the appropriateness of items used by way of downward extension would need to be demonstrated. Clinicians may then opt for the repeated use of selected measures from existing tests. This raises the question of practice effects as a confounding issue, which would limit conclusions that could be drawn from any measure. It would be important to review the manual and other available literature for any selected test to determine if this application was addressed in the development and validation of that test.

Attention is not a unitary phenomenon and is best seen as a continuum of skills, ranging from level of arousal, the ability to attend or respond to stimuli, span of attention, sustained attention and concentration, and the ability to selectively attend to relevant stimuli and ignore irrelevant stimuli (Yeates, 2000). Accordingly, a range of measures may be appropriate for measuring this construct, dependent on which aspect of attention is under investigation.

For measures of attention, several tests have selected measures that may be appropriate, depending on what particular aspect of attention is being considered. For example, the subtest Digit Span of the Wechsler Intelligence Scale for Children-Third Edition (WISC-III) (The Psychological Corp., 1992) requires the subject to repeat a series of digits (the initial task assesses for the greatest span of digits forward, the

second part of the task is the greatest span of digits in reverse order). A relatively simple continuous performance test (CPT), the "A" test for vigilance (Strub & Black, 1993) asks respondents to respond by tapping when they hear the letter "A" from a list of random letters read by the examiner. Although very simple in design, this task unfortunately has limited normative information for children, limiting its use to general information regarding patient status.

Several more complex, computer-administered, continuous performance measures are available, including the Conners' CPT (Conners, 1996) and the Gordon Diagnostic System (Gordon, 1996). The Conners' CPT is supplied as a software program to be installed on the examiner's computer, whereas the Gordon is a stand-alone unit. Both essentially are designed as a series of more complex tasks, beginning with simple reaction time tasks to conditional tasks.

The NEPSY (neuropsychological assessment of children) (Korkman et al., 1998) contains several tests for ages 3–12 that are appropriate for the measurement of attention: The Visual Attention task (versions covering ages 3–12) assesses speed and accuracy components for a visual search task (Korkman et al., 1998). The Statue task requires the child to maintain a predetermined, fixed posture for a 75-second period, inhibiting a response to distracters. The Auditory Attention and Response Set (ages 5–12) is essentially a CPT, assessing the child's ability to be vigilant and to maintain selective auditory attention and to shift response set in accord with changing instructions.

Language assessment devices typically are designed following a syndrome analysis model. As such, thorough measures (of a range of receptive and expressive language skills) or measures of a single skill typically are composed of items that are sensitive to dysfunction. Scores on such measures, then, represent an indication of the presence or absence of a particular disorder and can usually be used as well to indicate the relative severity of some aspect of language disturbance. Some critiques in the series of Mental Measurements Yearbooks (Plake and Impara, 2001) are critical of the limited availability of tests designed to assess language not only as a weakness or deficit, but also as a strength. However, most language screening measures have a limited ceiling and, as such, are not likely to produce a normal distribution of results. These tests, by design, are limited with regard to identification of language as a strength.

The Multilingual Aphasia Examination, Third Edition (MAE) is a comprehensive measure for the assessment of the presence and severity of aphasia (Benton et al., 1994). The MAE is comprised of nine subtests

(Visual Naming, Sentence Repetition, Controlled Oral Word Association, Oral Spelling, Written Spelling, Block Spelling, MAE Token Test, Aural Comprehension of Words and Phrases, and Reading Comprehension of Words and Phrases). Two rating scales allow for rating articulation and praxic features of writing. The availability of normative data (this test is appropriate for ages 6–69 years) is a strong feature of this battery.

Other commonly used tests for language assessment measure one aspect of receptive or expressive language. The Token Test for Children, for example, provides for the assessment of the subject's ability to follow a series of progressive more complex, verbally presented commands (DiSimoni, 1978). This task was normed on children ages 3–12 years and, as such, allows for assessment of auditory comprehension for a younger range of children than can be assessed with the MAE Token Test.

The Peabody Picture Vocabulary Test-III is a measure of receptive vocabulary that is appropriate for ages 2.5 years and above (Dunn et al., 1997). The subject is presented with groupings of four pictures and asked to point to the picture that best depicts the word provided by the examiner. Unlike some other language measures, this test does have a higher ceiling, allowing for the development of norm-based scores that will identify strengths (i.e., above average performance) for this receptive vocabulary task.

The Boston Naming Test is a visual confrontation naming task requiring the subject to name a series of large ink drawings (Kaplan et al., 1983). Originally developed for adults, norms have been collected for use with younger children.

The assessment of general intellectual functions is a standard part of more comprehensive neuropsychological assessments. These measures typically assess a variety of verbal and nonverbal (i.e., perceptual-organizational, perceptual-motor) skills that have been developed as an index of a more general factor of "intelligence." Individual subtests are reported, with some research addressing the issue of scatter among the various subtests, and these subtests are also combined for additional composite measures of verbal, nonverbal, or performance, and overall measures of intellectual functioning. Generally speaking, the individual subtests (and, as a result, the composite measures) each may tap into several skills (i.e., attention, auditory processing, expressive language) and, as such, do not tend to localize well with regard to brain-behavior relationships. This lessens the utility of the subtests and composite scores for frequent serial assessment, but they have a number of other applica-

tions. For example, measures of general intellectual functions tend to correlate strongly with academic experience/attainment and are useful in child cases as an aid in developing school-based interventions with children who have a developmental disorder. They also are helpful in addressing needs for transition back to school following an acquired illness. In combination with measures of achievement, they are also used as part of the process for identifying patterns of learning disorders.

The WISC-III measures general intellectual abilities in children ages 6–16 years of age (The Psychological Corp., 1992). The WISC-III contains 13 subtests grouped into verbal and performance domains. Of the six verbal measures, Information (general fund of information), Similarities (simple analogous reasoning), Arithmetic, Vocabulary, and Comprehension (social judgment) yield a Verbal composite measure, with Digit Span as a supplemental measure. Of the seven performance measures, Picture Completion (identifying the essential missing part of a picture), Coding (symbol substitution using a displayed key of symbol and number pairs), Picture Arrangement (arrangement of cartoons into logical sequences), Block Design (reproducing designs using a series of blocks), and Object Assembly (assembling jigsaw puzzles) yield a Performance composite measure, with Symbol Search (a visual search task for matching figures) and Mazes as supplemental measures. The combination of the Verbal and Performance composites in turn yield a Full Scale composite or IQ score.

The Wechsler Preschool and Primary Scale of Intelligence-Revised (WPPSI-R) is designed to measure general cognitive abilities in young children ages 3 to 7 years 3 months (Wechsler, 1989). The WPPSI-R contains 12 subtests grouped into verbal and performance domains. Of the six verbal measures, Information, Comprehension, Arithmetic, Vocabulary, and Similarities yield a Verbal composite measure, with Sentences (repetition of sentences) as a supplemental measure. Of the six performance measures, Object Assembly (placing pieces into a form board and assembling jigsaw puzzles), Geometric Design (selecting matching geometric designs and copying geometric designs), Block Design, Mazes (finding paths thorough a series of mazes), and Picture Completion yield a Performance composite measure, with Animal Pegs (placing colored pegs into the corresponding holes on a board) as a supplemental measure. The combination of the Verbal and Performance composite measures in turn yield a Full Scale composite measure. Nine of these subtests are similar in design to subtests of the

WISC-III, with three tests unique to the WPPSI-R (Sentences, Animal Pegs, and Geometric Design). This test essentially represents a downward extension of the WISC-III.

Executive function denotes the use of flexible strategies and planning (Denckla, 1986). As with the concept of attention, this is not a unitary phenomenon. It covers a wide range of complex abilities, including the capacity to adopt, maintain, and shift cognitive set; the ability to use organized search strategies' and the ability to plan, monitor, and adapt behavior secondary to changing demands. As such, some of the tasks from the NEPSY, mentioned earlier as aspects of complex attention/concentration, fit as well as measures of executive function (i.e., Auditory Attention and Response Set, Visual Attention, Statue). The Design Fluency task from the NEPSY, a task requiring the subject to generate a series of unique designs in rapid fashion, is an appropriate executive function task for 5- to 12-year-old children. The Knock and Tap, also ages 5–12, is considered a classic Lurian Go No-Go task, requiring the subject to follow a set of commands for rapid initiation of response to select stimuli, inhibit response to competing stimuli, and then break a routinized set of responses in accord with changing demands. Go No-Go tasks have long been part of bedside exams for adults and children. This task has the added benefit of norms, allowing for greater power with regard to interpretation of findings.

A final NEPSY task of executive function is the Tower, a variant of the Tower of London (Shallice, 1982). In this task, the subject is required to arrange colored balls on pegs to match a picture stimulus in as few moves as possible and within certain time limits. This task is appropriate for ages 5–12 years.

The Wisconsin Card Sorting Test was originally developed as a measure of abstract reasoning for adult populations (Heaton et al., 1993). The manual from Psychological Assessment Resources, Inc., and other publications provide norms for use of this task with children as young as 6.5 years. Briefly, this task, which can be administered by hand (and scored by hand or using scoring software) or by computer, consists of four stimulus cards and two sets of 64 response cards depicting combinations of four forms (circles, crosses, triangles, and stars), four colors (red, yellow, blue, and green), and four numbers (1–4). The subject is asked to sort the response card under one of the stimulus cards to match features. The features for correct sorting are not clearly identified, but the subject is provided with feedback after each sort. After a predetermined number of correct sorts, the features for correct sorting are changed, requiring the subject to shift response set. A number of scores are reported, including number of total correct category sorts, number of trials, number of errors, etc. The variety of scores available (software-based scoring is recommended) allows for a rich description of the typography of the subject's response style.

Memory is a complex domain including skills of acquisition, consolidation, and retrieval of information. From a developmental perspective, the diversity and complexity of information increases dramatically as a function of increased diversity and complexity of various sensory and motor skills. As children learn to operate more in their environment, the capacity to learn from experiences plays an increasingly important role in their overall development. Not surprisingly, a number of congenital and acquired conditions can adversely affect aspects of memory, which concomitantly can impact the child's further adaptation.

Among other tests, selected subtests from the NEPSY allow for the assessment of various aspects of learning/memory. Memory for Faces (ages 3–12) requires the child to remember faces in photographs that are sorted into two piles by gender (an attention-focusing task) using immediate and delayed trials. Memory for Names (ages 3–12) assesses memory for learning of names of eight line drawings over three trials with immediate and delayed trials. Narrative Memory (ages 3–12) assesses narrative memory with free and cued recall tasks.

The Children's Memory Scale (ages 5–16) consists of nine subtests that assess memory in three domains: auditory/verbal, visual/nonverbal, and attention/concentration (Cohen, 1998). Each domain contains two subtests with a third supplemental test. The test is designed to assess immediate and delayed recall (without any cueing) across auditory/verbal and visual/nonverbal domains, and cued recall/recognition, allowing the examiner to tease apart the various factors that may contribute to good (or poor) performance. This task has the unique feature of a linking sample. A subgroup of examinees were also administered either the WISC-III or the WPPSI-R, permitting exploration of relationships and discrepancies between memory and IQ.

Neither the structure nor development of the brain is independent of the context in which it operates (Edelman, 1987; Greenough et al., 1987). An appreciation for the dynamics of the reciprocal relationship between the organism and its environment furthers our appreciation of brain-behavior relationships in the normally developing child and in children who have been compromised by developmental and/or acquired conditions. A discussion of the field of Applied Behavior Analysis, briefly stated philosophically as an attempt to understand the interplay between behavior, the context or environment in which it exists, and its consequences (Malott et al., 1997), is beyond the scope of this chapter.

Although the functional analysis of behavior is not a standard part of neuropsychological assessment, some attention is paid to assessing behavior. In this context, rating scales/checklists address a particular aspect of behavior (e.g., Agitated Behavior Scale, Corrigan, 1989), attempt to identify the presence/absence of a broader range of disruptive behaviors and emotional states (e.g., Behavior Assessment System for Children, Reynolds & Kamphaus, 1992; and Child Behavior Checklist, Achenbach, 1994), or attempt to describe more pervasive personality and behavior tendencies (e.g., Personality Inventory for Children, Seat & Broen, 1977).

The Behavior Assessment System for Children-Revised is a series of parent and teacher completed rating scales (with self-report scales as well for ages 8–18) designed to aid in the identification and differential diagnosis of emotional/behavior disorders in children and adolescents for children ages 2.5–18.0. (Reynolds & Kamphaus, 1992). The informant rates the presence or absence of a series of behavioral and emotional descriptors (True/False for self-report scales and Never/Sometimes/Often/Always for parent and teacher versions). Domain scores are reported for Externalizing Problems (subscales including Aggression, Hyperactivity, and Conduct Problems), Internalizing Problems (Anxiety, Depression, and Somatization), School Problems (Attention Problems and Learning Problems), Atypicality, Withdrawal, and Behavioral Symptoms Index. The added domain of Adaptive Skills (Leadership, Social Skills, and Study Skills) represents an added dimension in comparison with older rating scales. The availability of parent and teacher ratings provides for an assessment of the typography of behavior across home and school environments, aiding in issues of differential diagnosis and treatment/intervention planning. Repeat administration of these scales also facilitates assessment of change/improvement with evolving conditions (e.g., TBI) and in addressing the effectiveness of interventions.

The Behavior Rating Inventory of Executive Function is a series of parent- and teacher-completed rating scales designed to assess impairment of executive function for children ages 5–18 (Gioia et al., 2001). The informant rates each of 86 items for the presence and frequency (never, sometimes, or often) of descriptors depicting aspects of executive function. The test yields two broad indices, Behavioral Regulation (reflecting subscales for inhibitory control, set shifting, and emotional control), and Metacognition (reflecting five subscales of task initiation, working memory, planning/organization, organization of materials, and self-monitoring) and also provides a Global Executive Composite score. The manual provides construct validity data correlating this measure with other behavior rating scales and also provides information about Behavior Rating Inventory of Executive Function profiles for various developmental and acquired conditions. Of interest will be future research comparing this observational report with objective findings of executive function deficits.

Neuropharmacology remains in great need of reliable rating scales for precision of classification of neural injury and for outcomes of pharmacological treatments. For adults there remains limited or no reliable way to predict efficacy in behavioral modification in acquired brain injury. This is even more evident where there have been far fewer studies in children (TOS) where most studies of drugs come from developmental and emotional/psychological disorders rather than from acquired organic brain injury (O'Dell et al., 1998). Application of adult medications, often not even approved for use in children (TOS), for childhood behavioral disorders secondary to neural deficits often ignores the differences in metabolisms due to varying body compartment spaces and maturation of renal and liver functions of children from adults.

Physiologic

The still elusive Holy Grail of Neurology is a reliable measure of tone and spasticity (Brown, 1993; Burry, 1972; Massagli 1991; Sehgal & McGuire, 1998; Task Force on Childhood Motor Disorders, 2001; Young & Wiegner, 1987). Just as for drugs and other medical interventions, the advent of selective dorsal rhizotomy, botulism toxin, and, even more so, for intrathecal baclofen pump has made effectiveness evaluations and research even more pertinent. The principal problem is that tone and spasticity are dynamic phenomena, changeable and varying from multifactorial influences, both internally and externally, such as time of day, emotional status, environmental temperature (cold often exaggerates tone), how much activity has occurred before testing (one tends to be stiffer after prolonged immobility like sleep), etc. The reliable measures of spasticity in children have long been problematic and, after attempted development of many instruments, still remain best done by clinical assessment. Ultimately, what is often overlooked in tone/spasticity measures is that it is not the score but how the person functions that matters to the person. One is not interested in one's Ashworth score first thing in the morning, but whether or not one can comb one's hair or cook one's breakfast. Direct electrophysiological measures (Sehgal & McGuire, 1998), indirect measures, and scoring of spasticity, such as by basal metabolic rate (BMR) and oxygen consumption measures, have also been attempted. Again, it must be recognized that these are time-isolated measures in an artificial environment and difficult to correlate with daily activities. A spasticity score and functional ability are not necessarily directly correlated (Damiano & Abel, 2000). Thus measures, such as the Functional Independent Measure for Children (WeeFIM) or the Pediatric Evaluation of Disability Inventory (PEDI), may have more clinical significance than a BMR or Ashworth Score. The former may be more important to the individual; the later more to simply document there was indeed a physical change. As a side issue, pain measures, QOL measures, and caregiver measures may be equally valuable measures in evaluating spasticity. Even if lessening spasticity does not improve function, QOL may, however, improve with less discomfort, improved positioning, and ease of handling by the caregiver for hygiene and dressing.

Test for Tone/Spasticity

Pendulum testing for spasticity, whether done qualitatively by observation (more subjective) or quantitatively instrumented using a light attached to a limb and recorded with an electrogoniometer and tachometer, which are more objective, are all controlled environment laboratory setting measures (Bajd & Vodovnik, 1984; Wartenberg, 1951). Also, most studies have been on adults and not on potentially more uncooperative children, raising questions of validity in younger ages.

Penn et al. (1989) has offered a Frequency of Spasms Score based on 10 adult patients with multiple sclerosis and 10 adults with SCI, but this has not been extensively validated, especially in children. Meythaler et al. (1997) has proposed the Reflex Score, again done initially in adults with hemiplegia from acquired brain injury and without extensive validation, especially not in children.

Although one of the most widely used measures of spasticity, the Ashworth Scale (Ashworth, 1964) until recently shared Sherkey's TOS. Most of the development and validation studies were on adults, one who was 17 years of age and the rest much older (Bohannon & Smith, 1987; Gregson et al., 1999; Katz et al., 1992; Meythaler et al., 1997, 1999; Penn et al., 1989; Skold et al., 1998). Researchers have developed various scales, such as the pendulum test, Frequency of Spasms, Reflexes Score, and the Ashworth Score, to report their results. Other researchers, then, have incorporated them into clinical reports of treatment results on children without evidence of scale validation for children. Even in adults, despite widespread use, validation, inter-relater reliability, and specificity questions have been raised (Damiano et al., 2002; Hass et al., 1996). Even more so, the Ashworth scale, often used as an outcome measure in treatment of children with cerebral palsy, appears to correlate only weakly with function (Damiano & Abel, 2000).

In April 2001 an interdisciplinary workshop was held at the National Institutes of Health to develop a consensus report on classification and definition of disorders causing hypertonia in childhood (Task Force on Childhood Motor Disorders, 2001). The consensus report (http://accessible.ninds.nih.gov/news_and_events/proceedings/Hypertonia_Meeting_2001.htm) provides an excellent overall review of the current measures of hypertonicity and dystonia and acknowledged the continuing difficulties in reaching consensus definitions and establishing consistent rating scales for a given diagnostic category. Reliability between different diagnostic categories is also at issue. The task force also acknowledged that functional ability measures, QOL measures, and impact on the functional limitations that are of direct concern to the child should be a central focus, with recommendations that rating scales for functional activity and societal participation be a part of their evaluations.

Functional

Scales for functional measures have been recognized as far back as 1945 (Deaver & Brown, 1945). One of the ongoing controversies is the relationship between spasticity and actual motor or functional performance, which dates back to the 1970s (Sahrmann & Norton, 1977). Unfortunately, many current studies of effectiveness of spasticity treatment fail to incorporate either the older studies of motor performance prognosis (Beals, 1966; Bleck, 1975; Molnar & Gordon, 1976) or even the functional scales like WeeFIM or PEDI to define function in life the critical goal for the patient. Instead focus may be on more esoteric parameters like BMR, oxygen consumption, or isolated rating of tone with instrumentation. A combination of both would seem more meaningful. Sir Edmund Hillary was supposedly once asked, "Why did you climb Mt. Everest?" He reputedly answered, "Because it was there." This has become known as the Everest Syndrome, to perform a procedure simply because a symptom exists, whether it truly enhances the patient's life outcome or not. Thus, to show a change alone is not sufficient in itself, such as a change in a BMR figure or Ashworth Score, but is the patient truly functionally improved (Brown, 1997; Butler & Campbell, 2000)? Therefore, several functional outcome measures have been developed and assessed for pediatrics (Campbell, 1996; Coster & Haley, 1992; Haley et al., 1991).

WeeFIM is a pediatric version of its better-known adult version, functional independence measure (FIM). It was developed by Uniform Data System for Medical Rehabilitation as a global functional measurement instrument. It is a proprietary instrument and requires subscription for use (Dittmar & Gresham, 1997; Grimby et al., 1996; Msall et al., 1993, 1994; Ottenbacher et al., 1996a, 1996b, 1997, 1999, 2000; Stineman et al., 1996). To participate, one must undergo periodic credentialing, which promotes greater uniformity and accuracy between various researchers and institutions not found in many other rating scales. Software along with national support and a databank permits multi-institutional comparisons. Both the Joint Commission on Accreditation of Healthcare Organizations under their ORYX initiative and the Commission on Accreditation of Rehabilitation Facilities have accepted the WeeFIM System as a performance measure system. The Health Care Financing Administration, now known as the Centers for Medicare & Medicaid, selected the adult FIM for Inpatient Rehabilitation Facility-Patient Assessment Instrument in 2001. The WeeFIM is applicable to children age 6 months to 7 years. However, it is said to be appropriate for children over 7 years, if their functional abilities as measured by the WeeFIM scores are below those expected of a nondisabled child. This allows the potential to transition data into the similar adult version, FIM, for long-term continuity studies as the child ages on into adulthood. It is a discipline-free test that can, with appropriate training and credentialing, be used by both clinicians and educators. It is reported to have excellent test-retest and inter-rater reliability. Uniform Data System is embarking on an effort to subdivide the reporting institutions

into three categories (Specialty Hospital: a children's hospital with a focus on particular services; Children's Hospital: a self-governing, not-for-profit children's hospital, including tertiary care hospitals; and General Hospital: a children's hospital within a hospital, or a hospital that does not fit in either of the other two categories). Hopefully, this would aid in comparison of outcomes and benchmarks between more compatible institutions. The WeeFIM is somewhat simpler than the PEDI. It consists of 18 items that measure functional performance in three domains. However, due to its smaller number of items, it may lack sensitivity to provide a comprehensive measure of all meaningful changes.

PEDI is a propriety clinical assessment scale of functional capabilities and performance of children 6 months to 7.5 years of age (Feldman et al., 1990; Haley et al., 1992; Nichols and Case-Smith, 1996; Nordmark et al., 2000; Reid et al., 1993). Under the auspices of Boston University, further details are readily available on their Web site at http://www.bu.edu/cre and an extensive reference list can be located at http://www.bu.edu/cre/pedi. This scale is standardized on a normative sample of children and can be used to describe the child's current function and to track changes over time. It may be used to detect functional limitations and disabilities, monitor progress, and evaluate programs within the same institution. It is not incorporated into a national database for multiple institutional comparisons nor does it require a periodic recredentialing process of the raters. It can be discipline-free so it can be used by both clinicians and educators. It consists of 197 functional skill items and 20 items that require caregiver assistance and modifications. It is said to have excellent inter-rater and inter-respondent reliability. Though perhaps more comprehensive, it tends to be more complex and difficult to administer and score. This factor coupled with the lack of periodic recredentialing may lead to questions about consistency of data between institutions.

A third pediatric functional scale has recently been developed through Rancho Los Amigos called the Functional Rehabilitation Evaluation of Sensori-Neurologic Outcomes (Roberts et al., 1999). Administration time is stated to be 45 minutes by a trained clinician or educator (discipline-free). Inter-rater reliability coefficient is stated at 0.87–0.93. As a newer scale, it lacks widespread use and has limited validation. Of the functional assessments available for children, WeeFIM and PEDI appear to be the most widely used.

	PEDI	WeeFIM
Age	6.0 mo–7.5 yr	6 mo–7 yr (18 yr)
Domains	Self-care	Self-care
	Social function	Cognition
	Mobility	Mobility
Testing time	45–60 min	20–30 min
	20–30 min if familiar with child	—
Inter-relater reliability	>0.90	0.95
Tester	Clinicians, educators	Clinicians, educators
National database	No	Yes
Periodic recredentialing	No	Yes

Quality of Life

Ultimately it is not the determination of whether a change was made by intervention, but whether the intervention was beneficial and for whom. Measures of QOL are becoming as important or perhaps more important than functional assessments (Brown, 1997; Butler, 1995; Harper, 1999; McLaughlin & Bjornson, 1998). One of the basic problems for children in this area is to clearly identify whom the decision-maker and/or reporter is. There may be subtle or even open discrepancies, especially in pediatrics, between the goals or perceptions of the professional doing the procedure or rating, the caregiver (usually the parents or family), and the patient. Their impressions and goals may not be identical. How often have we seen a child undergoing multiple painful surgeries and/or heavy braces to awkwardly walk to satisfy a caregivers' or professionals' goal of walking at all cost when a wheelchair as "a passport to freedom" would allow the child to zip along with peers? Yet, of course, the younger the child the more a second party must speak on behalf of the child.

As part of this overall domain, one must be able to measure the overall health status and function of children and their ability to cope with chronic medical conditions (Eisen et al., 1979; Hutchison, 1995; Simeonsson et al., 2000). A number of scales are available to measure health status in children, with some overlapping into QOL status (Kaplan et al.,

1976; Lewis et al., 1989; Starfield et al. 1993, 1995; Stein & Jessop, 1990; Stein et al., 1997). Three pediatric outcome questionnaires were developed by orthopedic and rheumatology clinics for children with musculoskeletal disorders to determine treatment outcomes, especially surgical outcomes. They include the following: the Activities Scale for Kids, the Child Health Questionnaire Parent Form, and the Pediatric Outcomes Data Collection Instrument (Pencharz et al., 2001). Although not designed or specifically tested for purely neurologic disorders, they may warrant future investigation for at least concomitant use in neurologic disorders with a motor dysfunction component.

QOL measures allow for the assessment of several aspects of the functional outcome of a condition (e.g., degree of success with adaptation to a condition, level of satisfaction with treatment) (Andreesen & Meyers, 2000; McSweeny & Creer, 1995; Spieth & Harris, 1996). As with other measures, serial or repeat assessment permits the identification of any significant change in those features as a function of time, additional treatments, etc.

There are several important considerations involved in the selection of a QOL measure. These include use of measures that are: generic versus disease-specific, questionnaires versus interviews, time-frame, etc. (Aaronson, 1988). Additional issues exist for the selection of measures for children, including the development or selection of measures completed by the child versus using parents as proxies, item selection appropriate to the child's level of understanding and comprehension, the child's capacity to comprehend various aspects of his or her condition, etc. (Connolly & Johnson, 1999).

The Child Attitude Toward Illness Scale is a short, self-report instrument for children with a chronic physical condition (Austin & Huberty, 1993). Thirteen items are contained in this measure, five with items progressing from negative to positive, eight with items progressing from positive to negative (i.e., each essentially represents a 5-point continuum). Scores are expressed on a 5-point scale. The scores are summed and divided by 13 to provide an average score.

The Play Performance Scale for Children with Cancer is a parent- or guardian-rated measure recording play activity of a child with cancer (Lansky et al., 1985). Analogous to the Karnofsky scale for adults, it is intended to provide a measure for a child's level of performance. A parent or guardian grades level of performance, with behavioral descriptors provided for various point levels for the preceding week.

Miscellaneous

A few scales that may be pertinent to the neurologist but are more peripheral will be noted here and referenced for further review if desired.

Spinal Cord Injuries

Although essentially developed for adult SCI, the ASIA International Standards for Neurological and Functional Classification of Spinal Cord Injury, Revised 2002 (American Spinal Injury Association, 2002) remains the principal classification of SCI. However, ASIA does not officially endorse or recommend the standards in children. Although every attempt is made to reflect best evidence-based medicine, the ASIA committee has tried to reach consensus between conflicting studies, such as the differences in dermatome pattern classifications, to yield a mutually agreed, standardized uniformity in reporting neurologic impairments for clinical management and research (Stover, 1992). Revisions continue. Because they are adult-based, many of the issues regarding application to children raised previously in this chapter can also be raised here (TOS). However, in line with the ASIA Committee's goal of consensus and recognition that the standards may not be exact and not endorsed by ASIA for children, so far this system may be the best rating system for children with SCI. With younger children, MMT (as previously noted for below 5 years old) and fine discrimination between normal sensation and hypo- or hypersensitivity, or even the level of absence, may be difficult, and bladder/bowel volitional continence in pretoilet trained children often remains questionable. Earlier the ASIA Standards were incorporated with Uniform Data System's FIM as a part of its standards, but with the use of multiple functional rating systems by different institutions this has been discontinued in the current addition. Although copyrighted, ASIA does allow copying of their forms for private use at http://www.asia-spinalinjury.org/publications/index.html.

Beyond acquired SCI, prenatal congenital SCI, most often as S/B, requires assessment. Often the ASIA guidelines, too, are used for S/B. However, some distinct clinical differences exist between acquired versus congenital SCI. Acquired SCI usually involves a previously physiologically uninvolved individual, with the remaining uninjured organs, at least initially, functioning normally. However, SCI may be associated with either recognized or unrecognized TBI). S/B at onset often has congenital deficits in other major body organs such as the brain and skeleton. Therefore, caution is necessary in using an instrument such as the ASIA score to compare different diagnoses and etiologies for broad overlapping outcomes. Again, ASIA does not endorse officially or recommend the use of the standards in nontraumatic SCI or S/B.

Several assessments have been proposed specifically for S/B. The Functional Activities (Sousa et el., 1976) measures activities of daily living within nine categories: five in self care, three in locomotion, and one in social interaction. These are compared with expectations for nonhandicapped children. The S/B children were divided into three groups based on the level of spinal deficit: sacral, L4/5, and L3 or above. The purpose was for rating the current functional status and to gauge the rate of progress. Sousa et al. (1983) reported an inventory of 166 items of seven categories: personal-social, eating, dressing, grooming, toileting, gross motor activities, and locomotion. Patients were divided into sacral (S1 or less), L4/5, L2–4, and L2 or greater levels of spinal cord deficit. By ascertaining varying factors beyond just level of paralysis, the scale could be used to predict the potential and time for learning appropriate developmental and functional skills. The Spina Bifida Neurological Scale, which uses a scoring system for motor function, reflexes, and bladder/bowel function to monitor positive or negative changes in neurologic status, serves as a predictor of future activities of daily living abilities (Oi & Matsumoto, 1992).

Technological Scales

Technologic procedures are increasingly being studied to produce rating scales and provide predictions for various adult and childhood disorders. As noted, BMR, oxygen consumption, and electromyography have been studied for spasticity measurement. However, there are significant difficulties in standardizing instrumentation, training of raters, and interpretation. Furthermore, the younger the child is the more difficult communication and cooperation is, which makes it harder to define what are strictly laboratory scores and what actually occurs in daily life. However, certain technology resources, (e.g., transcranial Doppler ultrasonography) are being explored for possible future rating scales in children (Adams et al., 1997; Seibert et al., 1998). Electrodiagnostic studies, such as somatosensory evoked potentials, are being explored to predict outcomes in severe brain injury in both adults and children (Beca et al., 1995; Carter & Butt,

2001; Carter et al., 1999; Wohlrab et al., 2001). To date, a definite rating scale along with title for these two areas still remains open, but possible rating criteria are available for review.

Clearance for Sports

Physicians are often approached for clearance for sports or recreational activities. However, very limited resources exist for factual guidelines. The Committee on Sports Medicine of the American Academy of Pediatrics has periodically provided recommendation guidelines of a broad and general nature (Committee on Sports Medicine, American Academy of Pediatrics, 1988, 2001; Committee on Sports Medicine and Fitness, American Academy of Pediatrics, 1994). In the latest (2001) and for the first time, deficits in judgment or cognition were recognized as a factor in decisions regarding noncontact sports. The only other widely recognized scale for sports return regarding neurologic issues is the Guidelines for the Management of Concussion in Sports, Revised, regarding return to contact/collision sports (Colorado Medical Society, Sports Medicine Committee, 1991).

Pain

Pain rating scales are becoming increasingly important in pediatric as well as adult management. This may be particularly true for spasticity research, chronic pain disorders, or paraesthesia disorders such as in SCI or phantom limb phenomena. The variability by age in children's ability to communicate or cooperate for assessment adds increased difficulty in the already complex debate of the interplay of psychological, psychosocial, and cultural influences of defining and rating pain. As with QOL measures, some of the considerations with regard to selection of pain measures include using the child as respondent (versus parents and/or other caregiver observations), item selection that adjusts for the child's level of understanding of what is being assessed, etc. In addition to self-report measures, some work in this area has focused on methods of caregiver observation/reporting of the behavioral and affective manifestations of pain in children (Bachanas & Blount, 1996; Graumlich et al., 2001; Jonas & Day, 1997).

The Modified Objective Pain Score is a modified version of the Objective Pain Score (adults) for use with children (Wilson & Doyle, 1996). Five parameters (crying, movement, agitation, posture, and verbal) allow for ratings from positive to negative (e.g., crying

0 for none, 1 for consolable, 2 for not consolable). A higher overall score connotes a greater pain experience for the child. The verbal measure includes parameters for complaints and/or ability to localize pain, perhaps limiting its use with preverbal children.

The Behavioral Approach-Avoidance and Distress Scale is designed to allow for measuring a child's distress and coping style during painful medical procedures (Hubert et al., 1988). Bachanas and Blount (1996) report on this measure as compared with other observational and subjective measures, describing high internal consistency and concurrent validity of the Distress subscale.

The FLACC Behavioral Scale for Postoperative Pain in Young Children (Merkel et al., 1997) is designed for use with young children who may not be able to verbalize postoperative pain and discomfort. Parameters including face, legs, activity, crying, and consolability (FLACC) allow for ratings from positive to negative, with higher scores indicating a higher degree of distress.

For the interested reader we would recommend Hain (1997), Franck et al. (2000), Merkel & Malviya (2000), and Summers (2001) for their reviews of current generalized pediatric pain assessments and ratings. Additionally for those working with neurologically impaired children, we would recommend Twycross et al. (1999), Fanurik et al. (1999), and Oberlander et al. (1999).

References

Aaronson NK Quantitative issues in health-related quality of life assessment. *Health Policy* 1988;10:217–30.

Achenbach TM. *Manual for the child behavior checklist.* Burlington, VT: Child Behavior Checklist, 1994.

Adams RJ, McKie VC, Carl EM, et al. Long-term stroke risk in children with sickle cell disease screened with transcranial Doppler. *Ann Neurol* 1997;42:699–704.

Adams W, Sheslow D. *WRAML manual.* Wilmington, DE: Jastak Associates, 1990.

Agre JC, Findley TW, McNally MC, et al. Physical activity capacity in children with myelomeningocele. *Arch Phys Med Rehabil* 1987;68:372–77.

Aitkens S, Lord J, Bernauer E, et al. Relationship of manual muscle testing to objective strength measurement. *Muscle Nerve* 1989;12:173–77.

Als H. *Naturalistic observation of newborn behavior (NONB).* Boston: Neonatal Individualized Developmental Care and Assessment Program Training Materials, Enders Ped Research Lab, Childrens' Hospital, 1981.

Als H, Lester BM, Tronick EZ, et al. Assessment of Preterm Infant Behavioral (APIB). In: Fitzgerald H, Joyner MW (eds.). *Theory & research in behavioral pediatrics*, vol. 1. New York: Plenum, 1982.

American Spinal Injury Association: *International standards for neurological classification of spinal cord injury, revised 2002*. Chicago: American Spinal Injury Association, 2002.

Amiel-Tison C, Grenier A. *Assessment for gestational age, neurological evaluation of the newborn and the infant*. New York: Mason, 1968.

Andressen EM, Meyers AR. Health-related quality of life outcomes measures. *Arch Phys Med Rehabil* 2000;81 (Suppl 2):S30–45.

Apgar V. A proposal for a new method of evaluation of the newborn infant. *Anesth Analg* 1953;32:260.

Ashworth B. Preliminary trial of carisoprodol in multiple sclerosis. *Practitioner* 1964;192:540–42.

Austin JK, Huberty TJ. Development of the child attitude toward illness scale. *J Pediatr Psychol* 1993;18:467–80.

Aylward GP. *Bayley infant neurodevelopmental screen manual*. San Antonio: Psychological Corp., 1992.

Ayres AJ. Tactile functions: their relation to hyperactive and perceptual motor behavior. *Am J Occup Ther* 1964;18:83–95.

Ayres AJ. *Sensory integration and the child*. Los Angeles: Western Psychological Services, 1979.

Ayres AJ. *Sensory integration and praxis tests*. Los Angeles: Western Psychological Services, 1989.

Bachanas PJ, Blount RL. The Behavioral approach-avoidance and distress scale: an investigation of reliability and validity during painful medical procedures. *J Pediatr Psychol* 1996;21:671–81.

Bailey DB Jr., Simeonsson RJ, Buysse V, et al. Reliability of an index of child characteristics. *Dev Med Child Neurol* 1993;35:806–15.

Bajd T, Vodovnik L. Pendulum testing of spasticity. *J Biomed Eng* 1984:6:9–16.

Barnerd KE. *Nursing child assessment satellite training and feeding scales (NCAST)*. Seattle: NCAST Publications, 1979.

Bax M. Aims and outcomes of therapy for the cerebral palsy child [editorial]. *Dev Med Child Neurol* 1986;28:695–96.

Bax M. "Controlled trial of physical therapy" at Johns Hopkins [editorial]. *Dev Med Child Neurol* 1988;30:285–86.

Bax M. What are we to measure? [editorial]. *Dev Med Child Neurol* 1993;35:565–66.

Bax M. Outcome studies [editorial]. *Dev Med Child Neurol* 1999;41:291–92.

Bayley N. *Manual for the Bayley Scales of Infant Development*. New York: The Psychology Corp., 1969.

Beals RK. Spastic paraplegia and diplegia: an evaluation of non-surgical and surgical factors influencing the prognosis for ambulation. *J Bone Joint Surg Am* 1966;48-A:827–46.

Beasley WC. Influence of method on estimates of normal knee extensor force among normal and postpolio children. *Phys Ther Rev* 1956;36:21–41.

Beasley WC. Quantitative muscle testing; principles and application to research and clinical services. *Arch Phys Med Rehabil* 1961;42:398–425.

Beca J, Cox PN, Taylor MK, et al. Somatosensory evoked potentials for prediction of outcome in acute severe brain injury. *J Pediatr* 1995;126:44–49.

Beery KE. *Developmental test of visual-motor integration (VMI)*. Cleveland: Modern Curriculum Press, 1989.

Benton AL, Hamsher deS, Sivan AB. *Multilingual aphasia examination*, 3rd. Iowa City: AJA Associates, 1994.

Berger E, Vavrik K, Hochgatterer P. Vigilance scoring in children with acquired brain injury: Vienna vigilance score in comparison with usual coma scales. *J Child Neurol* 2001;16:236–40.

Berglund K, Fugl-Meyer AR. Upper extremity function in hemiplegia: a cross-validation study of two assessment methods. *Scand J Rehab Med* 1986;18:155–57.

Berk RA, DeGangi GA. *DeGangi-Berk Test of Sensory Integration*. Los Angeles: Western Psychological Services, 1983.

Blair L. The role of the physical therapist in the evaluation studies of the poliomyelitis vaccine field trials. *Phys Ther Rev* 1957;37:437–47.

Blanche EI, Botticelli TM, Hallway MK. *Combining neurodevelopment treatment and sensory integration principles: approach to pediatric therapy*. Tucson, AZ: Therapy Skill Builders, 1995.

Bleck EE. Locomotor prognosis in cerebral palsy. *Develop Med Child Neurol* 1975;17:18–25.

Bobath B. The very early treatment of cerebral palsy. *Dev Med Child Neurol* 1967;9:373–90.

Bobath K. A neurophysiologic basis for the treatment of cerebral palsy. *Clin Dev Med* 1980;75:1–98.

Bohannon RW. Strength of lower limb related to gait velocity and cadence in stroke patients. *Physiother Can* 1986a;38:204–06.

Bohannon RW. Manual muscle test scores and dynamometer test scores of knee extension strength. *Arch Phys Med Rehabil* 1986b;67:390–92.

Bohannon RW, Smith MB. Interrater reliability of a modified Ashworth scale of muscle spasticity. *Phys Ther* 1987a;67:206–07.

Bohannon RW, Smith MB. Assessment of strength deficits in eight paretic upper extremity muscle groups of stroke patients with hemiplegia. *Phys Ther* 1987b;67:522–25.

Brander R, Kramer J, Dancsak M, et al. Inter-rater and test-retest reliabilities of the Movement Assessment of Infants. *Ped Phys Ther* 1993;5:9–15.

Braun MA, Palmer MM. A pilot study of oral-motor dysfunction in "at-risk" infants. *Phys Occup Ther Pediatr* 1985;5:13–25.

Brazelton TB. Neonatal Behavioral Assessment Scale. *Clinics in developmental medicine*, No. 50. Philadelphia: JB Lippincott Co., 1973.

Bricker D. *Assessment, evaluation and programming system for infants and children*. Baltimore: Paul H. Brookes Publishing Co., 1993.

Brigance AH: *Brigance inventory of early development.* North Billerica, MA: Curriculum Associates Inc., 1978.

Brink JD, Imbus C. Pediatric levels of consciousness: infants to 2 years, pre-school age 2 to 5 years and school-age 5 years and older. In: *Rehabilitation of head injured child and adult*. Downey, CA: Professional Staff Association of RLAMC, Inc., 1982.

Brown JK. Science and spasticity [editorial]. *Dev Med Child Neurol* 1993;35:471–72.

Brown K. They are improved, but are they better? [editorial]. *Dev Med Child Neurol* 1997;39:213.

Brown L, Sherbenou RJ, Johnson SK. *Test of nonverbal Intelligence* (3rd ed.). Austin, TX: PRO-ED, 1997.

Brown PJ, Marino RJ, Herbison GJ, et al. The 72-hour examination as a predictor of recovery in motor complete quadriplegia. *Arch Phys Med Rehabil* 1991;72:546–48.

Bruininks RH. *Bruininks-Oseretsky test of motor proficiency: examiners' manual.* Circle Pines, MI: American Guidance Services, 1978.

Bruininks RH, Woodcock RW, Wetherman RF, et al. *Scales of independent behavior (SIB)*. Allen, TX: DLM Teaching Resources, 1984.

Bruininks RH, Woodcock RW, Wetherman RF, et al. *Scales of independent behavior-revised (SIB-R)*. Itasca, IL: The Riverside Publishing Co., 1996.

Brunnstrom S. *Movement therapy in hemiplegia: a neurophysiological approach*. Hagerstown, MD: Harper & Row, 1970.

Burry HC. Objective measurement of spasticity. *Devel Med Child Neurol* 1972;14:508–23.

Butler C. Outcomes that matter [editorial]. *Dev Med Child Neurol* 1995;37:753–54.

Butler C, Campbell S. Evidence of the effects of intrathecal baclofen for spastic and dystonic cerebral palsy. *Dev Med Child Neurol* 2000;42:634–45.

Campbell SK. Quantifying the effects of interventions for movement disorders from cerebral palsy. *J Child Neurol* 1996;11 (Suppl 1):S61–70.

Campbell SK, Osten ET, Thubi H, et al. Development of the test of infant motor performance. *Phys Med Rehabil Clin N Am* 1993;4:541–50.

Capute AJ. Early neuromotor reflexes in infancy. *Pediatr Ann* 1986;15:217–18, 221–23, 226.

Carter BG, Butt W. Review of the use of somatosensory evoked potentials in the prediction of outcome after severe brain injury. *Crit Care Med* 2001;29:178–86.

Carter BG, Taylor A, Butt W. Severe brain injury in children: long-term outcome and its prediction using somatosensory evoked potentials (SEPS). *Intensive Care Med* 1999;25:722–28.

Case-Smith J, Bigsby R. *Posture and fine motor assessment of infants (PFMAI)*. San Antonio: The Psychological Corp., 2000.

Cauldwell B. *Home observation for measurement of the environment (HOME)*. Little Rock, AR: Center for Child Development and Education, University of Arkansas at Little Rock, 1984.

Chandler LS, Andrew MS, Swanson MW, et al. *Movement assessment of infants: a manual*. Seattle: Child Development and Mental Retardation Center, University of Washington, 1980.

Cohen MJ. *Children's memory scale*. San Antonio: The Psychological Corp., 1998.

Colarusso RP, Hammill DD. *Motor free visual perceptual test*. Novato, CA: Academic Therapy Publications, 1996.

Coley IL. *Pediatric assessment of self-care activities*. St. Louis: CV Mosby, 1978.

Colorado Medical Society, Sports Medicine Committee. *Guidelines for the management of concussion in sports, revised.* Denver: Colorado Medical Society, 1991.

Committee on Sports Medicine, American Academy of Pediatrics. Recommendations for participation in competitive sports. *Pediatrics* 1988;81:737–39.

Committee on Sports Medicine, American Academy of Pediatrics. Medical conditions affecting sports participation. *Pediatrics* 2001;107:1205–09.

Committee on Sports Medicine and Fitness, American Academy of Pediatrics. Medical conditions affecting sports participation. *Pediatrics* 1994;94:757–60.

Conners CK. *Conners' continuous performance test*. North Tonawanda, NY: Multi-Health Systems, Inc., 1996.

Connolly B: Testing in infants and children. In: Hislop HJ, Montgomery J (eds.). *Daniels and Worthingham's muscle testing: techniques of manual examination* (6th ed.). Philadelphia: WB Saunders Co., 1995.

Connolly MA, Johnson JA. Measuring quality of life in paediatric patients. *Pharmacoeconomics* 1999;16:605–25.

Corrigan JD. Development of a scale for assessment of agitation following traumatic brain injury. *J Clin Exp Neuropsychol* 1989;11:261–77.

Coryell J, Provost BM, Wilhelm IJ, et al. Stability of Bayley Motor Scale scores in the first two years. *Phys Ther* 1989;69:834–41.

Coster W, Deeney T, Haltiwanger J, et al. *School function assessment: user's manual.* San Antonio: The Psychological Corp., Therapy Skill Builders, 1998.

Coster WJ, Haley SM. Conceptualization and measurement of disablement in infants and young children. *Inf Young Children* 1992;4:11–22.

Coury DL. Training physicians for increased involvement with children with special needs. *Inf Young Children* 1990;2:51–57.

Damiano DL, Abel MF. Relationships among impairments, motor function, and perceived health status in spastic cerebral palsy: a multicenter collaboration [abstract]. *Dev Med Child Neurol* 2000;42 (Suppl 83):42.

Damiano DL, Quinlivan JM, Owen BF, et al. What does the Ashworth scale really measure and are instrumented measures more valid and precise? *Dev Med Child Neurol* 2002;44:112–18.

Deaver GG, Brown ME. *Physical demands of daily life.* New York: Institute for the Cripple and Disabled, 1945.

DeGangi G, Greenspan S. *Test of sensory functions in infants (TSFI).* Los Angeles: Western Psychology Services, 1989.

Delis D C, Kramer JH, Kaplan E, et al. *California verbal learning test, children's version.* San Antonio: The Psychological Corp., 1994.

Denckla MB. *A theory and model of executive function: a neuropsychological perspective.* G. R. Lyon and N. A. Krasnegor (eds.). Baltimore: Paul H. Brookes Publishing Co., 1986:263–78.

DiLalla LF, Thompson LA, Plomin R, et al. Infant predictors of preschool and adult IQ: a study of infant twins and their parents. *Dev Psychol* 1990;26:759–69.

DiSimoni, F. *The token test for children.* Allen, TX: DLM Teaching Resources, 1978.

Dittmar SS, Gresham GE. *Functional assessment and outcome measures for the rehabilitation health professional.* Gaithersburg, MD: Aspen Publications, 1997.

Donohoe M, Bleakney DA. Arthrogryposis multiplex congenita. In: Campbell SK (ed.). *Physical therapy in children.* Philadelphia: WB Saunders Co., 1994:261–77.

Dubowitz L, Dubowitz V. The neurological assessment of the preterm and full-term newborn infant. *Clinics in developmental medicine,* No. 79. Philadelphia: JB Lippincott Co., 1981.

Dubowitz L, Mercuri E, Dubowitz V. An optimality score for the neurologic examination of the term newborn. *J Pediatr* 1998;133:406–16.

Duncan PW, Propst M, Nelson SG. Reliability of the Fugl-Myer assessment of sensorimotor recovery following cerebrovascular accident. *Phys Ther* 1983;63:1606–10.

Dunn LM, Dunn LM, Williams KT, et al. *Peabody picture vocabulary test III.* Circle Pines, MN: American Guidance Service, Inc., 1997.

Dunn W. *Sensory profile.* San Antonio: The Psychological Corp., 1999.

Edelman GM. *Neural darwinism.* New York: Basic Books, 1987.

Eisen M, Ware JE Jr., Donald CA, et al. Measuring components of children's health status. *Med Care* 1979; 17:902–21.

Ellison PH, Horn JL, Browning CA. *Infant neurological international battery (INFINIB).* Tucson, AZ: Therapy Skill Builders, 1994.

Erhardt RP. *Developmental visual dysfunction assessment (EDVA).* Tucson, AZ: Therapy Skill Builders Communication Skill Builders, 1993.

Erhardt RP. *Developmental hand dysfunction theory assessment treatment (EDPA).* Tucson, AZ: Therapy Skill Builders Communication Skill Builders: 1994.

Evans P, Alberman E. Recording motor defects of children with cerebral palsy. *Dev Med Child Neurol* 1985;27:404.

Evans P, John A, Nutch L, et al. Report of the recording and reporting of cerebral palsy. *Dev Med Child Neurol* 1986;28:547.

Evans P, Johnson A, Mutch L, et al. Standardized recording and reporting of central motor deficit and associated sensory and intellectual deficits. *Dev Med Child Neurol* 1989;31:117.

Ewing-Cobbs L, Levin HS, Fletcher JM, et al. The Children's Orientation and Amnesia Test: relationship to severity of acute head injury and to recovery. *Neurosurgery* 1990;27:683–91.

Fanurik D, Koh JL, Schmitz ML, et al. Children with cognitive impairment: parent report of pain and coping. *J Dev Behav Pediatr* 1999;20:228–34.

Feldman AB, Haley SM, Coryell J. Concurrent and construct validity of the pediatric evaluation of disability inventory. *Phys Ther* 1990;70:602–10.

Field T, Dempsey J, Shuman HH. Bayley behavioral ratings of normal and high-risk infants: their relationship to Bayley mental scores. *J Pediatr Psychol* 1979; 4:277–83.

Filiatrault J, Arsenault AB, Dutil E, et al. Motor function and activities of daily living assessments: a study of three test for persons with hemiplegia. *Am J Occup Ther* 1991;45:806–10.

Fiorentino MR. *Reflex testing methods for evaluation C.N.S. development.* Springfield, IL: Charles C Thomas, 1963.

Fisher AG, Bundy AC. Sensory integration theory. In: Forssberg H, Hirschfeld H (eds.). *Movement disorders in children; medicine and sport science,* vol. 36. Basel: Karger, 1992:16–20.

Florence J, Pandya S, King W, et al. Intrarater reliability of manual muscle test (Medical Research Council Scale) grades in Duchenne muscular dystrophy. *Phys Ther* 1992;72:115–26.

Folio R, Fewell RR. *Peabody developmental motor scales and activity cards*. Hingham, MA: Teaching Resources Corporation, 1983.

Franck LS, Greenberg CS, Stevens B. Pain assessment in infants and children. *Pediatr Clin N Am* 2000;47:487–512.

Frankenburg WK, Dodds JB. The Denver Developmental Screening Test. *J Pediatr* 1967;71:181.

Frankenburg WK, Dodds JB, Fandal AW. *Denver developmental screening test, revised manual*. Denver: University of Colorado Medical Center, 1970.

Fugl-Meyer AR, Jaasko L, Leyman I, et al. The post-stroke hemiplegic patient: 1. A method for evaluation of physical performance. *Scand J Rehabil Med* 1975;7:13–31.

Furuno S, O'Reilly K, Hosaka C, et al. *Hawaii early learning profile (HELP)*. Palo Alto, CA: Vort Corp, 1988.

Gajdosik CG, Gajdosik RL. Musculoskeletal development and adaptation. In: Campbell SK (ed.). *Physical therapy for children*. Philadelphia: WB Saunders Co., 1994:105–26.

Gardner MF. *Test of visual-perceptual skills*. San Francisco: Health Publishing Company in affiliation with Children's Hospital of San Francisco, 1988.

Gardner MF. *Test of visual motor skills (TVMS-R)*. Hydesville, CA: The Psychological and Educational Publications, Inc., 1995.

Gesell AL, Amatruda CS. Developmental diagnosis. In: Knobloch H, Pasmanick B (eds.). *The infancy and early childhood*. New York: Harper & Row, 1974.

Gilfoyle E M, Grady AP, Moore JC. *Children adapt*. Thorofare, NJ: Charles B. Slack, 1981.

Gioia GA, Isquith PK, Guy SC, et al. *Behavior rating inventory of executive function*. San Antonio: The Psychological Corp., 2001.

Glascoe FP, Byrne KE, Ashford LG, et al. Accuracy of the Denver-II in developmental screening. *Pediatrics* 1992;89:1221–25.

Glover ME, Preminger JL, Sanford AR. *Early leaning accomplishment profile (E-LAP)*. Lewisville, NC: Kaplan School Supply Press, 1978.

Gordon M. *The Gordon diagnostic system*. DeWitt, NY: Gordon Systems, Inc., 1996.

Gormley ME Jr., Krach LE. Pediatric functional assessment: choosing the right tools is the key to compare outcomes. *Rehab Manag* 1997;10:32–35, 103.

Granger CV, Msall ME, Braum S, et al. *WeeFIM system clinical guide: version 5.01*. Buffalo, NY: University at Buffalo, 1998.

Graumlich SE, Powers SW, Byars KC, et al. Multidimensional assessment of pain in pediatric sickle cell disease. *J Pediatr Psychol* 2001;26:203–14.

Greenough WE, Black JE, Wallace CS. Experience and brain development. *Child Dev* 1987;58:539–59.

Gregson JM, Leathley M, Moore AP, et al. Reliability of the Tone Assessment Scale and the Modified Ashworth Scale as clinical tools for assessing poststroke spasticity. *Arch Phys Med Rehabil* 1999;80:1013–16.

Grimby G, Andren E, Holmgren E, et al. Structure of a combination of functional independence measure and instrumental activity measure items in community-living persons: a study of individuals with cerebral palsy and spina bifida. *Arch Phys Med Rehabil* 1996;77:1109–14.

Gross Motor Measure Group. *Gross motor function measures*. Hamilton, Ontario: Chedoke-McMaster Hospital, 1990, revised September 1993.

Hagen C, Malkmus D, Durham P. *Levels of cognitive functioning. Rehabilitation of the head injured adult: comprehensive physical management*. Downey, CA: Professional Staff Association of Rancho Los Amigos National Rehabilitation Center, 1974.

Hahn YS, Chyung C, Bartel MJ, et al. Head injuries in children under 36 months of age. *Child's Nerv Syst* 1988; 4:34–40.

Hain RD. Pain scales in children: a review. *Palliative Med* 1997;11:341–50.

Haley SM, Baryza MJ, Coryell J, et al. *Assessment of movement in infants*. Boston: Research Training Center in Childhood Trauma and Rehabilitation, 1989.

Haley SM, Coster WJ, Ludlow LH. Pediatric functional outcome measures. *Phys Med Rehabil Clin N Am* 1991; 2:689–723.

Haley SM, Coster WJ, Ludlow LH, et al. *Pediatric evaluation of disability inventory: development, standardization, and administration manual, version 1.0*. Boston: New England Medical Center, 1992.

Haley SM, Inacio C, Gans BM. *Tufts assessment of motor performance, pediatric clinical version*. Boston: New England Medical Center Hospital, 1991.

Hammill DD, Pearson NA, Voress JK. *Developmental test of visual perception (DVTR-2)*. Austin, TX: ProEd, 1993a.

Hammill DD, Pearson NA, Voress JK. *Test of visual motor integration (TVMI)*. Austin, TX: ProEd, 1993b.

Harper DC. Who does well—why? [editorial]. *Dev Med Child Neurol* 1999;41:579.

Harris SR, Daniels LE. Content validity of the Harris Infant Neuromotor Test. *Phys Ther* 1996;76:727–37.

Hass BM, Bergstrom E, Jamous A, et al. The inter rater reliability of the original and of the modified Ashworth Scale for the assessment of spasticity in-patients with spinal cord injury. *Spinal Cord* 1996;34:560–64.

Heaton RK, Chelune GJ, Talley JL, et al. *Wisconsin card sorting test, revised and expanded*. Lutz, FL: Psychological Assessment Resources, Inc., 1993.

Henderson S, Sugden DA. *Movement assessment battery for children (movement ABC)*. San Antonio: Psychological Corp., 1992.

Hinderer KA, Hinderer SR. Muscle strength development and assessment in children and adolescents. *Int Persp Phys Ther* 1993;8:93–140.

Hislop HJ, Montgomery J. *Daniels and Worthingham's muscle testing* (6th ed.). Philadelphia: WB Saunders Co., 1995.

Hoskins TA, Squires JE. Developmental assessment: a test for gross motor and reflex development. *Phys Ther* 1973;53:117–25.

Hubert NC, Jay SM, Saltoun M, et al. Approach avoidance and distress in children undergoing preparation for painful procedures. *J Clin Child Psychol* 1988;17:194–202.

Hutchison T. The classification of disability. *Arch Dis Child* 1995;73:91–99.

Iddings DM, Smith LK, Spencer WA. Muscle testing: part 2. Reliability in clinical use. *Phys Ther Rev* 1961;41:249–56.

Jebsen RH, Taylor N, Trieschmann RB, et al. An objective and standardized test of hand function. *Arch Phys Med Rehabil* 1969;50:311–19.

Jepson HA, Talashek ML, Tichy AM. The APGAR score: evolution, limitations, and scoring guidelines. *Birth* 1991;18:83–92.

Johnson-Martin NM, Jens KA, Attermeier SN, et al. *The Carolina curriculum for infants and toddlers with special needs* (2nd ed.). Baltimore: Paul H. Brookes Publishing Co., 1991.

Jonas D, Day A. Assessing pain in children. *Community Nurse* 1997;3:23, 26–28.

Juretschke LJ. Apgar scoring: its use and meaning for today's newborn. *Neonatal Netw* 2000;19:17–19.

Kaplan E, Goodglass H, Weintraub S. *The Boston naming test* (2nd ed.). Boston: Lea and Feibeger, 1983.

Kaplan RM, Bush JW, Berry CC. Health status: types of validity and the index of well-being. *Health Serv Res* 1976;11:478–507.

Katz RT, Rovai GP, Brait C, et al. Objective quantification of spastic hypertonia: correlation with clinical findings. *Arch Phys Med Rehabil* 1992;73:339–47.

Kaufman AS, Kaufman NL. *Kaufman assessment battery for children*. Circle Pines, MN: American Guidance Service, Inc., 1983.

Kaufman AS, Kaufman NL. *Kaufman brief intelligence test*. Circle Pines, MN: American Guidance Service, Inc., 1990.

Kendall FP, McCreary EK, Provance PG. *Muscles: testing and function* (4th ed.). Baltimore: Williams & Wilkins, 1993.

Kinsman SL. Predicting gross motor function in cerebral palsy. *JAMA* 2002;288:1399–1400.

Knoblock H, Stevens F, Malone AF. *Manual of development: the administration and interpretation of revised Gesell and Amatruda developmental examination*. Houston: Gesell Developmental Materials, Inc., 1987.

Knott M, Voss DE. *Proprioceptive neuromuscular facilitation: patterns and techniques* (2nd ed.). New York: Harper & Row, 1968.

Korkman M, Kirk U, Kemp S. *NEPSY: a developmental neuropsychological assessment*. San Antonio: The Psychological Corp., 1998.

Korner AF, Thom VA. *Neurobehavioral assessment of preterm infant (NAPI)*. San Antonio: Psychological Corp., 1990.

Kovacs M. *Children's depression inventory*. North Tonawanda, NY: Multi-Health Systems, Inc., 1982.

Landgraf JM, Abetz L, Ware JE. *Child health questionnaire (CHQ): a user's manual*. Boston: The Health Institute, New England Medical Center, 1996.

Lansky LL, List MA, Marcy A, et al. Toward the development of a play-performance scale for children (PPSC). *Cancer* 1985;56:1837–40.

Law M, Baptiste S, Carswell A, et al. *The Canadian occupational performance measure* (2nd ed.). Ottawa: CAOT Publications ACE, 1994.

Lazar RB, Yarkony GM, Ortolano D, et al. Prediction of functional outcome by motor capability after spinal cord injury. *Arch Phys Med Rehabil* 1989;70:819–22.

Lewis CC, Pantell RH, Kieckhefer GM. Assessment of children's health status: field test of new approaches. *Med Care* 1989;27(Suppl):S54–65.

Lilienfield AM, Jacobs M, Willis M. A study of the reproducibility of muscle testing and certain other aspects of muscle scoring. *Phys Ther Rev* 1954;34:279–89.

Linder T. *Transdisciplinary play based assessment*. Baltimore: Paul H. Brookes Publishing Co., 1990.

Lollar DJ, Simeonsson RJ, Nanda U. Measures of outcomes for children and youth. *Arch Phys Med Rehabil* 2000; 81(Suppl 2):S46–52.

Long TM. Measurement instruments frequently used by pediatric physical therapists (Table 2.2). In: Long TM, Cintas HL. *Handbook of Pediatric Physical Therapy*. Baltimore: Williams & Wilkins, 1995:55–79.

Long TM, Tieman B. Review of two recently published measurement tools: the AMIS and the T.I.M.E. *Pediatr Phys Ther* 1998;10:62–66.

Lovelace-Chandler V. Techniques of pediatric muscle testing. In: Reese NB (ed.). *Muscle and sensory testing*. Philadelphia: WB Saunders Co., 1999:338–76.

Lovett RW. *The treatment of infantile paralysis*. Philadelphia: P. Blakiston's Co., 1916.

Lowman CL. A method of recording muscle tests. *Am J Surg* 1927;3:588–91.

Majnemer AJ, Limperopoulos C. Importance of outcome determination in pediatric rehabilitation. *Dev Med Child Neurol* 2002;44:773–77.

Malott RW, Whaley DL, Malott ME. *Elementary principles of behavior* (3rd ed.). Upper Saddle River, NJ: Prentice Hall, 1997.

Markwardt FC. *Peabody individual achievement test-revised*. Circle Pines, MN: American Guidance Service, 1989.

Marosszeky JE, Batchelor J, Shores EA, et al. The performance of hospitalized, non-head-injured children on the Westmead PTA scale. *Clin Neuropsychol* 1993;7:85–95.

Marrin M, Paes BA. Birth asphyxia: does the APGAR score have a diagnostic value? *Obstet Gynecol* 1988;72:120–23.

Massagli TL. Spasticity and its management in children. *Phys Med Rehabil Clin N Am* 1991;2:867–89.

Matheny AP. Bayley's Infant Behavior Record: behavioral components and twin analysis. *Child Dev* 1980;51:1157–67.

Matti M, Sterling H, Spalding N. *Quick neurological screening test (QNST)*. Los Angles: Western Psychological Services, 1989.

McLaughlin JF, Bjornson KF. Quality of life and developmental disabilities [editorial]. *Dev Med Child Neurol* 1998;40:435.

McSweeny AJ, Creer TL. Health-related quality-of-life assessment in medical care. *Dis Mon* 1995;41:1–71.

Merkel S, Malviya S. Pediatric pain, tools, and assessment. *J Perianesth Nurs* 2000;15:408–14.

Merkel SI, Voepel-Lewus T, Shayevitz JR, et al. The FLACC: a behavioral scale for scoring postoperative pain in young children. *Pediatr Nurs* 1997;23:293–97.

Meythaler JM, Guin-Renfroe S, Hadley MN. Continuously infused baclofen for spastic/dystonic hemiplegia: a preliminary report. *Am J Phys Rehabil* 1999;78:247–54.

Meythaler JM, McCary A, Hadley MN. Prospective assessment of continuous intrathecal infusion of baclofen for spasticity caused by acquired brain injury: a preliminary report. *J Neurosurg* 1997;87:415–19.

Milani-Comparetti A, Gidoni EA. Pattern analysis of motor development and its disorders. *Dev Med Child Neurol* 1967a;9:625–30.

Milani-Comparetti A, Gidoni EA. Routine developmental examination in normal and retarded children. *Dev Med Child Neurol* 1967b;9:631–38.

Miller LJ. *Miller assessment of preschoolers*. Littleton, CO: Foundation for Knowledge in Development, 1982.

Miller LJ. *Infant toddler scale for every baby (ITSE)*. Englewood, CO: Foundation for Knowledge in Development, 1992.

Miller LJ. *Screening test for evaluating preschoolers (first steps)*. San Antonio: Psychological Corp., 1993.

Miller LJ, Roid GH. *The T.I.M.E. Toddler and Motor Evaluation*. Tucson, AZ: The Psychological Corp., 1994.

Molnar GE, Gordon SU. Cerebral palsy: predictive value of selected clinical signs for early prognostication of motor function. *Arch Phys Med Rehabil* 1976;57:153–58.

Molnar GE, Sobus KM. Growth and development. In: Molnar GE, Alexander MA (eds.). *Pediatric rehabilitation* (3rd ed.). Philadelphia: Hanley & Belfus, 1999:13–28.

Morgan AM, Koch V, Lee V, et al. Neonatal Neurobehavioral Examination: a new instrument for quantitative analysis of neonatal neurological status. *Phys Ther* 1988;68:1352–58.

Msall ME. Functional assessment in neurodevelopmental disabilities. In: Capute AJ, Accardo PJ (eds.). *Developmental disabilities in infancy and children*, vol. 1, 2nd ed. Baltimore: Paul H. Brookes Publishing, 1996.

Msall ME, DiGaudio K, Rogers BT, et al. The functional independence measure for children (WeeFIM): conceptual basis and pilot use in children with developmental disabilities. *Clin Pediatr (Phila)* 1994;33:421–30.

Msall ME, DiGaudio KM, Duffy LC. Use of functional assessment in children with developmental disabilities. *Phys Med Rehabil Clin N Am* 1993;4:517–27.

Mullen EM. *Mullen scales of early learning: AGS edition*. Circle Pines, MN: American Guidance Service, Inc., 1995.

Newborg J, Stock JR, Wnek L. *Battelle developmental inventory (BDI)*. Allen, TX: DML Teaching Resources, 1984.

Nichols DS, Case-Smith J. Reliability and validity of the pediatric evaluation of disability inventory. *Pediatr Phys Ther* 1996;8:15–24.

Nickel R, Renken C, Gallestein J. *The infant motor screen (INS)*. Eugene, OR: Crippled Children's Division, The Oregon Health Sciences University, 1989.

Nordmark E, Jarnlo G, Hagglund G. Comparison of the Gross Motor Function Measure and the Pediatric Evaluation of Disability Inventory in assessing motor function in children undergoing selective dorsal rhizotomy. *Dev Med Child Neurol* 2000;42:245–52.

Oberlander TF, O'Donnell ME, Montgomery CJ. Pain in children with significant neurological impairment. *J Dev Behav Pediatr* 1999;20:235–43.

O'Dell MW, Bell KR, Sandel ME. Brain injury rehabilitation. 2. Medical rehabilitation of brain injury. *Arch Phys Med Rehabil* 1998;79(Suppl):S10–15.

O'Donnell ME, Roxborough L. Evidence-based practice in pediatric rehabilitation. *Phys Med Rehabil Clin N Am* 2002;13:991–1005.

Oi S, Matsumoto S. A proposed grading and scoring system for spina bifida: Spina Bifida Neurologic Scale (SBNS). *Child's Nerv Syst* 1992;8:337–342.

Ottenbacher KJ, Hsu Y, Granger CV, et al. The reliability of the functional independence measure: a quantitative review. *Arch Phys Med Rehabil* 1996b;77:1226–32.

Ottenbacher KJ, Msall ME, Lyon NR, et al. Interrater agreement and stability of the functional independence measure for children (WeeFIM): use in children with developmental disabilities. *Arch Phys Med Rehabil* 1997;78:1309–15.

Ottenbacher KJ, Msall ME, Lyon N, et al. Measuring developmental and functional status in children with disabilities. *Dev Med Child Neurol* 1999;41:186–94.

Ottenbacher KJ, Msall ME, Lyon NR, et al. Functional assessment and care of children with neurodevelopmental disabilities. *Am J Phys Med Rehabil* 2000;79:114–23.

Ottenbacher KJ, Taylor ET, Msall ME, et al. The stability and equivalence reliability of the functional independence measure for children (WeeFIM). *Dev Med Child Neurol* 1996a;38:907–16.

Palisano RJ. Concurrent and predictive validities of the Bayley Motor scale and the Peabody Development Motor Scales. *Phys Ther* 1986;66:1714–1719.

Palisano RJ, Rosenbaum PL, Walter SD, et al. Development and reliability of a system to classify gross motor function in children with cerebral palsy. *Dev Med Child Neurol* 1997;39:214–23.

Parks S, Furuno S, O'Reilly KA, et al. *HELP … at home.* Palo Alto, CA: VORT Corporation, 1988.

Patrick DL, Connell FA, Edwards TC, et al. *Age-appropriate measure of quality of life and disability outcomes among children: the youth quality of life study.* Atlanta: Center for Disease Control and Prevention, 1998.

Paul SM, Kathirithamby DR. Exposure to childhood onset disabilities in pediatric residency training [abstract]. *Am J Phys Med Rehabil* 1991;70:229.

Pencharz J, Young NL, Owen JL, et al. Comparison of three outcome instruments in children. *J Pediatr Orthop* 2001; 21:425–32.

Penn RD, Savoy SM, Corcos D, et al. Intrathecal baclofen for severe spinal spasticity. *N Engl J Med* 1989;320:1517–21.

Piper MC, Darrah J. *Motor Assessment of the Developing Infant.* Philadelphia: WB Saunders, 1993.

Piper MC, Pinnell LE, Maguire T, et al. Construction and validation of the Alberta Infant Motor Scales (AIMS). *Can J Public Health* 1992;83(Suppl 2):S46–50.

Plake BS, Impara JC (eds.). *The fourteenth mental measurements yearbook.* Lincoln, NE: The University of Nebraska Press, 2001.

Prechtl HF. *The neurological examination of the full term newborn infant: clinics in developmental medicine, no. 63.* (2nd ed.). Philadelphia: JB Lippincott Co., 1977.

Raimondi AJ, Hirschauer J. Head injury in the infant and toddler: coma scoring and outcome scale. *Child's Brain* 1984;11:12–35.

Reese NB. *Muscle and sensory testing.* Philadelphia: WB Saunders Co., 1999.

Reid DT, Boschen K, Wright V. Critique of the pediatric evaluation of disability inventory (PEDI). *Phys Occup Ther Pediatr* 1993;13:57–93.

Reilly PL, Simpson DA, Sprod R, et al. Assessing the conscious level in infants and young children: a paediatric version of the Glasgow Coma Scale. *Child's Nerv Syst* 1988;4:30–33.

Reitan R. *Halstead-Reitan neuropsychological test battery for children.* Tucson, AZ: Reitan Neuropsychology Laboratory/Press, 1993a.

Reitan, R. *Halstead-Reitan neuropsychological test battery for older children.* Tucson, AZ: Reitan Neuropsychology Laboratory/Press, 1993b.

Reynolds CR, Kamphaus RW. *Behavior assessment system for children.* Circle Pines, MN: American Guidance Service, Inc., 1992.

Reynolds CR, Bigler ED. *Test of memory and learning.* Austin, TX: PRO-ED, 1994.

Reynolds G, Archibald, KC, Brunnstrom S, et al. Preliminary report on neuromuscular function testing of the upper extremity in adult hemiplegic patients. *Arch Phys Med Rehabil* 1958;39:303–10.

Robbins AR, Crowley J. Psychological assessment in pediatric rehabilitation. In: Molnar GE, Alexander MA (eds.). *Pediatric rehabilitation* (3rd ed.). Philadelphia: Hanley & Belfus, 1999:29–56.

Roberts SD, Wells RD, Brown IS, et al. The FRESNO: a pediatric functional outcome measurement system. *J Rehabil Outcomes Meas* 1999;3:11–19

Rogers DS, D'Eugenio DB. *Developmental programming for infants and young children, vol. 1. Assessment and application.* Ann Arbor, MI: University of Michigan Press, 1977.

Rosenbaum PL, Walter SD, Hanna SE, et al. Prognosis for gross motor function in cerebral palsy: creation of motor development curves. *JAMA* 2002;288:1357–63.

Russell DJ, Avery LM, Raina PS, et al. Improved scaling of the gross motor function measure for children with cerebral palsy: evidence of reliability and validity. *Phys Ther* 2000;80:873–85.

Russell DJ, Rosenbaum PL, Cadman DT, et al. The Gross Motor Function Measure: a means to evaluate the effects of physical therapy. *Dev Med Child Neurol* 1989; 31:341–52.

Russell JD, Rosenbaum PL, Lane M, et al. Training users in the Gross Motor Function Measure: methodological and practical issues. *Phys Ther* 1994;74:630–36.

Sahrmann SA, Norton BJ. The relationship of voluntary movement to spasticity in the upper motor neuron syndrome. *Ann Neurol* 1977;2:460–65.

Schmidt M. *Rey Auditory verbal learning test.* Los Angeles: Western Psychological Services, 1996.

Schwartz S, Cohen ME, Herbison GJ, et al. Relationship between two measures of upper extremity strength: manual muscle test compared to hand-held myometry. *Arch Phys Med Rehabil* 1992;73:1063–68.

Scull SA, Athreya B. Childhood arthritis. In: Goldberg B (ed.). *Sports and exercise for children with chronic health conditions.* Champaign, IL: Human Kinetics, 1995:135–48.

Seat PD, Broen WE. *Personality inventory for children-2.* Los Angeles: Western Psychological Services, 1977.

Sehgal N, McGuire JR. Beyond Ashworth: electrophysiological quantification of spasticity. *Phys Med Rehabil Clin N Am* 1998;9:949–79.

Seibert JJ, Glasier CM, Kirby RS, et al. Transcranial Doppler, MRA, and MRI as a screening examination for cerebrovascular disease in patients with sickle cell anemia: an 8-year study. *Pediatr Radiol* 1998;28:138–42.

Semans S. Specific Tests and evaluation tools for the child with central nervous system deficit. *J Am Phys Ther Assoc* 1965;45:456–62.

Semans S, Phillips R, Romanoli M, et al. A cerebral palsy assessment chart: instructions for administration of the test. *J Am Phys Ther Assoc* 1965;45:463–68.

Sepega AA. Muscle performance evaluation in orthopaedic practice. *J Bone Joint Surg Am* 1990;72-A:1562–74.

Shallice T. In: Broadbent DE, Weiskranz L (eds.). *Specific impairments in planning.* London: Royal Society, 1982:199–209.

Sheldon MP. A physical achievement record for use with crippled children. *Journal of Health, Physical Education, Recreation* 1935;6:30–31, 60.

Shevell MI. Neonatal neurologic prognostication: the asphyxiated term newborn. *Pediatr Neurol* 1999;21:776–84.

Shirkey H. Therapeutic orphans [editorial]. *J Pediatr* 1968; 72:119–20.

Shores EA, Marosszeky JE, Sandanam J, et al. Preliminary validation of a clinical scale for measuring the duration of post-traumatic amnesia. *Med J Aust* 1986;144:569–72.

Simeonsson RJ, Lollar D, Hollowell J, et al. Revision of the international classification of impairments, disabilities, and handicaps: developmental issues. *J Clin Epidemiol* 2000;53:113–24.

Skold C, Harms-Ringdahl K, Hulting C, et al. Simultaneous Ashworth measurements and electromyographic recordings in tetraplegic patients. *Arch Phys Med Rehabil* 1998;79:959–65.

Sneed RC, May WL, Stencel CS. Training of pediatricians in care of physical disabilities in children with special health care needs: results of a two-state survey of practicing pediatricians and national resident training programs. *Pediatrics* 2000;105:554–61.

Soderberg GL. Handheld dynamometry for muscle testing. In: Reese NB. *Muscle and sensory testing.* Philadelphia: WB Saunders Co., 1999:378–420.

Sousa JC, Gordon LH, Shurtleff DB. Assessing the development of daily living in patients with spina bifida. *Dev Med Child Neurol* 1976;18 (Suppl 37):134–42.

Sousa JC, Telzrow RW, Holm RA, et al. Developmental guidelines for children with myelodysplasia. *Phys Ther* 1983;63:21–29.

Sparrow SA, Balla DA, Cicchetti DV. *Vineland adaptive behavior scales. Interview edition.* Survey Form Manual. Circle Pines, MN: American Guidance Services, 1984.

Spieth LE, Harris CV. Assessment of health-related quality of life in children and adolescents: an integrated review. *J Pediatr Psychol* 1996;21:175–93.

Squires J, Bricker D. *Infant monitoring questionnaires.* Eugene, OR: Center on Human Development, University of Oregon, 1989.

Starfield B, Bergner M, Ensminger M, et al. Adolescent health status measurement: development of the Child Health and Illness Profile. *Pediatrics* 1993;91: 430–35.

Starfield B, Riley AW, Green BF, et al. The adolescent Child Health and Illness Profile: a population-based measure of health. *Med Care* 1995;33:553–66.

Steel KO, Glover J, Spasoff RA. The Motor Control Assessment: an instrument to measure motor control in physically disabled children. *Arch Phys Med Rehabil* 1991;72:549–53.

Stein RE, Jessop DJ. Functional Status II(R): a measure of child health status. *Med Care* 1990;28:1041–55.

Stein RE, Westbrook LE, Bauman LJ. The Questionnaire for Identifying Children with Chronic Conditions: a measure based on a noncategorical approach. *Pediatrics* 1997;99:513–21.

Stineman MG, Shea JA, Jette A, et al. The functional independence measure: test of scaling assumptions, structure, and reliability across 20 diverse impairment categories. *Arch Phys Med Rehabil* 1996;77:1101–08.

Stover SL. Classifications standards for SCI, revised 1992 [editorial]. *Arch Phys Med Rehabil* 1992;73:783.

Strub RL, Black FW. *The Mental Status Examination in* Neurology (4th ed). Philadelphia: FA Davis Company, 1993.

Stuberg W, Metcalf W. Reliability of quantitative muscle testing in healthy children and in children with Duchenne muscular dystrophy using hand held dynamometers. *Phys Ther* 1988;68:977–82.

Stuberg WA, White PJ, Miedaner JA, et al. Item reliability of the Milani-Comparetti Motor Development Screening Test. *Phys Ther* 1989;69:328–35.

Summers S. Evidence-based practice part 2: reliability and validity of selected acute pain instruments. *J Perianesth Nurs* 2001;16:35–40.

Sussman M. Why don't we know more about what we are doing? [editorial]. *Dev Med Child Neurol* 2001;43:507.

Taggart PJ, Aguilar, C. Pediatric motor assessment. In: Alexander MA, Molnar GE (eds.). *Physical Medicine and Rehabilitation: State of the Art Reviews: Pediatric Rehabilitation.* Philadelphia: Hanley & Belfus, 2000:185–96.

Talley JL. *Children's auditory verbal learning test-2.* Lutz, FL: Psychological Assessment Resources, Inc., 1993.

Tanner JM. *Growth at adolescence* (2nd ed.). New York: Appleton-Century-Crofts, 1966.

Tardieu G, Shentoub S, Delarue R. A la recherche diune technique de mesure de la spasticite. *Revue Neurologique* 1954;91:143–44.

Task Force on Childhood Motor Disorders. *Consensus report of a meeting at the National Institutes of Health,* April 22–24, 2001. (http://accessible.ninds.nih.gov/news_and_events/ proceedings/Hypertonia_Meeting_2001.htm).

Taylor N, Sand PL, Jebsen RH. Evaluation of hand function in children. *Arch Phys Med Rehabil* 1973;54:129–35.

The Psychological Corporation. *Wechsler intelligence scale for children* (3rd ed.). San Antonio: The Psychological Corp., 1992.

The Psychological Corporation. *Wechsler abbreviated scale of intelligence*. San Antonio: The Psychological Corp., 1999.

The Psychological Corporation. *Wechsler individual achievement test* (2nd ed.). San Antonio: The Psychological Corp., 2001.

The Psychological Corporation. The Bayley II. *Bayley scales of infant development* (2nd ed.). San Antonio: Harcourt Brace & Co., 1993.

Tiffin J, Asher EJ. The Purdue Pegboard: norms and studies of reliability and validity. *J Appl Psychol* 1948;32:234–47.

Twycross A, Mayfield C, Savoy J. Pain management for children with special needs: a neglected area? *Pediatr Nurs* 1999;11:43–45.

Wartenberg R. Pendulousness of the legs as a diagnostic test. *Neurology* 1951;1:18–24.

Wechsler D. *Wechsler preschool and primary scale of intelligence-revised*. San Antonio: The Psychological Corp., 1989.

Wilkinson GS. *Wide range achievement test 3*. Delaware: Wide Range, Inc., 1993.

Wilson GAM, Doyle E. Validation of three paediatric pain scores for use by parents. *Anaesthesia* 1996;51:1005–7.

Wohlrab G, Boltshauser E, Schmitt B. Neurological outcome in comatose children with bilateral loss of cortical somatosensory evoked potentials. *Neuropediatrics* 2001;32:271–74.

Yeates KO. *Pediatric neuropsychology: research, theory, and practice*. New York: The Guilford Press, 2000.

Young RY, Wiegner AW. Spasticity. *Clin Orthop* 1987;219: 50–62.

Amyotrophic Lateral Sclerosis Clinimetric Scales—Guidelines for Administration and Scoring

5

Benjamin Rix Brooks, M.D.

Amyotrophic lateral sclerosis (ALS) is a progressive degeneration of corticobulbar, corticospinal, brainstem, and spinal cord motor neurons whose clinical manifestations are weakness, muscle atrophy, hyperreflexia, and spasticity. Using the World Health Organization model for disease consequences, the *pathology* of ALS may be measured by motor neuron pathologic change, motor neuron loss, and corticospinal tract degeneration (Table 5-1). Disease-related *impairment* is defined by strength loss, respiratory insufficiency, spasticity, loss of fine motor coordination, and speech and swallowing difficulties. These impairments are measured by elements of the neurologic examination including manual muscle testing and functional testing (Brooks et al., 1989; Caroscio et al., 1987; Fallat, 1994; Fallat et al., 1979). These impairments result in *disability* that may be measured by a number of clinimetric scales (Table 5-2). The initial clinimetric scale used to evaluate the course of ALS was developed to assess the ergotropic effects of guanidine (Norris et al., 1974). It actually included both impairments and disabilities in five domains (bulbar, respiratory, arm, trunk, and leg) to weight the

different regional involvement of the nervous system in ALS. The evolution of clinimetric scales resulted in more quantitation of impairments and addition of further measures of disability maintaining the same regional weighting (Appel et al., 1987). In an attempt to define clinical impairment before it could be ascertained by manual muscle testing, isometric muscle testing was incorporated into clinimetric scales for the evaluation of the clinical course of ALS (Munsat et al., 1988; Ringel et al., 1993). Recent clinical trials of new therapies for ALS have used both the Appel scale and composite evaluations measuring impairments of isometric muscle strength or timed bulbar, respiratory, arm, and leg function [ALS Ciliary Neotrophic Factor (CNTF) Treatment Study (ACTS) Phase I–II Study Group, 1995a, 1995b, 1996; ALS CNTF Treatment Study (ACTS) Phase II–III Study Group, 1996; Miller et al., 1996b]. More important, the new composite evaluations have separated impairments from disabilities and permit separate evaluation of the effects of the ALS on impairments and the disabilities resulting from impairments due to ALS (see Table 5-2). The *handicap* to individual patients is in direct proportion to the accumulation of these ALS-related disabilities

Table 5-1. World Health Organization Disease Consequences—Amyotrophic Lateral Sclerosis

Domain	Substrate	Measurement
Pathology	Motor neuron pathologic change	Ubiquitin (+) motor neurons
		Neurofilament (+) motor neurons
	Motor neuron loss	
	Corticospinal tract	Glial fibrillary acidic protein (+)
	Degeneration	Corticospinal tract staining
Impairment	Strength loss	Manual muscle testing
	Arm	Maximal voluntary isometric contraction
	Leg	
	Breathing	Respiratory rate
		Vital capacity (forced, slow)
		Peak inspiratory flow rate
	Spasticity	Ashworth Spasticity Scale
		Walking velocity
	Fine coordination loss	Ashworth Spasticity Scale
Disability	Function loss	
	Speech	Intelligibility, PaTa velocity
		Speech ALS FRS
	Swallow	Deglutition
		Swallowing ALS FRS
	Breathing	Breathing ALS FRS
	Arm	Arm ALS FRS
	Leg	Leg ALS FRS
Handicap	Independence loss	Quality-of-life scales
	Work	Sickness Impact Profile
	Social integration	
	Self-care	Short Form 36
	Death	Survival

ALS FRS = Amyotrophic Lateral Sclerosis Functional Rating Scale.

and results in a decreased quality of life leading ultimately to accelerated death.

Muscle strength, pulmonary function, and mortality are being used in current clinical trials of treatments for ALS to measure the effects of treatment on ALS-determined impairments; however, the impact of potential new therapies on the activities of self-care must be captured by a disease-specific assessment of activities of daily living in patients with ALS. Previous clinimetric scales in ALS have combined measurements of impairments with measures of disability or handicap (Appel et al., 1987; Brooks et al., 1990, 1991, 1994; Norris et al., 1974). Mixture of impairment and disability elements in the same clinimetric scale leads to difficulty with regard to interpretation of the dynamic range of the total score or subscores of the clinimetric scale as measures of the health status in individuals or groups of individuals with ALS being studied and to difficulty concerning the statistical behavior of the total score or subscores of the clinimetric scale in individuals or groups of individuals over time (Feinstein, 1987; Streiner &

Table 5-2.   Comparison of Impairments and Disabilities in Norris Scale, Appel Scale, and ACTS ALS Evaluation

	Norris ALS Scale	Appel ALS Scale	ACTS ALS Evaluation
Bulbar			
Impairments	Fasciculations/atrophy	—	Speech PaTa
	Fatigue	—	—
	Jaw jerk	—	—
	Labile emotions		
Disabilities	Speech	Speech	Speech ALS FRS
	Swallowing	Diet	Swallow ALS FRS
	Chewing	—	Salivation ALS FRS
Respiratory			
Impairments	—	Vital capacity	Vital capacity
Disabilities	Breathing	—	Breathing ALS FRS
	Cough	—	—
Arm			
Impairments	Fasciculations/atrophy	Deltoid, biceps, triceps	Deltoid, biceps, triceps
	Fatigue	Wrist extensor/flexor	Isometric strength
	Biceps, brachial radialis	Finger extensor/flexor	—
	Triceps tendon reflexes	Manual muscle strength	—
	—	Grip isometric strength	Grip isometric strength
	—	Pinch isometric strength	—
	—	Timed propelling wheelchair	—
	—	Timed large block board	—
	—	Timed cutting Theraplast	—
	—	Timed pegboard	Timed pegboard
Disabilities	Change arm position	Dressing	Dressing ALS FRS
	Grip, lift self	Feeding	Feeding ALS FRS
	Lift book, lift utensil	—	—
	Writing	—	Writing ALS FRS
	Buttons, zipper	—	—
Trunk			
Impairments			
	Fasciculations/atrophy	—	—
	Fatigue	—	—
Disabilities	—	—	Turning in bed ALS FRS

(continued)

Table 5-2.   *(continued)*

		Norris ALS Scale	*Appel ALS Scale*	*ACTS ALS Evaluation*
Leg				
	Impairments	Fasciculations/atrophy	Timed walk 20 ft	Timed walk 15 ft
		Fatigue	Timed stand from lying	—
		Quadriceps, adductor, Achilles tendon reflexes	Timed stand from chair	—
			Timed climb stairs	—
		Plantar responses	—	—
		Leg rigidity	—	—
	Disabilities	Climb stairs	—	Climbing stairs ALS FRS
		Walk one block unassisted	AFO/cane/walker	Walking ALS FRS
		Walk one room unassisted	Occasional/constant wheelchair	—
		Stand	Climb stairs unassisted	—
		Change leg position	—	—

AFO = ankle-foot orthosis; ALS = amyotrophic lateral sclerosis; ALS FRS = Amyotrophic Lateral Sclerosis Functional Rating Scale.

Norman, 1989). Disease impairments may occur early in the disease process, but the time course of change in the degree of impairment may be quite different from the time course of change in the degree of disability (Brooks et al., 1990, 1991, 1994; Brooks, 1996). Both the Norris scale and the Appel scale have mixed impairments and disabilities in varying proportions (see Table 5-2). The Norris scale weights reflexes, fasciculations, and weakness as impairments and other self-reported items as disabilities in bulbar : respiratory : arm : trunk : leg domains in the ratio 3 : 1 : 5 : 2 : 5. The Appel scale weights bulbar : respiratory : arm : leg domains in the ratio 5 : 5 : 8 : 8. The different weighting of respiratory relative to other domains between the Appel and Norris scales is problematic. Moreover, within the Appel scale, there is duplication of the scale with respect to rating lower extremity function and use of aids. This duplication indicates that the same clinical information is added to the total scale more than once, causing increased autocorrelation (Feinstein, 1987; Streiner & Norman, 1989). In addition, the total Appel scale demonstrates nonlinearity over time during the early and late stages of the disease. This effect is amply demonstrated in several studies (Brooks et al., 1991; Italian ALS Study Group, 1993; Lange et al., 1996). Weighting of the five domains is arbitrary, but guidelines have now been developed to establish the ele-

ments measuring impairment, disability, and handicap that should be used in clinical trials of therapies for ALS (Subcommittee on Motor Neuron Diseases, 1995).

Recent and current clinical trials include the Amyotrophic Lateral Sclerosis Functional Rating Scale (ALS FRS), a clinimetric scale developed specifically to measure disease-related disability alone in ALS. This scale was developed because currently used clinimetric scales were contaminated with impairment measurements, did not measure the broad range of disabilities that result from ALS, and did not lend themselves to subscore analysis that was based entirely on disability components (Feinstein, 1987; Louwerse et al., 1990; Streiner & Norman, 1989). The ALS FRS is a synthesis of five elements from the Unified Parkinson's Disease Rating Scale, four elements from the Amyotrophic Lateral Sclerosis Severity Scale, and a new element concerning the breathing state of the ALS patient [ALS CNTF Treatment Study (ACTS) Phase I–II Study Group, 1996; Hillel et al., 1989, 1990]. The ALS FRS was developed as an internally consistent, reliable, and valid measure of disability in ALS patients as part of the ALS CNTF Treatment Study (ACTS Phase I–II Study Group, 1996). The ability of the ALS FRS to be responsive to change in the clinical status of ALS patients was evaluated cross-sectionally and prospectively over time in phase I and phase II studies of CNTF in ALS [ALS CNTF Treatment

Study (ACTS) Phase I–II Study Group, 1995a, 1995b, 1996; ALS CNTF Treatment Study (ACTS) Phase II–III Study Group, 1996].

Administration of Norris Amyotrophic Lateral Sclerosis Scale

The Norris Amyotrophic Lateral Sclerosis Scale was developed to follow clinical change in ALS patients after treatment (Brooks, 1994; Norris et al., 1974). This scale (Figure 5-1) measures both impairments and disabilities in a single patient. Both are regionally grouped under the *bulbar, respiratory, arm, trunk, leg,* and *general* domains. The Norris scale has evolved since its introduction in 1974 and can be performed with minimum equipment in a number of clinical situations by neurologists or well-trained research nurses (Table 5-3).

Administration of Appel Amyotrophic Lateral Sclerosis Scale

The total Appel ALS Scale score (Figure 5-2) consists of five domain subscores: *bulbar, respiratory, muscle strength, lower extremity function,* and *upper extremity function* (Table 5-4). The patients are graded in an ALS clinic. Those involved in the actual grading of the patients may include the neurologist (muscle strength testing), the occupational therapist (blocks, pegboard, grip, lateral pinch), the respiratory therapist (vital capacity), and the research nurse (remainder of rating scale). The examination could easily be performed by a neurologist (muscle strength testing) and a nurse (remainder of the rating scale). The important principle is that parts of the test be performed by the same person at each subsequent visit.

The bulbar subscore is determined by the ALS clinic team based on the recommendations given at that clinic visit from either the neurologist or dietitian. The patient may say he or she is taking a general diet but if the ALS clinic team recommends that the patient should have only chopped or ground foods and thickened liquids, the patient should receive a grade of 9 points for swallowing. If choking spells occur with regular liquids, thickened liquids should be recommended and the grade drops to 9 points.

The respiratory subscore is based on changes in the forced vital capacity (FVC) presented in terms of the predicted FVC for that patient based on gender, height, and age according to the Morris formula:

$$\text{Male predicted FVC} = [0.148 \times (\text{height in inches})] - [0.025 \times (\text{age})] - 4.241$$

$$\text{Female predicted FVC} = [0.115 \times (\text{height in inches})] - [0.024 \times (\text{age})] - 2.852$$

The FVC measurement should be performed with a nose clip and with the patient standing if possible. It is important to have masks available in case of poor lip seal. Each test should be performed at least twice to obtain a maximal effort. The best effort is recorded. If a patient with an FVC of 80% predicted receives respiratory medications, he or she should be recorded as 12 points (Fallat et al., 1979; Fallat, 1994; Glindmeyer et al., 1987; Norris & Fallat, 1988).

The muscle strength subscore consists of manual muscle testing according to the Medical Research Council grading system. Both the right and left deltoid, biceps, triceps, wrist extensors, wrist flexors, finger extensors, and finger flexors are tested. The sum of the right and left sides is determined and coded according to the algorithm in Table 5-4.

Handgrip is measured carefully. The handle of the Jamar dynamometer is adjusted to fit the subject's hand and allow metacarpophalangeal flexion. The subject rests his or her forearm on the desktop, but the dynamometer is not rested on the desktop. Maximal handgrip is measured twice, with a rest period between the two testing sessions (1–3 minutes). The sum of the right and left maximal handgrip is divided by two. The appropriate grade is assigned according to Table 5-4.

Lateral pinch is measured as the preceding, with an Osco pinch gauge between the tip of the pad of the thumb and the lateral surface of the index finger. The right and left pinch is measured once, summed, and divided by two. The appropriate score is assigned according to Table 5-4.

The lower extremity function subscore involves timed functional tests. Standing from sitting in a chair is timed from the start of standing until the patient reaches the erect posture. The examiner is not allowed to assist. If assistance is required, the patient is graded as "unable" and receives a score of 5 points. Standing from lying supine is timed in arising from a supine position of a standard examining table height to a standing position. The examiner is not allowed to assist. If a patient requires assistance, he or she is graded as "unable" and given a score of 6 points.

Norris ALS Scale

	3 Normal	2 Impaired	1 Trace	0 No Use
1. Hold up neck				
2. Chewing				
3. Swallowing				
4. Speech				
5. Roll over in bed				
6. Do a sit-up				
7. Bowel/bladder pressure				
8. Breathing				
9. Coughing				
10. Write name				
11. Work buttons, zippers				
12. Feed self				
13. Grip/lift self				
14. Grip/lift book/tray				
15. Grip/lift fork/pencil				
16. Change arm position				
17. Climb stairs – 1 flight				
18. Walk – 1 block				
19. Walk – 1 room				
20. Walk – assisted				
21. Stand up from chair				
22. Change leg position				

	Normal	Hyper/Hypo	Absent	Clonic
23. Stretch reflexes – arms				
24. Stretch reflexes – legs				

	Absent	Present	Hyperactive	Clonic
25. Jaw jerk				

	Flexor	Mute	Equivocal	Extensor
26. Plantar response – right				
27. Plantar response – left				

	None/Rare	Slight	Moderate	Severe
28. Fasciculation				
29. Atrophy – face, tongue				
30. Atrophy – arms, shoulders				
31. Atrophy – legs, hips				
32. Labile emotions				

		0 to Mild		Moderate to Severe
33. Fatigability				
34. Leg rigidity				

				PATIENT TOTAL SCORE
Patient Subtotals				
Normal Subtotals	96	4		

Figure 5-1. Norris Amyotrophic Lateral Sclerosis (ALS) Scale rating form.

Table 5-3. Guidelines for Administration/Scoring Norris Amyotrophic Lateral Sclerosis Scale

Item	Description	Score
1	Hold up head (test)—no problem	3
	Droops when tired, or unable to complete chin-test	2
	Always droops without support collar, only clears pillow supine	1
	Cannot clear pillow when supine	0
2	Chewing (history)—no problem	3
	Requires some soft or blenderized foods, some rest periods	2
	Completely soft/blenderized foods, frequent rest periods	1
	Food must be pushed to back of mouth	0
3	Swallowing (test)—no problem	3
	Aspirates some water but not saliva during entire examination	2
	Aspirates saliva occasionally, drools frequently	1
	Water runs out of mouth, aspirates saliva frequently	0
4	Speech (test)—normal throughout visit	3
	Any problem during visit	2
	Barely understandable simple phrases	1
	Grunts, groans, rare intelligible sounds	0
5	Roll over (test)—turn readily to at least one side from supine on examination table	3
	Any problems (may be due to severe arm weakness but score here also)	2
	Barely turns with great effort to just one side	1
	Needs assistance to turn	0
6	Sit up (test)—sit to full vertical from supine on examination table	3
	Clears head, shoulders, but not trunk, without pulling	2
	Clears head, but not shoulders, without pull/lift	1
	Requires lift of both head, trunk	0
7	Bowel/bladder pressure (history)—no apparent problem	3
	Problem bearing down; needs laxative or stool softener every week	2
	Needs laxative or softener more often, occasional enema	1
	Enema needed more often than not	0
8	Breathing (test)—no problem during entire visit	3
	Dyspnea arriving at office or during strength test	2
	Dyspnea in ordinary conversation	1
	Respiratory distress	0
9	Cough (test)—examiner unable to restrain lower chest in coughing (hold from behind)	3
	Cough effective but examiner able to restrain chest	2
	Cough usually ineffective (e.g., multiple shallow coughs after aspiration)	1
	Cough ineffective	0

(continued)

Table 5-3. *(continued)*

Item	Description	Score
10	Write (test)—write name, address; spouse confirms normalcy	3
	Any legibility problem with name, address	2
	Unable to complete name, address, or mainly illegible	1
	Only able to make marks	0
11	Buttons, zippers (test)—button shirt; may use both hands, time not limited but no assist devices, pull zipper closed	3
	Unable to complete above without aid	2
	Only able to do two buttons with assist devices, half of zipper	1
	Unable to perform above, near-full assistance needed	0
12	Feeding (history)—no problem or needs simple assist devices only, large handle	3
	Requires help cutting meat or needs more assist devices, finger splints, arm slings/pivots, etc.	2
	Unable to cut or use fork but can raise food to mouth	1
	Must be fed	0
13	Grip/lift self (test)—pulls self erect from supine position with one hand	3
	Above with great effort or both grips necessary	2
	Above using trunk flexors (examiner palpates abdomen)	1
	Requires lift or pull by examiner	0
14	Grip/lift book, tray (test)—lifts large book from lap to face level	3
	Clears lap but cannot lift to face	2
	Lifts paperback book from lap to face	1
	Clears lap with paperback book but cannot lift to face	0
15	Grip/lift fork, pencil (test)—holds pencil to write, legibility not considered	3
	Lifts pencil but unable to grip enough to mark	2
	Lifts pencil clear of table only briefly	1
	May move pencil but cannot lift clear	0
16	Change arm position (test)—lift both arms over head from lap	3
	Arms clear lap but not shoulders	2
	Moves both arms from lap to arm rests	1
	Wiggles arms but not enough to move from lap	0
17	Climb stairs (test)—climbs one flight without pausing or pulling	3
	Climbs one flight but resting or pulling on rail required	2
	Climbs two or more steps unaided	1
	Climbs less than two steps, probably needs lift onto examination table	0

Table 5-3. *(continued)*

Item	Description	Score
18	Walk (test)—walks one block (office corridor four times without pause), may wear favorable shoes, ankle brace, etc., <5 min	3
	Completes the distance with problems of any type or needs >5 min	2
	Completes only with assist or multiple rests	1
	Cannot complete	0
19	Walk one room (test 15 ft)—completes without difficulty	3
	Any problems	2
	Completes but needs minimal assist or is exhausted	1
	Cannot complete without substantial aid including cane/crutch	0
20	Walk assisted (test only if assist required above, score three if item 19 scores one or better)—completes one room using cane/crutch or holding examiner's arm	3
	Cannot complete without assistance	2
	Takes steps in transfer from chair to examination table	1
	Legs drag in assisted transfer	0
21	Stand (test)—stands readily from standard chair, no pushing with arms	3
	Any problem	2
	Actively assists but needs lift to complete rise	1
	Needs lifting throughout	0
22	Change leg position (test)—raises each leg to 45 degrees in supine position	3
	Clears table but one leg cannot reach 45 degrees	2
	Only clears table briefly, on one leg completely paralyzed	1
	Only ineffective wiggles	0
23	Biceps, brachioradialis, triceps muscle stretch reflexes (test)—all within the broad range of normal and symmetric	3
	Asymmetry or at least one clearly abnormal	2
	Any three absent, the remaining three only trace responses	1
	Any three clonic	0
24	Quadriceps, Achilles, internal hamstring muscle stretch reflexes (test)—as in item 23	
25	Jaw jerk (test)—absent	3
	Present	2
	Hyperactive	1
	Clonic	0
26, 27	Plantar responses (test)—flexor	3
	Mute	2
	Equivocal	1
	Extensor	0

(continued)

Table 5-3.   *(continued)*

Item	Description	Score
28	Fasciculation (observe throughout examination), patient stripped to standard underwear, no T-shirt; no neuromuscular function drugs—i.e., pyridostigmine—during the previous 24 hr	
	None/rare	3
	Slight	2
	Moderate	1
	Severe	0
29–31	Wasting—atrophy (observe)—normal bulk	3
	Mild loss of bulk	2
	Moderate loss of bulk	1
	Marked loss of bulk	0
32	Labile emotions (history and observation)—no problem, spouse confirms	3
	Occasional inappropriate weeping or giggling	2
	At least daily lability	1
	Weeping (rarely laughter) with most stimuli, entering office	0
33	Fatigability (test)—no abnormality ranging to occasional reduction in strength during examination with rapid recovery in minutes	2
	Frequent reduction in strength during examination or general decline in function with time	0
34	Leg rigidity (test)—muscle tone normal or slightly increased in both legs, or normal in one but moderate (resists gravity) in the other; no muscle relaxant in last 24 hr	2
	Moderate rigidity in both, or board-like rigidity in one, or worse	0

Adapted from Brooks BR. The Norris ALS score: Insight into the natural history of amyotrophic lateral sclerosis provided by Forbes Norris. In: Rose FC (ed.). *ALS—From Charcot to the present and into the future—The Forbes H. Norris (1928–1993) Memorial Volume.* London: Smith-Gordon, 1994:21–29. [Advances in ALS/MND, Vol. 3].

Timed walking 20 feet is timed from the first step through the first step across the finish line. The examiner is not allowed to assist but should accompany the patient for safety. If assistance is needed, the patient is graded as "unable" and receives a grade of 5 points. Climbing and descending four standard stairs are timed. The examiner is not allowed to assist. If it is found that it would be unsafe to perform this task, the patient is scored "unable" and receives a grade of 6 points. The hips and legs portion is determined after the previous tests have been completed.

The upper extremity function subscore involves timed functional tests. Propelling wheelchair 20 feet with arms is timed from the initiation of wheel turning through the first point at which the bottom of the wheel of the wheelchair crosses the finish line. No assistance may be given. The arms and shoulders test should be graded according to the most affected side. A patient who can raise his or her right arm above the head with no problem but can raise only his or her left arm above the head by flexing the elbow is given a score of 2 points. Cutting Theraplast requires the patient to use the dominant hand to cut Theraplast 0.25 inches thick and 4 inches in diameter. The knife is positioned in the hand at the beginning of the timing on the Theraplast. Timing is measured from the initial cut until the entire Theraplast is cut through. Pegboard testing requires the construction of peg units in sequence of a pin, followed by a washer, followed by a collar in 60 seconds by each hand. The construction of the peg unit should be demonstrated for the patient. The pegboard is placed on a table that allows the

Appel ALS Scale

Bulbar Subscore
6 – 30

Swallowing Grade   *3 – 15*

Speech Grade   *3 – 15*

Respiratory Subscore
6 – 30

Vital Capacity Grade   *6 – 30*

Muscle Strength Subscore
6 – 36

Upper Extremity Muscle Strength Grade   *2 – 14*

Lower Extremity Muscle Strength Grade   *2 – 14*

Hand Grip Grade   *1 – 4*

Lateral Pinch Grade   *1 – 4*

Lower Extremity Muscle Function Subscore
6 – 35

Stand from Chair Grade   *1 – 5*

Stand from Lying Grade   *1 – 6*

Walk 20 Feet Grade   *1 – 5*

Need for Assistive Devices Grade   *1 – 5*

Climb & Descend Four Standard Steps Grade   *1 – 6*

Hips and Legs Grade   *1 – 8*

Upper Extremity Muscle Function Subscore
6 – 33

Dress and Feed Self Grade   *1 – 5*

Propel Wheelchair 20 Feet Grade   *1 – 6*

Arms and Shoulders Grade   *1 – 6*

Cut Theraplast Grade   *1 – 6*

Pegboard Grade   *1 – 5*

Block Coordination Grade   *1 – 5*

TOTAL APPEL ALS SCALE SCORE

30 – 164

Figure 5-2. Appel Amyotrophic Lateral Sclerosis (ALS) Scale rating form.

Table 5-4. Guidelines for Administration/Scoring Appel Amyotrophic Lateral Sclerosis Scale

---

A. Bulbar subscore (6–30 points)

1. *Swallowing grade*

3 points	General diet
6 points	Soft diet (soft, cooked; eliminates popcorn, crumbly foods, etc.)
9 points	Mechanical soft diet (finely chopped or ground and thickened liquids)
12 points	Pudding consistency diet (strained, pureed, blended, thickened liquids)

The score is determined by the nurse based on the recommendations given at clinic visit from either the neurologist or dietitian. For example, the patient may still say he/she is taking a general diet, but if the team recommends that he/she should have only chopped or ground foods and thickened liquids, the patient receives a score of 9 points. Please note that if the patient can take a general diet or soft diet, he/she is taking regular liquids and has no need to use thickened liquids. If choking spells occur with regular liquids, thickened liquids should be recommended, and the bulbar subscore should be designated as 9 points.

2. *Speech grade*

3 points	Clear
6 points	Slightly slurred
9 points	Slurred
12 points	Unintelligible
15 points	None

The score is determined by the nurse. If in doubt, other members of the ALS team should be consulted.

Bulbar subscore (6–30 points) = Swallowing grade + speech grade

B. Respiratory subscore (6–30 points)

Vital capacity grade

6 points	Vital capacity within 80–100% of predicted value
12 points	Vital capacity within 60–79% of predicted value or incentive spirometry, medication, or chest physical therapy
18 points	Vital capacity within 40–59% of predicted value or intermittent positive pressure breathing or suctioning
24 points	Vital capacity <39% of predicted value or tracheostomy being considered
30 points	Tracheostomy

Respiratory subscore (6–30 points) = Vital capacity grade

C. Muscle strength subscore (6–36 points)

1. *Upper extremity muscle strength grade* (sum of right and left sides)

2 points	Sum of muscle strength is 70 (normal)
4 points	Sum of muscle strength is 62–69

Table 5-4.   *(continued)*

6 points	Sum of muscle strength is 54–61
8 points	Sum of muscle strength is 46–53
10 points	Sum of muscle strength is 32–45
12 points	Sum of muscle strength is 18–31
14 points	Sum of muscle strength is ≤17

2. *Lower extremity muscle strength grade* (sum of right and left sides)

2 points	Sum of muscle strength is 70 (normal)
4 points	Sum of muscle strength is 62–69
6 points	Sum of muscle strength is 54–61
8 points	Sum of muscle strength is 46–53
10 points	Sum of muscle strength is 32–45
12 points	Sum of muscle strength is 18–31
14 points	Sum of muscle strength is ≤17

3. *Handgrip grade* (sum of right and left handgrips in pounds) divided by 2

1 points	Sum divided by 2 is ≥60
2 points	Sum divided by 2 is 46–59
3 points	Sum divided by 2 is 20–45
4 points	Sum divided by 2 is <20

4. *Lateral pinch grade* (sum of right and left lateral pinch in pounds) divided by 2

1 points	Sum divided by 2 is ≥14
2 points	Sum divided by 2 is 10–13
3 points	Sum divided by 2 is 5–9
4 points	Sum divided by 2 is <5

Muscle strength   =   Upper extremity grade
subscore   + lower extremity grade
(6–36 points)   + handgrip grade
**   + lateral pinch grade**

D. Lower extremity muscle function subscore (6–35 points)

1. *Standing from chair grade* (best time)

1 points	Standing time is 0.0–1.0 sec
2 points	Standing time is 1.5–3.0 sec
3 points	Standing time is 3.5–5.0 sec
4 points	Standing time is <5.0 sec
5 points	Unable to stand

2. *Standing from lying supine grade* (best time)

1 points	Standing time is ≤2.0 sec
2 points	Standing time is 2.5–4.0 sec
3 points	Standing time is 4.5–6.0 sec

(continued)

Table 5-4.   *(continued)*

4 points	Standing time is 6.5–10.0 sec
5 points	Standing time is >10.0 sec
6 points	Unable to stand

3. *Walking 20 ft grade* (best time)

1 points	Walking time is ≤8.0 sec
2 points	Walking time is 8.5–12.0 sec
3 points	Walking time is 12.5–16.0 sec
4 points	Walking time is >16.0 sec
5 points	Unable to stand

4. *Need for assistive devices grade*

1 points	None
2 points	Ankle-foot orthosis/cane/boots
3 points	Walker, crutches, and/or occasional wheelchair (for long trips, etc.)
4 points	Wheelchair-bound or wheelchair most of the time
5 points	Bed confined

5. *Climbing and descending four standard steps grade* (best time)

1 points	Climbing time is ≤5.0 sec
2 points	Climbing time is 5.5–8.0 sec
3 points	Climbing time is 8.5–12.0 sec
4 points	Climbing time is 12.5–18.0 sec
5 points	Climbing time is >18.0 sec
6 points	Unable to climb stairs

6. *Hips and legs grade*

1 points	Walks and climbs stairs without assistance
2 points	Walks and climbs stairs with aid of railing
3 points	Cannot climb stairs but walks unassisted and rises from chairs
4 points	Cannot climb stairs but walks unassisted with either ankle-foot orthosis or cane
5 points	Cannot climb stairs but walks with minimal assistance or walks unassisted with crutches or walker
6 points	Cannot climb stairs but walks with crutches or walker with assistant or walks with total support
7 points	Is in wheelchair
8 points	Confined to bed

Lower extremity = **Standing from chair grade**
function   **+ standing from lying supine grade**
subscore   **+ walking 20-ft grade**
(6–35 points)   **+ need for assistive devices grade**
    + climbing/descending 4 standard steps grade
    + hips and legs grade

Table 5-4. *(continued)*

E. Upper extremity muscle function subscore (6–33 points)

1. *Dress and feed grade*

1 points	Independent
2 points	Independent with aids
	Button hooks, zipper pull, padded utensils, plate holder, etc., but patient does not need caretaker to assist
3 points	Minimal assist
	Patient needs caretaker to assist (cutting meat, buttons, shifting clothing, etc.)
4 points	Major assist
	Caretaker does majority of dressing and/or feeding
5 points	Dependent

The grade is based on questioning and the observed status.

2. *Propelling wheelchair 20-ft grade* (best time)

1 points	Propelling time is ≤11.0 sec
2 points	Propelling time is 11.5–20.0 sec
3 points	Propelling time is 20.5–30.0 sec
4 points	Propelling time is 30.5–40.0 sec
5 points	Propelling time is >40.0 sec
6 points	Unable to stand

One trial is performed. No assistance can be given.

3. *Arms and shoulders grade* (evaluate the most affected side)

1 points	Starting with arms at the sides, abducts the arms in a full circle until they touch above the head
2 points	Raises arms above the head only by flexing at the elbow or using accessory muscles
3 points	Cannot raise hands above the head but raises glass of water to mouth
4 points	Raises hands to mouth but cannot raise glass of water to mouth
5 points	Cannot raise hands to mouth but can use hands to hold articles
6 points	Cannot raise hands to mouth and has no useful function of hands

The most affected side is graded. If a patient can raise one arm above his/her head but cannot raise the other arm above his/her head without flexing his/her arm at the elbow, then the weaker arm determines that the grade is 2 points.

4. *Cutting Theraplast grade* (time for dominant hand)

1 points	Cutting time is ≤5.0 sec
2 points	Cutting time is 5.5–10.0 sec
3 points	Cutting time is 10.5–15.0 sec
4 points	Cutting time is 15.5–20.0 sec
5 points	Cutting time is >20.0 sec
6 points	Unable

(continued)

Table 5-4.   *(continued)*

The patient cuts a $^1/_4$-in.-thick piece of Theraplast that is set out on the board in the diameter of 4 in. Only the dominant hand is tested. The knife is positioned in the hand at the beginning of the timing.

5. *Pegboard grade* (sum of pegs constructed with right hand and left hand in 60 sec) divided by 2

1 points	Sum divided by 2 is 27–36
2 points	Sum divided by 2 is 22–26
3 points	Sum divided by 2 is 18–21
4 points	Sum divided by 2 is 1–17
5 points	Unable

The Model 32030 Purdue Pegboard is 18 in. by 11 in. with two parallel rows of 25 hoses running vertically down the center of the board. The rows are 1 in. apart, each hole is $^1/_3$ in. apart. The holes are $^1/_8$-in. diameter. At the base of the board are wells that hold the pegs that will be assembled. The fine motor test consists of forming the following construct of (1) a 1-in. pin ($^1/_8$-in. diameter), (2) a washer ($^3/_8$-in. diameter), and (3) a collar ($^1/_4$-in. long, $^3/_{16}$-in. diameter). The patient is instructed to assemble the construct as follows:

"Make as many constructs consisting of a pin, followed by a washer, followed by a collar as you can in 60 sec with one hand."

The command is followed by a demonstration for the patient, then the command is repeated. The timing begins with the patient holding his/her hand above the tray containing the 1-in. pins. There is no standard table height. Ideally, the table should be adjustable to allow the patient to easily rest his/her forearms on the table. The patient is given 60 sec to assemble as many units as he/she can and is given credit for each component added to a construct. If the patient completes 2 units of pin, washer, and collar plus 1 unit of pin and washer only, the score is $(2 \times 3) + 2 = 8$ in 60 sec.

6. *Block coordination grade* (sum of blocks turned with right hand and left hand in 60 sec) divided by 2

1 points	Sum divided by 2 is 75–95
2 points	Sum divided by 2 is 62–74
3 points	Sum divided by 2 is 43–61
4 points	Sum divided by 2 is 1–42
5 points	Unable

The block coordination grade is part of the Gonzalez Evaluation of Coordination. This part is derived from the standardized test, Minnesota Rate of Manipulation Test. It may be administered by the occupational therapist. The board is 3 ft long, with two horizontal rows of eight openings large enough to accommodate the round blocks (2.5- in. diameter and 0.75 in. wide). Each hand is tested. The patient is instructed to turn as many blocks over as he/she can in 1 min. When testing the right hand, the patient begins at the upper left-hand corner of the board and goes clockwise. When testing the left hand, the patient begins at the upper right-hand corner and goes counterclockwise.

Upper extremity = **Dress and feed grade**
function   **+ Propelling wheelchair 20-ft grade**
subscore   **+ arms and shoulders grade**
(6–33 points)   **+ cutting Theraplast grade**
                 + pegboard grade
                 + block coordination grade

Table 5-4. *(continued)*

F. Total Appel ALS score (30–164 points)

The grades for each subscore are determined. The subscores are then summed as described below to provide the total Appel ALS Scale.

$$
\begin{aligned}
\textbf{Total Appel} \quad = \quad &\textbf{Bulbar subscore} \\
\textbf{ALS Scale} \quad &+ \textbf{Respiratory subscore} \\
\textbf{(30–164 points)} \quad &+ \textbf{muscle strength subscore} \\
&+ \textbf{lower extremity function subscore} \\
&+ \textbf{upper extremity function subscore}
\end{aligned}
$$

Equipment list for Appel ALS Scale

Stopwatch	Pinch dynamometer
Theraplast	Grip dynamometer
Plastic knife	Chair
Pegboard	Stairs
Wheelchair	Standard examining table
Board with blocks	

Spirometer for vital capacity (see Table 5-5)

ALS = amyotrophic lateral sclerosis.
Adapted from *ALS—Cyclosporine Treatment Study Principal Investigators Procedure Manual* 1987.

---

patient to easily rest his or her forearms on the table. The Gonzalez Evaluation of Coordination subtest is derived from the standardized Minnesota Rate of Manipulation Test. Each hand is tested. The patient is instructed to turn as many blocks over as he or she can in 60 seconds. When testing the right hand, the patient begins at the upper left-hand corner of the board and goes clockwise. When testing the left hand, the patient begins at the upper right-hand corner and goes counterclockwise.

Administration of ACTS ALS Evaluation

The ACTS ALS Evaluation evolved from previous standardized clinimetric scales developed by Munsat and collaborators (Andres et al., 1986; Munsat et al., 1988, 1989) as well as Ringel and collaborators (1993). The ACTS ALS Evaluation separately assesses impairments and disabilities. Impairments are measured by (1) quantitative function tests; (2) quantitative strength tests; and (3) spasticity, fasciculation, atrophy, and cramp scales. Disabilities are measured by the ALS FRS, which was developed and then validated in three large multicenter clinical trials [ALS CNTF Treatment Study (ACTS) Phase I–II Study Group, 1995a, 1995b, 1996; ALS CNTF Treatment Study (ACTS) Phase II–III Study Group, 1996; Bradley et al., 1995].

The quantitative function tests include (1) speech diadochokinetic rates; (2) pulmonary function tests; (3) Purdue Pegboard tests; and (4) the 15-ft walk. Standardized normalized age- and gender-controlled data are available for all these clinical measures (Guiloff & Goonetilleke, 1994; Tourtellotte et al., 1965).

The quantitative strength tests include isometric muscle strength measurements in five upper extremity muscles including handgrip and five lower extremity muscles including ankle dorsiflexion (Sanjak et al., 1996; Tourtellotte et al., 1965).

The spasticity, fasciculation, atrophy, and cramp scales measure with ordinal scales the status of clinical features of the neurologic examination that relate to impairments specific to motor neuron diseases such as ALS [ALS CNTF Treatment Study (ACTS) Phase II–III Study Group, 1996; Ashworth 1964; Tourtellotte et al., 1965].

These procedures and methods are described in Tables 5-5 and 5-6, with explanations and descrip-

Table 5-5. Guidelines for Administration/Scoring ACTS ALS Evaluation

---

A. Quantitative function tests

1. *Speech diadochokinetic rates*

   Equipment: Sony M-330 Pressman microcassette recorder/tape/digital stopwatch

   The patient is seated and instructed to repeat the syllable "PaTa" as quickly and distinctly as possible until told to stop.

   Start the recorder. Make sure the recorder is set to normal (2.4) speed.

   State the patient's name, the date, and the trial number. Preset the timer at 5 sec. Timing begins when the subject begins speaking (after you say "start") and ends after 5 sec (when you say "stop"). The timer will beep after 5 sec has expired.

   Perform two trials. Play back the tape and count the number of PaTas in each 5-sec interval. Vary the speed as needed on playback, to slow (1.2) or fast (2.4), to determine the number of repetitions during each 5-sec interval.

2. *Pulmonary function tests*

   Equipment: PB 100 Portable Spirometer (Puritan-Bennett Renaissance Spirometry System) and PB110 Base Station/PB 130 Patient Data Memory Card/3-L Calibration Syringe/BD250 Bi-Directional Flow Sensors (Pneumo Tach)/nose clips and facemask (when indicated)/printer

   Refer to Renaissance Spirometry System operator's guide for installation and calibration of equipment. Before initial use, configure spirometer per operator's guide. Configuration will be retained in memory and should not have to be repeated until a protocol change.

   Turn on spirometer and printer; allow at least a 2-min warm-up period before use.

   Spirometer should be calibrated each day before use with the 3-L syringe provided. To calibrate, push the test button and then push button #4. Follow spirometer instructions. Repeat until error is <3%.

   Enter the new patient information data by pressing the new patient button. Follow spirometer instructions.

   Direct patient on how to perform the test. "The purpose of this test is to measure the biggest breath of air you can get in and out of your lungs on a single breath and also how fast you can get the air out of your lungs. The first thing I'll have you do is place your feet flat on the ground and sit up as straight as you can. Next, I will place this mouthpiece in your mouth, between your lips, and over your tongue (remove dentures if loose). Be sure your lips are sealed tightly around the outside of the mouthpiece—we don't want to lose any air."

   "I will close your nose with a noseclip. Hold your head up like you're playing the trumpet. When I tell you, take a deep breath in and blow all of your air out of your lungs as fast as you possibly can, like blowing the birthday candles out on your birthday cake."

   "Remember, the object of this test is to measure how much air you are able to blow out, along with how fast you can blow it out. From the very beginning, you'll want to use all the muscle groups you use to cough with, only don't cough, to try and get the air out as quickly as possible."

   "You can probably blow one continuous breath out for at least 8 seconds, but try and get most of the air out within the first second . . . like this [demonstrate]. Remember, you have to keep pushing all of the air out of your lungs, even though you can't feel it coming out. You can only feel about the first 80% coming out of your lungs, and I'll keep coaching you to keep on pushing and squeezing with your chest and stomach muscles to get the last 15–20% out." Perform the test at least three good times but not more than eight trials.

   Print out the report as per manual instruction.

3. *Purdue pegboard*

   Equipment: Purdue Pegboard/digital stopwatch

Table 5-5. *(continued)*

The pegboard is placed directly in front of the patient, 4 in. from the table's front edge, with at least 20 pegs in the exterior cup above the appropriate column. The pegboard may be moved closer or farther from the patient but may not be moved or aligned diagonally.

The patient is instructed to pick up one peg at a time from the cup and place it in order in the right hole column closest to the cup and tested side as quickly as possible. If the patient picks up two pegs, he/she must drop one of the pegs. When a peg is dropped intentionally or accidentally, the patient should not pick it up, but go on with another peg as quickly as possible.

Preset the timer at 30 sec. Say "Ready . . . start." Timing begins when the patient touches the first peg and ends when 30 sec has expired. The timer will beep. The number of pegs placed in the holes is recorded.

Perform the test on the right hand twice and then the left hand twice. The left column of holes and cup is used for the left hand. Record the number of pegs on the test report form provided.

4. *Fifteen-foot walk*

(This test should be performed only if the patient normally performs these tasks unassisted at home.)

Equipment: Measuring tape (15 ft minimum)/digital stopwatch

Fifteen feet of walking distance should be marked in the room or hallway using two clearly visible tapes or other marking device. This is the start and finish distance. Two tapes similar in color and length are placed 3 ft exterior to the 15 ft of tape. These are the target finish lines.

Instruct the patient to stand with feet touching the start line (the interior line) and to "walk as fast as you safely can to the target line" (but caution to not run or walk so fast as to risk falling). Clinical evaluator should walk slightly behind patient for safety.

Timing is started when the patient starts to move (not when you say to start) and ends as both feet cross the finish line.

Record the complete time to one decimal place (tenths of second) on scoring sheet.

B. Quantitative strength tests

1. *Isometric muscle strength testing*

Equipment: Standard examination table (180 cm long, 60 cm wide, 7.5 cm high)

Electronic strain gauge tensiometer (Interface and Advance Force Measurement, Scottsdale, AZ)/aluminum upright and adjustable rings/nylon straps

Macintosh Base Computerized Data Acquisition System and printer

MacAdios II Jr. (Data acquisition A/D Board, GW Instruments)

MacAdios ABD Analog Breakout System (GW Instruments)

SuperScope for data acquisition

Excel for data management and final reports production

Maximal voluntary isometric force is measured with an electronic strain gauge connected to a Macintosh Data Acquisition System. The patient is tested in the supine position for the upper extremities and ankle dorsiflexors, sitting upright at the end of the table for lower extremities (knee extensor testing), and semireclined with a wedge for lower extremities (hip flexor testing).

After attaching the strap to the joint being measured, the patient is encouraged to "push" or "pull" against the strap as hard as he/she can "with all your strength." Contraction should be held for 3–4 sec to ensure maximal effort is reached. Encouragement needs to be consistent with all patients. A minimum of 3 sec should elapse between trials. Patients should not stabilize themselves by holding onto the table. The clinical examiner should be alert for any signs of respiratory distress when the patient is in the supine position.

(continued)

Table 5-5. *(continued)*

To eliminate errors, the order of testing is always as follows:

1. Left shoulder extension	7. Left knee extension
2. Left elbow flexion	8. Right knee extension
3. Right shoulder extension	9. Right hip flexion
4. Right elbow flexion	10. Left hip flexion
5. Right ankle dorsiflexion	11. Right handgrip
6. Left ankle dorsiflexion	12. Left handgrip

2. *Specific muscle testing directions*

Shoulder extension

Patient is supine with shoulder at 90 degrees of flexion, neutral rotation. Strap is placed just proximal to the elbow. Examiner supports the arm before the test (no tension on the strap). Stabilization is superior on the shoulder so that the shoulder does not elevate during the test and the patient does not slide upward.

Elbow flexion

Patient remains supine with arm resting on table. Elbow is positioned at 90 degrees, forearm in neutral rotation. The strap is placed just proximal to the styloid process. Examiner secures the elbow from an inferior position and holds the shoulder from protracting as well.

Foot dorsiflexion

Patient is supine, with hips and knees extended and ankle in slight plantarflexion. Strap placed across metatarsals. Heels are over the edge of the table. A towel roll is placed under the ankle. Patient attempts maximal dorsiflexion without pelvis elevation. Stabilization is downward over the proximal tibia. The ankle should be in slight plantarflexion initially so that with contraction it is a neutral ankle position (90 degrees). If the patient is unable to maintain a neutral ankle position (90 degrees) but is in some plantarflexion at the initiation of the trial, the clinical evaluator may "pinch" the strap manually around the patient's foot to prevent the strap from sliding off the foot.

Knee extension

Patient is seated over the end of the table with knees at 90 degrees. Strap is placed just proximal to the malleoli. Femur is parallel to the table. Examiner provides stabilization by exerting downward force over the ipsilateral shoulder and contralateral hip or by exerting downward force over both shoulders if sitting behind the patient to prevent the hips from rising up off the table.

Hip flexion

Patient is semireclined with head and shoulders supported by a wedge. A towel roll for increasing tension may be used and is placed under test leg, which is at approximately 20 degrees of flexion at the hip. Knee is at 90 degrees of flexion. Strap is placed proximal to the knee joint. Strap not over patella or patient won't pull hard. The untested leg is supported by the tester with the hip and knee at 90 degrees of flexion to maintain pelvis in a posterior tilt. Patient attempts maximal hip flexion. Tension on the strain gauge should be enough at rest so that force is measured without actual elevation of the leg.

Handgrip

Handgrip is measured manually with an adjustable handgrip dynamometer. The seated patient is positioned with wrist resting on lap and elbow flexed at approximately 110 degrees. The handle of the dynamometer should be adjusted to position 3. Place the dynamometer in the tested hand with dial facing toward the evaluator. Examiner supports the dynamometer from the side and should not pull on it. The wrist should not be supported. The patient is instructed to squeeze with his/her tested hand as hard as possible. Grip tests are performed twice on the right hand and then twice on the left hand with dynamometer always set at 3. Measurements will be recorded in kilograms. Record score on test report form.

Table 5-5. *(continued)*

Equipment list for ACTS ALS evaluation

PB100 Portable Spirometer (Renaissance Spirometry System)	Puritan-Bennett Corporation
PB110 Base Station	
PB130 Patient Data Memory Card	
3-L Calibration Syringe	
Digital thermometer	
BD250 Disposable Bi-Directional Flow Sensors	
Facemasks	
Digital stopwatch with countdown timer capable of measuring to tenths of seconds	RadioShack
Purdue Pegboard	Lafayette Instrument Company Box 5729 Lafayette, IN 47903 (317) 423-1505
18-in. high chair with arms	
28-in. high desk or table	
Jamar Adjustable Hydraulic Hand Dynamometer (Model 2A)	Lafayette Instrument Company Box 5279 Lafayette, IN 47903 (317) 423-1505
Sony M-330 Pressman Microcassette Recorder and Tape	
Isometric strength testing table	
Standard treatment table	
Zimmer orthopedic bars and accessories	
18-in. single clamp bar	
27-in. plain bar	
66-in. swivel clamp bar	
85-in. plain bar	
96-in. plain bar (heavy duty)	
Cross clamp	
Trapeze clamp with D ring and S hook	
Connecting cables, straps	
S hooks	
Calibration weights (25 kg)	
SM-250 Super Mini Load Cell	Interface Corporation
20-ft cable	Scottsdale, AZ
Modular plug	(800) 947-5598
Two 28-thread eyebolts	
Macintosh Data Acquisition System Macintosh Ilsi, 9 MB RAM, 80 MB hard drive, Nubus card, Monochrome monitor/Microsoft Excel software	
MacAdios Analog to Digital System	GW Instruments
MacAdios II Jr.	35 Medford Street
12 mcs data acquisition board	Somerville, MA 02143 (617) 625-4096

(continued)

Table 5-5. *(continued)*

MacAdios ABO (analog breakout system)
    modified to accommodate a modular jack
      34-wire cable (10 ft)
      SuperScope Software, version 1.6.3

Printer

C. Spasticity, fasciculation, atrophy, and cramp scales

   1. *Spasticity scale:* Spasticity is assessed in the upper and lower extremities when the patients are seated. The grading is modified to be opposite to that previously reported (Ashworth, 1964).

Grading of spasticity

Modified Grade	Rating	Ashworth Grade
4	Normal	0
3	Slight catch; passive movement of limb, otherwise unimpeded	1
2	Definite resistance to passive movement	2
1	Increased tone sufficient to require effort on part of examiner to overcome resistance	3
0	Passive movement of joint impossible	4

Upper extremities: Spasticity is assessed by passive range of motion on pronation and supination of the forearm and flexion and extension of the forearm at the elbow. Pronation and supination, flexion, and extension should be performed at less than one movement per second and then increased to a higher rate above 5 per sec.

On the initial acceleration of the rate of movement above three cycles per second, if a single catch is felt with no passive movement of the limb impeded, then this is rated as a 3.

When the passive movement is restricted such that one or more catches are felt or the rate of movement cannot be increased as easily as in a limb without spasticity, then the limb is graded as 2.

In the forearm, rapid-alternating movements occurring at rates below 3.0 Hz (not explained by muscular atrophy) are usually associated with grade 2 spasticity. Occasionally, there may be limitation of full supination in patients with grade 2 spasticity, but this is usually limited to <160 degrees of supination.

If passive range of motion at less than one cycle per second is inhibited and increasing the rate of supination-pronation or flexion-extension at the elbow limits the full range of motion of the muscle group being tested, then give a rating of 1. Spasticity in the upper extremities associated with a rating of 1 usually is associated with a limitation of rapid alternating movements to supination at an angle between 120 and 160 degrees.

If passive range of motion of the arm during supination-pronation or flexion-extension is limited at one cycle per second, then give a grade of 0.

Lower extremities: The limb is elevated and supported by the hand under the knee, and the leg is moved in flexion-extension movement about the knee at less than one cycle per second. The movement is then accelerated to determine whether there is any spastic catch. Spastic catches may be noted particularly in the quadriceps muscle group but occasionally can be felt in the hamstring muscle group.

Table 5-5.   *(continued)*

When the acceleration is above 3 Hz, if one single catch is felt, then this is given a grade of 3.

If the acceleration of the limb is above 3 cycles per second and one feels one or more catches where there is resistance to movement through the entire range of movement, then this is given a grade of 2.

If, with acceleration of flexion-extension of the leg at the knee, more than three catches or continuous resistance is felt but the leg can still be moved, then this is given the score of 1.

If on passive movement at less than one cycle per second there is minimal movement, or if on acceleration full movement cannot be completed, then a score of 0 is given.

Flexion and extension of the foot at the ankle may also be used to assess spasticity. If there is one spastic catch on accelerating the dorsiflexion-plantar flexion movement of the foot to greater than three cycles per second, then a rating of 3 is given to that limb.

If on accelerating the rate of flexion-extension of the ankle on dorsiflexion there is more than one catch or increased resistance of forced dorsiflexion, then this is rated as 2.

If on accelerating the passive range of motion to above three cycles per second there is continuous resistance of movement, then this is given a rating of 1.

If the forced dorsiflexion creates clonus, then the rating is given as 0.

In the lower extremity, contractures are much more common in the hamstrings and the posterior leg compartment muscles. This may limit passive range of motion. The distinction between spasticity and contracture is determined by the lack of full range of motion at low-frequency passive range of motion.

2. *Fasciculation scale:* Fasciculations should be evaluated by both inspection and palpation.

Grading of fasciculations

Grade	Rating	Explanation
4	Absent	—
3	Rare	Felt only once during examination or reported by patient
2	Evident on inspection	Consistently seen after exercise
1	Obvious	Consistently seen before exercise
0	Continuous	—

The patient should be graded as no fasciculations if there is no report of fasciculations and there are no fasciculations observed on examination.

Continuous fasciculations are present regardless of activity and are graded 0. The rate of fasciculation is unimportant; whether they completely go away is the crucial determinant.

Bulbar muscles: The tongue should be observed in repose and on protrusion.

If fasciculations occur after protrusion when the tongue is at rest, fasciculations should be graded as 2 (evident on inspection).

Fasciculations noted at rest without protrusion of the tongue are graded as 1 (obvious).

Submentalis fasciculations are graded as 2 (evident on inspection after contraction) if they occur after facial testing with grimacing or blowing out the cheeks.

(continued)

Table 5-5.   *(continued)*

Submentalis fasciculations should be graded as 1 (obvious) if they occur spontaneously without exercise-induced production of fasciculation.

Arm and hand muscles:

If active or passive range of motion–induced fasciculations are palpated or observed, this is a 2 (evident on inspection after contraction).

If the fasciculations are present without active or passive range of motion of the arm, this is graded as 1 (obvious).

Trunk muscles: The trunk, shoulder, chest, abdomen, and rhomboids should be observed or palpated for fasciculations.

In the trunk region, rare fasciculations are those reported by the patient that may or may not be felt or observed once during the examination.

If only one fasciculation is noted, it should be graded as 3.

Leg and foot muscles: Fasciculation should be observed or palpated in the quadriceps, hamstrings, and posterior calf muscles and anterior compartment muscles.

Fasciculations are noted as 1 (obvious) if they are observed or palpated on examination before active or passive range of motion of the muscle.

Fasciculations are noted as 2 (evident on inspection) if they are present only after active or passive range of motion of the muscle.

3. *Atrophy scale:* Atrophy should be evaluated by both inspection and palpation.

Grading of atrophy

Grade	Rating	Explanation
4	None	—
3	Mild	Loss of normal muscle contour
2	Moderate	Shallowing of muscle belly in anatomical compartment
1	Severe but without complete loss of muscle bulk	Bony limits of muscle in anatomical compartment easily palpated
0	Complete loss of muscle bulk	No muscle palpated

Bulbar muscles: Atrophy is graded in the muscles innervated by the hypoglossal and facial cranial motor nerves.

Tongue atrophy is graded mild as 3 if there is only lateral furrowing.

Tongue atrophy is graded moderate as 2 if there is lateral furrowing and dimpling throughout the muscle mass.

Tongue atrophy is graded severe as 1 if there is extreme deepening of the central ridge and lateral furrowing.

Tongue atrophy is graded severe as 0 if there is marked dimpling and lateral furrowing with loss of bulk evident on attempted protrusion.

Tongue muscle bulk is graded as complete loss of muscle bulk when there is very little muscle mass usually smaller than the thumb of the patient with lateral furrowing, dimpling, and, in a late stage, even loss of fasciculation.

Facial atrophy is graded mild as 3 when the orbicularis oris cannot purse with lip protrusion.

Table 5-5.   *(continued)*

Facial atrophy is graded moderate as 2 when there is loss of muscle mass such that zygomatic dysfunction is lost with no elevation of the corners of the mouth, and the smile is not made as a flat smile over the entire breadth of the face but is only an oval smile.

Facial atrophy is graded severe as 1 when there is decreased elevation of the forehead, poor closure of the eyes, or incomplete closure of the eyes with poor burying of the eyelashes and loss of facial expression.

Facial atrophy is graded complete as 0 when muscle bulk is such that the lips cannot approximate and no facial expression is possible.

Arm and hand muscles:

Arm atrophy is noted as mild when the biceps or first dorsal interosseus has lost its normal contour.

Arm atrophy is noted as moderate when there is flattening of either of these muscles.

Arm atrophy is noted as severe when there is severe hollowing of the first dorsal interossei and the interosseus muscle or loss of the normal curvature of the biceps muscle.

Triceps muscle should not be assessed for atrophy. Forearm muscles may be assessed if the biceps and first dorsal interosseus cannot be assessed.

Trunk muscles:

Trunk atrophy is graded as mild when there is some decrease in the deltoid bulk bilaterally.

Trunk atrophy is graded as moderate when deltoid bulk is lost anteriorly but present laterally.

Trunk atrophy is graded as severe when there is easy palpation of the shoulder joint.

Trunk atrophy is graded as 0 with complete loss of muscle bulk when the shoulders are ptotic and the shoulder joint is visually apparent.

Spine extensor atrophy is graded as mild when muscle bulk is asymmetrically lost in a focal manner.

Spine extensor atrophy is graded as moderate when extensor muscles of the back are lost to palpation.

Spine extensor atrophy is graded as severe when there is marked bony prominence.

Spine extensor atrophy is graded as 0 when there is complete loss of muscle bulk, associated with extreme extensor weakness of the back.

Leg and foot muscles:

Lower extremity atrophy is graded as mild if there is flattening of the anterior compartment muscles.

Lower extremity atrophy is graded as moderate if there is shallowing of the anterior compartment muscles.

Lower extremity atrophy is graded as severe if there is easily apparent bony ridging of the anterior compartment.

Lower extremity atrophy is graded as 0 when there is complete loss of muscle bulk and is usually associated with complete footdrop and easy palpation of the ridge of the tibia with no apparent muscle (saber shins).

Posterior compartment muscles are most difficult to evaluate from the point of view of atrophy but may be affected. Mild atrophy is loss of the medial head of the gastrocnemius, moderate atrophy is decreased bulk in both heads, and severe atrophy is flattening of the posterior compartment muscle.

It is rare to see complete loss of posterior compartment muscle bulk.

4. *Cramp scale:* The patient should be asked if he/she has any cramps described as pain with contraction or tightness of muscle group either occurring spontaneously or brought on by exercise, which cause the patient to want to lengthen the muscle to relieve the pain or contraction.

(continued)

Table 5-5. *(continued)*

Patients sometimes confuse spasms due to spasticity with cramps and that has to be sorted out by history and topography. Patients may have cramps when they are stretching their legs at night or when they are getting up. They may have spasms, however, shortly after going to bed with extensor or flexor spasms. These spasms may or may not be painful. The cramps usually are painful. There is a diurnal variation in cramping with cramping being primarily in the supine position in some patients at night. Tongue cramps are very unusual in amyotrophic lateral sclerosis.

Grading of cramps

Grade	Rating	Explanation
4	None	—
3	Rare cramps, related to voluntary muscle activity	Induced by stretching or brisk stiff contractions or less than one cramp/week
2	Spontaneous cramps one to seven times weekly	Occur with or without movement but strong contractions not required to cause cramp
1	More than one cramp per day, or seven per week	Occur with or without movement but strong contractions not required to cause cramp
0	Activity interrupted by severe cramps on multiple occasions daily	—

Bulbar and neck muscles: The patient may describe that his/her tongue gets stuck, but it is not truly a cramp.

Neck cramps may be common particularly on extension but occasionally on flexion or rotation. These are usually induced by activity.

If they occur with every activity, they are graded as 0 (activity interrupted by severe cramps on multiple occasions daily). Most patients, however, have these cramps with some maneuvers and not with others. Temporal mandibular joint dislocation with or without forced yawning is not a cramp.

Arm and hand muscles: Upper extremity cramps are more common in the fingers of the hand and the forearm. Flexor cramps are much more common than extensor cramps. Biceps cramps occur commonly on lifting; triceps cramps are extremely rare.

Trunk muscles: Back or flank cramps are occasionally present on extension when yawning. The patient occasionally has abdominal cramps on sneezing or coughing. Chest wall cramps are unusual.

Leg and foot muscles: In the lower extremity, foot cramps are common at night when small intrinsic muscles of the foot contract with curling of the toes. There are also posterior compartment cramps that involve extension of the leg. It is rare to have anterior compartment cramps except on repetitive activity.

Anterior thigh compartment cramps are much less common than posterior compartment cramps, but they may occur. The grading of cramps is done by history and rarely by examination. A patient will usually report that there are no cramps, but sometimes further questioning is required to ascertain specifically in anatomical areas where there may be cramping when there is activity that the patient does not interpret as cramps.

Cramps may be rare, less than one per week, and occur only on voluntary muscle activity. These are rated as 3.

Spontaneous cramps that occur without voluntary activity are rated as 2. Sometimes it is difficult to sort out whether voluntary activity activates cramps. If the cramping is very frequent (one to seven times weekly), and it is unclear whether it is voluntary muscle activity–induced cramping or spontaneous cramping, rate it as a 2 nevertheless.

If there is more than one cramp per day or more than seven cramps per week due to voluntary or spontaneous activity about specific muscle groups, grade these cramps as 1.

Adapted from *ACTS Group Principal Investigator and Procedure Manuals* 1993.

Table 5-6. Guidelines for Administration/Scoring Amyotrophic Lateral Sclerosis Functional Rating Scale (ALS FRS)

Item	Description	Grade
1.	Speech	
	Normal speech processes	4
	Detectable speech disturbance	3
	Intelligible with repeating	2
	Speech combined with nonvocal communication	1
	Loss of useful speech	0
2.	Salivation	
	Normal	4
	Slight but definite excess of saliva in mouth; may have nighttime drooling	3
	Moderately excessive saliva; may have minimal drooling	2
	Marked excess of saliva with some drooling	1
	Marked drooling; requires constant tissue or handkerchief	0
3.	Swallowing	
	Normal eating habits	4
	Early eating problems—occasional choking	3
	Dietary consistency changes	2
	Needs supplemental tube feeding	1
	Nothing by mouth (exclusively parenteral or enteral feeding)	0
4.	Handwriting (with dominant hand before ALS onset)	
	Normal	4
	Slow or sloppy; all words legible	3
	Not all words are legible	2
	Able to grip pen but unable to write	1
	Unable to grip pen	0
5a.	Cutting food and handling utensils (patients without gastrostomy)	
	Normal	4
	Somewhat slow and clumsy but no help needed	3
	Can cut most foods, although clumsy and slow; some help needed	2
	Food must be cut by someone but can still feed slowly	1
	Needs to be fed	0
5b.	Cutting food and handling utensils (patients with gastrostomy)	
	Normal	4
	Clumsy but able to perform all manipulations independently	3
	Some help needed with closures and fasteners	2
	Provides minimal assistance to caregiver	1
	Unable to perform any aspect of task	0

(continued)

Table 5-6. *(continued)*

Item	Description	Grade
6.	Dressing and hygiene	
	Normal function	4
	Independent and complete self-care with effort or decreased efficiency	3
	Intermittent assistance or substitute methods	2
	Needs attendant for self-care	1
	Total dependence	0
7.	Turning in bed and adjusting bed clothes	
	Normal	4
	Somewhat slow and clumsy but no help needed	3
	Can turn alone or adjust sheets but with great difficulty	2
	Can initiate but not turn or adjust sheets alone	1
	Helpless	0
8.	Walking	
	Normal	4
	Early ambulation difficulties	3
	Walks with assistance (any assistive device including ankle-foot orthoses)	2
	Nonambulatory functional movement only	1
	No purposeful leg movement	0
9.	Climbing stairs	
	Normal	4
	Slow	3
	Mild unsteadiness or fatigue	2
	Needs assistance (including handrail)	1
	Cannot do	0
10.	Breathing	
	Normal	4
	Shortness of breath with minimal exertion (e.g., walking, talking)	3
	Shortness of breath at rest	2
	Intermittent (e.g., nocturnal) ventilatory assistance	1
	Ventilator dependent	0

Adapted from *ACTS Group Principal Investigator and Procedure Manuals* 1993.

tions of equipment as necessary. All clinical evaluators should adhere to these procedures so that measurement errors are minimized. It is important to remember throughout this study that there are always three sources of error that affect measurements: (1) observer error (minimized by understanding what is being measured and being consistent in measurements); (2) patient error (minimized by explaining what is expected from them at the beginning of each test session); and (3) instrument error (minimized by regular calibration) (Hulley & Cummings, 2001).

Administration of Amyotrophic Lateral Sclerosis Functional Rating Scale

The ALS FRS (Figure 5-3) may be administered by the physician, nurse coordinator, physical therapist, or a trained assistant to assess the patient's present ability to perform activities of daily living and functional improvement or decline at interval visits. The evaluator shall state to the patient (or spouse or other caregiver if the patient cannot communicate effectively):

"I now have a few questions I would like to ask you to help me better understand how you (or the patient) are functioning at home."

"Please answer each question to the best of your ability."

The evaluator then asks, "How are you doing at (...)?"

Record the patient's response, to the closest approximation available from the appropriate five-point (0–4) list. If the patient is unable to volunteer a satisfactory response, the evaluator may prompt, using one of the available choices (e.g., asking "Do you find that people are having trouble understanding your speech?"). Record the response on the case response form provided. Patients who become more independent because of the use of an assistive device, such as a wheelchair, walker, or elevator, cannot improve in their rating scores. The following examples elaborate on the scoring of patients who require assistance or assistive devices for ambulation: (1) walking score as "walks with assistance" or worse; (2) climbing stairs score as "needs assistance" or worse (requiring use of handrail equates to "needs assistance").

Comparison of Amyotrophic Lateral Sclerosis Clinimetric Scales

The clinical usefulness and robustness of clinimetric scales for ALS depend on their accuracy, sensitivity, reproducibility, and validity (Hulley & Cummings, 2001). The clinimetric scales described in this chapter vary in their accuracy, sensitivity, reproducibility, and validity. Moreover, practical issues are important in the choice of particular clinimetric scales. The Norris scale has historical precedence. The Appel scale has been used in fewer clinical trials, but it is the only clinimetric scale to date that has been instrumental in demonstrating a potential treatment effect of a neurotrophic factor in ALS (Lai et al., 1996; Lange et al., 1996). The ACTS ALS Evaluation consists of quantitative functional tests; quantitative strength tests; and associated spasticity, fasciculation, atrophy, and cramp ordinal scales that measure impairment. These measures of impairment are kept separate from measures of disability, evaluated by the ALS FRS, which has been validated by other standard techniques. The ALS FRS is a simple, accurate, sensitive, reproducible measure of disability resulting from ALS-related impairments that is validated and may be used easily in the primary physician's office, the consulting neurologist's office, the ALS multidisciplinary clinic, or clinical trials.

The Norris ALS Scale has been used in many studies from 1974 through 1993. Its properties have been well described (Brooks, 1994). It has many difficulties, including the mixing of impairments and disabilities in the same scale (Feinstein, 1987; Louwerse et al., 1990). The total Norris ALS score for the individual patient may have a variable course over time, but it generally shows stability or a linear decline. Similar behavior is noted for the Norris ALS score for groups of patients (Figure 5-4).

The Appel ALS Scale has been used in fewer studies from 1984 to the present. Its properties are less well described (Brooks et al., 1991; Haverkamp et al., 1995; Lai et al., 1996). To understand the properties of this scale, we have provided a summary of the changes in Appel subscores over time in 18 ALS patients who also had isometric muscle strength testing with the ACTS ALS Evaluation. We used time-to-failure analysis to permit comparison among the different subscores (Figure 5-5). It is clear that muscle strength testing, lower extremity muscle function, and upper extremity muscle function change more

ALS Functional Rating Scale

1). SPEECH
4 Normal speech processes.
3 Detectable speech disturbance.
2 Intelligible with repeating.
1 Speech combined with nonvocal communication.
0 Loss of useful speech.

2). SALIVATION
4 Normal.
3 Slight but definite excess of saliva in mouth; may have nighttime drooling.
2 Moderately excessive saliva; may have minimal drooling.
1 Marked excess of saliva with some drooling.
0 Marked drooling; requires constant use of tissue or handkerchief.

3). SWALLOWING
4 Normal eating habits.
3 Early eating problems — Occasional choking.
2 Dietary consistency changes.
1 Needs supplemental tube feeding.
0 NPO (exclusively parenteral or enteral feeding).

4). HANDWRITING
4 Normal.
3 Slow or sloppy; all words are legible.
2 Not all words are legible.
1 Able to grip pen but unable to write.
0 Unable to grip pen.

5a). CUTTING FOOD & HANDLING UTENSILS (w/o gastrostomy)
4 Normal.
3 Somewhat slow and clumsy, but no help needed.
2 Can cut most foods, although clumsy and slow; no help needed.
1 Food must be cut by someone, but can still feed self slowly.
0 Needs to be fed.

5b). CUTTING FOOD & HANDLING UTENSILS (with gastrostomy)
4 Normal.
3 Clumsy but able to perform all manipulations independently.
2 Some help needed with closures and fasteners.
1 Provides minimal assistance to caregiver.
0 Unable to perform any aspect of task.

6). DRESSING & HYGIENE
4 Normal function.
3 Independent and complete self-care with effort or decreased efficiency.
2 Intermittent assistance or substitute methods.
1 Needs attendant for self-care.
0 Total dependence.

7). TURNING IN BED & ADJUSTING BED CLOTHES
4 Normal.
3 Somewhat slow and clumsy, but no help needed.
2 Can turn alone or adjust sheets, but with great difficulty.
1 Can initiate, but not turn or adjust sheets alone.
0 Helpless.

8). WALKING
4 Normal.
3 Early ambulation difficulties.
2 Walks with assistance (any assistive device including ankle foot orthosis).
1 Nonambulatory functional movement only.
0 No purposeful leg movement.

9). CLIMBING STAIRS
4 Normal.
3 Slow.
2 Mild unsteadiness or fatigue.
1 Needs assistance (including handrail).
0 Cannot do.

10). BREATHING
4 Normal.
3 Shortness of breath with minimal exertion (e.g., walking, talking).
2 Shortness of breath at rest.
1 Intermittent (e.g., nocturnal) ventilator dependence.
0 Ventilator dependent.

☐ **Speech**

☐ **Salivation**

☐ **Swallowing**

☐ **Handwriting**

☐ **Cutting Food & Handling Utensils** *Gastrostomy* ☐

☐ **Dressing & Hygiene**

☐ **Turning in Bed & Adjusting Bed Clothes**

☐ **Walking**

☐ **Climbing Stairs**

☐ **Breathing**

Total Score ☐

Figure 5-3. Amyotrophic Lateral Sclerosis (ALS) Functional Rating Scale form.

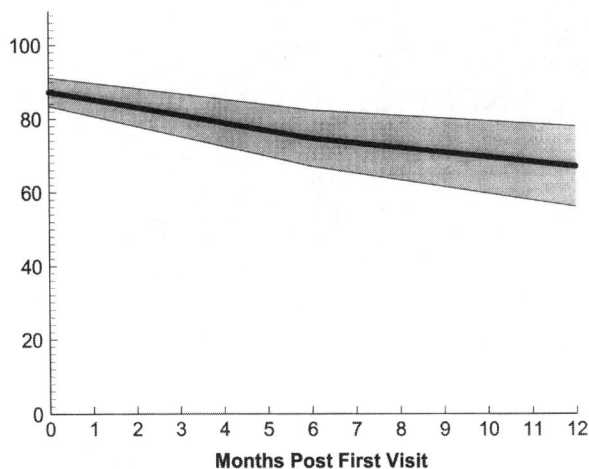

Figure 5-4. Norris Amyotrophic Lateral Sclerosis (ALS) Scale changes over 12 months. Mean ± 95% confidence limits of total Norris ALS Scale score in 18 ALS patients.

dramatically over time than the bulbar function or respiratory function subscores. It is clear, however, that isometric strength testing is much more sensitive than manual muscle testing that is used in the Appel ALS Scale (Figure 5-6). The functional scores for this group of ALS patients followed for up to 12 months demonstrate changes in upper extremity function by 3 months of follow-up compared with delayed changes in lower extremity function after 6 months of follow-up (Figure 5-7). These properties of the subscores of the Appel scale are instrumental in allowing the scale to demonstrate clinically significant changes that may occur in the active treatment arms of the clinical trial. More important, however, is the fact that the Appel ALS Scale still mixes impairments and disabilities in attempting to define a single score for the ALS patient. This problem makes interpretation of Appel scale score changes difficult. In the individual patient, the Appel ALS Scale provides sufficient follow-up information that is useful for clinical management. Its use in clinical trials has been demonstrated, but the interpretation of clinically significant improvement or stabilization is fraught by the difficulty in mixing impairments and disabilities.

The ACTS ALS Evaluation is based on Airlie House guidelines, prepared by the Subcommittee on Motor Neuron Diseases of the World Federation of Neurology Research Group on Neuromuscular Diseases (Subcommittee on Motor Neuron Diseases,

1995). It is divided into quantitative function tests, quantitative strength tests and ordinal scales of impairments, and a clinimetric disability scale [ALS CNTF Treatment Study (ACTS) Phase I–II Study Group, 1995a, 1995b, 1996]. The impairments measured by quantitative functional tests are specifically related to disability measured by the ALS FRS (Figure 5-8). In addition, the impairments measured by quantitative strength tests are specifically related to disability measured by the ALS FRS (Figure 5-9). The change over time in the isometric strength of specific muscles in ALS patients is a function of the anatomic location of the muscles tested (Figure 5-10). Proximal muscles are stronger overall as a percent of the normal predicted value for each patient. Distal muscles are weaker. These individual differences among muscles make it difficult to form a composite score of muscle strength because some muscles are further along in the disease process than others. Isometric strength measurements are crucial in the individual patient to identify significant changes in clinical strength not measurable by manual muscle testing (see Figure 5-6). This change over time is instrumental in providing information of progression required to increase the certainty of the diagnosis of ALS according to the El Escorial criteria (Subcommittee on Motor Neuron Diseases/Amyotrophic Lateral Sclerosis, 1994). Early diagnosis is enhanced by the use of isometric muscle strength changes over time in addition to other neurodiagnostic techniques. Isometric strength measurements are also important in determining treatment effects in short-term studies where survival or other clinimetric scales do not show changes during the shorter time period [ALS CNTF Treatment Study (ACTS) Phase II–III Study Group, 1996; Bradley et al., 1995; Miller et al., 1996a, 1996b).

The ALS FRS is a measure of disability in ALS patients. It has been validated against other quantitative measures of function and strength changes resulting from impairments caused by ALS. It is a sensitive, accurate, and reproducible measure of the clinical course of ALS. Its properties have been described in some detail (Brooks, 1996; Brooks et al., 1994). In this chapter, the authors present the course of disability due to ALS measured by ALS FRS subscores in a large group of ALS patients described in two different ways. The average score over time is contrasted with the probability of maintaining a specific ALS FRS subscore over time (Figure 5-11). In this manner, different disabil-

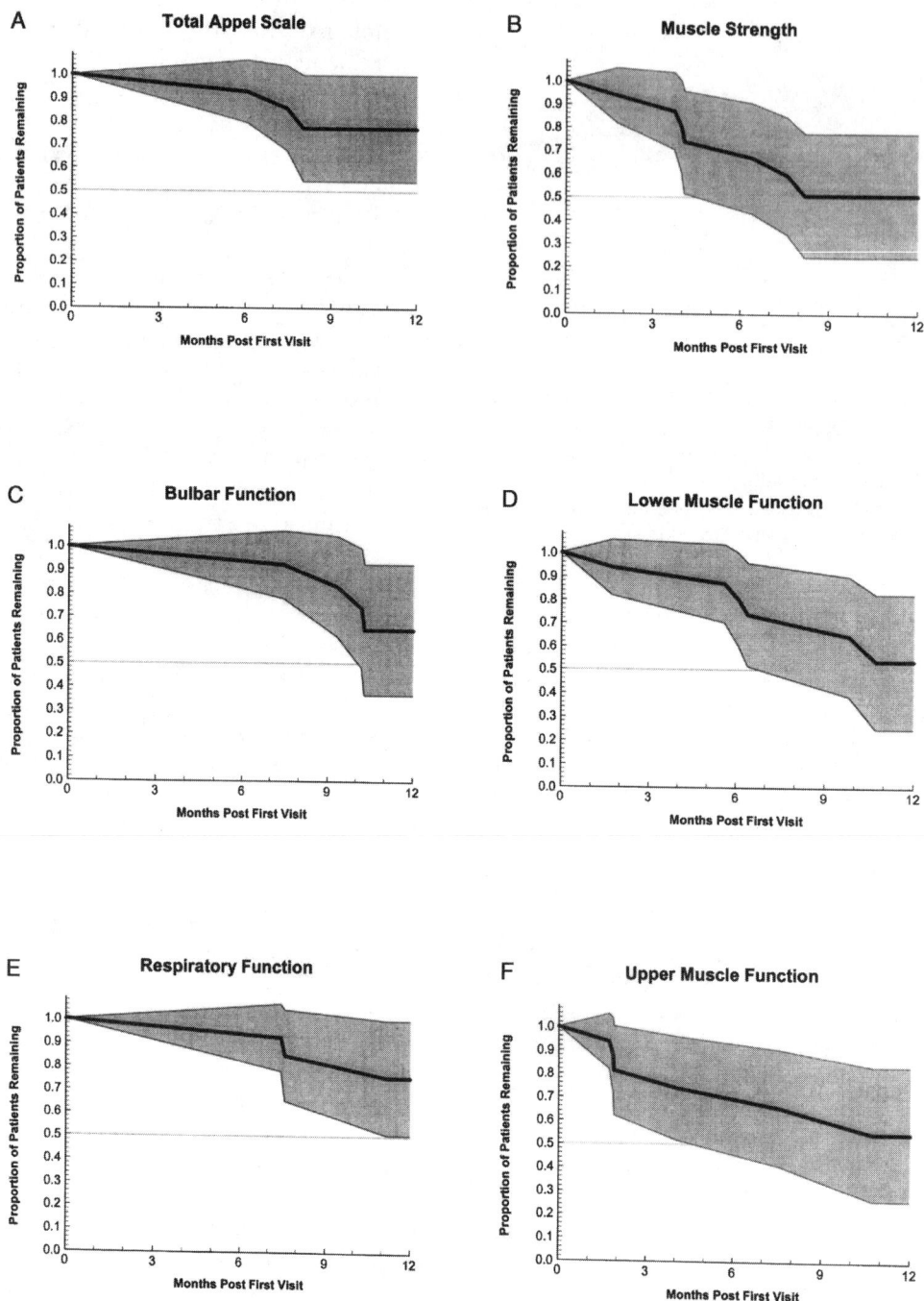

Figure 5-5. Time to failure for total Appel Amyotrophic Lateral Sclerosis (ALS) Scale score and subscores over 12 months. **A.** Proportion ± 95% confidence limits of 18 ALS patients maintaining total Appel ALS Scale score <103 points. **B.** Proportion ± 95% confidence limits of 18 ALS patients maintaining muscle strength Appel ALS Scale subscore <22 points. **C.** Proportion ± 95% confidence limits of 18 ALS patients maintaining bulbar Appel ALS Scale subscore <17 points. **D.** Proportion ± 95% confidence limits of 18 ALS patients maintaining lower extremity function Appel ALS Scale subscore <21 points. **E.** Proportion ± 95% confidence limits of 18 ALS patients maintaining respiratory Appel ALS Scale subscore <24 points. **F.** Proportion ± 95% confidence limits of 18 ALS patients maintaining upper extremity function Appel ALS Scale subscore <19 points.

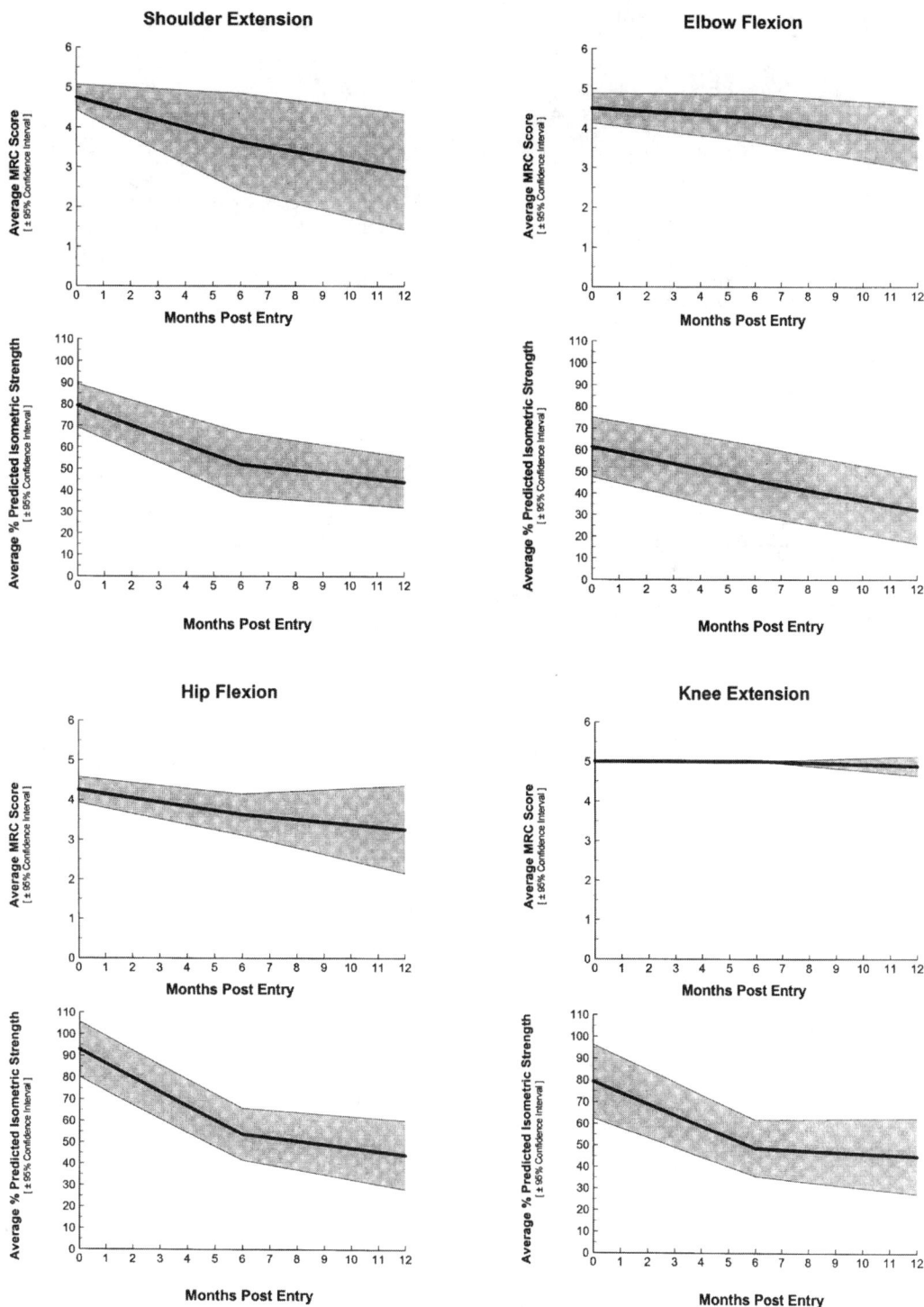

Figure 5-6. Comparison of change in Medical Research Council (MRC) score with change in isometric strength in amyotrophic lateral sclerosis patients. The average MRC score ± 95% confidence limits was compared over 12 months with the average percent predicted isometric muscle strength ± 95% confidence limits for the following right and left muscle groups of 18 amyotrophic lateral sclerosis patients: shoulder extension, elbow flexion, hip flexion, and knee extension.

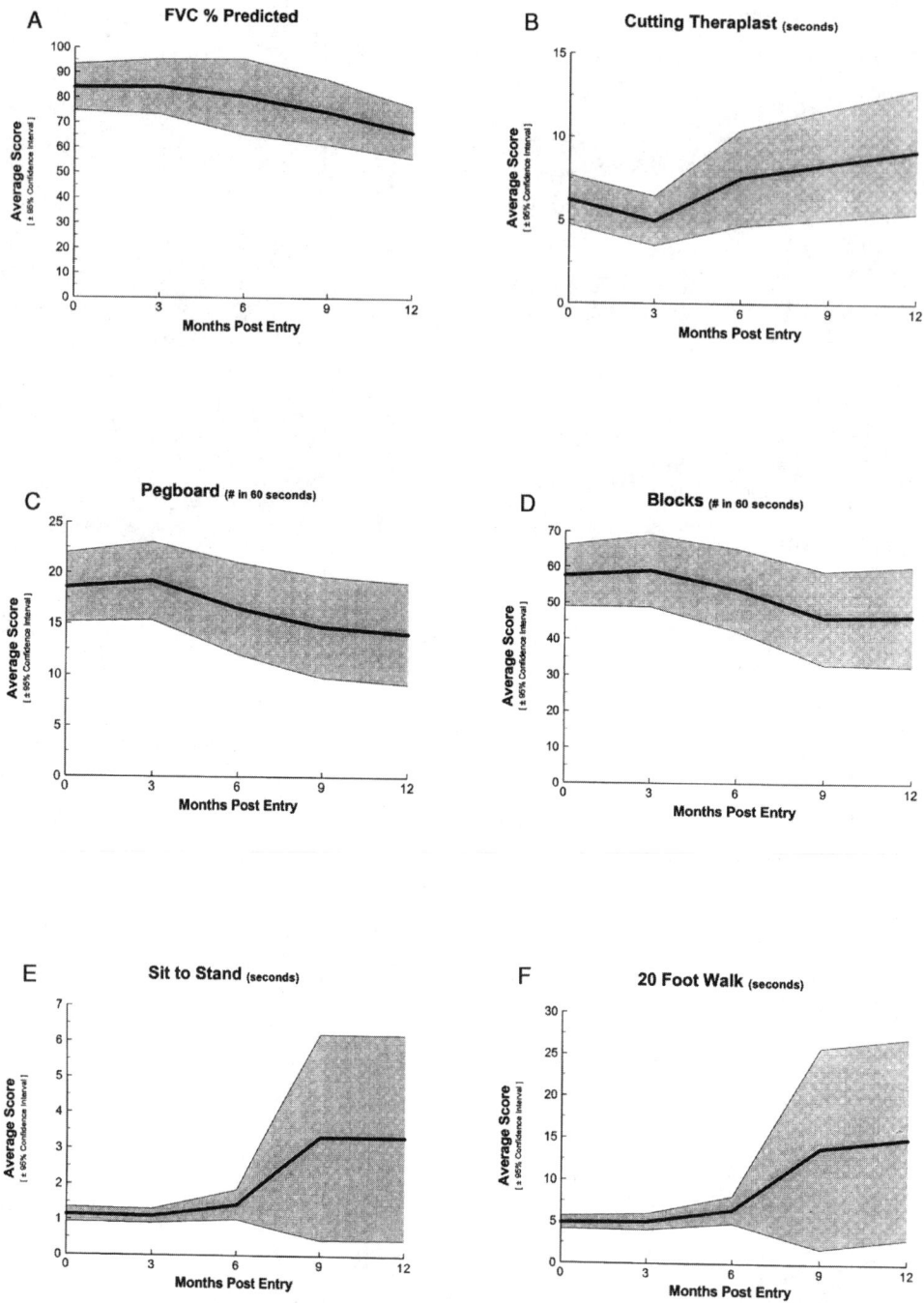

Figure 5-7. Average score for functional measurements in Appel Amyotrophic Lateral Sclerosis (ALS) Scale subscores. The average score ± 95% confidence limits for 18 ALS patients followed 12 months by the Appel ALS Scale was determined for the following respiratory, upper extremity, and lower extremity functions. **A.** Forced vital capacity percent predicted. **B.** Cutting Theraplast time. **C.** Pegboard constructs in time interval. **D.** Block turning in time interval. **E.** Standing from chair time. **F.** Twenty-foot walk time. Missing data imputed by the last value carried forward technique.

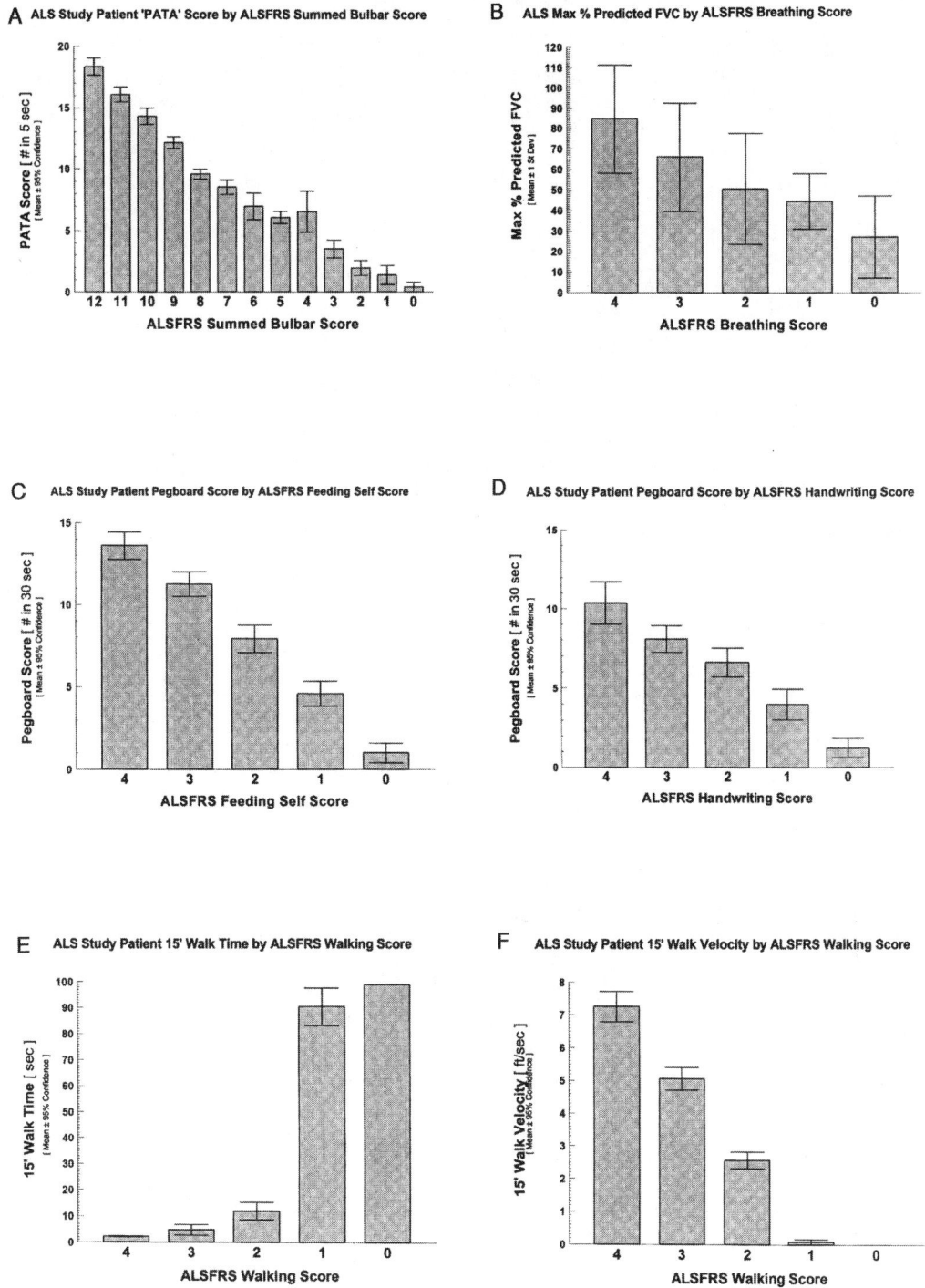

Figure 5-8. Comparison of functional measurements in ACTS ALS Evaluation with Amyotrophic Lateral Sclerosis Functional Rating Scale (ALSFRS) subscores. The average value ± 95% confidence limits for functional measurements in the ACTS ALS Evaluation of 132 ALS patients was compared with the ALSFRS subscore for the following functional measurements. **A.** Bulbar diadochokinetic [PaTa] score with ALSFRS summed bulbar subscore. **B.** Forced vital capacity percent predicted with ALSFRS breathing subscore. **C.** Pegboard constructs in time interval with ALSFRS feeding subscore. **D.** Pegboard constructs in time interval with ALSFRS handwriting subscore. **E.** Walking time with ALSFRS walking subscore. **F.** Walking velocity with ALSFRS walking subscore.

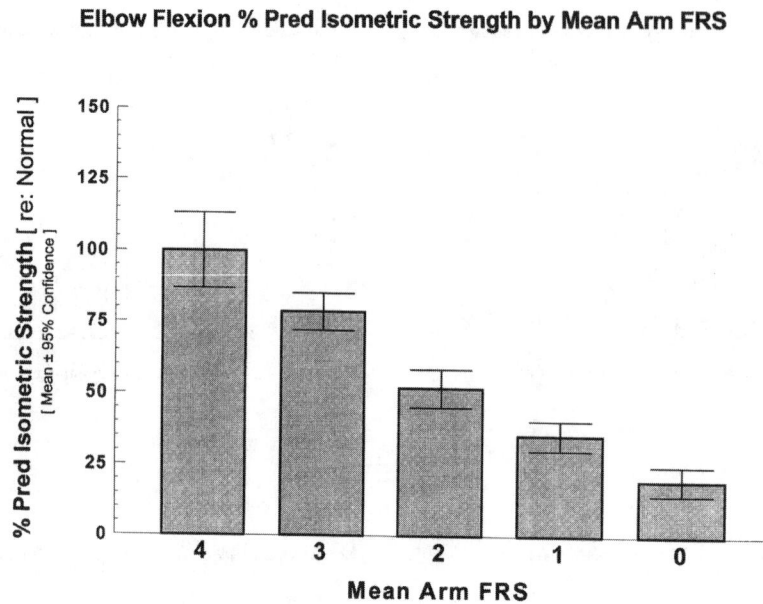

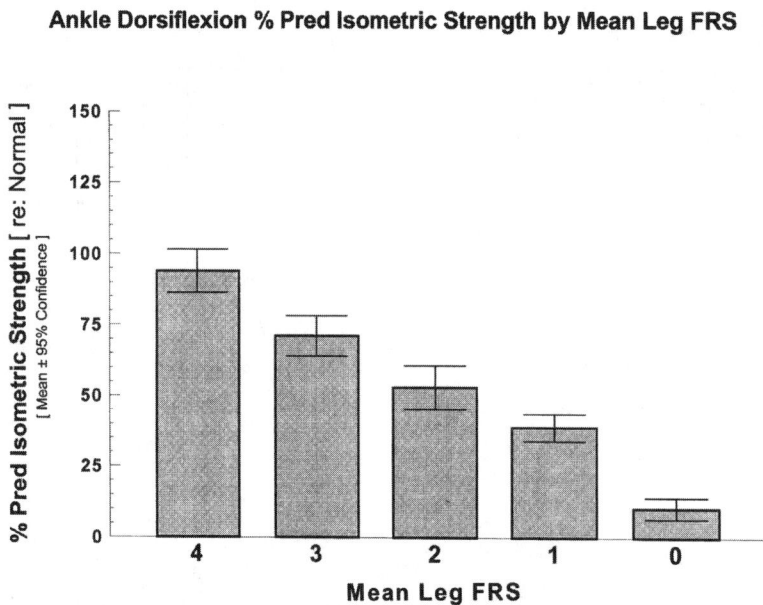

Figure 5-9. Comparison of isometric strength measurements in ACTS ALS Evaluation with Amyotrophic Lateral Sclerosis Functional Rating Scale (ALS FRS) subscores. The average value ± 95% confidence limits for right and left isometric strength (as percent predicted relative to normal) measurements in the ACTS ALS Evaluation of 132 ALS patients was compared with the ALS FRS subscore for the following muscle groups: elbow flexion and ankle dorsiflexion.

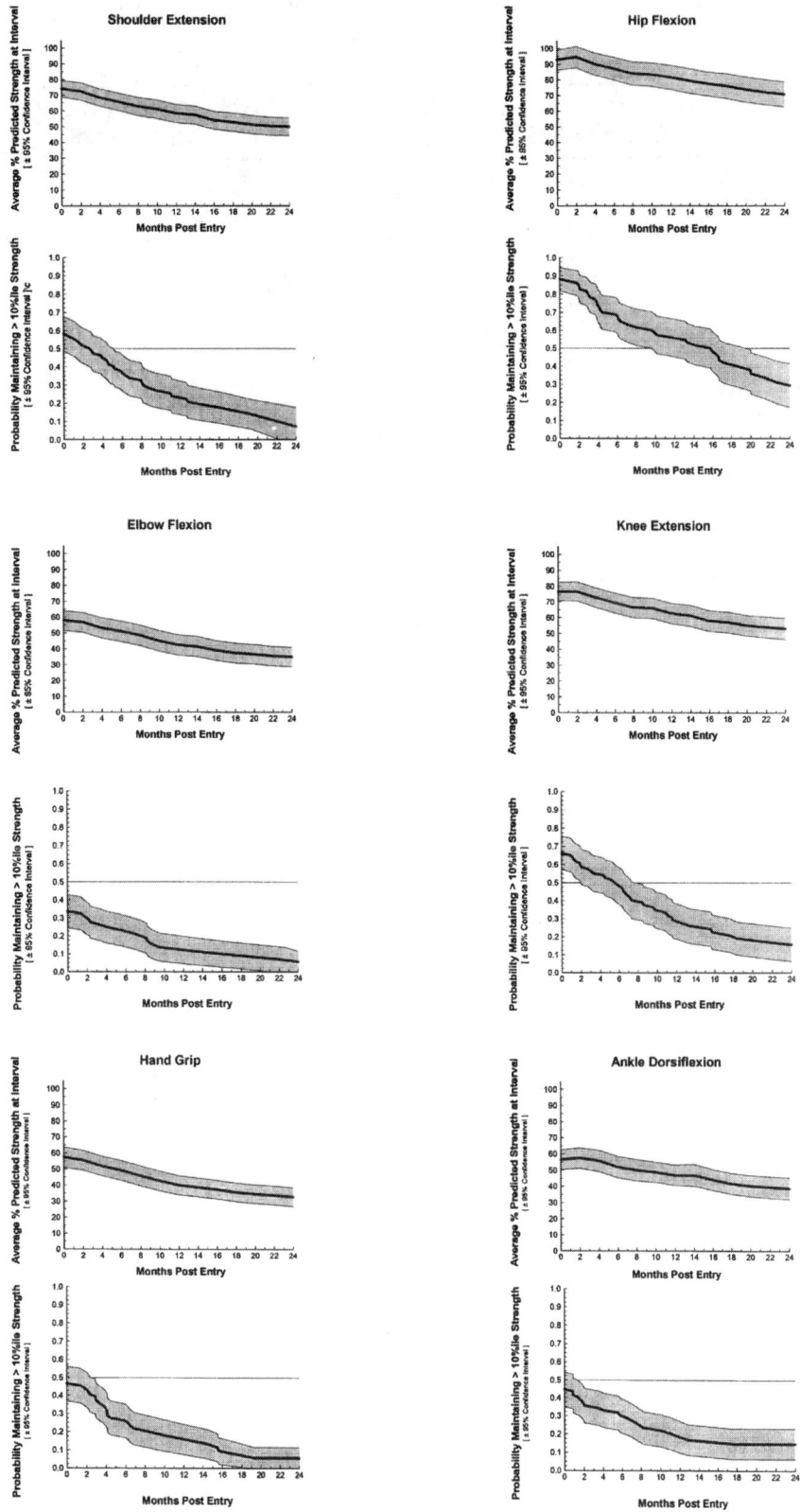

Figure 5-10. Isometric muscle strength changes over time in ACTS ALS Evaluation. The average value ± 95% confidence limits for right and left isometric strength (as percent predicted relative to normal) measurements over time in the ACTS ALS Evaluation of 132 amyotrophic lateral sclerosis patients was compared with time to failure (<10% predicted normal strength) for the following muscle groups: shoulder extension, hip flexion, elbow flexion, knee extension, handgrip, and ankle dorsiflexion.

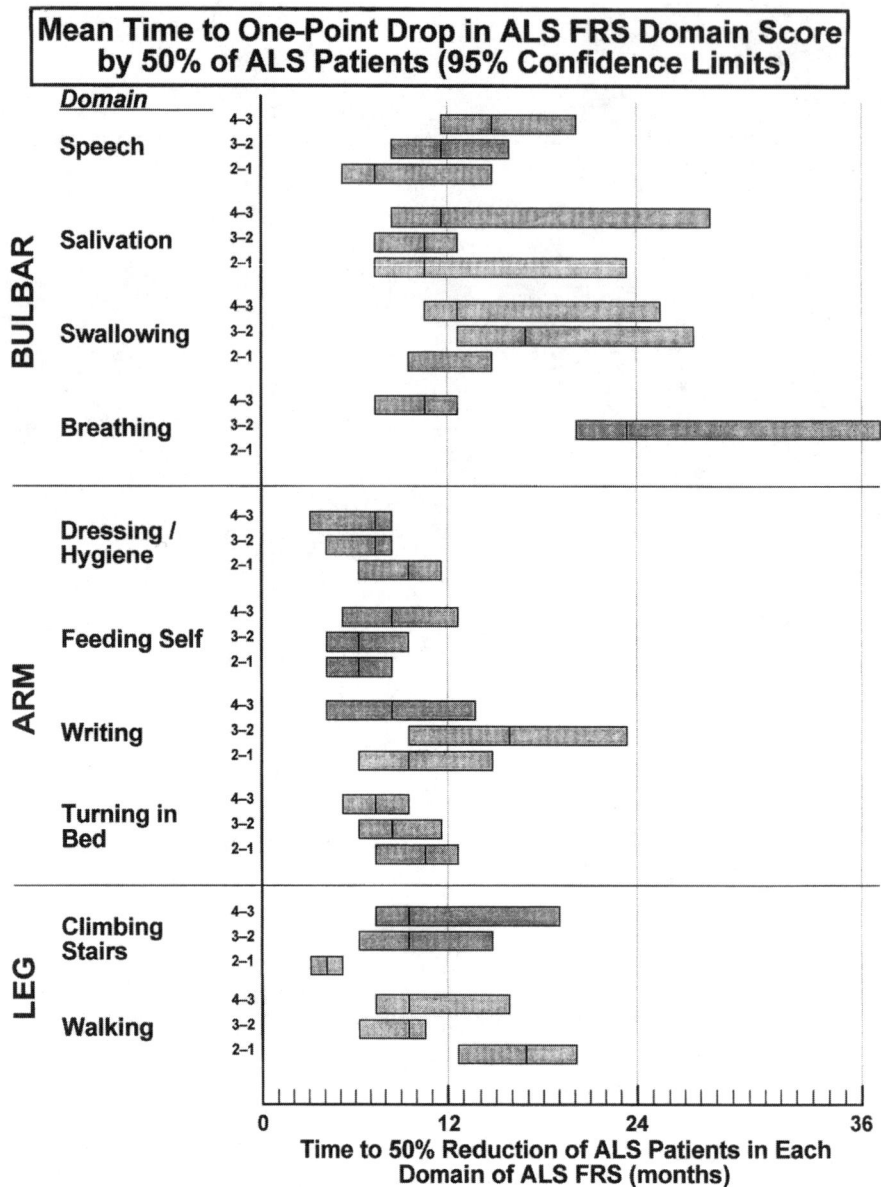

Figure 5-11. Amyotrophic Lateral Sclerosis Functional Rating Scale (ALS FRS) subscore changes over time in ACTS ALS Evaluation. The average value ± 95% confidence limits for individual subscore measurements over time in the ACTS ALS Evaluation of 132 ALS patients was compared with time to failure [by 1-point drop to lower score: 4 to 3 (*solid black line*), 3 to 2 (*thick horizontal dashed black line*), 2 to 1 (*thin vertical dashed line*)] for the following ALS FRS subscores: bulbar, speech, salivation, swallowing, arm, dressing and hygiene feeding self, writing, turning in bed, leg, climbing stairs, and walking.

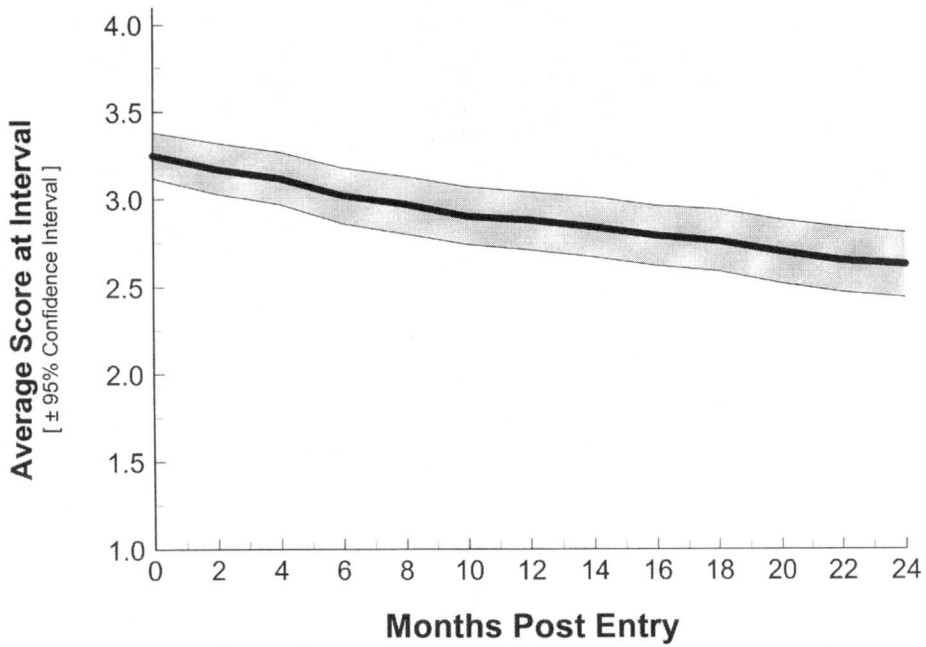

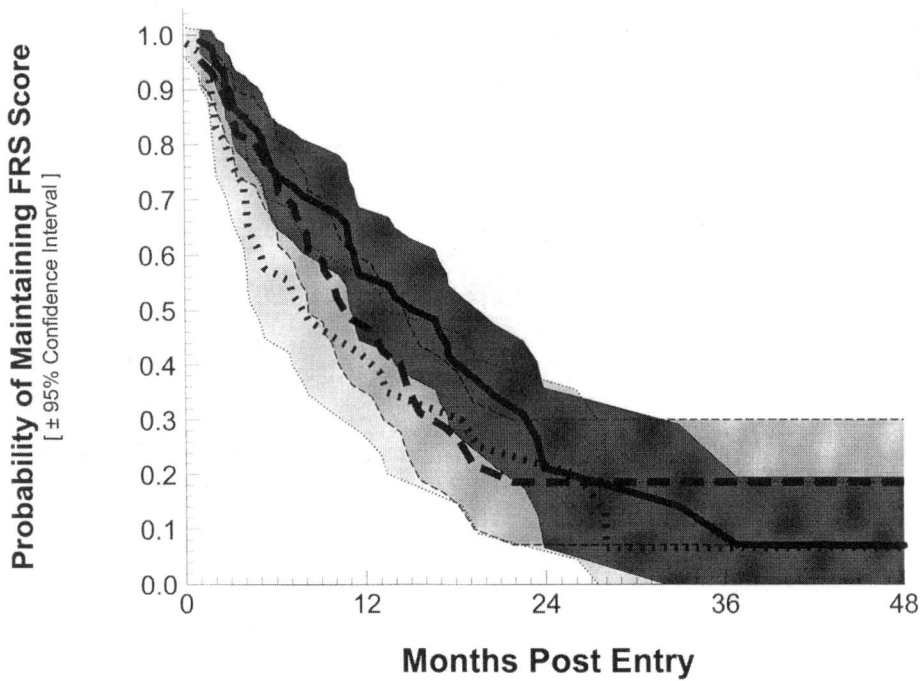

Figure 5-11a. Mean time to 1-point drop in Amyotrophic Lateral Sclerosis Functional Rating Scale (ALS FRS) domain score by 50% of ALS patients (95% confidence limits). The mean time in months ± 95% confidence limits for 1-point drop to lower score: 4 to 3 (*solid line*), 3 to 2 (*horizontal dash*), 2 to 1 (*diagonal dash*) for ALS FRS subscores.

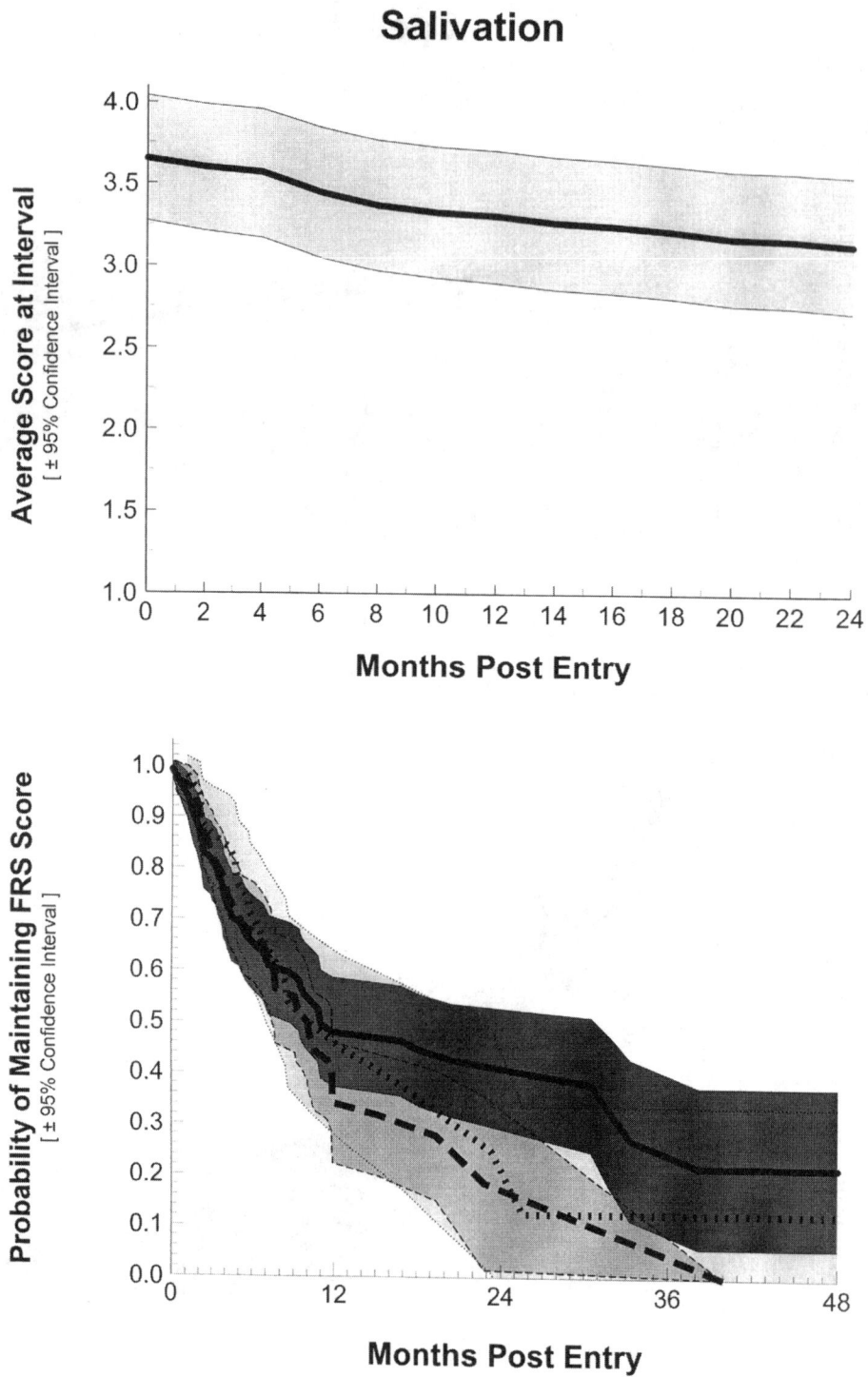

Figure 5-11b.

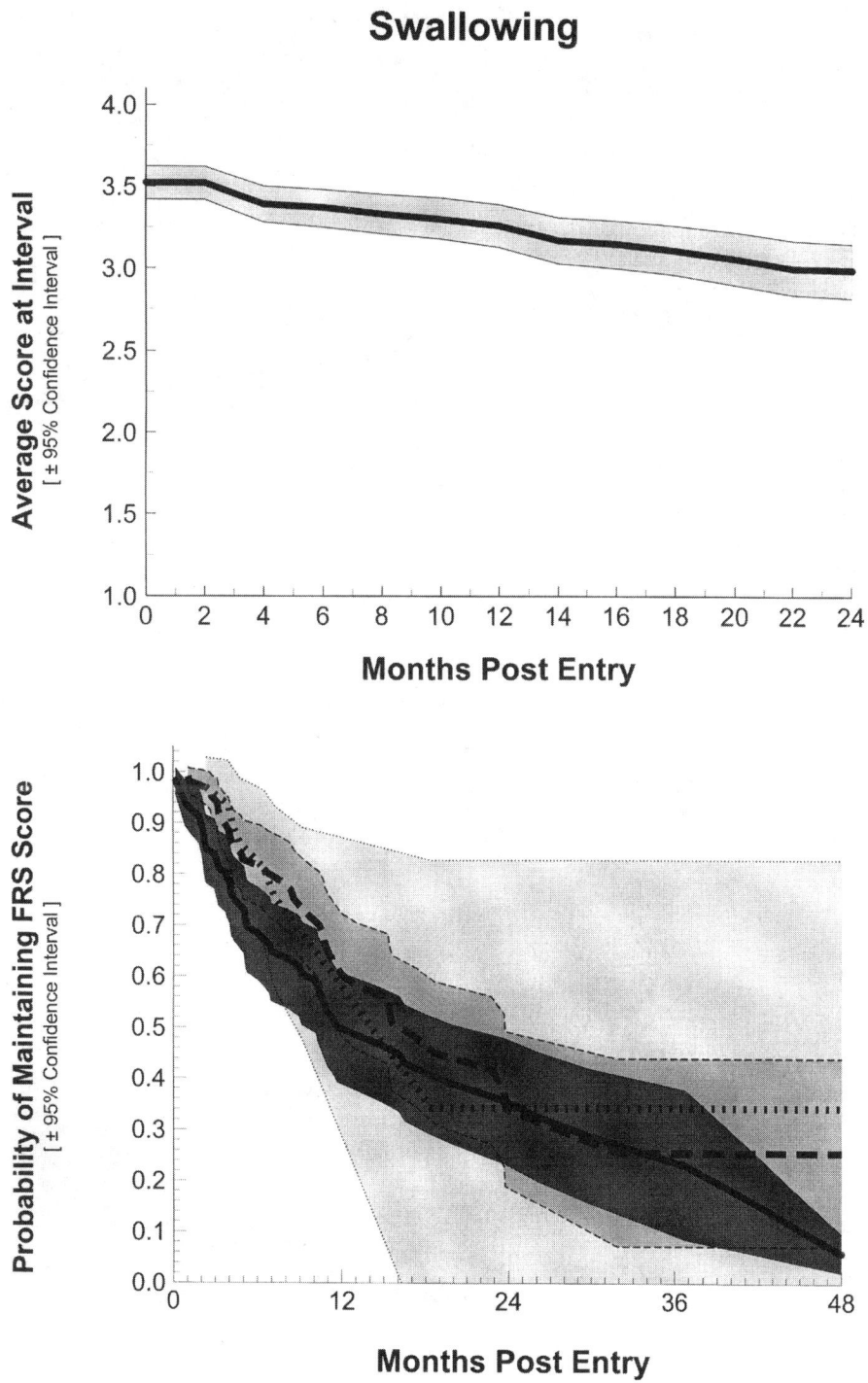

Figure 5-11c.

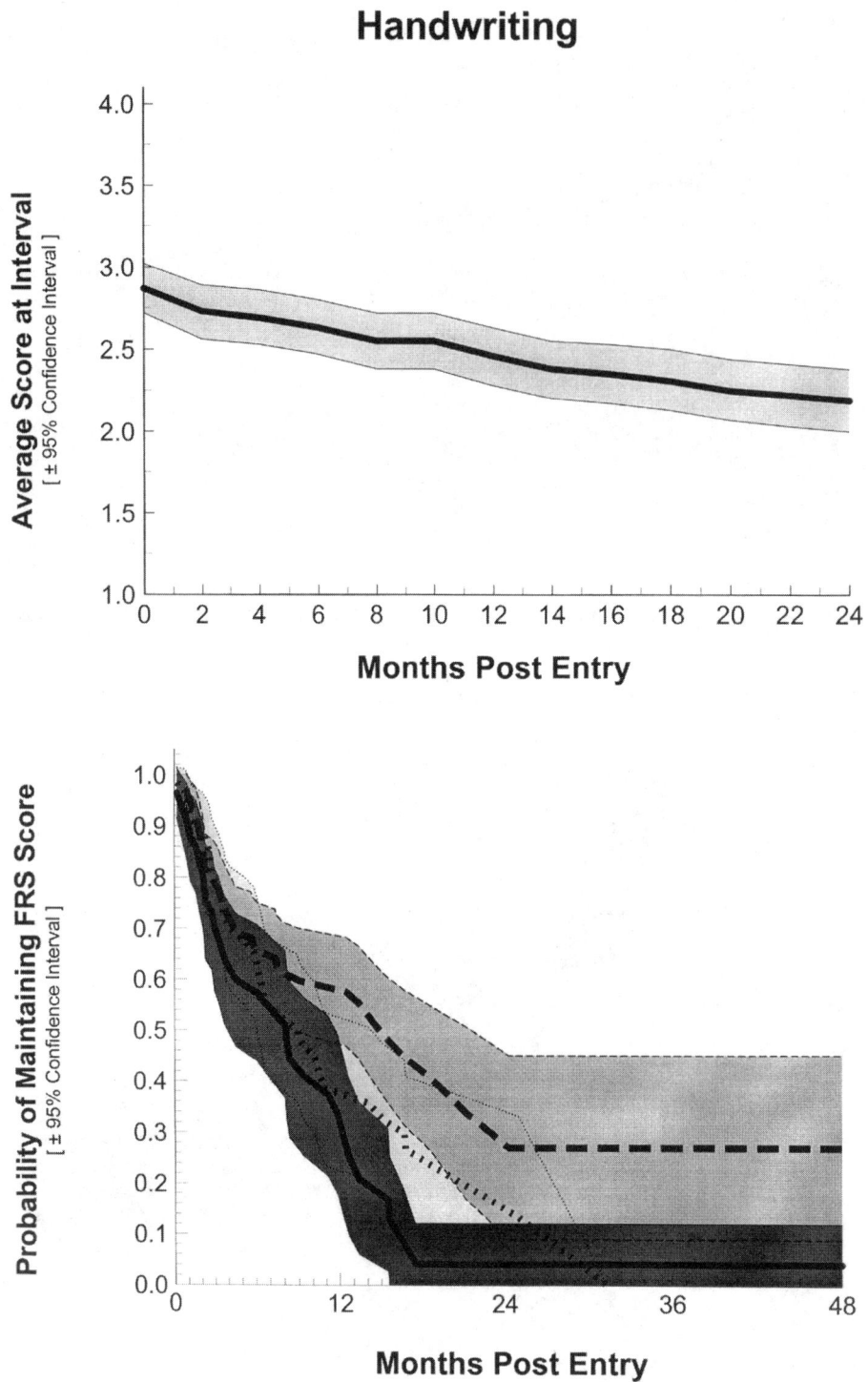

Figure 5-11d.

Feeding Self

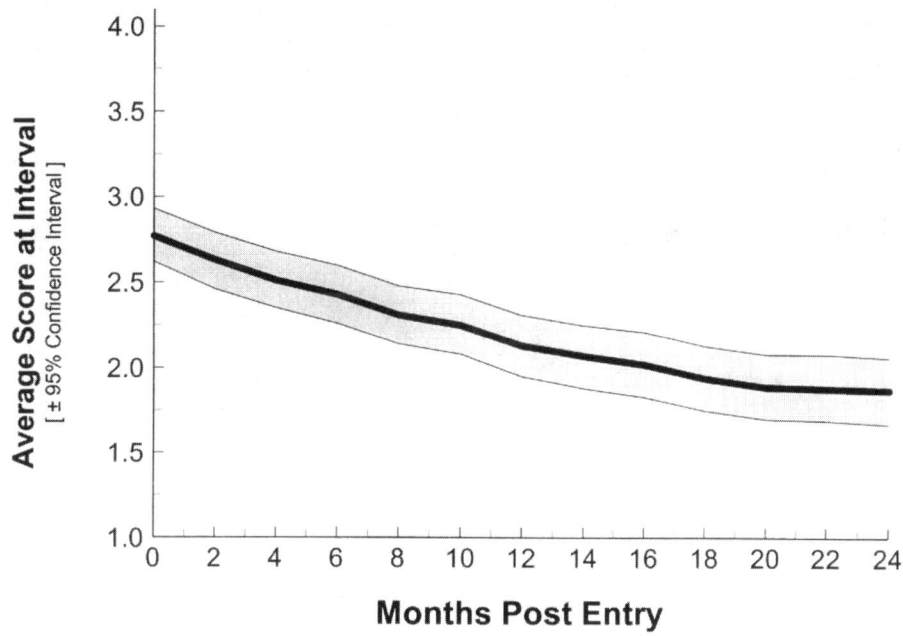

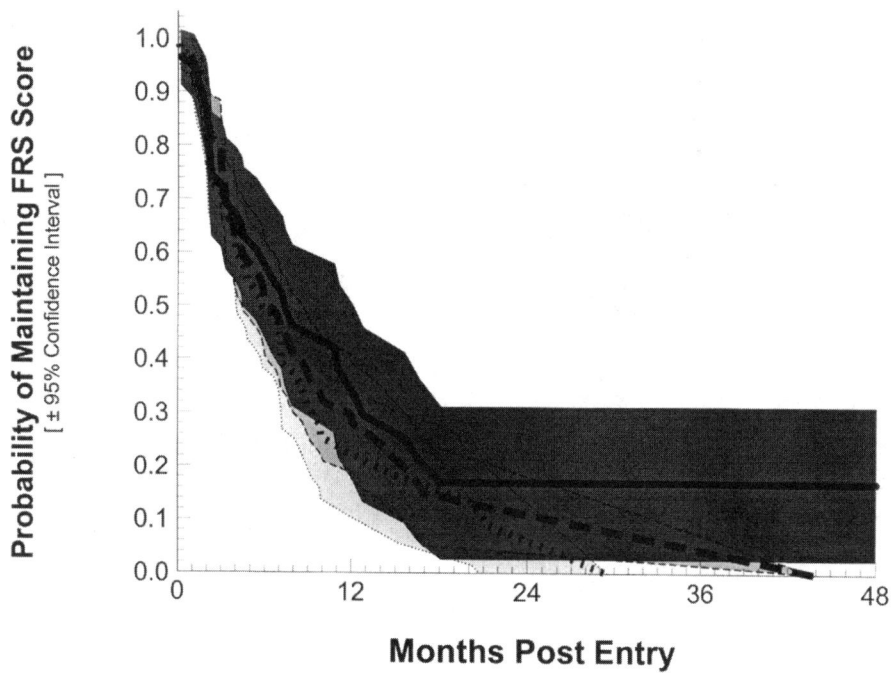

Figure 5-11e.

Dressing & Hygiene

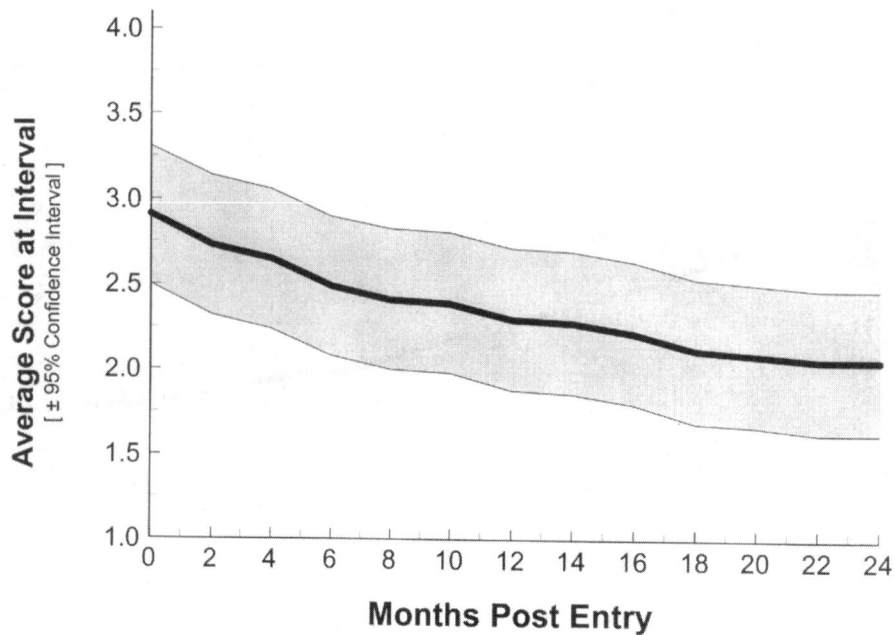

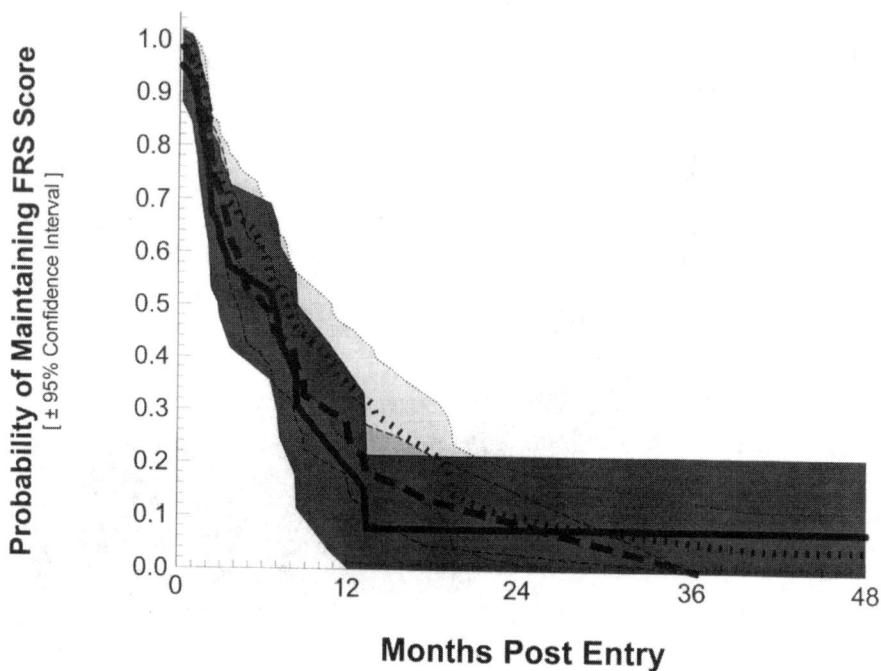

Figure 5-11f.

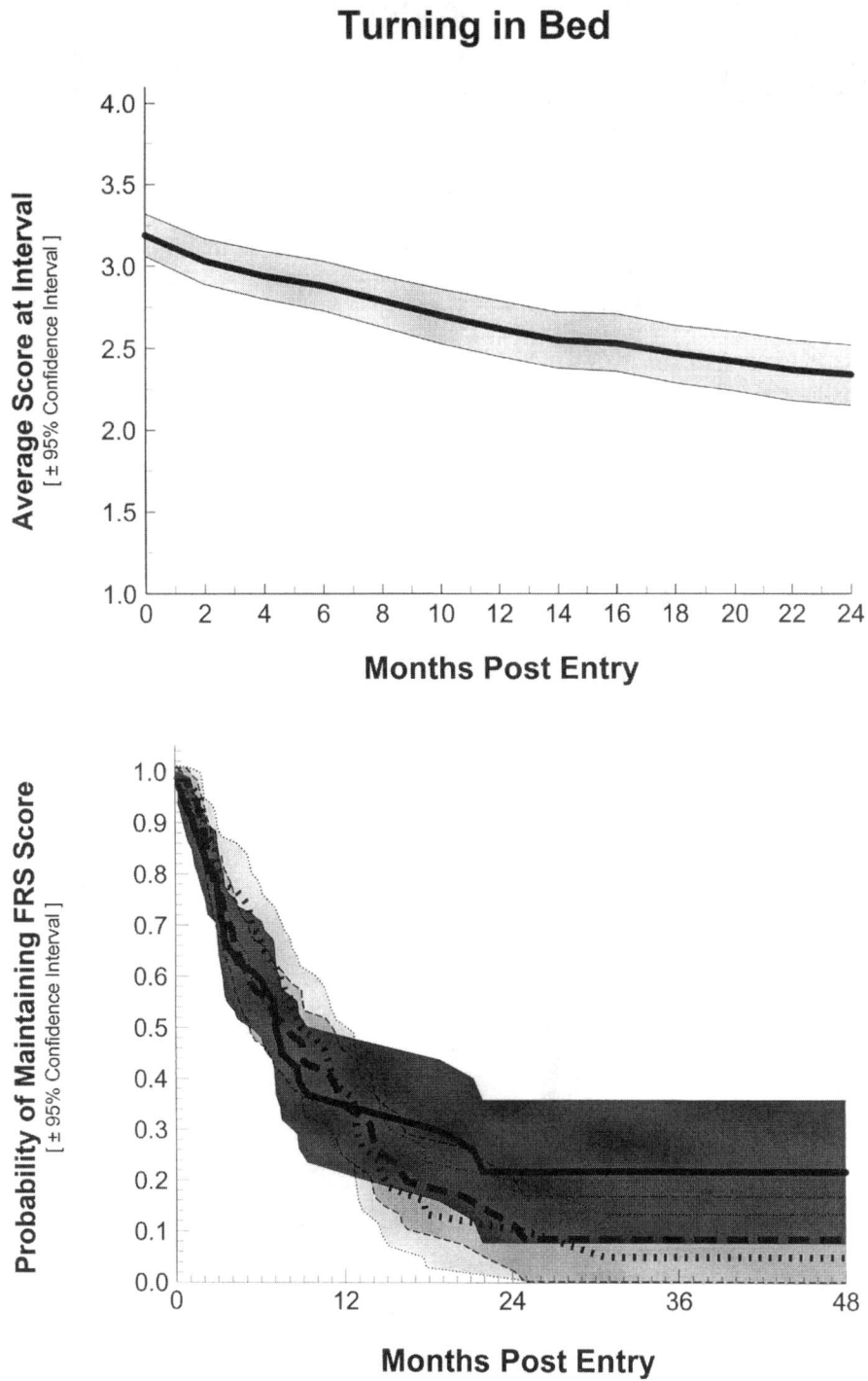

Figure 5-11g.

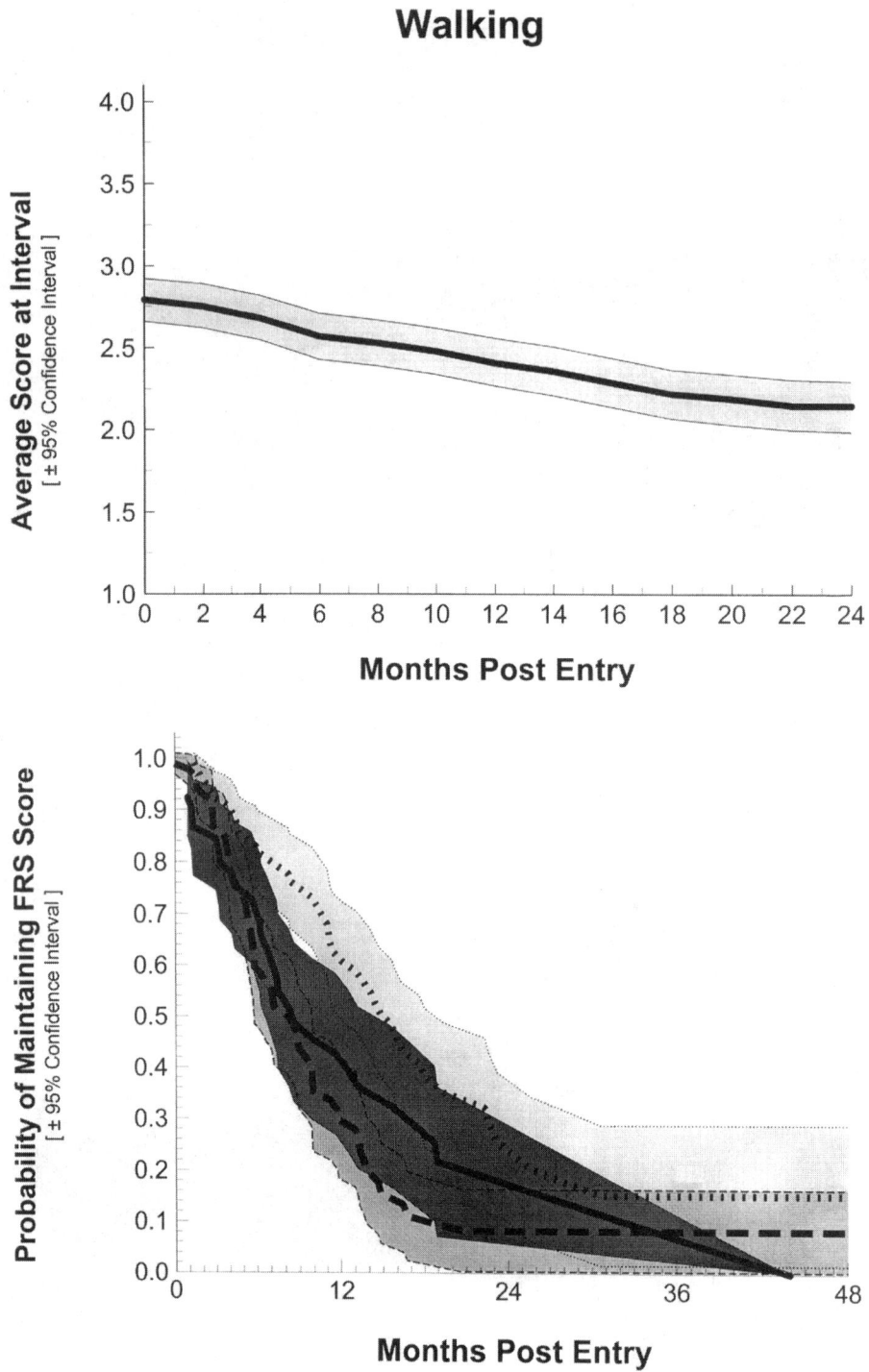

Figure 5-11h.

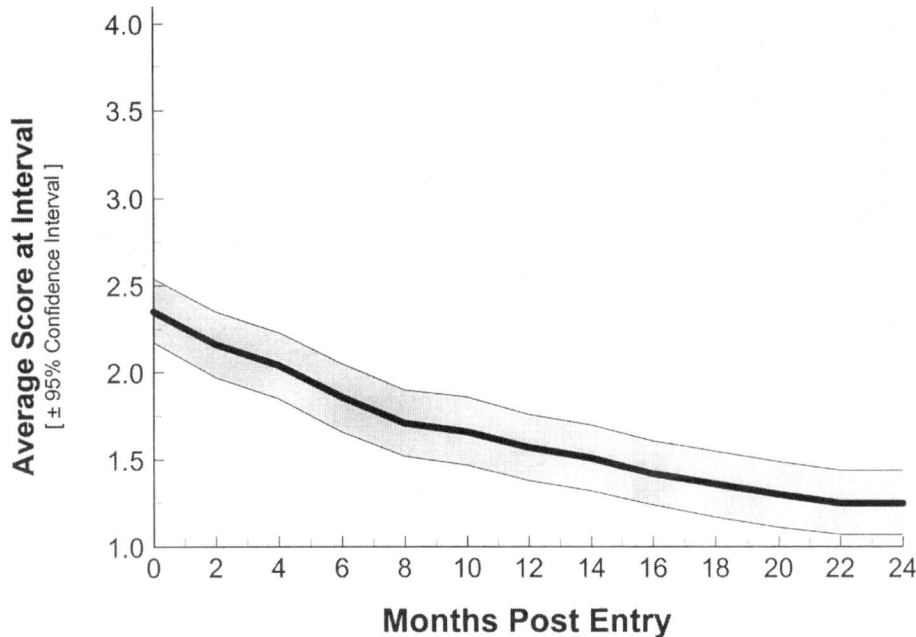

Figure 5-11i.

ity states may be seen in a population of ALS patients. There is a one-point drop from normal in the dressing and hygiene subscore in nearly all patients by 12 months, and handwriting and feeding subscores drop one point from normal between 12 and 24 months after entry. Climbing stairs and walking subscores drop one point from normal in this same time period, but the drop from grade 2 to grade 1 occurs in a shorter time span. Bulbar subscore measures do not drop one point from normal in the majority of patients until after 24 months from entry. The speech subscore changes in the majority of patients occur earlier than the salivation or swallowing subscores.

The ALS FRS permits a definition of the time spent in different disability states as a function of the time spent following entry before a one-point drop from normal (4 to 3), from mildly affected (3 to 2), from moderately affected (2 to 1), and from severely affected to moribund (1 to 0) (Figure 5-12). The range of the time spent in these different states is broad (Table 5-7). Nevertheless, this means of describing disability due to ALS permits a simple mode for obtaining clini-

cal information that allows follow-up of individual patients in different clinical settings, as well as application of sophisticated biomedical statistical methods for efficient and economical future clinical trials.

Acknowledgments

The information provided in this chapter derives from a cooperative effort of many collaborators at the ALS Clinical Research Center (Daryn Belden, Mohammed Sanjak, Jennifer Parnell, Christy Dewitt, John Wheat, and Kelly Wheat), the ALS Clinic (Kathryn Roelke, Andrew Waclawik, Barend Lotz, and Bradley Beinlich), and the Wisconsin Chapter of the Muscular Dystrophy Association (Paula McGuire).

Information obtained for this review was obtained during studies that were supported in part by the Muscular Dystrophy Association, Department of Veterans Affairs, Regeneron Pharmaceuticals, Amgen-Regeneron Partners, and Rhone-Poulenc Rorer Pharmaceuticals.

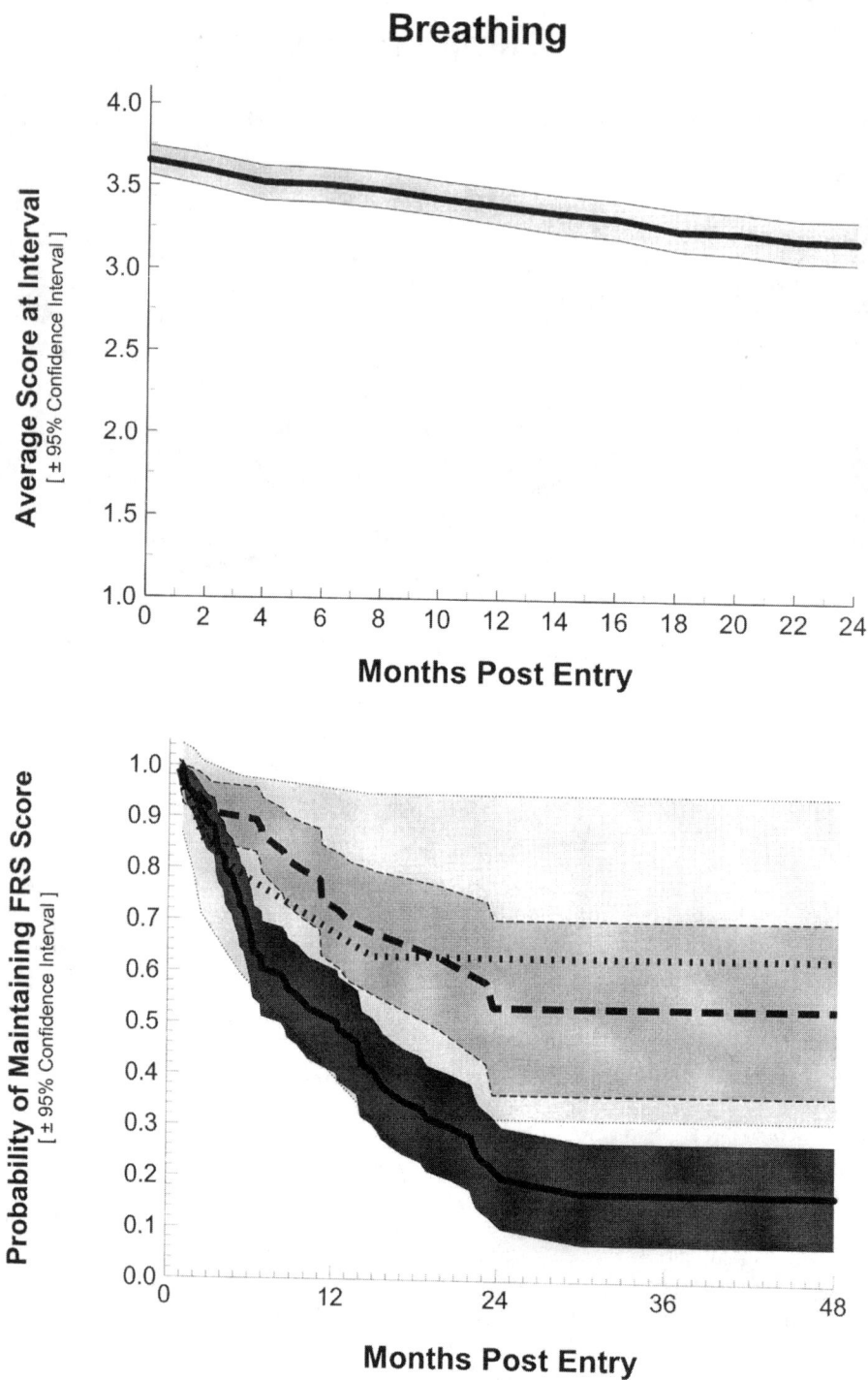

Figure 5-11j.

Climbing Stairs

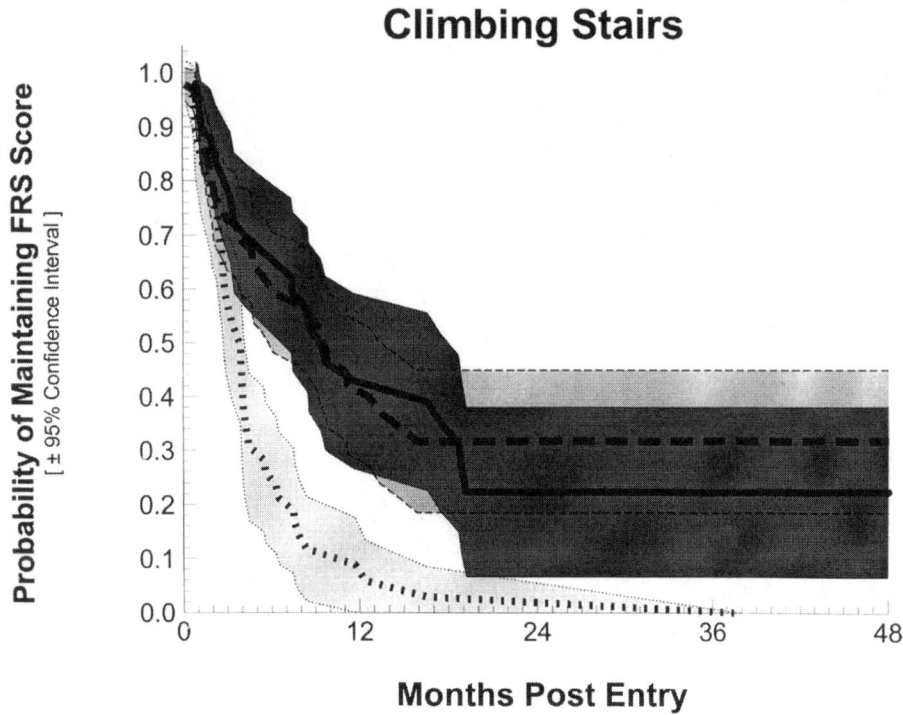

Figure 5-12.

Table 5-7. Mean Time to 1-Point Drop in Amyotrophic Lateral Sclerosis Functional Rating Scale (ALS FRS) Domain Score by 50% of Amyotrophic Lateral Sclerosis (ALS) Patients

Time to 50% Reduction of ALS Patients in Each Domain of ALS FRS (95% Confidence Limits)			
Score Change	*4 → 3*	*3 → 2*	*2 → 1*
Domain			
Bulbar			
Speech	14 mo	11 mo	7 mo
	Detectable	Repeating required	Nonverbal aids used
	(11–19)	(8–15)	(5–14)
Salivation	11 mo	10 mo	10 mo
	Nocturnal drooling	Mild saliva during day	Moderate saliva
	(8–27)	(7–12)	(7–22)
Swallow	12 mo	16 mo	14 mo
	Detectable, occasional choking	Soft diet	Supplemental tube feedings
	(10–24)	(8–15)	(9–Indeterminate)
Respiratory			
Breathing	10 mo	22 mo	Indeterminate
	Short of breath on exertion	Short of breath at rest	Bilevel positive airway pressure/continuous positive airway pressure
	(7–12)	(19–40)	(–)

(continued)

Table 5-7. *(continued)*

Time to 50% Reduction of ALS Patients in Each Domain of ALS FRS (95% Confidence Limits)

Score Change Domain	4 → 3	3 → 2	2 → 1
Arm			
Dressing/hygiene	7 mo Decreased efficiency (3–8)	7 mo Intermittent assistance (7–12)	9 mo With full assistance (7–22)
Feeding/cutting	8 mo Slow but full turn, unaided (5–12)	6 mo Clumsy, occasionally aided (4–9)	6 mo Cutting by aide (4–8)
Writing	8 mo Slow, legible (4–13)	15 mo Illegible (9–22)	9 mo Hold pen, not write (6–14)
Trunk			

Turning in bed	7 mo
	Slow, unaided
	
	(10–24)
		8 mo
		Worse but full turn,
		    unaided
		(8–15)
			10 mo
			Can initiate but not turn fully
			    without an aid
			(9–10)

Leg			
Climbing stairs	9 mo Slow, unaided (7–18)	9 mo Unsteady, unaided (6–14)	4 mo With hand rail or assistance (3–5)

Walking	9 mo
	Slow, unaided
	
	(7–15)
		9 mo
		Requires assistive device,
		    including ankle-foot
		    orthosis
		(6–10)
			16 mo
			Nonambulatory
			
			(12–19)

References

ALS CNTF Treatment Study (ACTS) Phase I–II Study Group. The pharmacokinetics of subcutaneously administered recombinant human ciliary neurotrophic factor (RHCNTF) in patients with amyotrophic lateral sclerosis—relation to parameters of the acute-phase response. *Clin Neuropharmacol* 1995a;18:500–14.

ALS CNTF Treatment Study (ACTS) Phase I–II Study Group. A phase I study of recombinant human ciliary neurotrophic factor (RHCNTF) in patients with amyotrophic lateral sclerosis. *Clin Neuropharmacol* 1995b;18:515–32.

ALS CNTF Treatment Study (ACTS) Phase I–II Study Group. The Amyotrophic Lateral Sclerosis Functional Rating Scale—assessment of activities of daily living in patients with amyotrophic lateral sclerosis. *Arch Neurol* 1996;53:141–47.

ALS CNTF Treatment Study (ACTS) Phase II–III Study Group. A double-blind placebo-controlled clinical trial of subcutaneous recombinant human ciliary neurotrophic factor (RHCNTF) in amyotrophic lateral sclerosis. *Neurology* 1996;46:1244–49.

Andres PL, Hedlund W, Finison L, et al. Quantitative motor assessment in amyotrophic lateral sclerosis. *Neurology* 1986;36:937–41.

Appel V, Stewart SS, Smith G, et al. A rating scale for amyotrophic lateral sclerosis: description and preliminary experience. *Ann Neurol* 1987;22:328–33.

Ashworth B. Preliminary trial of carisoprodol in multiple sclerosis. *Practitioner* 1964;192:540–42.

Bradley WG, BDNF Study Group. A phase I/II of recombinant human brain derived neurotrophic factor in amyotrophic lateral sclerosis [Works in Progress Abst 1]. *Ann Neurol* 1995;38:971.

Brooks BR. Natural history of ALS: Symptoms, strength, pulmonary function and disability. *Neurology* 1996; 47(Suppl 2):S71–82.

Brooks BR. The Norris ALS score: insight into the natural history of amyotrophic lateral sclerosis provided by Forbes Norris. In: Rose FC (ed.). *ALS—From Charcot to the present and into the future—The Forbes H. Norris (1928–1993) Memorial Volume.* London: Smith-Gordon, 1994: 21–29. [Advances in ALS/MND, Vol. 3].

Brooks BR, Lewis D, Rawling J, et al. The natural history of amyotrophic lateral sclerosis. In: William AC (ed.). *Motor neuron disease.* London: Chapman & Hall, 1994: 131–69.

Brooks BR, Sufit RL, DePaul R, et al. Design of clinical therapeutic trials in amyotrophic lateral sclerosis. In: Rowland LP (ed.). *Amyotrophic lateral sclerosis and other motor neuron diseases.* New York: Raven, 1991: 521–46.

Brooks BR, DePaul R, Tan YD, et al. Motor neuron disease. In: Porter RJ, Schoenberg BS (eds.). *Controlled clinical trials in neurological disease.* Boston: Kluwer Academic, 1990:249–81.

Brooks BR, Sufit RL, Clough JA, et al. Isokinetic and functional evaluation of muscle strength over time in amyotrophic lateral sclerosis. In: Munsat TL (ed.). *Quantification of neurologic deficit.* Boston: Butterworth, 1989:143–54.

Caroscio IT, Mulvihill MN, Sterling R, et al. Amyotrophic lateral sclerosis—Its natural history. *Neurol Clin* 1987: 1–8.

Fallat RJ. Pulmonary function in amyotrophic lateral sclerosis: caveats and value in clinical management and future clinical trials. In: Rose FC (ed.). *ALS—From Charcot to the present and into the future—The Forbes H. Norris (1928–1993) Memorial Volume.* London: Smith-Gordon, 1994:309–13. [Advances in ALS/MND, Vol. 3].

Fallat RJ, Jewitt B, Bass M, et al. Spirometry in amyotrophic lateral sclerosis. *Arch Neurol* 1979;36:74–80.

Feinstein AR. *Clinimetrics.* London: Yale University Press, 1987.

Glindmeyer HW, Jones RN, Barkman HW, et al. Spirometry: quantitative test criteria and test acceptability. *Am Rev Respir Dis* 1987;136:449–52.

Guiloff RJ, Goonetilleke A. Longitudinal clinical assessments in motor neurone disease. Relevance to clinical trials. In: Rose FC (ed.). *ALS—From Charcot to the present and into the future—The Forbes H. Norris (1928–1993) Memorial Volume.* London: Smith-Gordon, 1994: 73–82. [Advances in ALS/MND, Vol. 3].

Haverkamp LJ, Appel V, Appel SH. Natural history of amyotrophic lateral sclerosis in a database population—Validation of a scoring system and a model for survival prediction. *Brain* 1995;118:707–19.

Hillel AD, Miller RM, Yorkston K, et al. Amyotrophic Lateral Sclerosis Severity Scale. In: Rose FC (ed.). *Amyotrophic lateral sclerosis.* New York: Demos, 1990:93–97.

Hillel AD, Miller RM, Yorkston K, et al. Amyotrophic Lateral Sclerosis Severity Scale. *Neuroepidemiology* 1989;8:142–50.

Hulley S, Cummings R. *Designing clinical research.* Baltimore: Williams & Wilkins, 2001.

Italian ALS Study Group. Branched-chain amino acids and amyotrophic lateral sclerosis: a treatment failure. *Neurology* 1993;43:2466–70.

Lai EC, Felice K, Gawel M, et al. Amyotrophic lateral sclerosis disease progression in a historical database group accurately reflects the rate of decline of placebo controls in a phase III clinical trial for insulin-like growth factor [Abst S64.003]. *Neurology* 1996;46(Suppl 2):A469–70.

Lange DJ, Felice KJ, Festoff BW, et al. Recombinant human insulin-like growth factor-I in ALS: description of a double-blind, placebo-controlled study. *Neurology* 1996;47(Suppl 2):S93–95.

Louwerse ES, de Jong JMBV, Kuether G. Critique of assessment methodology in amyotrophic lateral sclerosis. In: Rose FC (ed.). *Amyotrophic lateral sclerosis.* New York: Demos, 1990:151–79.

Miller RG, Gelinas D, Moore M, et al. A placebo-controlled trial of gabapentin in amyotrophic lateral sclerosis [Abst S64.002]. *Neurology* 1996a;46(Suppl 2):A469.

Miller RG, Petajan JH, Byan WW, et al. A placebo-controlled trial of recombinant human ciliary neurotrophic (RHCNTF) factor in amyotrophic lateral sclerosis. *Ann Neurol* 1996b;39:256–60.

Munsat TL, Andres PL, Skerry LM. The use of quantitative techniques to define amyotrophic lateral sclerosis. In: Munsat TL (ed.). *Quantification of neurologic deficit.* Boston: Butterworth, 1989:129–42.

Munsat TL, Andres PL, Finison L, et al. The natural history of motoneuron loss in amyotrophic lateral sclerosis. *Neurology* 1988;38:409–13.

Norris FH, Fallat RJ. Staging respiratory failure in ALS. In: Tsubaki T, Yase Y (eds.). *Amyotrophic lateral sclerosis.* Amsterdam: Elsevier Excerpta Medica, 1988: 217–22.

Norris FH, Calanchini PR, Fallat R, et al. The administration of guanidine in amyotrophic lateral sclerosis. *Neurology* 1974;24:721–28.

Ringel SP, Murphy JR, Alderson MK, et al. The natural history of amyotrophic lateral sclerosis. *Neurology* 1993; 43:1316–22.

Sanjak M, Belden D, Cook T, Brooks BR. Muscle strength measurement. In: Lane RJM (ed.). *Handbook of muscle disease.* New York: Marcel Dekker, 1996:19–34.

Streiner DL, Norman GR. *Health measurement scales—A practical guide to their development and use.* Oxford: Oxford University Press, 1989.

Subcommittee on Motor Neuron Diseases/Amyotrophic Lateral Sclerosis of the World Federation of Neurology Research Group on Neuromuscular Disease and the El Escorial "Clinical Limits Amyotrophic Lateral Sclerosis" Workshop Contributors. El Escorial World Federation of Neurology Criteria for the Diagnosis of Amyotrophic Lateral Sclerosis. *J Neurol Sci* 1994;124(Suppl):96–107.

Subcommittee on Motor Neuron Diseases of the World Federation of Neurology Research Group on Neuromuscular Disease and the Airlie House "Therapeutic Trials in ALS" Workshop Contributors. Airlie House Guidelines—Therapeutic Trials in Amyotrophic Lateral Sclerosis. *J Neurol Sci* 1995;129(Suppl):1–10.

Tourtellotte WW, Haerer AF, Simpson JF, et al. Quantitative clinical neurological testing 1. A study of a battery of tests designed to evaluate in part the neurological function of patients with multiple sclerosis and its use in a therapeutic trial. *Ann N Y Acad Sci* 1965;122:480–505.

6 Scales for the Assessment of Movement Disorders

Stephen T. Gancher, M.D.

A variety of scales have been developed during the past several decades for measurement of the severity of various movement disorders. They vary from simple, limited assessments that are easily performed to comprehensive scales that may be time-consuming and take practice to administer.

One common feature of these scales is an emphasis on motor signs. Depending on the disease, various symptoms associated with the condition have also been used for rating, and some scales or portions of scales use descriptions of functional status and ability to perform self-care activities as a basis for rating disease. This chapter reviews the most widely used scales for Parkinson's disease, dystonia, tic disorders, and tardive dyskinesia, and a rating scale for Huntington's disease is referenced as well.

Parkinson's Disease

Before the development of levodopa treatment of Parkinson's disease, studies describing the efficacy of drug treatment or surgical therapy largely relied on an overall subjective impression of disease severity rather than formal ratings. With the advent of levodopa therapy, many drug trials were conducted and created a need to rate the severity of parkinsonism in a more standardized fashion.

One of the first widely used scales is a single-item assessment, reported by Drs. Margaret Hoehn and Melvin Yahr in a study of the natural history of Parkinson's disease (Hoehn & Yahr, 1967). Although this scale is mainly useful for broad classification of patients and is not sufficiently detailed to follow patients who exhibit motor fluctuations, it is easily administered and still widely used. Other early scales, such as the Northwestern University Disability Scale (Canter et al., 1961), evaluated functional status and both functional and objective tests (Webster, 1968; Schwab, 1960), and a scale developed at Columbia University (Yahr et al., 1969) was extensively used. These scales, as well as others, are comprehensively reviewed by Martinez-Martin (1993).

Because of the marked variability between scales and differences in weighting signs and symptoms, a committee chaired by Dr. Stanley Fahn was created in 1984 to develop a standardized scale. This scale, the

Unified Parkinson's Disease Rating Scale (UPDRS) (Fahn et al., 1987), is a composite of various previous scales and its use in the United States has largely supplanted other scales.

Unified Parkinson's Disease Rating Scale

The UPDRS (Table 6-1) is a composite scale consisting of six sections. Unless indicated otherwise, all items are rated from 0 (normal) to 4 (severely affected); each item is defined by a short sentence.

Part I of the UPDRS consists of four items that assess mentation, behavior, and mood. Although helpful as a general screen, these items are inadequate for measurement of dementia or depression, so other instruments should be used for their assessment.

Part II consists of 13 items and assesses the performance of activities of daily living. Items include assessment of difficulty with speech and swallowing, self-care, speaking, turning over in bed, and walking.

Two limitations should be mentioned in the use of this subscale. First, as it is based on symptoms, there may be disagreement between items that reflect bradykinesia and objective estimates of bradykinesia in the physical examination portion of the scale (part III). Also, because patients may perceive symptoms differently despite similar signs, it is possible for them to have different scores despite a similar degree of bradykinesia or tremor.

A second difficulty with this subscale relates to its use in comparing "on" and "off" states. Because many items are based on specific activities such as dressing or eating, in patients who time these activities to coincide with "on" states, a rating of functional difficulties performing these activities during "off" states may be artificial and difficult to interpret.

Part III is a 14-item rating of motor signs that is based on items in the Columbia disability scale. In addition to ratings of tremor and an assessment of facial and generalized bradykinesia, performance on several tasks is used to rate disease severity, including any difficulty noted while repeatedly tapping the index finger against the thumb, clenching and unclenching a fist, and arising from a chair. The definitions of difficulties with each task are straightforward, and the scale is reproducible. However, this motor scale does not take into account interference from dyskinesias or dystonias, which may present difficulty in motor performance in some patients.

Part IV rates complications of therapy. It includes several questions that attempt to quantify the duration and severity of dyskinesias and motor fluctuations and a three-item section concerning anorexia, sleep disturbance, and orthostatic hypotension. Unlike the previous sections, some items in this section are not graded, and it may be difficult to consistently rate patients who describe minor difficulties with sleep or minimal orthostatic dizziness.

Part V is a modified version of the Hoehn and Yahr staging system; overall disease severity is divided into unilateral (stage I), bilateral but without a gait or balance disorder (stage II), and bilateral disease with progressively more difficulty with mobility and balance (stage III–V); half points are allowed between stages I–II and II–III.

Part VI is a disability scale based on a scale reported by Schwab and England (Martinez-Martin, 1993). It is an estimation of the degree of interference with normal functioning and dependency due to parkinsonism; like other symptom-based scales, it reflects subjective perception, and patients with similar motor difficulties may sometimes report discrepant scores.

Core Assessment Program for Intracerebral Transplantation and Core Assessment Program for Surgical Interventional Therapies Rating System

The Core Assessment Program for Intracerebral Transplantation (CAPIT) and the Core Assessment Program for Surgical Interventional Therapies in Parkinson's Disease (CAPSIT-PD) were devised to standardize assessments of patients undergoing surgical therapies in Parkinson's disease, to allow comparison between study centers. In the CAPIT evaluation, the UPDRS, ratings for the duration and severity of dyskinesias, diary information, timed motor tasks, and evaluations before and after a dose of L-dopa are used to evaluate patients (Langston et al., 1992). The CAPSIT-PD evaluation is similar but also includes administration of a quality of life scale and more extensive cognitive and behavioral testing (Defer et al., 1999).

Diary Ratings

Another popular instrument for the assessment of motor fluctuations involves self-reporting of hourly status by patients. The patient is instructed to rate motor symptoms, averaging performance over each hour. In some centers, this information is visually conveyed by constructing a table such that each horizontal line represents a different day and each vertical line a block of time; blacking in the individual squares during either "on" or "off" states graphically conveys patterns that may be unapparent on a single day but may

Table 6-1. Unified Parkinson's Disease Rating Scale

I. Mentation, behavior, and mood

  1. Intellectual impairment

   0—None.

   1—Mild. Consistent forgetfulness with partial recollection of events and no other difficulties.

   2—Moderate memory loss, with disorientation and moderate difficulty handling complex problems. Mild but definite impairment of function at home with need of occasional prompting.

   3—Severe memory loss with disorientation for time and often to place. Severe impairment in handling problems.

   4—Severe memory loss with orientation preserved to person only. Unable to make judgments or solve problems. Requires much help with personal care. Cannot be left alone at all.

  2. Thought disorder (due to dementia or drug intoxication)

   0—None.

   1—Vivid dreaming.

   2—"Benign" hallucinations with insight retained.

   3—Occasional to frequent hallucinations or delusions; without insight; could interfere with daily activities.

   4—Persistent hallucinations, delusions, or florid psychosis. Not able to care for self.

  3. Depression

   0—Not present.

   1—Periods of sadness or guilt greater than normal, never sustained for days or weeks.

   2—Sustained depression (1 wk or more).

   3—Sustained depression with vegetative symptoms (insomnia, anorexia, weight loss, loss of interest).

   4—Sustained depression with vegetative symptoms and suicidal thoughts or intent.

  4. Motivation/initiative

   0—Normal.

   1—Less assertive than usual; more passive.

   2—Loss of initiative or disinterest in elective (nonroutine) activities.

   3—Loss of initiative or disinterest in day-to-day (routine) activities.

   4—Withdrawn, complete loss of motivation.

II. Activities of daily living (determine for "on/off")

  5. Speech

   0—Normal.

   1—Mildly affected. No difficulty being understood.

   2—Moderately affected. Sometimes asked to repeat statements.

   3—Severely affected. Frequently asked to repeat statements.

   4—Unintelligible most of the time.

  6. Salivation

   0—Normal.

   1—Slight but definite excess of saliva in mouth; may have nighttime drooling.

   2—Moderately excessive saliva; may have minimal drooling.

(continued)

Table 6-1.   *(continued)*

      3—Marked excess of saliva with some drooling.

      4—Marked drooling; requires constant tissue or handkerchief.

  7. Swallowing

      0—Normal.

      1—Rare choking.

      2—Occasional choking.

      3—Requires soft food.

      4—Requires nasogastric tube or gastrotomy feeding.

  8. Handwriting

      0—Normal.

      1—Slightly slow or small.

      2—Moderately slow or small; all words are legible.

      3—Severely affected; not all words are legible.

      4—The majority of words are not legible.

  9. Cutting food and handling utensils

      0—Normal.

      1—Somewhat slow and clumsy, but no help needed.

      2—Can cut most foods, although clumsy and slow; some help needed.

      3—Food must be cut by someone, but can still feed slowly.

      4—Needs to be fed.

10. Dressing

      0—Normal.

      1—Somewhat slow, but no help needed.

      2—Occasional assistance with buttoning, getting arms in sleeves.

      3—Considerable help required, but can do some things alone.

      4—Helpless.

11. Hygiene

      0—Normal.

      1—Somewhat slow, but no help needed.

      2—Needs help to shower or bathe, or very slow in hygienic care.

      3—Requires assistance for washing, brushing teeth, combing hair, going to bathroom.

      4—Foley catheter or other mechanical aids.

12. Turning in bed and adjusting bed clothes

      0—Normal.

      1—Somewhat slow and clumsy, but no help needed.

      2—Can turn alone or adjust sheets, but with great difficulty.

      3—Can initiate, but not turn or adjust sheets alone.

      4—Helpless.

Table 6-1.   *(continued)*

13. Falling (unrelated to freezing)

    0—None.

    1—Rare falling.

    2—Occasionally falls, less than once per day.

    3—Falls an average of once daily.

    4—Falls more than once daily.

14. Freezing when walking

    0—None.

    1—Rare freezing when walking; may have start-hesitation.

    2—Occasional freezing when walking.

    3—Frequent freezing. Occasionally falls from freezing.

    4—Frequent falls from freezing.

15. Walking

    0—Normal.

    1—Mild difficulty. May not swing arms or may tend to drag leg.

    2—Moderate difficulty, but requires little or no assistance.

    3—Severe disturbance of walking, requiring assistance.

    4—Cannot walk at all, even with assistance.

16. Tremor

    0—Absent.

    1—Slight and infrequently present.

    2—Moderate; bothersome to patient.

    3—Severe; interferes with many activities.

    4—Marked; interferes with most activities.

17. Sensory complaints related to parkinsonism

    0—None.

    1—Occasionally has numbness, tingling, or mild aching.

    2—Frequently has numbness, tingling, or aching; not distressing.

    3—Frequent painful sensations.

    4—Excruciating pain.

III. Motor examination

18. Speech

    0—Normal.

    1—Slight loss of expression, diction, and/or volume.

    2—Monotone, slurred but understandable; moderately impaired.

    3—Marked impairment, difficult to understand.

    4—Unintelligible.

(continued)

Table 6-1.   *(continued)*

19. Facial expression

   0—Normal.

   1—Minimal hypomimia, could be normal "poker face."

   2—Slight but definitely abnormal diminution of facial expression.

   3—Moderate hypomimia; lips parted some of the time.

   4—Masked or fixed facies with severe or complete loss of facial expression; lips parted 0.25 in. or more.

20. Tremor at rest

   0—Absent.

   1—Slight and infrequently present.

   2—Mild in amplitude and persistent or moderate in amplitude, but only intermittently present.

   3—Moderate in amplitude and present most of the time.

   4—Marked in amplitude and present most of the time.

21. Action or postural tremor of hands

   0—Absent.

   1—Slight; present with action.

   2—Moderate in amplitude, present with action.

   3—Moderate in amplitude with posture holding as well as action.

   4—Marked in amplitude; interferes with feeding.

22. Rigidity (judged on passive movement of major joints with patient relaxed in sitting position; cogwheeling to be ignored)

   0—Absent.

   1—Slight or detectable only when activated by mirror or other movements.

   2—Mild to moderate.

   3—Marked, but full range of motion easily achieved.

   4—Severe, range of motion achieved with difficulty.

23. Finger taps (patient taps thumb with index finger in rapid succession, with widest amplitude possible, each hand separately)

   0—Normal.

   1—Mild slowing and/or reduction in amplitude.

   2—Moderately impaired. Definite and early fatiguing. May have occasional arrests in movement.

   3—Severely impaired. Frequent hesitation in initiating movements or arrests in ongoing movement.

   4—Can barely perform the task.

24. Hand movements (patient opens and closes hand in rapid succession with widest amplitude possible, each hand separately)

   0—Normal.

   1—Mild slowing and/or reduction in amplitude.

   2—Moderately impaired. Definite and early fatiguing. May have occasional arrests in movement.

   3—Severely impaired. Frequent hesitation in initiating movements or arrests in ongoing movement.

   4—Can barely perform the task.

Table 6-1. *(continued)*

25. Rapid alternating movements of hands (pronation-supination movements of hands, vertically or horizontally, with as large an amplitude as possible, both hands simultaneously)

    0—Normal.

    1—Mild slowing and/or reduction in amplitude.

    2—Moderately impaired. Definite and early fatiguing. May have occasional arrests in movement.

    3—Severely impaired. Frequent hesitation in initiating movements or arrests in ongoing movement.

    4—Can barely perform the task.

26. Foot agility (patient taps heel on ground in rapid succession, picking up entire foot; amplitude should be approximately 3 in.)

    0—Normal.

    1—Mild slowing and/or reduction in amplitude.

    2—Moderately impaired. Definite and early fatiguing. May have occasional arrests in movement.

    3—Severely impaired. Frequent hesitation in initiating movements or arrests in ongoing movement.

    4—Can barely perform the task.

27. Arising from chair (patient attempts to arise from a straight-back wood or metal chair with arms folded across chest)

    0—Normal.

    1—Slow; or may need more than one attempt.

    2—Pushes self up from arms of seat.

    3—Tends to fall back and may have to try more than one time, but can get up without help.

    4—Unable to arise without help.

28. Posture

    0—Normal erect.

    1—Not quite erect, slightly stooped posture; could be normal for older person.

    2—Moderately stooped posture, definitely abnormal; can be slightly leaning to one side.

    3—Severely stooped posture with kyphosis; can be moderately leaning to one side.

    4—Marked flexion with extreme abnormality of posture.

29. Gait

    0—Normal.

    1—Walks slowly, may shuffle with short steps, but no festination or propulsion.

    2—Walks with difficulty but requires little or no assistance; may have some festination, short steps, or propulsion.

    3—Severe disturbance of gait, requiring assistance.

    4—Cannot walk at all, even with assistance.

30. Postural stability (response to sudden posterior displacement produced by pull on shoulders while patient erect with eyes open and feet slightly apart; patient is prepared)

    0—Normal.

    1—Retropulsion but recovers unaided.

    2—Absence of postural response; would fall if not caught by examiner.

    3—Very unstable, tends to lose balance spontaneously.

    4—Unable to stand without assistance.

(continued)

Table 6-1.   *(continued)*

31. Body bradykinesia and hypokinesia (combining slowness, hesitancy, decreased arm swing, small amplitude, and poverty of movement in general)

    0—None.

    1—Minimal slowness, giving movement a deliberate character; could be normal for some persons. Possibly reduced amplitude.

    2—Mild degree of slowness and poverty of movement which is definitely abnormal. Alternatively, some reduced amplitude.

    3—Moderate slowness, poverty or small amplitude of movement.

    4—Marked slowness, poverty or small amplitude of movement.

IV. Complications of therapy (in the past week)

    A. Dyskinesias

32. Duration: What proportion of the waking day are dyskinesias present? (historical information)

    0—None.

    1—1–25% of day.

    2—26–50% of day.

    3—51–75% of day.

    4—76–100% of day.

33. Disability: How disabling are the dyskinesias? (historical information; may be modified by office examination)

    0—Not disabling.

    1—Mildly disabling.

    2—Moderately disabling.

    3—Severely disabling.

    4—Completely disabling.

34. Painful dyskinesias: How painful are the dyskinesias?

    0—No painful dyskinesias.

    1—Slight.

    2—Moderate.

    3—Severe.

    4—Marked.

35. Presence of early morning dystonia (historical information)

    0—No.

    1—Yes.

    B. Clinical fluctuations

36. Are any "off" periods predictable as to timing after a dose of medication?

    0—No.

    1—Yes.

Table 6-1.   *(continued)*

37. Are any "off" periods unpredictable as to timing after a dose of medication?

    0—No.

    1—Yes.

38. Do any of the "off" periods come on suddenly (e.g., over a few seconds)?

    0—No.

    1—Yes.

39. What proportion of the waking day is patient "off" on average?

    0—None.

    1—1–25% of day.

    2—26–50% of day.

    3—51–75% of day.

    4—76–100% of day.

C. Other complications

40. Does the patient have anorexia, nausea, or vomiting?

    0—No.

    1—Yes.

41. Does the patient have any sleep disturbances (e.g., insomnia or hypersomnolence)?

    0—No.

    1—Yes.

42. Does the patient have symptomatic orthostasis?

    0—No.

    1—Yes.

V. Modified Hehn and Yahr staging

    Stage 0—No signs of disease.

    Stage 1—Unilateral disease.

    Stage 1.5—Unilateral plus axial involvement.

    Stage 2—Bilateral disease, without impairment of balance.

    Stage 2.5—Mild bilateral disease with recovery on pull test.

    Stage 3—Mild to moderate bilateral disease; some postural instability; physically independent.

    Stage 4—Severe disability; still able to walk or stand unassisted.

    Stage 5—Wheelchair-bound or bedridden unless aided.

VI. Modified Schwab and England Activities of Daily Living Scale

    100%—Completely independent. Able to do all chores without slowness, difficulty, or impairment. Essentially normal. Unaware of any difficulty.

    90%—Completely independent. Able to do all chores with some degree of slowness, difficulty, and impairment. Might take twice as long. Beginning to be aware of difficulty.

(continued)

Table 6-1. *(continued)*

80%—Completely independent in most chores. Takes twice as long. Conscious of difficulty and slowness.

70%—Not completely independent. More difficulty with some chores. Three to four times as long in some. Must spend a large part of the day with chores.

60%—Some dependency. Can do most chores, but exceedingly slowly and with much effort. Errors; some impossible.

50%—More dependent. Help with half, slower, etc. Difficulty with everything.

40%—Very dependent. Can assist with all chores, but few alone.

30%—With effort, now and then does a few chores alone or begins alone. Much help needed.

20%—Nothing alone. Can be a slight help with some chores. Severe invalid.

10%—Total dependent, helpless. Complete invalid.

0%—Vegetative functions such as swallowing, bladder and bowel functions are not functioning. Bedridden.

become obvious over 3–5 days of assessment. In some versions, the patient is asked to distinguish between "on" and "on with dyskinesias."

Although patient diaries can be helpful, a number of problems are encountered with diary information. The major one is that in some patients a poor correlation may be noted between their self-reports and objective assessment of parkinsonism. This may be due to several factors. First, in patients with diphasic or peak-dose dyskinesias, motor functioning may be impaired by dyskinesias, and it may be difficult for patients to reliably distinguish between "on" and "off" states. An additional problem is compliance; patients may fill out diaries retrospectively, and their recall of performance may be inaccurate; the chapter authors' group has noted a relatively poor correlation between nursing rating of parkinsonism under controlled conditions in a research ward and patient self-reports. Although these problems represent a serious limitation in their usefulness, patient diaries may be a simple and effective way of reporting a number of symptoms, including prolonged "off" periods, levodopa dose failures, and severe dyskinesias that otherwise may prove difficult to quantify and can be useful in both patient care and drug studies.

Validation

Until recently, little effort was made to estimate the variability either in the assessments between individual raters (inter-rater reliability) or in the reproducibility of scales over time. In recent years, several studies have validated scales in Parkinson's disease using a variety of methods.

In a study by Richards and colleagues (Richards et al., 1994), 24 patients with Parkinson's disease were rated by two of three neurologists with experience in the use of this scale. Overall, ratings agreed between raters (the correlation coefficient, r, was 0.8), suggesting good inter-rater reliability. Selected items such as speech ($r = 0.29$) and facial akinesia ($r = 0.07$) were less reliable. One potential cause for the latter is that a score of 1 is assigned to patients with equivocal impairment. For example, a facial hypokinesia score of 1 reflects an appearance possibly within normal limits for an older person, and the authors suggested that this ambiguity hinders agreement between different raters.

A second, large study evaluated the test-retest reliability of the UPDRS (Siderowf et al., 2002). Four hundred patients with early-stage Parkinson's disease who participated in a clinical trial were assessed on two occasions two weeks apart. The UPDRS was very reproducible; the overall correlation coefficient was 0.92 between the first and second ratings. Some individual items varied more between ratings; the correlation coefficient for items rating mental impairment was 0.76 (Siderowf et al., 2002).

A third study assessed 111 patients with Parkinson's disease using the UPDRS and the Hoehn and Yahr staging system, using a single rating physician (van Hilten et al., 1994). This study found a close correlation between the two measures but found that some items in the UPDRS dealing with activities of daily living correlated poorly. It also found that some items appeared to be redundant and could be omitted without adverse effects on the overall scale.

A fourth study validated the UPDRS by assessing 40 patients with multiple raters and by a single neurologist's assessment of 127 patients over four hospitals in different regions (Martinez-Martin et al., 1994).

They found good agreement between different raters (overall $r = 0.98$). The least reliable items were facial expression, estimating the severity of sensory symptoms, and estimating overall bradykinesia. Using the Hoehn and Yahr stage as an independent variable, this study found a significant correlation ($r = 0.71$) between the UPDRS and the Hoehn and Yahr stage, also noting that six items in the UPDRS accounted for most of the correlation.

Other studies have also tried to identify the most meaningful items in the UPDRS to shorten the test. In one study involving 65 patients, three raters compared different disability ratings. Six items from part II of the UPDRS were internally consistent; were reproducible between different raters; and correlated well with the Hoehn and Yahr scale, the Columbia University Rating Scale, and the Webster Rating Scale (Martinez-Martin et al., 2000). Another study compared an abbreviated scale to the UPDRS. In this scale, which the authors termed the *Short Parkinson's Evaluation Scale*, each item is rated on a three-point scale. The evaluation of mentation was shortened to three items, the evaluation of activities of daily living shortened to eight items, the motor examination shortened to eight items, and the complications of therapy section shortened to four items. This scale was found to be very reproducible between different raters and equally reliable to the full UPDRS and was faster to use (Rabey et al., 1997).

Finally, a number of studies have demonstrated that metabolic changes in the basal ganglia, seen in patients with Parkinson's disease using positron emission tomography or single-photon emission computed tomography, correlate to a rough extent with clinical markers of disease severity (Benamer et al., 2000; Eidelberg et al., 1995; Rinne et al., 1999; Seibyl et al., 1995).

Taken together, these studies demonstrate that ratings of Parkinson's disease are generally reliable, reproducible, and reflect biochemical markers of disease severity from functional imaging studies.

Administration

The UPDRS is administered by a combination of patient interview and physical examination. It can be administered by a physician, a nurse experienced in Parkinson's disease, or a trained technician. Depending on the skill of the rater and interactions with the patient, the UPDRS requires approximately 20–30 minutes to administer; in one of the previous studies, the UPDRS took an average of 17 minutes to administer. In practice,

the motor portion of the UPDRS is the briefest to administer, particularly in mildly affected patients.

Dyskinesia

Description

A dyskinesia scale appropriate for Parkinson's disease was reported by Goetz and colleagues (1994) using a scale based on videotaped ratings of performance of motor tasks (Table 6-2). Patients are videotaped performing four tasks (walking, drinking from a cup, putting on a coat, and buttoning), and an overall severity score is assigned (0–5). The different types and most severe dyskinesias are also identified.

Validation

The description of the scale also included validation measures. Videotapes of 20 patients were reviewed on two occasions by multiple raters, including physicians and study coordinators. Agreement between raters on the severity, type of dyskinesia, and severity of dyskinesia was good for both groups of raters ($r = 0.8$–0.9). Ratings were also reproducible within individual raters.

Administration

The dyskinesia scale is easily performed by either a physician or a trained technician and may be used either during an interview or from a videotape. One advantage of this scale is that the rating is clearly defined relative to physical appearance and by performance of a motor task, features that reduce subjectivity.

Although it is useful, there are some limitations to this scale. First, it does not assess the distribution or amplitude of movements and may not be appropriate for some studies or uses. Second, many dyskinesias occur only at specific times of the day and may not be readily observed during office evaluations. Finally, the intensity of pain or other symptoms is not estimated on this scale. Nonetheless, the scale can be performed reasonably quickly and may be useful as an adjunct to the UPDRS.

Dystonia

A number of scales have been developed for dystonia, including scales for assessment of generalized dystonia and torticollis. Separate scales for craniocervical

Table 6-2. Dyskinesia Rating Scale

Directions

1. View the patient walk, drink from a cup, put on a coat, and button clothing.

2. Rate the severity of dyskinesias. These may include chorea, dystonia, and other dyskinetic movements in combination. Rate the patient's worst function.

3. Check which dyskinesias are observed (more than one response possible).

4. Check the type of dyskinesia that is causing the most disability on the tasks seen on the tape (only one response is permitted).

Severity rating code

0   Absent

1   Minimal severity, no interference with voluntary motor acts

2   Dyskinesias may impair voluntary movements but patient is normally capable of undertaking most motor acts

3   Intense interference with movement control, and daily life activities are greatly limited

4   Violent dyskinesias, incompatible with any normal motor task

Dyskinesias present
(more than one choice possible)

	Chorea (C)	Dystonia (D)	Other (List)	Most Disabling Dyskinesia (Choose One)		
Severity of worst dyskinesia observed	(0–4)	(0–4)	(0–4)	C	D	Other

dystonia and writer's cramp have also been devised (Weiner & Lang, 1989).

Description

A scale for generalized dystonia was devised by Fahn and Marsden in 1981, originally for use in a therapeutic trial of trihexyphenidyl. It has been subsequently used in a variety of genetic and pharmacologic studies (Burke et al., 1985). The scale (Table 6-3) rates the severity of movements affecting different body parts, each on a 5-point scale. The appearance of dystonic movements in each body part is also rated in relationship to the amount of activity required to produce the movements: 1 represents dystonia appearing only with action; 4 is assigned to persistent dystonia at rest. Truncal and limb movements are assigned a weight of 1, and cranial or cervical movements are assigned a weight of 0.5, for a maximal total score of 120. There is also a separate, disability scale.

Two brief scales have been described for rating spasmodic torticollis. In the Spasmodic Torticollis Rating Scale (developed by Fahn et al., see Weiner et al.,

1989), the degree of turn and tilt is rated from 0 to 6 and sagittal movements (antecollis or retrocollis) are rated from 0 to 3. These are added for a maximal score of 15 and multiplied by a severity factor from 0 to 4, for a maximum score of 60 (Table 6-4). The Torticollis Severity Scale (Tsui et al., 1986) rates rotation, tilt, and sagittal movements each on a 0–3 scale, for a maximum of 9. Head tremor is also rated from 0 to 2. Each of these items is multiplied by a duration score from 0 to 2, and shoulder elevation is also rated from 0 to 3, for a total possible score of 25 (Table 6-5).

More recently, other standardized scales have been devised to rate the severity of cervical dystonia. The Toronto Western Spasmodic Torticollis Rating Scale (TWSTRS) (Consky & Lang, 1994) is a composite scale. Part I is based on physical findings, part II rates disability, and part III rates pain. It is currently available on a Web site, http://www.wemove.org, which contains a detailed description and forms for the scale. A second scale, named the *Cervical Dystonia Severity Scale* is similar to the short, spasmodic torticollis rating scale presented in Table 6-5. In the Cervical Dystonia Severity Scale, a protractor and wall chart are used to

Table 6-3. Dystonia Movement Scale

Region	Provoking Factor		Severity Factor	Weight	Product
Eyes	0–4	X	0–4	0.5	0–8
Mouth	0–4	X	0–4	0.5	0–8
Speech/swallowing	0–4	X	0–4	1.0	0–16
Neck	0–4	X	0–4	0.5	0–8
Right arm	0–4	X	0–4	1.0	0–16
Left arm	0–4	X	0–4	1.0	0–16
Trunk	0–4	X	0–4	1.0	0–16
Right leg	0–4	X	0–4	1.0	0–16
Left leg	0–4	X	0–4	1.0	0–16

Sum: (maximum = 120)

I. Provoking factor

    A. General

        0—No dystonia at rest or with action

        1—Dystonia on particular action

        2—Dystonia on many actions

        3—Dystonia on action of distant part of body or intermittently at rest

        4—Dystonia present at rest

    B. Speech and swallowing

        1—Occasional, either or both

        2—Frequent either

        3—Frequent one and occasional other

        4—Frequent both

II. Severity factors

    Eyes

        0—No dystonia present

        1—Slight: occasional blinking

        2—Mild: frequent blinking without prolonged spasms of eye closure

        3—Moderate: prolonged spasms of eyelid closure, but eyes open most of the time

        4—Severe: prolonged spasms of eyelid closure, with eyes closed at least 30% of the time

(continued)

Table 6-3.   *(continued)*

Mouth

    0—No dystonia present

    1—Slight: occasional grimacing or other mouth movements (e.g., jaw open or clenched; tongue movements)

    2—Mild: movement present <50% of the time

    3—Moderate dystonic movements or contractions present most of the time

    4—Severe dystonic movements or contractions present most of the time

Speech and swallowing

    0—Normal

    1—Slightly involved; speech easily understood or occasional choking

    2—Some difficulty in understanding speech or frequent choking

    3—Marked difficulty in understanding speech or inability to swallow firm foods

    4—Complete or almost complete anarthria, or marked difficulty swallowing soft foods and liquids

Neck

    0—No dystonia present

    1—Slight: occasional pulling

    2—Obvious torticollis, but mild

    3—Moderate pulling

    4—Extreme pulling

Arm

    0—No dystonia present

    1—Slight dystonia: clinically insignificant

    2—Mild: obvious dystonia, but not disabling

    3—Moderate: able to grasp, with some manual function

    4—Severe: no useful grasp

Trunk

    0—No dystonia present

    1—Slight bending, clinically insignificant

    2—Definite bending, but not interfering with standing or walking

    3—Moderate bending, interfering with standing or walking

    4—Extreme bending of trunk preventing standing or walking

Leg

    0—No dystonia present

    1—Slight dystonia, but not causing impairment; clinically insignificant

    2—Mild dystonia: walks briskly and unaided

    3—Moderate dystonia: severely impaired walking or requires assistance

    4—Severe: unable to stand or walk on involved leg

Table 6-3. *(continued)*

Disability scale

A. Speech

    0—Normal

    1—Slightly involved; easily understood

    2—Some difficulty in understanding

    3—Marked difficulty in understanding

    4—Complete or almost complete anarthria

B. Handwriting (tremor or dystonia)

    0—Normal

    1—Slight difficulty; legible

    2—Almost illegible

    3—Illegible

    4—Unable to grasp to maintain hold on pen

C. Feeding

    0—Normal

    1—Uses "tricks"; independent

    2—Can feed, but not cut

    3—Finger food only

    4—Completely dependent

D. Eating/swallowing

    0—Normal

    1—Occasional choking

    2—Chokes frequently; difficulty swallowing

    3—Unable to swallow firm foods

    4—Marked difficulty swallowing soft foods and liquids

E. Hygiene

    0—Normal

    1—Clumsy; independent

    2—Needs help with some activities

    3—Needs help with most activities

    4—Needs help with all activities

F. Dressing

    0—Normal

    1—Clumsy, independent

    2—Needs help with some activities

    3—Needs help with most activities

    4—Helpless

G. Walking

    0—Normal

    1—Slightly abnormal; hardly noticeable

    2—Moderately abnormal; obvious to naïve observer

    3—Considerably abnormal

    4—Needs assistance to walk

    6—Wheelchair-bound

rate the severity of head deviation in three planes of motion (rotation, antecollis-retrocollis, and tilt).

Validation

The scale for evaluation of primary torsion dystonia has been validated by assessment of videotapes. In this evaluation (Burke et al., 1985), 10 patients were rated on a simple global evaluation scale (0–5) and by the Dystonia Movement Scale; in addition, patients were rated twice by two examiners. A close correlation ($r = 0.9$) was found in ratings between different raters, and an almost 100% correlation between repeated ratings, demonstrat-

ing both good inter-rater and intra-rater reliability; both trained and untrained raters performed consistently.

There have been fewer published studies describing the reliability of focal dystonia scales. The Cervical Dystonia Severity Scale was evaluated by assessing 42 patients with cervical dystonia, rated by two different raters at each of four centers, twice in the same day. The scale was very reproducible within and between different raters, with correlations ranging from 0.79 to 0.94 (O'Brien et al., 2001).

There are no published studies of verification of the TWSTRS scale, but it has been widely used to evaluate the effects of botulinum toxin, and improvements

Table 6-4. Spasmodic Torticollis Rating Scale*

A. Turn/tilt + sagittal

    Rate degrees of turn (chin to side of turn) plus degrees of tilt (ear down toward shoulder)

        0—0 degrees

        1—1–15 degrees

        2—15–30 degrees

        3—30–45 degrees

        4—45–60 degrees

        5—60–75 degrees

        6—75–90 degrees

    Add rating for sagittal deviation (antecollis/retrocollis)

        0—Absent

        1—Mild

        2—Moderate

        3—Severe

	Left	*Right*
Turn		
Tilt		
Sagittal		
Total		

B. Severity factor

    0—None

    1—Occasional deviation only

    2—Mild: deviation present <50% of time

    3—Moderate: excursions to maximal deviation present 50–75% of time *or* deviation present most of the time, but excursions largely submaximal

    4—Severe: excursions to maximal deviation present 75–100% of time

Score (A) turn/tilt + sagittal × (B) severity factor = total score

    Add rating for dystonia elsewhere (Fahn-Marsden Scale).

    Also record duration able to hold head in fixed central position; taken to first twitch of movement in direction of torticollis: maximum = 60 sec (mean of two trials).

*Some torticollis rating scales include a separate score for shoulder elevation.

Table 6-5. Torticollis Severity Scale

A. Amplitude of sustained movements:
  1. Rotation: 0 = absent, 1 = <15 degrees, 2 = 15–30 degrees, 3 = >30 degrees
  2. Tilt: 0 = absent, 1 = <15 degrees, 2 = 15–30 degrees, 3 = >30 degrees
  3. Anterograde/retrograde: 0 = absent, 1 = mild, 2 = moderate, 3 = severe

Combined A score—

B. Duration of sustained movements: 1 = intermittent, 2 = constant

C. Shoulder elevation: 0 = absent, 1 = mild and intermittent, 2 = mild and constant or severe and intermittent, 3 = severe and constant

D. Tremor severity: 1 = mild, 2 = severe

Duration:
  1 = occasional, 2 = continuous
  Severity + duration = D score
  Total score = (A × B) + C + D

after this treatment are reflected by changes in the TWSTRS score. One study, however, did not find a good correlation between motor findings from the brief Torticollis Severity Scale (indicated in Table 6-5) and pain and disability sections of the TWSTRS scale in 64 patients receiving botulinum toxin injections (Lindeboom et al., 1998). In this study, the nonmotor assessments changed more after injections, and the authors suggested that measurements of pain and disability may be more meaningful than motor examinations in patients with cervical dystonia.

Administration

The scales for both generalized dystonia and torticollis can be administered by either a physician or a technician trained in evaluation and recognition of dystonia. Both scales are brief and quick to administer.

Special Considerations

One feature of dystonia is that in some patients a variety of sensory "tricks" (*geste antagoniste*), such as touching the chin or talking, may partially or completely suppress the dystonic movements, and

patients should be instructed to not use such maneuvers while they are being evaluated. Other patients with task-specific dystonias may exhibit involuntary movements only under specific situations, such as writing; such triggering factors should be used for rating these patients.

Tourette's Syndrome

Among the movement disorders, tic disorders can be the most difficult to evaluate and assess quantitatively. Patients may exhibit a large variety of simple and complex motor and phonic tics that may appear and disappear over time.

Many patients also experience psychological symptoms such as obsessions, and many complex motor tics may blend into compulsive behaviors and make distinction between tics and compulsions arbitrary.

Several scales have been devised in an effort to quantify tics and associated behaviors. These include rating instruments based on a symptom checklist, an objective tic rating, or both. One symptom checklist that has been extensively used is the Tourette Syndrome Symptom List, which was developed at Yale to assist parents in assessing tic behaviors (Cohen et al., 1984); similar scales have been described by other investigators, ranging from simple, such as the Hopkins Motor/Vocal Tic Scale (Walkup et al., 1992), to complex, such as the Tourette's Syndrome Global Scale (TSGS).

Objective tic ratings are included in several scales. A scale described by Goetz and colleagues (1987) is based on tic counts from a short videotaped protocol. Other tic ratings are included in composite scales; these include the TSGS, described by Harcherik and colleagues in 1984 (Harcherik et al., 1984), and the Shapiro Tourette's Syndrome Severity Scale (Leckman et al., 1988). Many of these investigators also participated on a committee to develop a standardized scale, the Unified Tic Rating Scale, which is under development.

Description

The TSGS (Table 6-6) is a composite scale, roughly divided into two sections. The first section rates the frequency of simple motor tics, complex motor tics, simple phonic tics, and complex phonic tics on a scale of 1–5 (1 is one or fewer tics in 5 minutes, 5 is virtually uncountable), and the degree of disruption is graded on a scale of 1–5 (1 is easy to camouflage, 5 is disruptive to the point of making it impossible to

Table 6-6.   Tourette's Syndrome Global Scale

Name_____	Date_____	Rater_____

Code for Frequency	Frequency (F)	Disruption (D)
1 = 1 or less in 5 min		
2 = 1 in 2.0–4.9 min		
3 = from 1 in 1.9 min to 4 in 1 min		
4 = 5 or more in 1 min		
5 = virtually uncountable		
Simple motor (SM): Nonpurposeful tics, jerks, and/or movements	1 2 3 4 5	1 2 3 4 5 F × D =
Complex motor (CM): Purposeful, thoughtful actions (systematic actions), rituals, touching self, others, or objects	1 2 3 4 5	1 2 3 4 5 F × D =
Simple phonic (SP): Nonpurposeful noises, throat clearing, coughing	1 2 3 4 5	1 2 3 4 5 F × D =
Complex phonic (CP): Purposeful, insults, coprolalia, words, distinguishable speech	1 2 3 4 5	1 2 3 4 5 F × D =

Behavior (B) (conduct)

   0   No problem

   5   Subtle problems; normal peer, school, and family relations

  10 Some problems, at least one relationship area impaired

  15 Clear impairment in more than one area

  20 Serious impairment, affects all areas

  25 Unacceptable social behavior, constant supervision

School and learning problems

   0   No problem

   5   Low grades

  10 Should be or in some special classes, or repeated

  15 All special classes

  20 Special school

  25 Unable to remain in school, homebound

Motor restlessness (MR)

   0   Normal movement

   5   Adventitial movements, visible, no problem

  10 Increased motor restlessness, clearly visible, some problem

  15 Clear motor restlessness, moderate problem

  20 Mostly in motion but occasionally stops, impaired functioning

  25 Nonstop motion, clearly cannot function

Work and occupation problems

   0   No problem

   5   Stable job, some difficulty

  10 Serious problems

  15 Lost lots of jobs

  20 Almost never employed

  25 Unemployed

([SM + CM]12) = ([SP + CP]/2) + ([B + MR + school or work problems] × 2/3) = global score

(continued)

Table 6-6. *(continued)*

Severity rating scales

  Motor tics

    0—Absent

    1—Minimal; could be normal

    2—Mild; limited to a single muscle group

    3—Moderate; limited to a single body part

    4—Severe; involving more than one body part

    5—Extreme; complex behavior

  Vocalizations

    0—Absent

    1—Minimal; could be normal

    2—Mild; single words or sounds, separated by at least one breath or 4 sec

    3—Moderate; words or sounds repeated two or three times in series or single obscenities separated by at least one breath or 4 sec

    4—Severe; words or sounds repeated four or more times in series or obscenities repeated two or three times in series

    5—Extreme; obscenities repeated four or more times in series

otherwise function). Each of these is multiplied and is added and averaged. A second section uses a simple 0–25 scale for behavior, motor restlessness, school/learning or work/occupational problems, and these three items are also averaged; they are then weighted for a composite total score.

A second scale is described by Goetz and colleagues (1987) and uses videotape ratings. Patients are recorded for 2 minutes, seated at rest, without the examiner present; segments taped at near and at far are obtained. They are scored on a five-point motor tic and vocal tic scale, identifying tics in 11 different body parts. Tics are counted for 1 minute.

Validation

Twenty patients with Tourette's syndrome were compared using the TSGS, Tourette Syndrome Symptom List, Hopkins Motor/Vocal Tic Scale, Clinical Global Impression (reviewed in Leckman et al., 1988), and Child Behavior Checklist, using three raters and an hour-long, structured interview. This study found excellent inter-rater reliability for all scales, as well as good reliability between tests. The study found that the ratings of tics did not correlate with the presence of attention-deficit/hyperactivity disorder or obsessive-compulsive symptoms (Walkup et al., 1992). Similar results were obtained in a separate study of the TSGS (Leckman et al., 1988).

The videotape protocol was also validated (Goetz et al., 1987). Thirty patients were evaluated at 3-week intervals while taking placebo tablets as part of a controlled trial of clonidine. The scale was found to be highly reliable between raters (Pearson's ranged from $r = 0.8$ to $r = 0.98$ for evaluation of motor and vocal tic frequency and severity, and $r = 0.6$ for tic distribution). A moderate agreement ($r = 0.5–0.6$) was found after repeated evaluations, suggesting some waxing and waning of tic severity. This study also found that although rating of motor tic severity and frequency correlated with each other closely ($r = 0.8$), as did vocal tics ($r = 0.9$), there was a poor correlation between these two different tic types ($r = 0.4$), suggesting that a single summary measure is inadequate. A second portion of the study compared the tic counts to the TSGS in 12 patients and found a moderate correlation (motor tics, $r = 0.5$, vocal tics, $r = 0.6$). Finally, nine patients given neuroleptics for tics demonstrated a significant improvement in videotape tic counts.

Administration

Although portions of these scales may be administered by a trained technician, assessment and distinction between tics and other movements or sounds are difficult and require special expertise and training; they are best performed by a physician or an experienced research nurse. Many items are rated by answers to structured interviews, also requiring internal consistency in quantifying answers.

A quiet room is required for video recording; if more than one assessment is obtained, it is best to standardize the conditions under which video recordings are obtained.

Time to Administer

Unlike other movement disorders, the assessment of Tourette's syndrome is time-consuming. Even the simpler scales may take 30–45 minutes to administer, and evaluation by the Unified Tic Rating Scale may take more than an hour. This scale also requires special training; many items are obtained by structured interview, and interpretation of answers to questions by patient, spouse, or parents at times may be subjective.

Although the previously described scales have been validated and appear to be integrally reliable and consistent, the evaluation of Tourette's syndrome is difficult and affected by a variety of factors. These include waxing and waning of signs, a poor correlation between symptoms and motor signs, and a poor correlation between psychological and physical symptoms, and the overall clinical usefulness of ratings in a clinic setting is uncertain. If a rating is used, a simple rating of motor and vocal tic frequency and severity, such as the TSGS, is more quickly performed and therefore may be of greater practical use than more comprehensive scales.

Tardive Dyskinesia

A number of scales have been developed to evaluate extrapyramidal side effects seen in patients treated with dopaminergic antagonists. Of these, the Abnormal Involuntary Movement Scale (AIMS), described in the 1970s, is the most widely used and has been used to assess choreic movements in other disorders, including Parkinson's and Huntington's diseases (Guy, 1976). A second scale, the St. Hans Rating Scale for extrapyramidal syndromes, was also developed in the 1970s and has been widely applied (Gerlach et al., 1993).

Description

The AIMS (Table 6-7) consists of rating the severity of movements in seven regions, each on a 5-point scale, ranging from 0 (none) to 4 (severe), and a separate rating of the overall severity of the abnormal

movements, judged on the amplitude of movements, incapacitation, and patient awareness of movements. Specific postures and positions, including sitting in the chair, opening the mouth, tapping the thumb against each finger, holding the hands outstretched, and standing and walking, are included. Dental status is also rated as the presence or absence of problems with teeth or dentures (this latter assessment is included because edentulous individuals may sometimes exhibit involuntary movements without exposure to drugs).

Validation

Thirty-three patients were rated by two experienced and two inexperienced psychiatrists on at least two occasions. Significant correlations of moderate degree were found between raters (r ranged from 0.5 to 0.8 depending on body region). In general, the experienced raters were more consistent over time and had greater agreement (Lane et al., 1985).

A second study compared the AIMS to the St. Hans Rating Scale for the assessment of tardive dyskinesia (Gerlach et al., 1993). In this study, 30 patients were evaluated three times, once from a live examination and two additional times from review of a videotape from the same examination. Seven raters (two experienced, two with less experience, three naïve) performed the examinations and ratings. Intra-rater reliability was generally good; correlations ranged from 0.7 to 0.9 and did not differ between experienced and inexperienced raters. Inter-rater reliability also was good, with the experienced raters showing slightly greater agreement. There was good agreement between the two scales.

Administration

The AIMS is simple to administer, taking 10 minutes or less to perform. It may be performed by either a physician or a nurse trained in evaluation of involuntary movements.

Huntington's Disease Rating Scale

The Unified Huntington's Disease Rating Scale is a research tool developed by the Huntington's Study Group. This is a composite measure that includes a motor section and sections assessing cognitive function, behavioral abnormalities, and functional impairment. The original version is published (Huntington Study Group, 1996); the rating scale was revised in 1999 and is copyrighted. The rating scale has been

Table 6-7. Abnormal Involuntary Movement Scale

Definitions of 0–4 scale

Rate highest severity observed. Rate movements that occur on activation one less than those observed spontaneously. Use the following scale:

0 = none

1 = minimal

2 = mild

3 = moderate

4 = severe

Movement ratings

Muscles of facial expression

Examples: movements of forehead, eyebrows, periorbital area, cheeks; include frowning, blinking, smiling, grimacing

Lips and periorbital area

Examples: puckering, pouting, smacking

Jaw

Examples: biting, clenching, chewing, mouth opening, lateral movement

Tongue

Examples: rate only increase in movements, both in and out of mouth, *not* inability to sustain movement

Upper extremities

Examples: choreic movements (i.e., rapid, objectively, purposeless, irregular, spontaneous), athetoid movements (i.e., slow, irregular, complex, serpentine); do *not* include tremor (i.e., repetitive, regular, rhythmic)

Lower extremities

Examples: lateral knee movement, foot tapping, heel dropping, foot squirming, inversion and eversion of foot

Trunk

Examples: rocking, twisting, squirming, pelvic gyrations

Global judgment

Patient's awareness of abnormal movements

0 = none

1 = aware, no distress

2 = aware, mild distress

3 = aware, moderate distress

4 = aware, severe distress

Either before or after completing the examination procedure, observe the patient unobtrusively at rest (e.g., in waiting room). The chair to be used in this examination should be a hard, firm one without arms.

1. Ask patient whether there is anything in his/her mouth (e.g., gum, candy) and if there is to remove it.

2. Ask patient about the current condition of his/her teeth. Ask patient if he/she wears dentures.

(continued)

Table 6-7.   *(continued)*

3. Ask patient whether he/she notices any movements in mouth, face, hands, or feet. If yes, ask to describe and to what extent they currently bother patient or interfere with his/her activities.

4. Have patient sit in chair with hands on knees, legs slightly apart, and feet flat on floor. (Look at entire body for movements while in this position.)

5. Ask patient to sit with hands hanging unsupported. If male, between legs, and if female and wearing a dress, hanging over knees. (Observe hands and other body areas.)

6. Ask patient to open mouth. (Observe tongue at rest within mouth.) Do this twice.

7. Ask patient to protrude tongue. (Observe similarities of tongue movement.) Do this twice.

8. Ask patient to tap thumb with each finger, as rapidly as possible for 10–15 sec; separately with right hand, then with left hand. (Observe facial and leg movements.)

9. Flex and extend patient's left and right arm (one at a time).

10. Ask patient to stand up. (Observe in profile. Observe all body parts again, hips included.)

11. Ask patient to extend both arms outstretched in front with palms down. (Observe trunk, legs, and mouth.)

12. Have patient walk a few paces, turn, and walk back to chair. (Observe hands and gait.) Do this twice.

Scoring system instructions

Complete examination procedure before making ratings.

Movement ratings: Rate highest severity noted. Rate movements that occur on activation one less than those observed spontaneously.

Code: 0 = none; 1 = minimal may be extreme normal; 2 = mild; 3 = moderate; 4 = severe

(Circle one)

Facial and oral movements

1. Muscles of facial expression (e.g., movements of forehead, eyebrows, periorbital area, cheeks; include frowning, blinking, smiling, grimacing)	0	1	2	3	4
2. Lips and periorbital area (e.g., puckering, pouting, smacking)	0	1	2	3	4
3. Jaw (e.g., biting, clenching, chewing, mouth opening, lateral movement)	0	1	2	3	4
4. Tongue: rate only increase in movement both in and out of mouth, *not* inability to sustain movement	0	1	2	3	4

Extremity movements

5. Upper (arms, wrist, hands, fingers): include choreic movements (i.e., rapid, objectively, purposeless, irregular, spontaneous), athetoid movements (slow, irregular, complex, serpentine). Do *not* include tremor (i.e., repetitive, regular, rhythmic)	0	1	2	3	4
6. Lower (legs, knees, ankles, toes; e.g., lateral knee movement, foot tapping, heel dropping, foot squirming, inversion and eversion of foot)	0	1	2	3	4

Table 6-7. *(continued)*

Trunk movements					
7. Neck, shoulders, hips (e.g., rocking, twisting, squirming, pelvic gyrations)	0	1	2	3	4
Global judgments					
8. Severity of abnormal movements	0	1	2	3	4
9. Incapacitation due to abnormal movements					
10. Patient's awareness of abnormal movements					
Dental status					
11. Current problems with teeth and/or dentures	No	0			
	Yes	1			
12. Does patient usually wear dentures?	No	0			
	Yes	1			

extensively tested for internal consistency within the various sections and between different sections; it has also been found to change with disease progression in a large cohort of patients.

Conclusion

A number of scales for the assessment of movement disorders are presented in this chapter. Most have been demonstrated to be reasonably reproducible and to correlate well with each other. In the case of the UPDRS, a good correlation has been seen between the extent of loss of dopaminergic nerve terminals and the motor score, suggesting that for this scale (and presumably others), the disease severity score does reflect the pathologic abnormalities seen in the disease.

Practical issues, such as the ease of use and availability of the scale, should be emphasized in selecting a scale. For patient care, these scales sometimes add little, and their routine use should not be viewed as mandatory—for example, the appearance of tics may not correlate well with the patient's perception of interference with daily activities, and quantification of these diseases may not be helpful. However, quantitative assessment of other diseases, such as Parkinson's disease or dystonia, may allow comparison of different patients and may reveal trends in symptom patterns that may otherwise not be apparent. For Parkinson's disease, the motor section of the UPDRS is quickly performed, and its inclusion in a patient clinic visit

may be useful. Similarly, one of the brief assessments of dystonia may be useful in a variety of settings; assessment of torticollis by a brief scale, for example, may aid not only in the overall assessment of disease severity but also in the selection of different muscles for injection.

References

Benamer HT, Patterson H, Wyper DJ, et al. Correlation of Parkinson's disease severity and duration with 1231-FP-CIT SPECT striatal uptake. *Mov Disord* 2000;15: 692–98.

Burke RE, Fahn S, Marsden CD, et al. Validity and reliability of a rating scale for the primary torsion dystonias. *Neurology* 1985;35:73–77.

Canter CJ, de la Torre R, Mier M. A method of evaluating disability in patients with Parkinson's disease. *J Nerv Ment Dis* 1961;133:143–47.

Cohen DJ, Leckman JF, Shaywitz BA. The Tourette syndrome and other tics. In: Shaffer D, Ehirhardt AA, Greenwill L (eds.). *The clinical guide to child psychiatry.* New York: Free Press, 1984.

Consky ES, Lang AE. Clinical assessments of patients with cervical dystonia. In: Jankovic J, Hallett M (eds.). *Therapy with botulinum toxin.* New York: Marcel Dekker 1994:211–37.

Defer GL, Widner H, Marie RM, et al. Core Assessment Program for Surgical Interventional Therapies in Parkinson's Disease (CAPSIT-PD). *Mov Disord* 1999;14: 572–84.

Eidelberg D, Moeller JR, Ishikawa T, et al. Assessment of disease severity in parkinsonism with fluorine-18-fluorodeoxyglucose and PET. *J Nucl Med* 1995;36:378–83.

Fahn S, Elton RL, Members of the UPDRS Development Committee. In: Fahn S, Marsden CD, Calne DB, et al. (eds.). *Recent developments in Parkinson's disease.* Vol. 2. Fiorham Park, NJ: Macmillan Health Care Information, 1987:153–64.

Gerlach I, Korsgaard S, Clemmensen P, et al. The St. Hans Rating Scale for extrapyramidal syndromes: reliability and validity. *Acta Psychiatr Scand* 1993;87:244–52.

Goetz CG, Stebbins GT, Shale HM, et al. Utility of an objective dyskinesia rating scale for Parkinson's disease: Inter- and intrarater reliability assessment. *Mov Disord* 1994;9:390–94.

Goetz CG, Tanner CM, Wilson RS, et al. A rating scale for Gilles de La Tourette's syndrome: description, reliability, and validity data. *Neurology* 1987;37:1542–44.

Guy W. *ECDEU assessment manual for psychopharmacology.* DHEW publication, No. 76–338. Washington: U.S. Government Printing Office, 1976:534–37.

Harcherik DF, Leckman JF, Detlor J, et al. A new instrument for clinical studies of Tourette's syndrome. *J Am Acad Child Adolesc Psychiatry* 1984;23:153–60.

Hoehn MM, Yahr MD. Parkinsonism: onset, progression, and mortality. *Neurology* 1967;17:427–42.

Huntington Study Group. Unified Huntington's disease rating scale: reliability and consistency. *Mov Disord* 1996;11:136–142.

Lane RD, Glazer WM, Hansen TE, et al. Assessment of tardive dyskinesia using the Abnormal Involuntary Movement Scale. *J Nerv Ment Dis* 1985;173:353–57.

Langston JW, Widner H, Goetz CG, et al. Core Assessment Program for Intracerebral Transplantations (CAPIT). *Mov Disord* 1992;7:2–13.

Leckman JF, Towbin KE, Ort SI, et al. Clinical assessment of tic disorder severity. In: Cohen DJ, Bruun RD, Leckman JE (eds.). *Tourette's syndrome and tic disorders.* New York: Wiley, 1988:55–78.

Lindeboom R, Brans JW, Aramideh M, et al. Treatment of cervical dystonia: a comparison of measures for outcome assessment. *Mov Disord* 1998;13:706–712.

Martinez-Martin P. Rating scales in Parkinson's disease. In: Jankovic J, Tolosa E (eds.). *Parkinson's disease and movement disorders.* Baltimore: Williams & Wilkins, 1993:281–92.

Martinez-Martin P, Fontan C, Frades Payo B, et al. Parkinson's disease: quantification of disability based on the Unified Parkinson's Disease Rating Scale. *Neurologia* 2000;15:382–87.

Martinez-Martin P, Gil-Nagel A, Gracia LM, et al. Unified Parkinson's Disease Rating Scale characteristics and structure. *Mov Disord* 1994;9:76–83.

O'Brien C, Brashear A, Cullis P, et al. Cervical Dystonia Severity Scale reliability study. *Mov Disord* 2001;16:1086–90.

Richards M, Marder K, Cote L, et al. Interrater reliability of the Unified Parkinson's Disease Rating Scale Motor Examination. *Mov Disord* 1994;9:89–91.

Rabey JM, Bass H, Bonuccelli U, et al. Evaluation of the Short Parkinson's Evaluation Scale: a new friendly scale for the evaluation of Parkinson's disease in clinical drug trials. *Clin Neuropharmacol* 1997;20:322–37.

Rinne JO, Ruottinen H, Bergman J, et al. Usefulness of a dopamine transporter PET ligand [(18)F]beta-CFT in assessing disability in Parkinson's disease. *J Neurol Neurosurg Psychiatry* 1999;67:737–41.

Schwab RS. Progression and prognosis in Parkinson's disease. *J Nerv Ment Dis* 1960;130:556–66.

Seibyl JP, Marek KL, Quinlan D, et al. Decreased single-photon emission computed tomographic [123I]beta-CIT striatal uptake correlates with symptom severity in Parkinson's disease. *Ann Neurol* 1995;38:589–98.

Siderowf A, McDermott M, Kieburtz K, et al. Test-retest reliability of the Unified Parkinson's Disease Rating Scale in patients with early Parkinson's disease: results from a multicenter clinical trial. *Mov Disord* 2002;17:758–63.

Tsui JK, Eisen A, Mak E, et al. Double-blind study of botulinum toxin in spasmodic torticollis. *Lancet* 1986;2:245–47.

van Hilten JJ, van der Zwan AD, Zwinderman AH, et al. Rating impairment and disability in Parkinson's disease: evaluation of the Unified Parkinson's Disease Rating Scale. *Mov Disord* 1994;9:84–88.

Walkup IT, Rosenberg LA, Brown J, et al. The validity of instruments measuring tic severity in Tourette's syndrome. *J Am Acad Child Adolesc Psychiatry* 1992;30:472–77.

Webster DD. Critical analysis of the disability in Parkinson's disease. *Mod Treatment* 1968;5:257–82.

Weiner WI, Lang AE. *Movement disorders: a comprehensive survey.* Mount Kisco, NY: Futura, 1989.

Yahr MD, Duvoisin RC, Schear MJ, et al. Treatment of parkinsonism with levodopa. *Arch Neurol* 1969;21:343–54.

7 Multiple Sclerosis and Demyelinating Diseases

Robert M. Herndon, M.D., and Jeffrey I. Greenstein, M.D.

Selection and evaluation of patients with multiple sclerosis (MS) for clinical trials present a continuing challenge. It has long been recognized that accurate diagnosis is critical both for understanding the natural history of MS and for treatment. The earliest known diagnostic criteria for MS were those of Charcot (1877) and were intended for clinical purposes. Attempts to codify diagnostic criteria for clinical trials required more stringent criteria primarily because of the frequency with which other diseases have been mistakenly diagnosed as MS. Because enlisting misdiagnosed cases in clinical trials can seriously confound the results, formal diagnostic criteria were developed. The first such criteria, to our knowledge, were developed by a committee that met at the University of Wisconsin in May 1960, chaired by George Schumacher, and the criteria became known as the Schumacher criteria (Schumacher et al., 1965). These were revised and updated at a meeting in Washington, D.C., in April 1983 chaired by Charles Poser and variously known as the Washington conference criteria or Poser criteria (Poser et al., 1983). More recently, they were further revised and updated by an international committee that met in London (McDonald et al., 2001).

The earliest published attempts to develop rating scales in MS appear to be those of Arkin et al. (1950) and Alexander (1951). The Kurtzke disability status scale was published in 1955 and appears to be an outgrowth of these earlier scales. It was revised and expanded as the Extended Disability Status Scale (EDSS) in 1983 (Kurtzke, 1983). Despite severe limitations, it became the *de facto* standard for MS clinical research.

A number of major problems make development of scales to assess MS particularly difficult. These include (1) the large variety of noncommensurate signs and symptoms seen in the disease, (2) the difficulty in identifying boundaries in a continuum of physical signs and symptoms, and (3) the difficulty in developing standards with good intra- and inter-rater reliability in a disease with so many different signs and symptoms. How does one put such noncommensurate items as some minor hand incoordination, optic disk pallor with a small paracentral scotoma, internuclear ophthalmoplegia, facial numbness, and paraplegia on a single scale? In fact, in many instances we probably shouldn't attempt to have all these items on a single scale. The facial numbness and optic disk pallor don't belong on a disability scale, although the visual impairment may. The attempt to be comprehensive and include all signs and symptoms in the scales is often inappropriate and can degrade sensitivity. Even though each represents an underlying pathology, its significance in measures designed for a particular purpose must be considered. In a treatment trial, the objective is to detect change with a high degree of sensitivity and a minimum of false positives. In this situation, a new sign, such as a new internuclear ophthalmoplegia or new facial weakness, which has essentially no impact on disability, can still be a valuable indication of new or continuing disease activity. This has little to do with disability but is an indication of further demyelination. On the other hand, a change in mobility can also be an indication of disease activity and also affects disability and handicap.

The difficulty in identifying boundaries in a continuum of motor strength, coordination, or altered sensation that will be agreed upon by different observers and that will not shift over time for the same examiner presents a major challenge. Some fairly clear boundaries can be identified in some systems, but overall this presents a severe problem for reproducibility. It can be avoided in some situations by using quantitative measures such as timed gait, quantitative strength assessment using a dynamometer, and timed upper extremity tests, etc. This was done with the quantitative neurologic assessment in the ACTH trial (Rose et al., 1968), and this approach was subsequently expanded (Potvin et al., 1975). Nevertheless, there remain important findings in most situations in which there is no reasonable alternative to subjective assessment.

The third major problem is that scales, designed for a single purpose, are used and even considered a standard for a variety of different purposes once they become accepted. This has rarely been discussed. Scales used for clinical trials in early exacerbating remitting MS, scales for assessment of change during an attack, scales used for trials in late progressive MS, scales used for assessment of symptomatic therapies, and scales for assessment of disability and rehabilitation have different requirements. Failure to recognize the difference in requirements has led to the use of existing, widely accepted scales for purposes for which they are ill suited.

The Kurtzke scale is widely regarded as the gold standard in MS trials, so much so that a research proposal for an MS trial will almost automatically be turned down if it does not include assessment using the Kurtzke scale. It is used in widely varying kinds of trials—from trials designed for attack prevention,

symptomatic therapy, and rehabilitation. It is poorly adapted to trials in the middle and higher disability range where it lacks sensitivity and where more objective measures of upper and lower extremity function are more sensitive, reliable, and reproducible. In the lower ranges, many of the boundaries are ambiguous, but it is quite sensitive to new neurologic events. Basically, it changes from a multi-item impairment scale to a mobility scale around the 3.5 level. This led Weiss and Stadlan (1992) to conclude that only patients with a Kurtzke EDSS of less than 3.5 should be included in clinical trials.

In our opinion, this is the wrong conclusion. It is based on the assumption that the Kurtzke scale is the "gold standard" in clinical trials. The appropriate conclusion is that we need scales that are more sensitive and specific in the middle and more advanced stages of the disease. Goodkin et al. (1995) demonstrated in their methotrexate trial that better scales for clinical trials are possible. They showed a clear effect of methotrexate in more advanced progressive MS using a composite scale and a relatively small cohort of 60 patients—30 in each arm of a controlled clinical trial. Subsequently, this led to a detailed analysis of cohorts and tests from a number of clinical trials resulting in the Multiple Sclerosis Functional Composite (MSFC) scale (Rudick et al., 1997). This development effort is continuing, with the aim of adding a visual function component to the Multiple Sclerosis Composite (Balcer et al., 2000, 2003). Although it has distinct advantages, this approach also has drawbacks. For example, there are significant ceiling effects with the ambulation component, which becomes uninformative when the patient can no longer walk 25 ft.

Some effort has been made to develop scales targeted to specific types of trials, but the complexity of the task and the wide acceptance of the Kurtzke EDSS have discouraged new scale development. Many clinicians and investigators still believe that, if you can't show an effect on the Kurtzke EDSS, it is not a clinically meaningful effect. The insensitivity to change is illustrated by the fact that the development of weakness in one arm in a person with a Kurtzke score of 4–6 might not affect the EDSS and might not even show on the pyramidal functional scale. Even complete loss of function in one arm might not affect the EDSS at this level. The result of nearly exclusive dependence on the EDSS is that trials are larger, longer, and more expensive than necessary.

Many trials have depended on counting new attacks of MS as a simple and easy approach, but it is fraught with dangers as detailed below. MS presents a particularly difficult problem for measurement because so many of the findings are noncommensurate. Whether for clinical trials, prognostic purposes, assessment of rehabilitation, or for outcomes research, there is no satisfactory scale. Part of the problem is expecting too much from a scale by expecting it to serve too many purposes. A scale suitable for treatment trials has very different requirements and characteristics from one aimed at assessing rehabilitation or one intended for outcomes research. Even a scale designed for treatment trials aimed at preventing attacks will have different characteristics from one designed to prevent disease progression or disability. A scale for a treatment trial of an agent to prevent attacks should be sensitive to essentially any new neurologic sign. For this reason standard neurologic examination is usually used and compared with the previous examination. On the other hand, some trials have used the EDSS or the Scripps neurologic rating scale for this purpose to provide a value for attack severity. By contrast, if the goal of the trial is to prevent disease progression and disability, accurate measurement of extremity function, vision, and cognition assumes greater importance.

In the early stages of MS, there are often a number of minor symptoms and impairments that have very little impact and would not even register on a disability scale but are detectable and represent a real underlying pathology. In the later stages with ataxia, paraplegia, or quadriplegia, one has impairment, disability, and handicap. One could use a combination of ambulation and upper extremity measures, but this ignores other important functions, such as vision and cranial nerve signs, which can be used to detect disease activity.

Willoughby and Paty (1988) proposed the following criteria for a new MS scale: "(1) Component subscales should be based as far as possible on signs elicited in a standard neurologic examination rather than on symptoms; (2) grades within each 'functional system' should be clearly described (more precise, for example, than mild, moderate, and severe); (3) selection of 'functional systems' . . . should be based primarily on ease and reliability of clinical assessment . . .; (4) increasing impairment should be accompanied by an increasing score; and (5) the method of combining the subscales to form an overall scale should be clear and simple." Although we agree that these are good criteria for an impairment scale, we believe such a scale is unlikely to prove as efficient, sensitive, or specific for clinical trials as a more quantitative scale, such as the MSFC.

A good scale for clinical trials needs to be as objective as possible with sensitivity and specificity over the full range to be tested in the trial. If the scale does not cover the full range of the disease, the clinical trial will need to restrict entry level on the scale being used and require a scale that is sensitive to change in patients within the entry level window. For clinical trials, combining simple, quantitative, individual, upper-extremity functional tests, such as the Nine-Hole Peg Test and/or Box and Blocks Test, with an ambulation test, such as a timed 10-m walk, timed tandem gait, or the Hauser ambulation index, provides excellent test-retest reliability. Adding a test of vision should increase range and sensitivity. Addition of an assessment of oculomotor function and assessment of the other cranial nerves might provide superior specificity and sensitivity for clinical trials where the object is to reliably detect new or continuing disease activity but is likely to prove uninformative in most trial situations. In principle, scales used in clinical trials, aside from quality of life scales, should not include symptoms unless they can be objectified on examination.

By contrast, scales for routine use in the clinic need to be efficient, reproducible with little intra- and inter-observer variability, and responsive to change in the patient. The EDSS and the MS functional composite are too cumbersome for general office use. A simpler scale that appears efficient and responsive is the Cambridge Multiple Sclerosis Basic Score. It has had very limited use, to date, but appears to have many of the properties needed for an office scale (Mumford & Compston, 1993; Sharrack et al., 1999). The Scripps Neurological Rating Scale, since it is based on the standard neurologic examination, would also appear adaptable for general office use (Sipe et al., 1984; Sharrack et al., 1999).

For rehabilitation purposes in MS, handicap scales such as the Barthel index or the Functional Independence Measure are more appropriate than the Kurtzke EDSS.

Diagnostic Criteria

Published diagnostic criteria include the Schumacher committee criteria, the Washington conference criteria (Poser et al., 1983), and the international panel criteria (McDonald et al., 2001). The first two were designed to provide a clear definition of MS for use in evaluating patients for clinical trials. The international panel crite-

Table 7-1. Washington Conference Diagnostic Criteria for Multiple Sclerosis

Category	Attacks	Clinical Evidence	Paraclinical Evidence	CSF, OB/IgG
Clinically definite				
CDMS A1	2	2	—	—
CDMS A2	2	1 and	1	—
Laboratory-supported definite				
LSDMS B1	2	1 or	1	+
LSDMS B2	1	2	—	+
LSDMS B3	1	1 and	1	+
Clinically probable				
CPMS C1	2	1	—	—
CPMS C2	1	2	—	—
CPMS C3	1	1 and	1	—
Laboratory-supported probable				
LSPMS D1	2	—	—	+

CDMS = clinically definite multiple sclerosis; CPMS = clinically probable multiple sclerosis; CSF = cerebrospinal fluid; IgG = immunoglobulin G; LSDMS = laboratory-supported definite multiple sclerosis; LSPMS = laboratory-supported probable multiple sclerosis; OB = oligoclonal bands.
Attack (bout, episode, exacerbation): The occurrence of a symptom or symptoms of neurologic dysfunction, with or without objective confirmation, lasting >24 hr.
Historical information: The description of symptoms by the patient.
Clinical evidence of a lesion: Signs of neurologic dysfunction demonstrable by neurologic examination. This includes signs no longer present if they were previously found on examination by a competent examiner.
Paraclinical evidence of a lesion: This includes such items as high signal areas on magnetic resonance imaging, abnormal evoked responses, and other tests that establish the presence of a lesion in the central nervous system.
Separate lesions: Separate signs or symptoms that cannot be explained on the basis of a single lesion.
Laboratory support: For purposes of these criteria includes evidence of elevated IgG synthesis on cerebrospinal fluid examination and oligoclonal bands.
From Poser CM, Paty DW, Scheinberg L, et al. New diagnostic criteria for multiple sclerosis: guidelines for research protocols. *Ann Neurol* 1983;13:227.

ria were intended for clinical use, and it was suggested that they could be modified or adapted for research use. Because the Schumacher criteria are mainly of historic interest, they have not been included in this edition. The Washington Conference (Poser) Criteria have been used in a number of recently completed clinical trials and are included for that reason.

Washington Conference (Poser) Criteria

The Washington conference criteria were designed to classify diagnostic status in known and suspected MS patients for purposes of clinical trials (Table 7-1). They

are, to a considerable extent, an expansion and refinement of the Schumacher criteria incorporating laboratory and imaging tests.

Description

This is a set of diagnostic criteria used to classify MS patients into one of two groups, definite and probable, each with two major subgroups. The traditional *possible MS* was not included because these patients were deemed unsuitable for clinical trials.

Validation

The criteria have obvious face validity because they formalize common clinical diagnostic criteria.

Formal validation would presumably require a large autopsy series to prove diagnosis pathologically. Such validation has never been reported.

How Administered

Determination of which criteria an individual meets is accomplished by the physician's history and examination in conjunction with review of any diagnostic procedures that have been carried out.

Time to Administer

The criteria require 45–60 minutes of history, neurologic examination, and record review. For established patients, it may require as little as 5–10 minutes to determine which diagnostic level the individual meets.

Advantages

These are useful criteria that use modern imaging and laboratory testing to add to the certainty of diagnosis. They became the standard criteria to establish diagnosis for clinical trials but have been largely superseded by the International Panel (McDonald) criteria.

Disadvantages

The criteria will exclude many progressive MS patients and will generally not be satisfactory for patients with relatively late-onset progressive spinal MS where the spinal fluid is often normal or borderline and there is no evidence of a lesion outside the spinal cord. Some investigators believe that these cases represent a different disease process and should be treated separately. Other investigators consider it to be simply MS with a different disease pattern.

Summary

These were the standard for MS diagnosis for clinical trials until the recent publication of the International Panel (McDonald) criteria. They are relatively straightforward and will result in inclusion of very few incorrectly diagnosed patients while excluding only a small number who do have the disease. In general, except in special purpose trials, only clinically or laboratory definite patients are suitable for inclusion in a clinical trial.

International Panel Diagnostic Criteria

The international panel criteria supersede the Washington conference criteria (Table 7-2). They eliminate the *laboratory-supported, clinically definite,* and the *probable MS* categories and formalize the use of magnetic resonance imaging (MRI) in the diagnosis. They are likely to undergo further revision as new information becomes available. They are based on a combination of clinical, laboratory, and MRI findings. Assessment adds little time to the standard work-up for MS. The criteria shown here are based on what evidence is available and what additional information is needed to meet the criteria. The caveat of "no better explanation" continues to apply.

Advantages

The international panel criteria allow for earlier diagnosis of MS in that MRI criteria can be used as evidence for dissemination in time or location. They are a significant update and improvement on the previous (Poser) criteria. They are quite conservative, so there will be very few false positives.

Disadvantages

The international panel criteria are quite complex, and few radiologists will report the MRI in enough detail to determine if the MRI meets the criteria. In most cases, the neurologist will need to make this determination. The criteria are quite conservative and many individuals with MS will not meet criteria for definite MS. If used for treatment decision, it could delay treatment in some patients who clearly have the disease.

Summary

The international panel criteria are revised and updated. Although reportedly designed for clinical use, because of their complexity, they are not likely to be widely used clinically. They are adaptable for research use and are likely to be used primarily in the research setting. They should be revisited and updated more frequently than such criteria have been reassessed in the past.

Scales and Measures for Evaluation of Multiple Sclerosis Patients

Attack Number or Frequency

Counting attacks is widely used in MS trials and is acceptable to the U.S. Food and Drug Administration.

Table 7-2. International Panel Diagnostic Criteria

Criterion No. 1

Two attacks, objective evidence of two or more lesions

Additional evidence needed

None

Criterion No. 2

Two attacks, objective evidence of one lesion

Additional evidence needed

Dissemination in space by MRI, or

Positive CSF and two or more MRI lesions consistent with MS, or

Further clinical attack involving a different site

Criterion No. 3

One clinical attack and two or more objective lesions

Additional evidence needed

Dissemination in time by MRI, or

Second clinical attack

Criterion No. 4

Monosymptomatic (clinically isolated syndrome)

Additional evidence needed

Dissemination in space by MRI, or

Positive CSF and two or more MRI lesions consistent with MS, and

Dissemination in time by MRI or second clinical attack

Criterion No. 5

No attacks, progression from onset

Additional evidence needed

Positive CSF and

Dissemination in space by MRI evidence of nine or more T2 brain lesions, or

Two or more cord lesions or four to eight brain lesions and one cord lesion, or

Positive VEP with four to eight MRI lesions, or

Positive VEP with fewer than four brain lesions and one cord lesion, or

Dissemination in time by MRI or continued progression for 1 yr

Definitions used with the International Panel Criteria

Positive MRI—three out of four of the following

One gadolinium-enhancing lesion or nine T2 hyperintense lesions if no enhancing lesion

One or more infratentorial lesions

One or more juxtacortical lesions

Three or more periventricular lesions

Note—One cord lesion can substitute for one brain lesion.

MRI evidence of dissemination in time

One gadolinium-enhancing lesion in a scan done at least 3 mo after onset of the clinical attack at a site different from the attack, or

In absence of an enhancing lesion at 3-mo scan, follow-up scan after an additional 3 mo showing enhancing lesion or new T2 lesion

Positive CSF

Oligoclonal bands in CSF, not in serum, or

Elevated IgG index

Positive VEP

Delayed but well-preserved VEP wave form

CSF = cerebrospinal fluid; IgG = immunoglobulin G; MRI = magnetic resonance imaging; MS = multiple sclerosis; VEP = visual evoked potential.
From McDonald WI, Compston A, Edan G, et al. Recommended diagnostic criteria for multiple sclerosis: guidelines from the International Panel on the Diagnosis of Multiple Sclerosis. *Ann Neurol* 2001;50:121–127.

It is usually done by having the patient report the attack to the unblinded treating physician in a trial who then sends the patient to a blinded examining physician to confirm the presence of objective change on the examination. It may be done using time to first exacerbation, attack frequency, or some other scale based on number or frequency of attacks. Often, some measure of attack severity, such as the Scripps scale, will be added so attack severity can be used.

Validation

To the authors' knowledge no attempt at formal validation of this measure has been done. It has fairly good face validity, but there are, in fact, good reasons to doubt its reliability as detailed below.

Administration

Testing requires the patient to contact the study site for a brief evaluation by the treating neurologist and subsequent confirmation by an examining neurologist who is presumably blind to treatment. Depending on the scale used by the examining neurologist, it may involve doing an EDSS and/or a Scripps scale. It is administered by a neurologist and involves a neurologic examination. Estimated time to administer is 15–45 minutes depending on the requirements for confirmation and the scale(s) used in the confirmation examination.

Attack or Attack Frequency

The number of verified attacks occurring in a set period, usually 1 year, is used. Alternatively, time to first attack following institution of therapy may be used.

Advantages

Advantages include simplicity, familiarity, and wide acceptance.

Disadvantages

Despite its familiarity and wide acceptance, this is a very poor and highly unreliable measure. If the patients and treating physicians are not really blind to treatment because of side effects, as in the phase III Betaseron trial or because the treatments differ such that blinding is not possible, as in the EVIDENCE trial (Panitch et al., 2002), you have an unblinded study. Reporting these studies as *double-blind* or even *single-blind* is patently wrong. Patients who think they are on therapy rather than placebo or think they are on a

stronger or weaker drug may differentially report attacks. Unreported attacks are unlikely to be detected. Unblinded physicians may differentially send patients for further examination again leading to unblinding. Finally, the examining physician knows the patient thinks he or she is having an attack and this may bias the examination results.

Summary

This is a widely accepted, and simple, yet to the authors an extremely poor measure. It is subject to multiple sources of bias. Unless the patient, treating physician, and examining physician are all blind to treatment, it cannot be legitimately considered double blind.

Kurtzke Extended Disability Status Scale

The Kurtzke Disability Status Scale was first published in 1955 (Kurtzke, 1955) and revised and updated in 1983 as the EDSS (Kurtzke, 1983) as a means of assessing progression of disability in MS (Table 7-3). The EDSS is a composite scale with a range from 0 to 10 in 0.5-point steps except that there is no 0.5. There are subscales for pyramidal, cerebellar, brainstem, sensory, bowel and bladder, visual, cerebral, and other functions (Table 7-4). Zero is normal without neurologic signs or symptoms. From 1 to 4, the score is derived from the subscales by a fairly complex, nonadditive method. At a level of 4 the scale becomes increasingly and then solely dependent on mobility. Seven is wheelchair-bound but able to self-transfer, and 10 represents death from MS. It has been widely used in MS clinical trials.

Validation

Reliability has been assessed and is fair. A two-point change appears to reflect a real difference (Noseworthy et al., 1990). With training an intra-rater reliability of one step and an inter-rater reliability of 1.5 steps was found within the range of 1.0–3.5. Testing was done on a single day, so it is not entirely clear that training will necessarily result in long-term performance at this level (Goodkin et al., 1992). There is greater sensitivity and reproducibility at higher levels where ambulatory distance and use of walking aids make assessment more objective and a 0.5 change may be detected with fairly good reliability.

Table 7-3.   Kurtzke Extended Disability Status Scale

0.0	Normal neurologic examination (all grade 0 in FS*).
1.0	No disability, minimal signs in one FS* (i.e., grade 1).
1.5	No disability, minimal signs in more than one FS (more than one grade 1).
2.0	Minimal disability in one FS (one FS grade 2, others 0 or 1).
2.5	Minimal disability in two FS (two FS grade 2, others 0 or 1).
3.0	Moderate disability in one FS (one FS grade 3, others 0 or 1) or mild disability in three or four FS (three or four FS grade 2, others 0 or 1) although fully ambulatory.
3.5	Fully ambulatory but with moderate disability in one FS (one grade 3) and one or two FS grade 2; or two grade 3 (others 0 or 1) or five grade 2 (others 0 or 1).
4.0	Fully ambulatory without aid, self-sufficient, up and about some 12 hr/day despite relatively severe disability consisting of one FS grade 4 (others 0 or 1), or combination of lesser grades exceeding limits of previous steps, and the patient should be able to walk >500 m without assist or rest.
4.5	Fully ambulatory without aid, up and about much of the day, may otherwise require minimal assistance; characterized by relatively severe disability usually consisting of one FS grade 4 (others 0 or 1) or combinations of lesser grades exceeding limits of previous steps and walks >300 m without assist or rest.
5.0	Ambulatory without aid for at least 50 m; disability severe enough to impair full daily activities (e.g., to work a full day without special provision). (Usual FS equivalents are one grade 5 alone, others 0 or 1; combinations of lesser grades.) Patient walks >200 m without aid or rest.
5.5	Ambulatory without aid for at least 50 m; disability severe enough to preclude full daily activities. (Usual FS equivalents are one grade 5 alone, others 0 or 1; or combinations of lesser grades.) Enough to preclude full daily activities. (Usual FS equivalents are one grade 5 alone, others 0 or 1; or combinations of lesser grades.) Patient walks >100 m without aid or rest.
6.0	Intermittent or unilateral constant assistance (cane, crutch, brace) required to walk at least 100 m. (Usual FS equivalents are combinations with more than one FS grade 3.)
6.5	Constant bilateral assistance (canes, crutches, braces) required to walk at least 20 m. (Usual FS equivalents are combinations with more than one FS grade 3.)
7.0	Unable to walk at least 5 m even with aid, essentially restricted to wheelchair; wheels self and transfers alone; up and about in wheelchair some 12 hr/day. (Usual FS equivalents are combinations with more than one FS grade 4+; very rarely pyramidal grade 5 alone).
7.5	Unable to take more than a few steps; restricted to wheelchair; may need aid in transfer; wheels self but cannot carry on in wheelchair a full day. (Usual FS equivalents are combinations with more than one FS grade 4+; very rarely pyramidal grade 5 alone.)
8.0	Essentially restricted to chair or perambulated in wheelchair but out of bed most of day; retains many self-care functions; generally has effective use of arms. (Usual FS equivalents are combinations, generally grade 4+ in several systems.)
8.5	Essentially restricted to bed most of day; has some effective use of arm(s); retains some self-care functions. (Usual FS equivalents are combinations generally 4 in several systems.)
9.0	Helpless bed patient; can communicate and eat. (Usual FS equivalents are combinations, mostly grade 4+.)
9.5	Totally helpless bed patient; unable to communicate effectively, eat, or swallow. (Usual FS equivalents are combinations almost all grade 4+.)
10.0	Death due to multiple sclerosis.

FS = functional system.
*A mental function grade of 1 does not enter in FS scores for disability status score steps.

Table 7-4. Functional Scale (FS) Definitions for the Extended Disability Status Scale (EDSS)

FS1—pyramidal functions

0   Normal.

1   Abnormal signs without weakness.

2   Mild weakness (4+).

3   Moderate paraparesis or hemiparesis (strength 4/5 or 4–/5); or severe monoparesis—grade >3/5.

4   Severe paraparesis or hemiparesis, moderate quadriparesis, or monoplegia; there still may be movement somewhere; there may be severe weakness in three limbs—grades 3 or 2.

5   Paraplegia, hemiplegia, or marked quadriparesis; there is no movement in the limbs. For example, both lower extremities or there is movement or severe weakness in four but not three limbs.

6   Quadriplegia; no movement in four limbs.

7   Not testable.

8   Unknown.

FS2—cerebellar functions

Use finger-to-nose test, heel-to-shin test, rapid alternating movements, and gait. You are testing cerebellar function of trunk and limbs—not weakness. If one or more limbs cannot be tested for cerebellar dysfunction (e.g., paraplegia or hemiplegia) but the remaining limbs can be tested, score only the remaining limbs.

0   Normal—no evidence of cerebellar dysfunction. This may be used if one or more limbs are incoordinated due to weakness, apraxia, or sensory loss but not due to cerebellar dysfunction (but also use X and code 1, line 40).

1   Abnormal signs without disability—slight abnormality on formal testing but does not interfere with activities of daily living.

2   Mild ataxia (see definitions)—limb or gait ataxia in any or all limbs adequate to noticeably interfere with function when the targeted function is stressed, including stressed gait hopping, toes, heels; physical or mechanical adaptation of the targeted activity is not necessary.

3   Moderate ataxia—use this if there is moderate ataxia in any or all limbs, in gait, or stressed gait. This is also used if there is severe ataxia of one limb. A moderate ataxia requires some physical or mechanical adjustment for the targeted activity to be completed (e.g., the patient must hold the wall to hop or be steadied by the examiner).

4   Severe ataxia—more than two limbs for routine activities and/or routine gait, but still functional, albeit with difficulty (e.g., may still be able to walk with aids and feed self). Use also if only remaining testable limb(s) is severely ataxic.

5   Unable to perform coordinated limb or routine gait movements due to ataxia. Use also if only remaining testable limb(s) is unable to perform coordinated movement due to ataxia.

7   Not testable.

8   Unknown—used after any number (0–5) to indicate that weakness (grade 3 or more on pyramidal) interfered with testing of any extremity.

FS3—brainstem functions

0   Normal.

1   Signs only (unsustained nystagmus, detectable impairment of saccadic pursuit or ocular dysmetria).

2   Sustained conjugate nystagmus, incomplete internuclear ophthalmoplegia, or other mild disability.

3   Dysconjugate nystagmus (internuclear ophthalmoplegia) or severe extraocular weakness, or moderate disability of other cranial nerves.

4   Severe dysarthria or other severe disability of other cranial nerves.

5   Inability to swallow or speak.

6   Not testable.

7   Unknown.

(continued)

Table 7-4. *(continued)*

FS4—sensory function

0   Normal.

1   Detectable vibration or figure-writing decrease only in one or two limbs.

2   Mild decrease in touch or pain or position sense and/or moderate decrease in vibration in one or two limbs, or vibratory decrease alone in three or four limbs.

3   Moderate decrease in touch or pain or position sense, and/or essentially lost vibration in one or more limbs; mild decrease in touch or pain and/or moderate decrease in all proprioceptive tests in three of four limbs.

4   Marked decrease in touch or pain or loss of nociception, alone or combined, in one or two limbs; or moderate decrease in touch or pain and/or severe proprioceptive decrease in more than two limbs.

5   Loss (essentially) of sensation in one or two limbs, or moderate decrease in touch or pain and/or loss of proprioception for most of the body below the head.

6   Sensation essentially lost below the head.

7   Not testable.

8   Unknown.

FS5—bladder and bowel function—ask about both bladder and bowel; score the worst, as follows

Bladder

0   Normal bladder function.

1   Bladder symptoms but no incontinence.

2   Incontinence less than once per week.

3   Incontinence more than once per week but less than daily.

4   More than daily incontinence.

5   Indwelling bladder catheter.

6   Grade 5 bladder function plus grade 5 bowel function.

7   Not testable.

8   Unknown.

Bowel

0   Normal bowel function.

1   Mild constipation but no incontinence.

2   Severe constipation but no incontinence.

3   Rare (once per week) bowel incontinence.

4   Frequent (more than weekly but less than daily) bowel incontinence.

5   No bowel control.

6   Grade 5 bladder function plus grade 5 bowel function.

7   Not testable.

8   Unknown.

FS6—visual function (all visual acuity is best corrected)

0   Normal visual acuity better than 20/30 and no sign of optic nerve disease.

1   Visual acuity (corrected) better than or equal to 20/30 with signs of optic nerve disease (e.g., if there is an afferent pupil defect).

2   Worse eye with maximal visual acuity (corrected) of 20/40 or 20/50.

Table 7-4. *(continued)*

3	Worse eye with maximal visual acuity (corrected) of 20/70; check both eyes.
4	Worse eye with maximal visual acuity (corrected) of 20/100 or 20/200.
5	Worse eye with maximal visual acuity (corrected) worse than 20/200 and maximal acuity of better eye of 20/60 or better.
6	Grade 5 plus maximal visual acuity of better eye of 20/60 or worse.
7	Not testable.
8	Unknown.

FS7—cerebral (or mental) function

0	Normal.
1	Mood alteration only (does not affect disability status scale score).
2	Mild decrease in mentation.
3	Moderate decrease in mentation.
4	Marked decrease in mentation (chronic brain syndrome—moderate).
5	Dementia or chronic brain syndrome—severe or incompetent.
6	Not testable.
7	Unknown.

FS8—other functions (any other neurologic findings attributable to multiple sclerosis)

Spasticity

0	None.
1	Mild (detectable only).
2	Moderate (minor interference with function).
3	Severe (major interference with function).
4	Not testable.
5	Unknown.

Other

0	None.
1	Any other neurologic findings attributed to multiple sclerosis; specify.
2	Unknown.

Definitions for motor and ataxia scales

Mild	A measurable abnormality in function that is noticeable to the patient and examiner but does not require any compensatory activity or assistive equipment to complete the tasks required.
Moderate	As above, but some compensation, whether physical or mechanical, is necessary to complete activity required.
Severe	Activity measured can be initiated but not consistently completed even with physical or mechanical adaptation.

Note: EDSS steps <4.5 refer to patients who are fully ambulatory, and the precise step is defined by the Functional System score(s). EDSS steps from 5 up are defined largely or entirely based on ambulation and mobility. Although functional system scores may still be done, they are provided as additional information and contribute to the EDSS only insofar as they affect mobility functions between EDSS 4.5 and 8.
From Kurtzke JF. Rating neurologic impairment in multiple sclerosis: an expanded disability status scale (EDSS). *Neurology* 1983; 33:1444–52.

Administration

The test is administered by a neurologist and involves a neurologic examination. Estimated time to administer is 15–25 minutes.

Special Considerations

At levels 4.0–6.5 you have to actually walk the patient to get a valid score because patients' estimates of how far they can walk are unreliable. Interpretation of steps is fairly complex and, for purposes of clinical trials, expanded definitions and scoring rules are necessary. In one recent trial, a 15-page explanation of how to score the Kurtzke was used.

Advantages

The scale has wide acceptance and is still the *de facto* standard for MS trials. It is widely understood so that most neurologists who work with MS patients have a general idea of how disabled someone with a particular score is.

Disadvantages

The Kurtzke scale has a number of important disadvantages. For the purpose of clinical trials, it is poorly responsive to change (Sharrak et al., 1999). Beyond the level of 5.5, an optic neuritis leaving the patient blind in one or both eyes would not affect the score. This has led to the unfortunate recommendation that only patients with scores less than 3.5 be included in clinical trials in MS, which excludes most patients and severely complicates recruitment for trials. It is not an impairment or a disability scale but a mixture. The distribution of patients on the scale in the hands of most investigators is bimodal (Willoughby & Paty, 1988) although Kurtzke insists that, in his hands, it is Gaussian (Kurtzke, 1989). Additionally, the sensory and the bowel and bladder scales are largely subjective, which makes them of limited suitability in clinical trials.

Summary

The Kurtzke scale has been widely used and regarded as the "gold standard." Its main current use should be for comparing current trials with previous trials that used the scale. Because of its poor inter-rater and intra-rater reliability, more quantitative scales, such as the MS Functional Composite Scale, are likely to be more useful in future clinical trials.

Scripps Neurological Rating Scale

The Scripps scale is basically an impairment scale and is scored from a standardized neurologic examination with inclusion by inquiry of mentation and mood and of bowel and bladder function (Table 7-5). It has a theoretical scoring range from 100 (normal) to –10 although in practice, scores below zero are unlikely to occur. This range results from giving negative scores for bowel and bladder dysfunction, whereas all other scores are subtracted from a maximum score for the particular function. It is weighted somewhat toward visual and motor functions.

Validation

In the initial report, four neurologists scored five examinations done by a single examining neurologist with a range of variability of less than 2.6%. Because the various functions are graded as normal, mild, moderate, or severe by the examining physician, this does not address the overall variability or validity. It does have reasonable face validity and responsiveness (Koziol et al., 1999), but correlation with the Kurtzke EDSS was poor, and in nine of 48 cases the direction of change was inconsistent (Koziol et al., 1997).

Time to Administer

It is scored from a standardized neurologic examination that should take approximately 20 minutes with approximately 5 minutes to derive the score from the examination.

Advantages

Because it is based on the neurologic examination, the Scripps scale can be scored from a routine standardized neurologic examination sheet. It assesses each extremity independently except for coordination where the upper extremities are scored together and the lower extremities are scored together. It appears more sensitive to change than the Kurtzke scale and is probably about as reliable.

Disadvantages

The Scripps scale still has not been adequately validated, and its reliability has not been adequately established. It does have face validity in that it is based on a standard neurologic examination, but its sensitivity and specificity in clinical trials have not been adequately established.

Table 7-5. Scripps Neurological Rating Scale

System Examined	Maximum Points	Degree of Impairment			
		Normal	Mild	Moderate	Severe
Mentation and mood	10	10	7	4	0
Cranial nerves	21				
Visual acuity		5	3	1	0
Fields, disks, pupils		6	4	2	0
Eye movements		5	3	1	0
Nystagmus		5	3	1	0
Lower cranial nerves	5	5	3	1	0
Motor	20				
RU		5	3	1	0
LU		5	3	1	0
RL		5	3	1	0
LL		5	3	1	0
DTRS	8				
UE		4	3	1	0
LE		4	3	1	0
Babinski R, L (2 each)	4	4	0	0	0
Sensory	12				
RU		3	2	1	0
LU		3	2	1	0
RL		3	2	1	0
LL		3	2	1	0
Cerebellar	10				
UE		5	3	1	0
LE		5	3	1	0
Gait, trunk, balance	10	10	7	4	0
Special category bladder/ bowel/sexual					
Dysfunction	0	0	−3	−7	−10
Totals	**100**				

DTRS = deep tendon reflexes; LE = lower extremity; LL = left lower; LU = left upper; RL = right lower; RU = right upper; UE = upper extremity.
From Sipe JC, Knobler RL, Braheny SL, et al. A neurologic rating scale (NRS) for use in multiple sclerosis. *Neurology* 1984;34:1368–1372.

Summary

The Scripps scale is a fairly straightforward scoring system for the neurologic examination but it has not been adequately validated. Inter- and intra-rater reliability have not been reported beyond the initial report. The fact that it correlates poorly with the Kurtzke EDSS is a point of concern.

Hauser Ambulation Index

The Hauser index (Table 7-6) is a straightforward historical and observational assessment of ambulation with a range from 0 (normal) to 9 (wheelchair; unable to transfer independently) (Hauser et al., 1983).

Validation

The test as a direct measure of mobility has face validity. Little further validation would appear necessary.

Administration

Assessment is generally done by a physician or nurse. At the lowest levels it is dependent on a history from the patient or family members describing interference with athletic activity or episodic imbalance. At levels 3–9 it is basically an observational assessment of mobility.

Time to Administer

The Hauser test is quite brief, involving observation of the patient walking and timing an 8-m walk.

Advantages

The test is extremely simple with little opportunity for intra- or inter-observer variability.

Disadvantages

It is inadequate as an overall measure of neurologic dysfunction in MS but can represent a useful component of an overall assessment.

Summary

The Hauser Ambulation Index is a simple and useful measure of independent mobility.

Table 7-6. Hauser Ambulation Index

Level	Assessment
0	Asymptomatic; fully active.
1	Walks normally, but reports fatigue that interferes with athletic or other demanding activities.
2	Abnormal gait or episodic imbalance; gait disorder is noticed by family and friends; able to walk 25 ft in 10 sec or less.
3	Walks independently; able to walk 25 ft in 20 sec or less.
4	Requires unilateral support (cane or single crutch) to walk; walks 25 ft in 20 sec or less.
5	Requires bilateral support (canes, crutches, or walker) and walks 25 ft in 25 sec or less; or requires unilateral support but needs >20 sec to walk 25 ft.
6	Requires bilateral support and >20 sec to walk 25 ft, may use wheelchair on occasion.
7	Walking limited to several steps with bilateral support; unable to walk 25 ft; may use wheelchair for most activities.
8	Restricted to wheelchair; able to transfer self independently.
9	Restricted to wheelchair; unable to transfer self independently.

From Hauser SL, Dawson DM, Lehrich JR, et al. Intensive immunosuppression in progressive multiple sclerosis: a randomized three-arm study of high dose intravenous cyclophosphamide, plasma exchange and ACTH. *N Engl J Med* 1983;308:173–80.

Box and Block Test and Nine-Hole Peg Test

The Box and Block and Nine-Hole Peg Tests are two simple, timed tests of upper extremity function that will be dealt with together (Mathiowetz et al., 1985; Goodkin et al., 1988; Oxford et al., 2003). The box and blocks apparatus consists of a box of specified dimensions divided into two sections and 2.5-cm hardwood blocks. Using one hand, the object is to move as many blocks as possible, one at a time, from one side of the divider to the other in 1 minute. Each hand is tested separately. The Nine-Hole Peg Test consists of a block with nine holes and nine pegs. The time taken to insert all nine pegs and then remove them is measured.

Validation

Both tests have face validity as tests of upper extremity dexterity. At first glance, both would seem to be measuring the same function but the Nine-Hole Peg Test requires finer dexterity. Goodkin et al. (1988) has shown that better sensitivity is obtained if both are used. Intra- and inter-rater reliability is extremely high. A 20% change in time has been shown to occur by chance less than 5% of the time. Norms for each have been published (Mathiowetz et al., 1985; Oxford et al., 2003).

Administration

The two tests can be administered by anyone after a few minutes of instruction.

Time to Administer

Depending on the individual's dexterity, both tests can be administered in 5–7 minutes.

Advantages

These highly reliable tests can be administered by anyone and give a reliable measure of upper extremity fine and gross dexterity.

Disadvantages

The tests require special equipment.

Summary

These tests are very useful quantitative measures of upper extremity function. Both test kits are available from http://www.westons.com/acatalog/Online_Catalogue_Dexterity_1460.html.

Multiple Sclerosis Functional Composite Scale

This test is a combination of a timed 8-m walk, Nine-Hole Peg Test done with each hand and the Paced Auditory Serial Addition Test (PASAT), 3-second version. Test results are converted to Z-scores that allow the use of parametric statistics with this scale. The test was developed by a committee under the auspices of the National MS Society to improve test reliability and objectivity in MS clinical trials (Rudick et al., 1997).

Validation

Test development was based on data from control patients in multiple clinical trials. The attempt was to find simple, quantitative, and reliable measures that would allow smaller clinical trials. Further validation was accomplished with the International MS Secondary Progressive Avonex Controlled Trial in secondary progressive MS in which the EDSS failed to show a significant change but the MSFC scale showed a significant change in hand function and a borderline change in cognitive function (Cohen et al., 2002). Although it has poor face validity, construct validity appears better than the EDSS in the range between EDSS 4 and 9 where the EDSS is almost exclusively dependent on mobility because it includes a measure of upper extremity and cognition as well as a measure of lower extremity function. Neither cognitive function nor upper extremity function is captured at all well by the EDSS.

Administration

This is done by a trained technician and requires a stopwatch, a tape player with a paced PASAT tape, recording sheets, and equipment for the Nine-Hole Peg Test.

Time to Administer

The test takes 15–25 minutes.

Multiple Sclerosis Functional Composite

1. Timed 8-m walk—the patient may use any walking aids needed and is timed over an 8-m course twice, with the times averaged.
2. Nine-Hole Peg Test (see Box and Block Test and Nine-Hole Peg Test).
3. Three-second PASAT—The patient listens to a tape in which a single-digit number is called out every 3 seconds. The task is to add the last two digits spoken. This involves stating the sum of the first two digits, dropping the sum and adding the second and third digits and repeating this with the next spoken digit.

Advantages

This is a simple, extremely reliable (Kalkers et al., 2004) measure of change in MS, which is easily done by a trained technician. Its advantages include its efficiency, reliability, and reproducibility. It also simplifies the statistics that can be used to assess the data.

Disadvantages

It requires equipment—that is, a nine-hole peg-board and pegs, stopwatch, PASAT tape, and player with recording sheets. It does not yet include a measure of vision though attempts are being made to update it with a visual measure. Although it covers the entire range of the disease, ambulation becomes uninformative when the patient can no longer walk 8 meters. It requires initial patient training, particularly on the PASAT, to minimize learning effects. Finally, scoring is complicated because it requires averaging the baseline values of the patients and determining the standard deviation in each patient cohort to arrive at the base Z-score against which change is measured. Many patients find the PASAT unpleasant and the refusal rate can be a significant problem.

Availability

Details, including a manual on its use, are available online from the National MS Society at http://www.nationalmssociety.org.

Summary

This is a highly reliable and efficient scale. It is much more sensitive and precise than the Kurtzke EDSS. It is more difficult to use in that Z-scores must be calculated and the clinical interpretation of the Z-score is not intuitively obvious as it is for the EDSS. The precision should allow the use of smaller numbers of patients in clinical trials relative to the EDSS. It is unlikely to find a place in office use although the Nine-Hole Peg Test and timed gait components are used in the office setting in some clinics.

Contrast Letter Acuity

When the selection of tests for the MSFC was made it was recognized that vision was a dimension that needed to be included. However, the visual measures available were not sufficiently informative. Contrast letter acuity has since been explored as a potential test for inclusion in the MSFC as this detects visual impairment even with 20/20 vision (Balcer et al., 2000; Balcer et al., 2003). Binocular contrast letter acuity using Sloan charts (Precision Vision, LaSalle, IL) has been used to provide a measure of overall visual function. The charts have a standardized format, and each corresponds to a dif-

ferent contrast level (these are gray shade letters on a white background at 100%, 2.5%, and 1.25% contrast). The total score for each chart is the number of letters correctly read until five letters in succession are not identified. The Sloan chart scores are converted to Z-scores based on the number of standard deviations from the mean baseline score for a study group. This Z-score can be incorporated into an MSFC score (MSFC-4 Z-score).

Validation

Test development was done using individuals with other forms of visual impairment. It has since been used in various groups with MS. Inter-rater reliability has been shown to be very high. Concurrent validity is being tested with cerebral MRI measures and with Optical Coherence Tomography. Predictive validation is being evaluated in the IMPACT study and in studies using natalizumab in relapsing MS.

Administration

This is done using a defined protocol by a trained technician and requires a Sloan Low-Contrast Letter Chart with appropriately standardized lighting.

Time to Administer

The test takes 10 minutes.

Advantages

This is an easily administered and reliable test of low-contrast vision. In other conditions it has proven reliable and reproducible. It has the potential to add an independent dimension to the MSFC.

Disadvantages

Testing must be done using a trained technician with equipment and standardized lighting. Visual acuity must be corrected by refraction prior to testing and Snellen visual acuities must be 20/200 or better. The data require manipulation similar to the other MSFC components.

Summary

This test appears to be a reliable measure of the impact of visual pathway involvement in MS that is more sensitive to change than visual acuity and much easier and more rapid than formal visual field testing. It is likely that it will be added to the MSFC in the near future.

Cambridge Multiple Sclerosis Basic Score

The Cambridge Multiple Sclerosis Basic Score is a composite score consisting of four items (a) disability and impairment, (b) relapse, (c) progression, and (d) handicap. Each is scored on a 1 to 5 basis. It is a simple rapid test suitable for office use (Mumford & Compston, 1993) (Table 7-7).

Validation

The psychometric properties of the Cambridge Multiple Sclerosis Basic Score was evaluated in comparison with the Kurtzke EDSS, the Scripps Neurological Rating Scale, the Functional Independence Measure, and the Hauser Ambulation Index. The Cambridge Multiple Sclerosis Basic Score was found to be "reliable (all four domains) and responsive (relapse and progression domains) but had limited validity (handicap domain)" (Sharrack et al., 1999).

Advantages

This is a short, reliable measure with good sensitivity suitable for office use and for following changes in disease progression and disability. It has had limited use to date, mainly in the United Kingdom.

Disadvantages

Despite apparently good reliability and sensitivity, its suitability for clinical trials is not at all clear. It appears particularly limited in the areas of disability and handicap.

Multiple Sclerosis Neuropsychological Screening Questionnaire

The Multiple Sclerosis Neuropsychological Screening Questionnaire is a short, self-administered screening questionnaire designed to identify those patients at risk for cognitive impairment. It comes in two forms—one for patients and one for a family member or caregiver.

Administration

Both forms are self-administered and should not require more than 1 or 2 minutes to complete. Scoring is simple and requires less than a minute.

Validation

The final set of questions was derived from 80 items reduced by Rasch analysis to the 15 items in the questionnaire (Benedict et al., 2003, 2004). The questionnaire has good face and construct validity. The patient questionnaire correlated with depression but not with objective tests of cognitive function, whereas the caregiver questionnaire correlated with objective tests of cognitive function. Upon testing, using a cut-off score of 27 gave a sensitivity of 0.83 and a specificity of 0.97 when compared with a neuropsychological summary score encompassing processing speed and memory. The questionnaire is copyright protected. It has been distributed by the National MS Society and can be found in the literature (Benedict et al., 2003).

Advantages/Disadvantages

This is an effective and efficient screening test for cognitive problems in MS patients. It is not a test of cognition but rather a screening instrument, and those with caregiver scores above the cut-off level of 27 should receive formal cognitive testing.

Quality-of-Life Measures for Multiple Sclerosis

The symptoms resulting from disease in MS may have a substantial impact on a patient's overall perception of well-being. However, perceptions of well-being are not readily quantified by traditional outcome measures (Fischer et al., 1999). Health-related quality of life (HRQL) is a multidimensional construct that assesses patients' perceptions of their overall health and physical functionding as well as their psychological and social/role functioning (Miller et al., 2001; Miller, 2003). Assessment of HRQL can help evaluate the impact of a disease and the effect of treatment on a patient's ability to perform physical and social activities.

HRQL measures are available as generic and disease-specific assessments. The Medical Outcomes Study Short Form-36 (SF-36) (Ware et al., 1993, 1995) is a widely accepted generic measure. The profile and subscales are considered in Chapter 14. Normative data are available for different disease groups. The scale has been used to study the impact of disease on patients with MS and to compare them with individ-

Table 7-7. Cambridge Multiple Sclerosis Basic Score

Disability

− Patient's disability unknown.

1 Fully independent patient with no disturbance of vision, sensation, sphincters, arm function, or mobility.

2 Patient with one only of mild fatigue, visual blurring but able to read, minor sensory symptoms, minor sphincter disturbance, altered arm function, or mild difficulty with walking.

3 Patient with one or more of frequent or permanent assistance with continence, significant visual symptoms preventing reading, inability to use one or both arms, significant pain or dysesthesia, requirement for bilateral assistance with walking, significant intellectual impairment.

4 Patient who is wheelchair-bound or has other major disability severely restricting daily activities.

5 Bed-bound or totally dependent on others for all care.

Relapse

− Relapse status cannot be assigned.

1 Quiescent or nonrelapsing pattern of illness.

2 Subjectively worse than baseline state but improving or objectively unchanged.

3 Subjectively worse than baseline state and continuing to deteriorate.

4 Significantly worse than usual as a result of established relapse.

5 Major deterioration necessitating hospital admission and increased dependency on caregivers.

Progression

− No knowledge of natural history of illness up to present time.

1 Apart from any recent acute changes, clinical condition has not changed in past year.

2 Minor deterioration in clinical condition over past year.

3 Significant increase in handicap or disability in past year.

4 Rapid increase in handicap or disability in past year.

5 Devastating progression in past year (i.e., "malignant" form of disease).

Handicap

Ask the patient to mark the line below to obtain a score for handicap.

"Role in life"

"How severely does your condition affect your ability to perform a normal role in life? Make a mark on one digit on the line below to indicate this. A mark on the figure 1 would indicate that your condition has no effect on your role in life, your occupation, or your ability to support your family. A mark on the figure 5 would mean that the condition renders you completely incapable of any useful role in life, and totally prevents you from fitting into your normal social role (e.g., ability to do your job, ability to take a normal part in family life). You may make a mark on any digit on the line."

| 1 | 2 | 3 | 4 | 5 |

uals with other conditions (Brunet et al., 1996; Norvedt et al., 1999; Freeman et al., 1996). The utility of the scale is limited to an extent in MS because of ceiling and floor effects (Freeman et al., 2000). There are a number of different quality of life inventories for MS. We present two of these that are based on the SF-36 with additional, disease-specific items that appear well validated: the Multiple Sclerosis Quality of Life–54 (MSQOL-54) and the Multiple Sclerosis Quality of Life Inventory (MSQLI). We have also included the Multiple Sclerosis Impact Scale in this section, which is a well-validated, self-report scale on the impact of MS on daily activities. A number of other scales, such as the Functional Assessment of Multiple Sclerosis (Cella et al., 1996), although reasonably well validated, have not been included as they are less widely used.

Multiple Sclerosis Quality of Life–54

The MSQOL-54 is a 54-item quality of life index based on the SF-36 with 18 additional disease-specific items (Vickrey et al., 1995). Thus, it has generic items, which are used across disease types, and items specifically directed at elucidating common problems seen in MS.

Validation

The SF-36, a widely used and extremely well-validated generic health scale, forms the basis of the MSQOL-54. The total scale was initially tested in a sample of 179 adults with clinically definite MS and with disease status that ranged from newly diagnosed to severely impaired. It has good face validity. Construct validity is based on associations with symptom severity, role function, mental health, and ambulatory status. As pointed out by Coulthard-Morris (2000), much of this is due to the SF-36 component of the scale.

Administration and Scoring

This is a self-administered scale, although more handicapped patients may require assistance in filling out the form. It typically requires 11–18 minutes for completion, although more time may be required for more handicapped patients. The scale and scoring and composite weighting information are available in the MSQOL-54 manual (Vickrey BG, MSQOL-54: Instructions and scoring manual, 1998, UCLA Department of Neurology C-128 RNRC Box 951769, Los Angeles, CA 90095-1769).

Advantages

This is a well-validated quality-of-life inventory for MS. It is relatively efficient and is based on the SF-36 that permits easy comparison of MS with other diseases.

Disadvantages

The SF-36 on which it is based is proprietary and requires permission/license from the Rand Corporation. Its length may limit repeated use. Little information has been published regarding its responsiveness over time.

Multiple Sclerosis Quality of Life Inventory

The MSQLI was developed by the Consortium of Multiple Sclerosis Centers in collaboration with the National Multiple Sclerosis Society (Ritvo et al., 1997; Fischer et al., 1999) as a measure of MS-specific HRQL. It includes the SF-36 as a core measure as well as a number of subscales that reflect the broad range of disease-specific symptoms and components of disability.

Multiple Sclerosis Quality of Life Inventory
Health Status Questionnaire (SF-36): 36 items
Modified Fatigue Impact Scale (MFIS): 21 items
MOS Pain Effects Scale: 6 items
Sexual Satisfaction Scale: 5 items
Bladder Control Scale: 4 items
Impact of Visual Impairment Scale: 5 items
Perceived Deficits Questionnaire: 20 items
Mental Health Inventory: 18 items
MOS Modified Social Support Survey: 18 items

Most of these scales with over six items have validated, short, five-item versions.

Validation

The inventory has been validated for content, reliability, construct validity, and item reduction (Ritvo et al., 1997). Each of the subscales has been thoroughly validated. Details of the method of question selection and validation are available in the MSQLI manual available through the National MS Society Web site at http://www.nationalmssociety.org.

Administration

The MSQLI is completed by the subject. It can generally be administered in 45 minutes.

Advantages

The MSQLI provides a comprehensive assessment of disease-specific HRQL. It has been used to evaluate treatment effects (Miller et al., 2001) and the impact of rehabilitation treatment on disease (Bethoux, 2001). It does not require hands-on investigator time and can be administered in the office, at a clinic, or at the patient's home. The fact that it includes the SF-36 makes it possible to use it to compare quality of life in different diseases.

Disadvantages

The scale does not provide a single number to capture overall quality of life, which makes comparisons between groups a bit more difficult. It is quite long and the length of time necessary to complete the MSQLI may limit the frequency with which it can be incorporated into a study. Insufficient data are available on longitudinal responsiveness of the measure. The SF-36 on which it is based is proprietary and requires permission/license for use.

Summary

This is an excellent quality of life scale that has been thoroughly validated. It is longer than the MSQOL-54 but has the advantage of having a number of well-validated subscales that can be used separately to assess particular aspects of disease or therapy.

Multiple Sclerosis Impact Scale

The Multiple Sclerosis Impact Scale is a 29-item, self-report scale developed at Queen Square Hospital under the auspices of the British National Health Service R&D Health Technology Assessment Program (Table 7-8). It was developed based on interviews of 30 patients with MS regarding the impact of MS on their lives, literature review, and expert opinion. Using this information, 129 questions were generated. These were sent out to 1,530 randomly selected members of the UK MS Society. The items were then studied for their psychometric properties and reduced to a total of 29.

Validation

After development and item reduction, the 29 questions were sent to 1,250 MS patients in a postal survey to assess data quality, scaling assumptions, acceptability, and reliability. They were tested for responsiveness in 55 patients hospitalized for rehabilitation and steroid treatment for relapses. Although designed and developed using information from patients with relapsing-remitting, secondary progressive, and primary progressive disease, as a new scale, its applicability in other populations will require further testing. Validation methodology used in development of this scale is detailed by Hobart et al. (2004). This excellent article is recommended for review and study by anyone wishing to develop a new scale, especially a self-report scale.

Administration

This is a self-administered test and took from 1 minute 45 seconds to 4 minutes 26 seconds in a sample of patients tested. A scoring manual is available from Dr. Jeremy Hobart, Consultant Neurologist, Peninsula Medical School, Department of Clinical Neurosciences, Derriford Hospital, Plymouth PL6 8DH, UK.

Advantages

This is a very carefully developed, rapid, self-report instrument that should prove useful in surveys of MS population and looks likely to be quite responsive to changes in patient condition.

Disadvantages

It is a very new test and has not been used widely, so norms are limited, and it has not been tested in populations outside the United Kingdom.

Summary

This is a new but well-validated scale suitable for population surveys. The article by Hobart et al. (2004) should be required reading for anyone interested in developing scales of this general type.

Fatigue in Multiple Sclerosis

Fatigue is a common and often troubling symptom of MS. It can significantly impair ability to function in day-to-day activities and, in some instances, affects employability. Several scales have been developed to

Table 7-8.   Multiple Sclerosis Impact Scale

The following questions ask for your views about the impact of multiple sclerosis (MS) on your day-to-day life during the past 2 wk. For each statement, please circle the one number that best describes your situation. Please answer all questions.

	Not at All	A Little	Moderately	Quite a Bit	Extremely
In the past 2 wk, how much has your MS limited your ability to					
1. Do physically demanding tasks?	1	2	3	4	5
2. Grip things tightly (e.g., turning on taps)?	1	2	3	4	5
3. Carry things?	1	2	3	4	5
In the past 2 wk, how much have you been bothered by					
4. Problems with your balance?	1	2	3	4	5
5. Difficulties moving about indoors?	1	2	3	4	5
6. Being clumsy?	1	2	3	4	5
7. Stiffness?	1	2	3	4	5
8. Heavy arms and/or legs?	1	2	3	4	5
9. Tremor of your arms or legs?	1	2	3	4	5
10. Spasms in your limbs?	1	2	3	4	5
11. Your body not doing what you want it to do?	1	2	3	4	5
12. Having to depend on others to do things for you?	1	2	3	4	5
In the past 2 wk, how much have you been bothered by					
13. Limitations in your social and leisure activities at home?	1	2	3	4	5
14. Being stuck at home more than you would like to be?	1	2	3	4	5
15. Difficulties using your hands in everyday tasks?	1	2	3	4	5
16. Having to cut down the amount of time you spent on work or other daily activities?	1	2	3	4	5
17. Problems using transport (e.g., car, bus, train, taxi, etc.)?	1	2	3	4	5
18. Taking longer to do things?	1	2	3	4	5
19. Difficulty doing things spontaneously (e.g., going out on the spur of the moment)?	1	2	3	4	5
20. Needing to go to the toilet urgently?	1	2	3	4	5
21. Feeling unwell?	1	2	3	4	5
22. Problems sleeping?	1	2	3	4	5
23. Feeling mentally fatigued?	1	2	3	4	5
24. Worries related to your MS?	1	2	3	4	5
25. Feeling anxious or tense?	1	2	3	4	5
26. Feeling irritable, impatient, or short tempered?	1	2	3	4	5
27. Problems concentrating?	1	2	3	4	5
28. Lack of confidence?	1	2	3	4	5
29. Feeling depressed?	1	2	3	4	5

From Hobart JC, Riazi A, Lamping DL, et al. Improving the evaluation of therapeutic interventions in multiple sclerosis: development of a patient-based measure of outcome. *Health Technol Assess* 2004;8:1–48.

assess fatigue. These include the Fatigue Severity Scale, Fatigue Impact Scale (FIS), and MFIS. Visual analogue scales have also been used.

Fatigue Severity Scale

The Fatigue Severity Scale is a nine-item, self-report, Likert scale with seven levels of agreement with each statement (Table 7-9). It was developed by the reduction of a 29-item questionnaire. It was initially tested in two populations—MS patients and systemic lupus erythematosus patients. It was able to clearly differentiate the fatigue of these two diseases from that in a normal population.

Administration

The test is self-administered and should not take more than 2–5 minutes.

Validation

The scale has good face validity and would be expected to have reasonable test-retest reliability.

Advantages

This is a straightforward, self-report scale which has better reliability and sensitivity than previously used analogue scales.

Disadvantages

There are no substantial disadvantages to the test.

Summary

The scale is a simple, straightforward scale that appears useful in assessing patient fatigue.

Modified Fatigue Impact Scale

The MFIS is a 21-item Likert scale—a modified version of the FIS (Fisk et al., 1994)—that looks at the effect of fatigue on daily activity over the previous 4 weeks (Table 7-10). Scoring of each item ranges from 0 (no impact) to 4 (almost always) with a maximum score of 84.

Administration

This is a self-administered test and should take 1–2 minutes to complete.

Table 7-9. Fatigue Severity Scale

Please indicate your level of agreement with each of the following statements, with 1 indicating strong disagreement and 7 strong agreement.

1. My motivation is lower when I am fatigued.
2. Exercise brings on my fatigue.
3. I am easily fatigued.
4. Fatigue interferes with my physical functioning.
5. Fatigue causes frequent problems for me.
6. My fatigue prevents sustained physical functioning.
7. Fatigue interferes with carrying out certain duties and responsibilities.
8. Fatigue is among my three most disabling symptoms.
9. Fatigue interferes with my work, family, or social life.

Validation

Gottschalk et al. (2005) correlated the FIS, MFIS, and a visual analogue scale of fatigue showing good criterion-related validity. The MFIS correlated better with the visual analogue scale than did the FIS. Kos et al. (2005) assessed the scale in four European countries, and they found no cultural or linguistic differences for Belgian, Italian, Slovenian, or Spanish versions.

Advantages

The MFIS is a short, well-validated measure of fatigue in MS. It forms a part of the MSQLI and is a useful self-report measure.

Disadvantages

Like all fatigue scales, the MFIS is entirely subjective. The score may be affected by mood—particularly depression—and an evaluation of depression should be included in studies using fatigue scales.

Summary and Conclusions

There is much yet to be done in developing better scales for clinical trials in MS. The development of the MS Functional Composite by a committee of the National MS Society represents a major advance. It has proven to be more sensitive to change and to have excellent concurrent and predictive validity. It is not a

Table 7-10.   Modified Fatigue Impact Scale

Following is a list of statements that describe how fatigue may affect a person. Fatigue is a feeling of physical tiredness and lack of energy that many people experience from time to time. In medical conditions like multiple sclerosis, feelings of fatigue can occur more often and have a greater impact than usual. Please read each statement carefully and then circle the one number that best indicates how often fatigue has affected you in this way in the *past 4 wk.* (If you need help in marking your responses, tell the interviewer the number of the best response.) *Please answer every question.* If you are not sure which answer to select, please choose the one answer that comes closest to describing you. The interviewer can explain any words or phrases that you do not understand.

Because of My Fatigue during the Past 4 Wk	Never	Rarely	Sometimes	Often	Almost Always
1. I have been less alert.	0	1	2	3	4
2. I have had difficulty paying attention for long periods of time.	0	1	2	3	4
3. I have been unable to think clearly.	0	1	2	3	4
4. I have been clumsy and uncoordinated.	0	1	2	3	4
5. I have been forgetful.	0	1	2	3	4
6. I have had to pace myself in my physical activities.	0	1	2	3	4
7. I have been less motivated to do anything that requires physical effort.	0	1	2	3	4
8. I have been less motivated to participate in social activities.	0	1	2	3	4
9. I have been limited in my abilities to do things away from home.	0	1	2	3	4
10. I have had trouble maintaining physical effort for long periods.	0	1	2	3	4
11. I have had difficulty making decisions.	0	1	2	3	4
12. I have been less motivated to do anything that requires thinking.	0	1	2	3	4
13. My muscles have felt weak.	0	1	2	3	4
14. I have been physically uncomfortable.	0	1	2	3	4
15. I have had trouble finishing tasks that require thinking.	0	1	2	3	4
16. I have had difficulty organizing my thoughts when doing things at home or at work.	0	1	2	3	4
17. I have been less able to complete tasks that require physical effort.	0	1	2	3	4
18. My thinking has been slowed down.	0	1	2	3	4
19. I have had trouble concentrating.	0	1	2	3	4
20. I have limited my physical activities.	0	1	2	3	4
21. I have need to rest more often or for longer periods.	0	1	2	3	4

substitute for the EDSS in that it is not as easily interpreted in clinical terms. It has ceiling effects in that ambulation becomes uninformative in the wheelchair patient. It also does not stage the disease, and one cannot easily estimate overall level of function based on the Z-score. Addition of a visual component, if successful, will enhance the scale's overall usefulness. Despite some limitations, the MSQLI-54 and other quality of life scales and the Multiple Sclerosis Impact Scale have the potential for adding an additional dimension of patient-generated assessment of MS therapeutic trials. A quality of life scale should be incorporated in most clinical studies to allow the measurement of different dimensions of the impact of the disease.

References

Alexander L. New concept of critical steps in course of chronic debilitating neurologic disease in evaluation of therapeutic response. *Arch Neurol Psychiatry* 1951;66: 253–58.

Arkin H, Sherman IC, Weinberg SL. Tetraethylammonium chloride in the treatment of multiple sclerosis. *Arch Neurol Psychiatry* 1950;64:536–45.

Balcer LJ, Baier ML, Pelak VS, et al. New low-contrast vision charts: reliability and test characteristics in patients with multiple sclerosis. *Multiple Sclerosis* 2000;6:163–71.

Balcer LJ, Baier ML, Cohen JA, et al. Contrast letter acuity as a visual component for the Multiple Sclerosis Functional Composite. *Neurology* 2003;61:1367–73.

Benedict RHB, Munschauer F, Linn R, et al. Screening for multiple sclerosis cognitive impairment using a self-administered 15-item questionnaire. *Multiple Sclerosis* 2003;9:95–101.

Benedict RHB, Cox D, Thompson LL, et al. Reliable screening for neuropsychological impairment in multiple sclerosis. *Multiple Sclerosis* 2004;10:675–78.

Bethoux F. Randomized, controlled trial of rehabilitation following acute relapse of MS. *Multiple Sclerosis* 2001;7: 137–42.

Brunet DG, Hopman WM, Singer MA, et al. Measurement of health-related quality of life in multiple sclerosis patients. *Can J Neurol Sci* 1996;23:99–103.

Cella DF, Dineen K, Arnason B, et al. Validation of the functional assessment of multiple sclerosis quality of life instrument. *Neurology* 1996;47:129–39.

Charcot JM. *Lectures on diseases of the nervous system* (Trans. G. Sigerson). First series lectures 6, 7, 8 delivered 1868. London: The New Sydenham Society, 1877:157.

Cohen JA, Cutter GR, Fischer JS, et al. Benefit of interferon beta-1a on MSFC progression in secondary progressive MS. *Neurology* 2002;59:679–87.

Coulthard-Morris L. In: Burks JS, Johnson KP (eds.). *Multiple sclerosis: diagnosis, medical management and rehabilitation.* New York: Demos Publishing Co., 2000.

Fischer JS, LaRocca NG, Miller DM, et al. Recent developments in the assessment of quality of life in multiple sclerosis (MS). *Multiple Sclerosis* 1999;5:251–59.

Fisk JD, Ritvo PG, Ross L, Haase DA, et al. Measuring the functional impact of fatigue: initial validation of the Fatigue Impact Scale. *Clin Infect Dis* 1994;18 (Suppl 1):S79–83.

Freeman JA, Langdon DW, Hobart JC, et al. Health-related quality of life in people with multiple sclerosis undergoing inpatient rehabilitation. *J Neurol Rehab* 1996;10: 185–94.

Freeman JA, Hobart JC, Langdon DW, et al. Clinical appropriateness: a key factor in outcome measure selection: the 36 item short form health survey in multiple sclerosis. *J Neurol Neurosurg Psychiat* 2000;68:150–56.

Goodkin DE, Cookfair D, Wende K, et al. Inter- and intrarater scoring agreement using grades 1.0–3.5 of the Kurtzke Expanded Disability Status Scale (EDSS). *Neurology* 1992;42:859–63.

Goodkin DE, Hertsgaard D, Seminary J. Upper extremity function in multiple sclerosis: improving assessment sensitivity with box-and-block and nine-hole peg tests. *Arch Phys Med Rehabil* 1988;69:850–54.

Goodkin DE, Rudick RA, Vanderbrug Medendorp S, et al. Low-dose oral methotrexate reduces the rate of progression in chronic progressive multiple sclerosis. *Ann Neurol* 1995;37:30–40.

Gottschalk M, Kumpfel T, Flachenecker P, et al. Fatigue and regulation of the hypothalamo-pituitary-adrenal axis in multiple sclerosis. *Arch Neurol* 2005;62:277–80.

Hauser SL, Dawson DM, Lehrich JR, et al. Intensive immunosuppression in progressive multiple sclerosis: a randomized three-arm study of high dose intravenous cyclophosphamide, plasma exchange and ACTH. *N Engl J Med* 1983;308:173–80.

Hobart JC, Riazi A, Lamping DL, et al. Improving the evaluation of therapeutic interventions in multiple sclerosis: development of a patient-based measure of outcome. *Health Technol Assess* 2004;8(9):1–48.

Kalkers HJ, Barkhof F, Uitdehaag B, et al. Outcome measures for multiple sclerosis clinical trials: relative measurement precision of the Expanded Disability Status Scale and Multiple Sclerosis Functional Composite. *Mult Scler* 2004;10:41–46.

Kos D, Kerckhofs E, Carrea I, et al. Evaluation of the Modified Fatigue Impact Scale in four different European countries. *Mult Scler* 2005;11:76–80.

Koziol JA, Frutos A, Sipe JC, et al. A comparison of two neurologic scoring instruments for multiple sclerosis. *J Neurol* 1997;244:60–61.

Koziol JA, Lucero A, Sipe JC, et al. Responsiveness of the Scripps neurologic rating scale during a multiple sclerosis clinical trial. *Can J Neurol Sci* 1999;26:283–89.

Kurtzke JF. A new scale for evaluating disability in multiple sclerosis. *Neurology* 1955;5:580–83.

Kurtzke JF. Rating neurologic impairment in multiple sclerosis: an expanded disability status scale (EDSS). *Neurology* 1983;33:1444–52.

Kurtzke JF. The disability status scale for multiple sclerosis: apologia pro DSS sua. *Neurology* 1989;39:291–302.

Mathiowetz V, Volland G, Kashman N, et al. Adult norms for the box and block test of manual dexterity. *Am J Occup Ther* 1985;39:386–91.

McDonald WI, Compston A, Edan G, et al. Recommended diagnostic criteria for multiple sclerosis: guidelines from the International Panel on the Diagnosis of Multiple Sclerosis. *Ann Neurol* 2001;50:121–27.

Miller DM, Cohen JA, Tsao E, et al. Health-related quality of life in secondary progressive MS patients: results from the IMPACT study. *Multiple Sclerosis* 2001;7(Suppl 1): S15.

Miller DM. Health-related quality of life assessment in multiple sclerosis. In: Cohen JA, Rudick RA (eds.). *Multiple sclerosis therapeutics* (2nd ed.). London and New York: Martin Dunitz, 2003:61–79.

Mumford, CJ, Compston A. Problems with rating scales for multiple sclerosis: a novel approach—the CAMBS score. *J Neurol* 1993;240:209–15.

Noseworthy JH, Vandervoort MK, Wong CJ, et al. Interrater variability with the Expanded Disability Status Scale (EDSS) and functional systems (FS) in a multiple sclerosis clinical trial. The Canadian Cooperation MS Study Group. *Neurology* 1990;40:971–75.

Norvedt MW, Riise T, Myhr KM, et al. Quality of life in multiple sclerosis: measuring the disease effects more broadly. *Neurology* 1999;53:1098–1103.

Oxford GK, Vogel KA, Le V, et al. Adult norms for a commercially available nine-hole peg test for finger dexterity. *Am J Occup Ther* 2003;57:570–73.

Panitch H, Goodin DS, Chang P, et al. Randomized, comparative study of interferon beta-1a treatment regimens in MS: the EVIDENCE trial. *Neurology* 2002;59: 1496–1506.

Poser CM, Paty DW, Scheinberg L, et al. New diagnostic criteria for multiple sclerosis: guidelines for research protocols. *Ann Neurol* 1983;13:227.

Potvin AR, Tourtellotte WW, Henderson WG, et al. Quantitative examination of neurologic function: reliability and learning effects. *Arch Phys Med Rehabil* 1975; 56:439–42.

Ritvo PG, Fischer JS, Miller DM, et al. *Multiple sclerosis quality of life inventory: a user's manual.* New York: National Multiple Sclerosis Society, 1997.

Rose AS, Kuzma JW, Kurtzke JF, et al. Cooperative study in the evaluation of therapy in multiple sclerosis: ACTH vs. placebo in acute exacerbations. *Neurol* 1968;18(6 Suppl):1–10.

Rudick R, Antel J, Confavreux C, et al. Recommendations from the National Multiple Sclerosis Society Clinical Outcomes Assessment Task Force. *Ann Neurol* 1997; 42(3):379–82.

Schumacher GA, Beebe G, Kibler RF, et al. Problems of experimental trials of therapy in multiple sclerosis: report by the panel on the evaluation of experimental trials of therapy in multiple sclerosis. *Ann N Y Acad Sci* 1965;122:552–68.

Sharrack B, Hughes RA, Soudain S, et al. The psychometric properties of clinical rating scales use in multiple sclerosis. *Brain* 1999;122:141–59.

Sipe JC, Knobler RL, Braheny SL, et al. A neurologic rating scale (NRS) for use in multiple sclerosis. *Neurology* 1984;34:1368–72.

Vickrey BG, Hays RD, Harooni R, et al. A health related quality of life measure for multiple sclerosis. *QOL Res* 1995;4:187–206.

Ware JEJ, Snow KK, Kosinski M, et al. SF-36 *Health survey: user's manual and interpretation guide.* Boston: The Health Institute, New England Medical Center, 1993.

Ware JEJ, Kosinski M, Bayliss MS, et al. Comparison of methods for the scoring and statistical analysis of SF-36 health profile and summary measures: summary of results from the Medical Outcomes Study. *Med Care* 1995;33(Suppl 4):AS264–79.

Weiss W, Stadlan EM. Design and statistical issues related to testing experimental therapy in multiple sclerosis. In: Rudick RA, Goodkin DE. *Treatment of multiple sclerosis: trial design, results, and future perspectives.* London: Springer-Verlag, 1992:91–112.

Willoughby EW, Paty DW. Scales for rating impairment in multiple sclerosis: a critique. *Neurology* 1988;38:1793–98.

8 Assessment of the Elderly with Dementia

Richard Camicioli, M.D., and Katherine Wild, Ph.D.

D ementia is a syndrome of persistent cognitive dysfunction caused by impairment in multiple domains (Cummings & Benson, 1992). A number of formal definitions are available including the *Diagnostic and Statistical Manual* (most recently DSM-IV-TR; American Psychiatric Association, 2000). Dementia has numerous causes, some of which are amenable to treatment when identified by laboratory investigations (Clarfield, 1988; Hejl et al., 2002). Neuroimaging, in particular, can identify contributions to dementia that might not be evident from clinical assessment (Massoud et al., 2000). The most common type of dementia is Alzheimer's disease (AD) (McKhann et al., 1984), but other causes of dementia, including vascular dementia (Chui et al., 1992; Knopman et al., 2003; Roman et al., 1993), dementia with Lewy bodies (McKeith et al., 2000b), Parkinson's disease with dementia, and frontotemporal dementia (McKhann et al., 2001), account for a significant subset of cases (Stevens et al., 2002). Although there is currently no cure for AD or the other causes of dementia, optimal management and counseling require an accurate diagnosis. Early diagnosis facilitates future planning by families and allows treatable entities to be uncovered before the accumulation of excess disability (Knopman et al., 2001). Clearly, accurate diagnosis is critical for recruitment into clinical trials. The scales to be discussed can be used to rate change over time in the context of a clinical trial, once a diagnosis has been made.

Despite the importance of dementia as a public health problem, standardized approaches to assessment are not widely used in clinical practice (Brodaty et al., 1994). Among the possible reasons for this may be the lack of recognition of the utility of standardized assessment, lack of familiarity with available instruments, the limitations of commonly used instruments, and time constraints of busy clinical practices. Objective evaluation allows the clinician to compare performance at different times in a standardized and reliable fashion and has been shown to be superior to clinician's impressions (Cooper et al., 1992; Knopman & Gracon, 1994a; Wind et al., 1994). In mild dementia documented objective change on a standardized instrument may allow early detection of dementia in an appropriate clinical context. Once the diagnosis is established standardized tools allow better evaluation of changes over time and improved assessment of acute change (Galasko et al., 1991).

In this chapter, we discuss the use of selected scales for detecting and following progression in patients with dementia. We consider scales that measure: (a) cognitive function, (b) functional status, (c) global function, and (d) aspects of behavior. We discuss the strengths and weaknesses of each and will explain how to use selected instruments. For the current chapter, the scales for this section were chosen from the literature using PubMed, Medline, and PsychInfo searches for specific scales and clinic trials in dementia (Table 8-1). Some published books on assessment of dementia are also reviewed (Burns et al., 1999; McKeith et al., 1999). This compilation is a selective one, and readers should refer to the secondary sources and the primary literature for a comprehensive review. The scales are relatively simple to administer and are in wide use. Validity and reliability data have been published and are discussed.

Table 8-1 summarizes the scales selected along with data regarding effect size in some clinical trials that allow its calculation. Of note, some studies do not provide sufficient data for assessing effect sizes. The effect sizes noted to date in clinical dementia trials are modest and similar across domains assessed.

Cognitive Assessment Instruments

Several brief scales are available for the assessment of cognitive function in patients with dementia. One must keep in mind that dementia is defined by involvement of more than one cognitive domain (Table 8-2). The brief scales discussed test limited domains and, therefore, they should be supplemented by historical information and/or additional testing to reach a diagnosis of dementia or to exclude such a diagnosis.

The Mini-Mental State Examination (MMSE) is a widely used mental status scale (Folstein et al., 1975). Numerous studies have demonstrated its test characteristics (Tombaugh & McIntyre, 1992). The Short Orientation-Memory-Concentration (Short-OMC) test is another instrument that is somewhat briefer than the MMSE (Katzman et al., 1983). Other brief instruments suitable for office use include the Short Test of Mental Status (Kokmen et al., 1991), the Short Portable Mental Status Questionnaire (Pfeiffer, 1975), and the Mental Status Questionnaire (Kahn et al., 1960), but these have not been commonly used in clinical trials and won't be considered further.

Table 8-1. Observed Treatment Effects Based on Scales Used in Recent Clinical Trials

Scale	Effect Size
Cognitive scales	
Mini-Mental Status Examination	0–0.78
Blessed Information-Memory-Concentration Test	NA
Alzheimer Disease Assessment Scale—Cognitive	0–0.41
Functional scales	
Activities of Daily Living	NA
Functional Assessment Staging	0.31
Disability Assessment for Dementia	0.23–0.31
ADCS-ADLI	0.25–0.32
Global scales	
Clinical Dementia Rating	NA
Global Deterioration Scale	0.21
Clinician Interview Based Impression of Change	0.27–0.88
Behavioral	
BEHAVE-AD	0.10
CERAD-B	NA
Neuropsychiatric Inventory	0.05–0.25
Cohen-Mansfield Agitation Inventory	NA
Cornell Depression Rating Scale	0–0.68
Geriatric Depression Scale	NA

ADCS-ADLI = Alzheimer Disease Cooperative Study Unit—Activities of Daily Living Inventory; BEHAVE-AD = Behavioral Pathology in Alzheimer's Disease Rating Scale; CERAD-B = Consortium to Establish a Registry for Alzheimer's Disease Behavioral Rating Scale for Dementia; NA = not applicable or data are not available.
Note: Summary of scales discussed and estimated minimum and maximum treatment effect size from some recent clinical trials reporting standard deviations and change scores. Negative scores indicate worsening and positive scores indicate improvement.

The problem of low sensitivity for early detection of dementia can be circumvented in several ways. Some authors have modified the MMSE (Mayeux et al., 1981; Teng & Chui, 1987) by adding items that have greater sensitivity (Katzman & Rowe, 1992). Others have developed brief batteries of tests

Table 8-2. Elements of the Mental Status Examination Relevant for the Diagnosis of Dementia

Cognitive Domain	Tests (Examples)
Memory	3, 4, 10 or longer word list: registration, recall, and recognition
Orientation	To person, place, time
Attention	Digit span (forward, reverse)
	Serial subtractions
	Reversals (days of the week, months of the year, etc.)
Visuospatial	Clock drawing
	Figure drawing and copying
Language	Fluency, grammar, and content of spontaneous
	Speech
	Naming
	Repetition
	Comprehension
	Reading
	Writing
Praxis	Multiple step commands
Executive function and reasoning	Calculations
	Similarities and differences
	Proverb interpretation
	Problem solving
	Judgment

that emphasize sensitivity (Fuld, 1978; Knopman & Ryberg, 1989), some of which are based on pre-existing neuropsychological tests (Eslinger et al., 1984).

Expanded cognitive testing instruments offer the potential of early detection of dementia and better response to change over the course of longitudinal follow-up. The Mattis Dementia Rating Scale (Mattis, 1976), the Alzheimer's Disease Assessment Scale (ADAS) (Rosen et al., 1984), the Neurobehavioral Cognitive Status Exam (Kiernan et al., 1987), the Dementia Assessment Battery (Teng et al., 1989), and the Cambridge Cognitive Assessment Scale (Cullum et al., 2000) are five such instruments, among others (Lezak, 1995). In general they take longer to perform and require the purchase or construction of special mate-

rials, which may be justified in a clinical practice or study focusing on the elderly with dementia.

Scales that incorporate measures of executive function and frontal abilities have been published (Dubois et al., 2000; Mathuranath et al., 2000). These may find utility in clinical practice and clinical trials of disorders that have prominent impairment of frontal function (e.g., frontotemporal dementia, Parkinson's disease with dementia, dementia with Lewy bodies, and vascular dementia).

Formal neuropsychological testing, which usually includes tests of multiple cognitive domains, is the best approach to evaluate mildly impaired patients when a diagnosis is in question. Specific test combinations that are particularly useful in detecting or tracking changes in dementia have been published (Lezak, 1995; Locascio et al., 1995; Morris et al., 1989; Parks et al., 1993). Psychometric tests with well-defined properties may offer the best way of documenting progression in dementia, although the briefer instruments have been used for the same purpose. Development and validation of neuropsychological batteries that can be used in longitudinal studies will be important for future clinical trials (Randolph et al., 1998). Psychometric batteries that minimize ceiling effect are necessary for patients with mild cognitive impairment.

A disadvantage of many instruments used to assess dementia is that severely impaired subjects may not be able to perform the test. At the extremes of the scoring range, the patient's disease may progressively worsen without detectable change in scores—the floor effect (i.e., a patient cannot score worse than 0). Approaches to deal with severely impaired patients are not as well worked out, but several tools that are sensitive to change in severely impaired patients have been described (Albert et al., 1992; Cole & Dastoor, 1987; Saxton et al., 1990) and have been reviewed (Boller et al., 2002). Functional, global, and behavioral scales, discussed in subsequent sections of this chapter, are essential in tracking meaningful change in severely impaired patients. In this section, we will focus our discussion on the MMSE, the Blessed scales, and the ADAS and their modifications as the most commonly used instruments in clinical trials.

Mini-Mental State Examination and Modified Mini-Mental State Examination

The MMSE was developed as a brief tool for grading the level of cognitive impairment in the elderly (Folstein et al., 1975). It is currently used for this purpose, as well as in screening for dementia (Fratiglioni et al., 1992; Ganguli et al., 1993; Paykel et al., 1994). It has been used in clinical trials for AD as a tool to grade initial dementia severity as well as to measure the effect of medications, although it may not be sensitive enough to change for the latter use (Knopman & Gracon, 1994a). Other measures, such as the ADAS, may be better suited to detect change. Nevertheless, the established properties of this scale, its widespread use, and its brevity make it an excellent choice for office use. Hence, it is often used as a secondary measure in clinical trials.

Description

The MMSE is a 30-point scale, consisting of several orientation questions (10 points), a registration and recall task (6 points), an attention task (5 points), a multistep command (3 points), two naming tasks (2 points), a repetition task (1 point), a reading comprehension task (1 point), a written sentence (1 point), and a visual construction task (1 point). The reading comprehension task involves the patient reading the sentence, "Close your eyes," and performing this command. The construction task involves copying interlocking pentagons. These items are generally printed on the form used to facilitate administration of the test.

Administration

The patient is asked the questions directly by the examiner. A watch, a plain piece of paper, and a pencil are the only equipment required.

Time

The MMSE takes 5–10 minutes to administer.

Reliability and Validity

The MMSE has been validated in a number of ways. It has face validity in that it tests cognitive domains important to the diagnosis of dementia: orientation, language, memory, attention, and construction abilities. It has convergent validity as indicated by the high correlation with other brief instruments, including the Short-OMC (Murden et al., 1991). Scores on the MMSE and the Short-OMC correlate with the pathologic changes at autopsy in patients with AD (Terry et al., 1991).

Internal consistency of the MMSE is quite good with Cronbach's alpha, ranging from 0.54 to 0.96 (Tombaugh & McIntyre, 1992), depending on the patient population. Test-retest and inter-rater reliability are also

excellent. There is a practice effect with repeated administration of the MMSE or the Short-OMC (Galasko et al., 1993). Publication of a standardized approach to administration may improve reliability (Molloy 1999; Molloy et al., 1991; Molloy & Standish, 1997).

Special Considerations

As with all mental status tests, optimal patient cooperation should be obtained. At the outset the patient should be made comfortable with the examiner. A conversation regarding recent events and autobiographical details usually puts the patient at ease. It is useful to provide the patient with a nonthreatening introduction to the formal testing. For example, one could say: "Now I am going to ask you some questions that test your memory and thinking. Some of the questions are very easy, whereas others are harder for everyone. Please do the best that you can, but don't worry if you can't get an answer."

Demographic factors, such as age, socioeconomic group, race (Murden et al., 1991), gender, and education (Uhlmann et al., 1991) all affect performance on mental status tests, including the MMSE (Crum et al., 1993). Age-appropriate norms have been developed internationally (Grigoletto et al., 1999). With less than 9 years of education the cutoff for suspecting dementia on the basis of mental status tests alone should be adjusted downward from 23/24 to 21/22 to minimize false-positive classification (Liu et al., 1994). The MMSE has been translated and adapted for use with Spanish- and Chinese-speaking people (Liu et al., 1994; Mungas et al., 1996).

Advantages

The MMSE is quite easy to administer and takes minimal training. It has been validated in numerous studies (Tombaugh & McIntyre, 1992) and has been used in studies examining subjects longitudinally (Doody et al., 2001). Although up to 20% of patients with dementia in some studies may score above the recommended cutoff of 23/24, the MMSE is more sensitive to dementia than routine clinical judgment. Follow-up of patients (Braekhus et al., 1995) and appropriate reliance on clinical history should increase its diagnostic accuracy.

A validated version of the MMSE is available for administration by telephone (Roccaforte et al., 1992). Overall, the MMSE makes an excellent choice for office use. By keeping its limitations in mind, clinicians can use it to advantage in assessing cognitive status in dementia.

Disadvantages

One disadvantage of the MMSE is its insensitivity to the early changes of dementia. This is due, in part, to its heavy weighting towards orientation and memory, which makes the test especially insensitive in cases that present with difficulties in cognitive domains other than memory. The test relies on verbal responses, which is a problem in patients with language disorders, such as aphasia or dysarthria, due to motor problems as seen in motor neuron disease. Compared with usual practice, however, it represents a considerable improvement.

The MMSE is insensitive to cognitive impairment in cerebrovascular disease (Grace et al., 1995), multiple sclerosis (Swirsky-Sacchetti et al., 1992), and Parkinson's disease (Rothlind & Brandt, 1993). It fails to assess cognitive functions that are often impaired in these diseases, such as executive function and attention, which are best tested using different instruments (Royall, 1994). Currently, the use of the MMSE as developed by Folstein has been copyrighted (http://harcourtassessment.com) as has the standardized MMSE. Modified versions of the 30-point instrument are in wide use. Although expanded versions may be useful in clinical trials settings, their longitudinal properties should be assessed. The Modified MMSE has been used as a screening instrument, suggesting a similar sensitivity (79%) and specificity (56%) to the MMSE (Hogan & Ebly, 2000). We reproduce the Modified MMSE and highlight the items that form part of the 30-item MMSE (Figure 8-1).

Short Orientation-Memory-Concentration Test and Blessed Information-Memory-Concentration Test

Blessed et al. (1968) were among the first to examine the relationship between cognitive measures and neuropathologic changes in dementia. The scale that they developed to measure cognitive and functional status has been subsequently modified for use in numerous clinical studies. Modified versions of the cognitive aspects of their scale are quite useful in clinical practice (Katzman & Rowe, 1992). We will discuss the use of a Short-OMC (Figure 8-2) because it provides a brief alternative to the MMSE, and its psychometric properties have been well documented. It is contrasted with the longer Blessed Information-Memory-Concentration Test (BIMC), which was adapted for use in the United States (Fuld, 1978) from the original version. Activities of daily living (ADL) are addressed by the complete Blessed Dementia Rating Scale (Figure 8-3).

Description

The Short-OMC consists of six items, compared with 26 items in the full-length BIMC (Figure 8-4). There are three orientation items, one of which is administered along with two additional distracters between a registration and recall task. The distracter tasks also test concentration. Each item is given a weighting that allows the calculation of a total possible range of 0–28, with higher scores indicating maximal impairment. The long BIMC includes additional orientation, memory, and attention items for a total of 33 items that can be scored. The original version's top score is 37, with 0 indicating no errors and 37 indicating errors on every item of the test, with some items weighted for more than 1 point. ADL are assessed by questioning an informant regarding performance on specific tasks. Cognitive sub-items of the Blessed Dementia Rating Scale have been separately validated from the ADL items. The ADL items have reasonable face validity.

Administration

The scale is administered directly to the patient in an interview setting as part of a mental status evaluation. No special equipment is needed, but autobiographical information, queried on the long version, would have to be corroborated with a reliable informant.

Time

The Short-OMC administration takes about 5 minutes. The BIMC takes approximately 15 minutes to administer. The additional ADL items take approximately 15 minutes to apply.

Reliability and Validity

Katzman et al. (1983) have validated the scale in a population admitted to a skilled nursing facility. Results on the short test ($r = 0.54$; $p < .001$) and the long version ($r = 0.59$; $p < .001$) both correlate with the autopsy findings of AD. The Blessed scales have been shown to correlate with the Clinical Dementia Rating scale (CDR), an integrated rating of overall function (Davis et al., 1990). Longitudinal assessment using the Blessed scales suggests that they might be useful in longitudinal assessment (Katzman et al., 1988; Stern et al., 1992). These two stud-

ID Number: _____   Date: _____

The Modified Mini-Mental State (3MS) Examination

SCORE SHEET

Rater _____   Protocol _____

_____

	3MS	MMS
DATE AND PLACE OF BIRTH Year:_____ Month: _____ Day: _____ Town: _____ State: _____ 5		
REGISTRATION (No. of presentations: _____) Shirt, Brown, Honesty (or: Shoes, Black, Modesty) (or: Socks, Blue, Charity) 3		3
MENTAL REVERSAL 5 to 1 Accurate 2 1 or 2 errors/ misses 0 1 DLROW 0 1 2 3 4 5 7		5
FIRST RECALL Spontaneous recall 3 After "Something to wear" 2 "Shoes, Shirt, Socks" 0 1 Spontaneous recall 3 After "A color" 2 "Blue, Black, Brown" 0 1 Spontaneous recall 3 After "A good personal quality" 2 "Honesty, Charity, Modesty" 0 1 9		3

TEMPORAL ORIENTATION
Year
   Accurate   8
   Missed by 1 year   4
   Missed by 2–5 years   0   2
Season
   Accurate or within 1 month   0   1
Month
   Accurate within 5 days   2
   Missed by 1 month   0   1
Day of Month
15
		5

Figure 8-1. (Adapted from Teng EL, Chui HC. The Modified Mini-Mental State [3MS] examination. *J Clin Psychiatry* 1987; 48[8]:314–18. Copyright 1987, Physicians Postgraduate Press.)

Accurate		3	
Missed by 1 or 2 days		2	
Missed by 3–5 days	0	1	
Day of week			
Accurate	0	1	

SPATIAL ORIENTATION				
State	0	2		
County	0	1		
City (town)	0	1	5	5
Hospital/ Office Building/ Home ?	0	1		

NAMING (MMS: Pencil _____ Watch _____)			
Forehead _____ Chin _____ Shoulder _____			
Elbow _____ Knuckle _____		5	2

FOUR LEGGED ANIMALS (30 seconds) 1 point each		
	10	

SIMILARITIES			
Arm-Leg			
Body part; limb; etc.		2	
Less correct answer	0	1	
Laughing-Crying			
Feeling; emotion		2	6
Other correct answer	0	1	
Eating-sleeping			
Essential for life		2	
Other correct answer	0	1	

REPETITION				
"I would like to go home/ out."		2		
1 or 2 missed/ wrong words	0	1	5	1
"No IFS – ANDS – OR BUTS –"				

READ AND OBEY "CLOSE YOUR EYES"				
Obeys without prompting		3		
Obeys after prompting		2		
Reads aloud only	0	1	3	1
(spontaneously or by request)				

WRITING (1 minute)		
(I) Would like to go home/out.		
(MMS: Spontaneous sentence: 0 1)	5	1

Figure 8-1. *continued*

ID Number: _____   Date: _____

COPYING TWO PENTAGONS (1 minute)			
	Each Pentagon		
5 approximately equal sides	4 4		
5 unequal (>2:1) sides	3 3		
Other enclosed figure	2 2		
2 or more lines	0 1 0 1	10	1
	Intersection		
4 corners	2		
Not-4-corner enclosure	0 1		
THREE-STAGE COMMAND			
_____ Take this paper with your left/ right hand			
_____ Fold it in half, and			
_____ Hand it back to me		3	3
SECOND RECALL			
(Something to wear)	0 1 2 3		
(Color)	0 1 2 3		
(Good personal quality)	0 1 2 3	9	
	TOTAL SCORE	100	30

Figure 8-1. *continued*

ies, which scored subjects' cognitive performance from 0 to 33, found a mean change of about 4+/–4 points in one study (Stern et al., 1992) with a range of 2–5 points per year depending on the level of initial severity and living situation of the patients (Katzman et al., 1988). Unfortunately, sensitivity, specificity, and population-based predictive values have not been reported.

Advantages

The use of a reproducible, valid instrument is advantageous. The Short-OMC scale is much briefer than the MMSE by virtue of the elimination of a large number of questions that address orientation. As it is presented, subjects don't have to use their limbs. This allows it to be used with patients with no motor component except speech. It has been adapted for a telephone interview (Kawas et al., 1995).

Disadvantages

This test has both floor and ceiling effects, as with the MMSE. It cannot be used to make the diagnosis of dementia because it only tests a limited number of cognitive domains. It must be supplemented with tests in other domains to establish a diagnosis. It contains no items that specifically assess executive function or visuospatial performance. Katzman and Rowe (1992) recommend using it in conjunction with tests of specific cognitive domains, namely, a construction task, such as clock drawing (Mendez et al., 1992; Spreen & Strauss, 1991; Tuokko et al., 1992); a verbal fluency task, such as listing as many animals as possible in one minute (Spreen & Strauss, 1991); a multistep command, such as taking a piece of paper, folding it, placing it in an envelope, and preparing the envelope for mailing; and a test of naming, such as naming a pen and its component parts or naming body parts. Together with the

ID Number: _____   Date: _____

Short Orientation-Memory-Concentration Test (Short-OMC)

SCORE SHEET

Rater _____   Protocol _____

Instructions:
To facilitate consistent administration of the Short-OMC, the examiner should pose questions as worded below. Please note instructions specific to each test item in italics.

Question	Maximum Error	Error Score	Weight	Weighted Sub Score	Maximum Weighted Score
1. What year is it now ?	(1)		X 4 =		4
2. What month is it now ?	(1)		X 3 =		3
Memory Phrase: Please repeat this phrase after me and try to remember it: John Brown 42 Market Street Chicago Number of Trials: _____					
3. About what time is it without looking at your watch ? *(within an hour)* Response: _____ Actual Time: _____	(1)		X 3 =		3
4. Count backwards from 20 to 1. *(Draw a line through carefully correctly sequenced numerals. Score 1 point for 1 error; score 2 points for 2 more errors).* 20 19 18 17 16 15 14 13 12 11 10 9 8 7 6 5 4 3 2 1	(2)		X 2 =		4
5. Say the months of the year in reverse order. *(Draw a line through correct months. Score 1 point for 1 error; score 2 points for 2 or more errors)* D N O S A JL JN MY AP M F J	(2)		X 2 =		4
6. Repeat the name and address I asked you to remember. *(Draw a line through each segment of the phrase correctly repeated. Score 1 point for each error)* John Brown 42 Market Street Chicago	(5)		X 2 =		10
TOTAL WEIGHTED SCORE (0 – 28) =					

Figure 8-2.   (From Katzman R, Brown T, Fuld P, et al. Validation of a short Orientation-Memory-Concentration Test of cognitive impairment. *Am J Psychiatry* 1983;140[6]:734–39, with permission. Copyright 1983, the American Psychiatric Association; http://ajp.psychiatryonline.org.)

ID Number: _____   Date: _____

The Blessed Dementia Scale (BDS)

SCORE SHEET

Rater _____   Protocol _____

0 = Competent   1/2 = Partial Competence   1 = Total Incompetence in Activity

The Blessed Dementia Scale

	Changes in Performance of Everyday Activities			
1	Inability to perform household tasks	1	½	0
2	Inability to cope with small sums of money	1	½	0
3	Inability to remember short list of items (e.g., in shopping)	1	½	0
4	Inability to find way about indoors	1	½	0
5	Inability to find way about familiar streets	1	½	0
6	Inability to interpret surroundings (e.g., to recognize whether in hospital, or at home, to discriminate between patients, doctors and nurses, relatives and hospital staff, etc.)	1	½	0
7	Inability to recall recent events	1	½	0
8	Tendency to dwell in the past	1	½	0

	Changes in Habits	
9	Eating:	
	Cleanly with proper utensils	0
	Messily with spoon only	2
	Simple solids (e.g., biscuits)	2
	Has to be fed	3
10	Dressing:	
	Unaided	0
	Occasionally misplaced buttons, etc.	1
	Wrong sequence, commonly forgetting items	2
	Unable to dress	3
11	Complete sphincter control	0
	Occasional wet beds	1
	Frequent wet beds	2
	Doubly incontinent	3

	Changes in Personality, Interests, Drive	
	No change	0
12	Increased rigidity	1

Figure 8-3.   (From Blessed G, Tomlinson BE, Roth M. Association between quantitative measures of dementia and of senile change in the cerebral grey matter of elderly subjects. *Br J Psychiatr* 1968;114:797–811, with permission.)

ID Number: _____   Date: _____

13	Increased egocentricity	1
14	Impairment of regard for feelings of others	1
15	Coarsening of affect	1
16	Impairment of emotional control (e.g., increased petulance and irritability)	1
17	Hilarity in inappropriate situations	1
18	Diminished emotional responsiveness	1
19	Sexual misdemeanour (appearing *de novo* in old age)	1
	Interests retained	0
20	Hobbies relinquished	1
21	Diminished initiative or growing apathy	1
22	Purposeless hyperactivity	1

	Total	

Figure 8-3.   *continued*

clinical history, these provide a reasonable overall assessment of cognitive function. The Blessed Dementia Rating Scale has not been used as an outcome measure in the major published clinical trials.

Alzheimer's Disease Assessment Scale

The ADAS (Figure 8-5) is the most widely used scale in clinical dementia trials. In its original conception it was divided into cognitive and noncognitive subsections, but the cognitive section is most widely used and will be described here. It was initially designed to assess patients with AD (Rosen et al., 1984), but it has been used in clinical trials of vascular dementia (Erkinjuntti et al., 2002; Orgogozo et al., 2002; Wilcock et al., 2002), and has been validated in different languages (Inzitari et al., 1999) and in patients with a low level of education (Liu et al., 2002).

Description

The test is administered to the patient by a trained evaluator. Scores range from 0, where patients make no errors, indicating maximally good performance, to 70, indicating poor performance. There are 11 cognitive domains tested in the most widely used version of the test: memory (3 items), orientation (1 item), language (5 items), and praxis (2 items).

Administration

The ADAS is administered directly to the patient as part of the mental status evaluation. An approach to standardized administration of the ADAS has been published (Standardized Alzheimer's Disease Assessment Scale [SADAS]) (Standish et al., 1996).

Time

This test takes 20–30 minutes to administer.

Reliability and Validity

Inter-rater reliability for the conventional and standardized version are both excellent (intraclass correlation coefficient: ADAS, 0.90, and SADAS, 0.91) as is intra-rater reliability (intraclass correlation coefficient: ADAS, 0.86, and SADAS, 0.88). It correlates significantly with other cognitive tests, indicating convergent validity. Sensitivity for detecting longitudinal change is greater for the ADAS compared with the Short-OMC (Stern et al., 1994).

Advantages

This scale tests cognitive domains similar to those tested by other scales discussed. The test has a performance range that may be broader than the MMSE and the BIMC and clearly superior to the Short-OMC, which offers only a limited performance range. It has

Blessed Information-Memory-Concentration Test (BIMC)

	Information-Memory-Concentration Test		
Information Test			
1	Name		1
2	Age		1
3	Time (hour)		1
4	Time of day		1
5	Day of week		1
6	Date		1
7	Month		1
8	Season		1
9	Year		1
10	Place -	Name	1
		Street	1
		Town	1
11	Type of place (e.g., home, hospital, etc.)		1
12	Recognition of persons (cleaner, doctor, nurse, patient, relative; any two available)		2

		Total	

Memory			
	1. Personal		
13		Date of birth	1
14		Place of birth	1
15		School attended	1
16		Occupation	1
17		Name of sibs or Name of wife	1
18		Name of any town where patient had worked	1
19		Name of employers	1
	2. Non Personal		
20		Date of World War I[1]	1
21		Date of World War II[2]	1
22		Monarch[3]	1
23		Prime Minister[3]	1
	3. Name and address (5-minute recall)		
24	- Mr. John Brown - 42 West Street - Gateshead		5

		Total	

Figure 8-4. [1]0.5 point for approximation within 3 years. [2]Note: For Europeans and Canadians, World War II is 1939–1945; for U.S., 1941–1945. [3]In the United States, use President and Governor. (From Blessed G, Tomlinson BE, Roth M. The association between quantitative measures of dementia and of senile change in the cerebral grey matter of elderly subjects. *Br J Psychiatry* 1968;114[512]:797–811, with permission.)

ID Number: _____   Date: _____

Concentration				
25	Months of year backwards		2 1 0	
26	Counting 1–20		2 1 0	
27	Counting 20–1		2 1 0	

		Total		

		TOTAL SCORE =		

Figure 8-4.   *continued*

been widely used in clinical trials, and sufficient data regarding predicted change and variability is available to allow sample size calculations. It has been recently used in clinical trials of vascular dementia and has been shown to be sensitive to change in response to medications (Erkinjuntti et al., 2002; Orgogozo et al., 2002; Wilcock et al., 2002; Wilkinson et al., 2003).

Disadvantages

The test was designed for patients with AD and consequently does not contain items for assessing frontal/executive function. The test is biased to testing memory. Patients who have more focal impairment may do well on these items, yet be significantly impaired. Other patient characteristics may be related to responsiveness on this scale (Doraiswamy et al., 1997). This test needs to be validated in other populations to test its overall utility, but experience in the vascular dementia population suggests that it may be useful in groups other than patients with AD. Approaches to expand the scale to include items to test other domains have been suggested (Mohs et al., 1997). To our knowledge it has not been validated with respect to pathologically confirmed cases.

Functional Status Instruments

Functional status is a patient-based measure that refers to a person's ability to perform tasks in the real world.

Functional assessment is usually divided into ADL and Instrumental Activities of Daily Living (IADL; Table 8-3; Figure 8-6). These tasks are a necessary part of daily living, so that, if a patient cannot perform them, they must be performed by a caregiver. ADLs refer to basic self-care tasks such as dressing or eating. These tasks are impaired only in more severely affected patients. IADLs are more complex tasks such as using the telephone or cooking. These are more cognitively demanding and, consequently, are impaired earlier in the course of dementia. Impairment in IADLs has been used as an early indicator of dementia (Barberger-Gateau et al., 1992, 1993). Cognitive and physical impairments can both affect performance in ADLs and IADLs. It is important for both practical and research purposes to determine which aspect of a person's illness is contributing to impairment in daily life functioning. Some may be amenable to remediation at the individual or environmental level.

Determining a person's functional status can be achieved through direct questioning of a patient or caregiver, testing in a clinic, or observation in the home or other setting. Because patient's self-reported function is unreliable (Kiyak et al., 1994), the most practical approach for the medical practitioner is to question a caregiver. In some cases consultation with an occupational or physical therapist can be invaluable in determining how a patient performs in a simulated or actual home environment (Zanetti et al., 1998). One should distinguish what the patient actually does from what the patient can do. Both are important. The

ID Number: _____   Date: _____

The Alzheimer's Disease Assessment Scale - Cognitive (ADAS-Cog)

SCORE SHEET

Rater _____   Protocol _____

_____

Cognitive Behavior

1. Spoken language ability _____

2. Comprehension of spoken language _____

3. Recall of test instructions _____

4. Word-finding difficulty _____

5. Following commands _____

6. Naming: objects, fingers

High:	1	2	3	Fingers: Thumb
Medium:	1	2	3	Pinky Index
Low:	1	2	3	Middle Ring

RATING SCALE
x = Not assessed
0 = Not present
1 = Very mild
2 = Mild
3 = Moderate
4 = Moderately severe
5 = Severe

7. Constructions: drawing _____

   Figures correct: 1   2   3   4

   Closing in: Yes _____   No _____

8. Ideational praxis _____

   Step correct: 1   2   3   4   5

9. Orientation _____

   Day _____   Year _____   Person _____   Time of day _____

   Date _____   Month _____   Season _____   Place _____

10. Word recall: mean error score _____

11. Word recognition: mean error score _____

                                        Cognition Total: _____

Figure 8-5. (From Rosen WG, Mohs RC, Davis KL. A new rating scale for Alzheimer's disease. *Am J Psychiatry* 1984; 141[11]:1356–64, with permission. Copyright 1984, the American Psychiatric Association; http://ajp.psychiatryonline.org.)

Table 8-3. Examples of Items in a Functional Assessment: Activities of Daily Living and Instrumental Activities of Daily Living

Activities of Daily Living	Instrumental Activities of Daily Living
Rising from bed	Using the telephone
Walking	Transportation (beyond residence)
Dressing	
Bathing or showering	Shopping
Grooming (combing or brushing hair, shaving, brushing teeth, etc.)	Cooking meals
	Housework and home maintenance
Eating	Handling money
Toileting	Hobbies and employment
	Taking medications

former refers to real needs (which the caregiver is providing for), whereas the latter is a measure of that which might potentially be achieved (e.g., through rehabilitation).

Although many scales are available to assess function, few validated scales have been developed for use in patients with dementia. Some available scales include: the Barthel Activities of Daily Living Scale (Wade, 1992), the Blessed Dementia Scale (Blessed et al., 1968), the Bristol Activities of Daily Living Scale; (Bucks et al., 1996; Byrne et al., 2000), the Cleveland Scale of Activities of Daily Living (Mace et al., 1993; Patterson et al., 1992), the Direct Assessment of Functional Status (Loewenstein et al., 1989), the Katz Activities of Daily Living Scale (Wade, 1992), the Physical Self-Maintenance and IADL Scale of Lawton and Brody (Lawton & Brody, 1969; Reed et al., 1989), the Rapid Disability Rating Scale-2 (Linn & Linn, 1982), the Scale of Functional Capacity (Pfeffer et al., 1982), the Structured Assessment of Independent Living (Mahurin et al., 1991), and the Geriatric Evaluation by Relatives Rating Instrument (Schwartz, 1983).

We discuss two brief scales selected on the basis of documented validity, reliability, and ease of administration: the Older Americans Resources and Services Procedures (OARS) functional assessment scale (Fillenbaum & Duke University, 1988) and the Functional Assessment Staging (FAST) test (Sclan & Reisberg, 1992). We will also discuss two longer scales that have found use in clinical trials, the Disability

Assessment for Dementia Scale (DAD) and the Alzheimer's Disease Cooperative Study-Activities of Daily Living Inventory (ADCS-ADLI). The latter are comprehensive and offer advantages over older instruments. There are several comprehensive scales available for the rehabilitation or research setting that may be more appropriate for specific disorders, which we will not discuss.

Modified Older Americans Resources and Services Procedures Instrument

A modification of an extensive multidimensional assessment instrument that was validated for practical use (Fillenbaum, 1985) is described below to illustrate the assessment of ADLs (Figure 8-6). Subscales of this instrument focus on ADLs and IADLs (Fillenbaum & Duke University, 1988). Assessment of ADLs are more useful in moderately or severely demented patients (Reed et al., 1989).

Description

In applying the modified OARS instrument, questions should be addressed to caregivers of patients with dementia. The scale, as formulated, addresses the capabilities of the patient, as assessed by a caregiver. There are nine items that address ADLs and seven items that address IADLs, each on a 3-point scale. A score of 0 indicates complete independence on an item, a score of 1 indicates slight impairment or need for help, and a score of 2 indicates full dependence on the assistance of others. The exception to this approach is the question regarding incontinence as an ADL, which is graded with respect to severity. Each part has been validated.

Administration

The caregiver is usually questioned separately from the patient to facilitate honest responses without distressing the patient. For example, the caregiver is asked if the patient can use the telephone without help. If the answer is negative the score on that item is either 1 or 2. The criterion for independence should be applied strictly. For instance, if someone needs assistance or needs reminding to take medicines, the score is 1. Next, one asks if the task can be performed with slight or full assistance. If the patient cannot perform the task at all, even with full assistance, the score is 2.

ID Number: _____   Date: _____

ACTIVITIES OF DAILY LIVING (ADL) AND INSTRUMENAL ACTIVITIES OF DAILY LIVING (IADL)

SCORE SHEET

Rater_____   Protocol _____

INSTRUCTIONS: Elicit complete descriptions of functional ability by providing examples like those in italics below. If patient/subject is able to perform activity but requires prompting or reminders from the caregiver, score 1 for Slight Assistance Needed.

Activities of Daily Living – ADL

Tester should try to evaluate what subject is functionally capable of doing, not what (s)he actually does. Sample probes in italics below.

Assistance Needed

1. Eating *(needs food cut up, reminder to eat)?* _____

2. Dressing and undressing *(needs clothing set out for him/her, help with buttons)?* _____

3. Combing hair and shaving *(needs to be reminded)?* _____

4. Walking _____

5. Getting in and out of bed _____

6. Bathing or showering *(needs prompting or reminders; needs assistance with part of task, i.e., washing hair)?* _____

7. Toileting *(needs reminder or help with cleaning self after toileting)?* _____

8. Incontinence

Score:	
0	Never or less than once a week
1	Once or twice/week
2	Three or more times/week

_____

Unless otherwise specified, Score:	
0	None
1	Slight
2	Full

9. Needs help with shopping, bathing, housework, and/or getting around? _____

Total ADL Score: _____

Instrumental Activities of Daily Living – IADL

Tester should try to evaluate what subject is functionally capable of doing, not what (s)he actually does. Sample probes in italics below

Assistance Needed

1. Using telephone *(does subject look up phone numbers or answer phone)?* _____

2. Traveling by car, bus, or taxi _____

3. Shopping for food and clothing *(able to choose appropriate items)?* _____

4. Preparing meals *(needs ingredients set out or other supervision)?* _____

5. Doing housework _____

6. Taking own medicine _____

7. Handling own money *(receives correct change, writes checks)?* _____

Unless otherwise specified, Score:	
0	None
1	Slight
2	Full

Total IADL Score: _____

Figure 8-6. (From Fillenbaum GG. Activities of Daily Living [ADL] and Instrumental Activities of Daily Living [IADL]. Screening the elderly. A brief instrumental activities of daily living measure. *J Am Geriatr Soc* 1985;33[10]:698–706, with permission of Blackwell Publishing.)

Time

Five to 10 minutes are required for asking about ADLs and IADLs.

Reliability and Validity

The OARS scale has been extensively validated with a sample of more than 6,000 people (Fillenbaum, 1985; Fillenbaum & Duke University, 1988). A physical therapist examined patients in their homes to determine their self-care capacity, which was compared with the instrument, showing an excellent agreement between approaches (Kendall's tau = .83; $r = 0.89$). The OARS scale incorporates items from Lawton and Brody's scale for IADL and the Physical Self-Maintenance Scale (Lawton & Brody, 1969; Reed et al., 1989), suggesting concurrent validity. The latter scales are also used in clinical trials but are not considered further.

Test-retest reliability and inter-rater reliability data have both been published. Overall, the reliability coefficient for ADLs is 0.84 (Fillenbaum & Duke University, 1988) whereas that for IADLs is 0.87. The scale has obvious content validity in that the items selected are relevant to daily self-care and the ability to live independently.

Special Considerations

It is important to not ask these questions of demented patients directly. Although mildly impaired patients may be accurate, one cannot be sure of their accuracy without asking a caregiver.

Advantages

The scale has been very well studied in a wide range of individuals with a broad spectrum of disabilities. It is valid and reliable. The scales from which this tool has been derived are widely used.

Disadvantages

It is critical to have a reliable caregiver or patient for the administration of this scale. It has not been validated on a population with AD, although it has been used in a broad spectrum of people, including patients with cognitive impairment. By asking caregivers about the patient's capabilities, the scale may be biased toward overestimating function. Other scales may avoid this bias by addressing actual performance (Wade, 1992).

Functional Assessment Staging

The FAST is a scale that was developed specifically for functional assessment of elderly people with dementia (Sclan & Reisberg, 1992; Figure 8-7).

Description

The FAST is an ordinal scale ranging from 1, indicating normal function, to 7, indicating severe dementia. Levels 6 and 7 are divided into specific subscales, yielding 16 possible ratings (Sclan & Reisberg, 1992). Each level is indicated by a functional description with adequate detail for clinical scoring.

Administration

The FAST score is derived from a caregiver interview.

Time

Administration of the FAST takes 15–20 minutes.

Reliability and Validity

The FAST was developed by clinicians experienced in the care of patients with dementia. It has face validity as well as convergent validity with psychometric measures and other clinical measures (Sclan & Reisberg, 1992). The intra-class correlation coefficient for inter-rater agreement was 0.86 ($p <.01$), which represents a high rate of agreement. Correlation with psychometric tests is high with a range from –0.60 to –0.79 ($p <.001$) (Reisberg et al., 1994). The correlation with the MMSE is 0.83 (Reisberg et al., 1992). The coefficient of reproducibility was 0.99, indicating excellent reliability (Sclan & Reisberg, 1992). Progression of disease can be assessed with the FAST.

Special Considerations

By emphasizing functional elements in everyday performance, the FAST allows the clinician to identify areas of difficulty that may be related to caregiving. It is possible that individual patients would not progress in an orderly, hierarchical fashion. The staging mixes items that are cognitive with those that are more functionally relevant. This may be appropriate in addressing the hierarchical loss of domains in the course of dementia, but it addresses behaviorally distinct constructs.

ID Number: _____   Date: _____

Functional Assessment Staging (FAST)

SCORE SHEET

Rater _____   Protocol _____

Informant Name _____   Relationship with Subject _____

_____

[If an item is assessed as being due to other causes apart from dementia (e.g., paralysis, arthritis, etc.), please check "No" and note these other causes next to the item.]

#	Question	Yes	Months[1]	No
1	No difficulties, either subjectively or objectively.			
2	Complains of forgetting location of objects; subjective work difficulties.			
3	Decreased job functioning evident to coworkers; difficulty in traveling to new locations.			
4	Decreased ability to perform complex tasks (e.g., planning dinner for guests; handling finances; marketing).			
5	Requires assistance in choosing proper clothing.			
6a	Difficulty putting clothing on properly.			
6b	Unable to bathe properly; may develop fear of bathing.			
6c	Inability to handle mechanics of toileting (i.e., forgets to flush, doesn't wipe properly).			
6d	Urinary incontinence.			
6e	Fecal incontinence.			
7a	Ability to speak limited (1 to 5 words a day).			
7b	All intelligible vocabulary lost.			
7c	Non-ambulatory.			
7d	Unable to sit up independently.			
7e	Unable to smile.			
7f	Unable to hold head up.			

Comments: _____

_____

_____

Figure 8-7.   Note: Functional staging score = highest ordinal value. [1]Number of months FAST stage deficit has been noted. (From Reisberg B. Functional assessment staging [FAST]. *Psychopharmacol Bul* 1988;24[4]:653–59, with permission of Med-Works Media.)

Advantages

This scale provides reliable ratings for the early stages of dementia but remains sensitive to differences between subjects in the severe range of cognitive performance, an advantage shared with other functional scales that measure ADL. The FAST can be used to stage patients whose behavioral symptoms interfere with cognitive testing. It has been used to stage patients for selection in some clinical trials (Feldman et al., 2001b).

Disadvantages

Its application to non-AD dementia has been studied to a limited extent. The relationship between the FAST and other functional scales is not clear, as studies examining convergent validity are not widely available.

Disability Assessment for Dementia

The DAD is a scale that was developed specifically for functional assessment of elderly people with dementia (Gelinas et al., 1999; Figure 8-8).

Description

The DAD is a 40-item ordinal scale that addresses a variety of functional domains (including hygiene, dressing, continence, eating, meal preparation, telephoning, going on an outing, finance, correspondence, medication, leisure, and housework). Scores can range from 0 to 40. Each item is rated as 0 if the patient is unable to perform the described task and 1, indicating normal function. Like the FAST, each level is indicated by a functional description with adequate detail for clinical scoring.

Administration

The DAD score is derived from a caregiver interview.

Time

Administration of the DAD takes 15–20 minutes.

Reliability and Validity

The DAD was developed by clinicians experienced in the care of patients with dementia, including individuals with physical and occupational therapy expertise. It has face validity as well as convergent validity with psychometric measures and other clinical measures, including the Global Deterioration Scale (GDS) (Gelinas et al., 1999). Internal consistency was high ($r = 0.957$). Intraclass correlation coefficients for inter-rater agreement was 0.96, which represents a high rate of agreement, with excellent test-retest reliability (intraclass correlation coefficient = 0.96). There was no evidence for differences between men and women. The DAD has been used to document change in clinical trials (Gelinas et al., 2000).

Special Considerations

By emphasizing functional elements in everyday performance, the DAD allows the clinician to identify areas of difficulty that may be related to caregiving. As noted, the scale shows sensitivity to change in clinical trials, but long-range changes are not studied as yet.

Advantages

This scale includes a range of functional abilities from basic to IADLs and, hence, may be useful across a range of dementia severity. Recent trials assessed the performance of the scale in clinical AD patients, including those with moderate to severe impairment (Blesa et al., 2003; Feldman et al., 2001a; Feldman et al., 2003; Raskind et al., 2000; Wilcock et al., 2000).

Disadvantages

Its application to non-AD dementia has been studied to a limited extent, but by incorporating questions about initiation, the scale has the potential to be useful in studies of disorders that predominantly affect executive function. The relationship between the DAD and other specific cognitive functional scales is not clear.

Alzheimer's Disease Cooperative Study-Activities of Daily Living Inventory

The ADCS-ADLI is a comprehensive assessment scale which was developed specifically for functional assessment of elderly people with AD (Galasko et al., 1997; Figure 8-9).

Description

The ADCS-ADLI is an ordinal scale that, in a pilot study, addressed over 30 items in a comprehensive

ID Number: _____   Date: _____

The Disability Assessment for Dementia (DAD)

SCORE SHEET

Rater _____   Protocol _____

_____

During the past two weeks, did (name) · _____ , without help or reminder

SCORING: YES = 1 NO = 0 N/A = NOT APPLICABLE	Initiation	Planning & Organization	Effective Performance
HYGIENE			
Undertake to wash himself/herself or to take a bath or shower		■	■
Undertake to brush his/her teeth or care for his/her dentures		■	■
Decide to care for his/her hair (wash and comb)		■	■
- Prepare the water, towels, and soap for washing, taking a bath or a shower	■		■
- - Wash and dry completely all parts of his/her body safely	■	■	
- - Brush his/her teeth or care for his/her dentures appropriately	■	■	
- - Care for his/her hair (wash and comb)	■	■	
DRESSING			
Undertake to dress himself/herself		■	■
- Choose appropriate clothing (with regard to the occasion, neatness, the weather and color combination)	■		■
- Dress himself/herself in the appropriate order (undergarments, pant/dress, shoes)	■		■
- - Dress himself/herself completely	■	■	
- - Undress himself/herself completely	■	■	
CONTINENCE			
Decide to use the toilet at appropriate times		■	■
- - Use the toilet without "accidents"	■	■	
EATING			
Decide that he/she needs to eat		■	■
- Choose appropriate utensils and seasonings when eating	■		■
- - Eats his/her meals at a normal pace and with appropriate manners	■	■	
MEAL PREPARATION			
Undertake to prepare a light meal or snack for himself/herself		■	■
- Adequately plan a light meal or snack (ingredients, cookware)	■		■
- - Prepare or cook a light meal or a snack safely	■	■	

Figure 8-8. (From Gelinas I, Gauthier L, McIntyre M, et al. Development of a functional measure for persons with Alzheimer's disease: the Disability Assessment for Dementia. *Am J Occup Ther* 1999;53[5]:471–81, with permission. Copyright 1999 by the American Occupational Therapy Association, Inc.)

ID Number: _____   Date: _____

During the past two weeks, did (name) _____, without help or reminder

	Initiation	Planning & Organization	Effective Performance
SCORING: YES = 1 NO = 0 N/A = NOT APPLICABLE			
TELEPHONING			
Attempt to telephone someone at a suitable time	☐	■	■
- Find and dial a telephone number correctly	■	☐	■
- - Carry out an appropriate telephone conversation	■	■	☐
- - Write and convey a telephone message adequately	■	■	☐
GOING ON AN OUTING			
Undertake to go out (walk, visit, shop) at an appropriate time	☐	■	■
- Adequately organize an outing with respect to transportation, keys, destination, weather, necessary money, shopping list	■	☐	■
- - Go out and reach a familiar destination without getting lost	■	■	☐
- - Safely take the adequate mode of transportation (car, bus, taxi)	■	■	☐
- - Return from the store with the appropriate items	■	■	☐
FINANCE AND CORRESPONDENCE			
Show an interest in his/her personal affairs such as his/her finances and written correspondence	☐	■	■
- Organize his/her finance to pay his/her bills (cheques, bankbook, bills)	■	☐	■
- Adequately organize his/her correspondence with respect to stationery, address, stamps	■	☐	■
- - Handle adequately his/her money (make change)	■	■	☐
MEDICATIONS			
Decide to take his/her medications at the correct time	☐	■	■
- - Take his/her medications as prescribed (according to the right dosage)	■	■	☐
LEISURE AND HOUSEWORK			
Show an interest in leisure activity(ies)	☐	■	■
Take an interest in household chores that he/she used to perform in the past	☐	■	■
- Plan and organize adequately household chores that he/she used to perform in the past	■	☐	■
- - Complete household chores adequately as he/she used to perform in the past	■	■	☐
- - Stay safely at home by himself/herself when needed	■	■	☐

Comments: _____

_____

SUB TOTAL / # applicable items	/ /	
DAD TOTAL / # applicable items	/	
DAD TOTAL in %		

Figure 8-8. *continued*

ID Number: _____   Date: _____

23 Items from the Alzheimer's Disease Cooperative Study Activities of Daily Living Inventory (ADCS-ADLI)

SCORE SHEET

Rater _____   Protocol _____

Information obtained through: ☐ Informant Visit   ☐ Telephone Call

---

Instructions: For each question, use the subject's name where {S} appears. Before beginning, read the questionnaire guidelines to the informant.

---

1. Regarding **eating**:
   Which best describes {S} usual performance during the past 4 weeks ?
   ☐ ate without physical help, and used a knife
   ☐ used a fork or spoon, but not a knife, to eat
   ☐ used fingers to eat
   ☐ {S} usually or always was fed by someone else

2. Regarding **walking** (or getting around in a wheelchair), in the past 4 weeks, which best describes his/her **optimal** performance:
   ☐ mobile outside of home without physical help
   ☐ mobile across a room without physical help
   ☐ transferred from bed to chair without help
   ☐ required physical help to walk or transfer

3. Regarding bowel and bladder function **at the toilet**, which best describes his/her **usual** performance in the past 4 weeks:
   ☐ did everything necessary without supervision or help
   ☐ needed supervision, but no physical help
   ☐ needed physical help, and was usually continent
   ☐ needed physical help, and was usually incontinent

4. Regarding **bathing**, in the past 4 weeks, which best describes his/her usual performance:
   ☐ bathed without reminding or physical help
   ☐ no physical help, but needed supervision/reminders to bathe completely
   ☐ needed minor physical help (e.g., with washing hair) to bathe completely
   ☐ needed to be bathed completely

5. Regarding **grooming**, in the past 4 weeks, which best describes his/her **optimal** performance:
   ☐ cleaned and cut fingernails without physical help
   ☐ brushed or combed hair without physical help
   ☐ kept face and hands clean without physical help
   ☐ needed help for grooming of hair, face, hands and fingernails

Figure 8-9. (From D Galasko, D Bennett, M Sano, et al. An inventory to assess activities of daily living for clinical trials in Alzheimer's disease. The Alzheimer's Disease Cooperative Study. *Alzheimer Dis Assoc Disord* 1997;11[Suppl 2]:S33–S39, with permission.)

ID Number: _____   Date: _____

6. Regarding **dressing, in the past 4 weeks**:
    A. Did {S} <u>select</u> his/her first set of clothes for the day ?
       If yes, which best describes his/her usual performance:
       - ❏ without supervision or help
       - ❏ with supervision
       - ❏ with physical help

	Yes	No	Don't Know
	❏	❏	❏

    B. Regarding physically getting dressed, which best describes his/her usual performance in the past 4 weeks:
       - ❏ dressed completely without supervision or physical help
       - ❏ dressed completely with supervision, but without help
       - ❏ needed physical help only for buttons, clasps, or shoelaces
       - ❏ dressed without help if clothes needed no fastening or buttoning
       - ❏ always needed help, regardless of the type of clothing

7. In the past 4 weeks, did {S} <u>use a telephone</u> ?
    If yes, which best describes his/her **highest** level of performance:
    - ❏ made calls after looking up numbers in white and yellow pages, or by dialing directory assistance
    - ❏ made calls <u>only</u> to well-known numbers, <u>without</u> referring to a directory or list
    - ❏ made calls <u>only</u> to well-known numbers, <u>by using</u> a directory or list
    - ❏ answered the phone; did not make calls
    - ❏ did not answer the phone, but spoke when put on the line

	Yes	No	Don't Know
	❏	❏	❏

8. In the past 4 weeks, did {S} <u>watch television</u> ?
    If yes, ask all questions:
    Did {S}:
    a. usually select or ask for different programs or his/her favorite show ?
    b. usually talk about the content of a program while watching it ?
    c. talk about the content of a program within a day (24 hrs) after watching it ?

	Yes	No	Don't Know
	❏	❏	❏
	❏	❏	❏
	❏	❏	❏
	❏	❏	❏

9. In the past 4 weeks, did {S} ever appear to <u>pay attention to conversation or small talk</u> for at least 5 minutes ?
    Note: {S} did not need to initiate the conversation.
       If yes, which best describes his/her usual degree of participation:
       - ❏ <u>usually</u> said things that were related to the topic
       - ❏ <u>usually</u> said things that were not related to the topic
       - ❏ rarely or never spoke

	Yes	No	Don't Know
	❏	❏	❏

10. Did {S} clear the dishes from the table after a meal or snack ?
    If yes, which best describes how he/she usually performed:
    - ❏ without supervision or help
    - ❏ with supervision
    - ❏ with physical help

	Yes	No	Don't Know
	❏	❏	❏

11. In the past 4 weeks, did {S} usually manage to <u>find his/her personal belongings</u> at home ?
    If yes, which best describes how he/she usually performed:
    - ❏ without supervision or help
    - ❏ with supervision
    - ❏ with physical help

	Yes	No	Don't Know
	❏	❏	❏

Figure 8-9.   *continued*

ID Number: _____   Date: _____

12. In the past 4 weeks, did {S} <u>obtain a hot or cold beverage</u> for him/herself ?
   (A cold beverage includes a glass of water)
   If yes, which describes his/her highest level of performance
      ❑ made a hot beverage, usually without physical help
      ❑ made a hot beverage, usually if someone else heated the water
      ❑ obtained a cold beverage, usually without physical help

Yes	No	Don't Know
❑	❑	❑

13. In the past 4 weeks, did {S} make him/herself a meal or snack at home ?
   If yes, which describes his/her highest level of food preparation:
      ❑ cooked or microwaved food, with little or no help
      ❑ cooked or microwaved food, with extensive help
      ❑ mixed or combined food items for a meal or snack, without cooking
         or microwaving (e.g., made a sandwich)
      ❑ obtained food on his/her own, without mixing or cooking it

Yes	No	Don't Know
❑	❑	❑

14. In the past 4 weeks, did {S} <u>dispose of garbage or litter</u> in an appropriate place or container at home ?
   If yes, which best describes how he/she usually performed:
      ❑ without supervision or help
      ❑ with supervision
      ❑ with physical help

Yes	No	Don't Know
❑	❑	❑

15. In the past 4 weeks, did {S} <u>get around</u> (or travel) <u>outside of his/her home</u> ?
   If yes, which best describes his/her **optimal** performance:
      ❑ alone, went at least 1 mile away from home
      ❑ alone, but remained within 1 mile of home
      ❑ only when accompanied and supervised, regardless of the trip
      ❑ only with physical help, regardless of the trip

Yes	No	Don't Know
❑	❑	❑

16. In the past 4 weeks, did {S} ever <u>go shopping</u> ?
   If yes, ask A and B:
   A. Which one best describes how {S} usually <u>selects</u> items:
      ❑ without supervision or physical help ?
      ❑ with some supervision or physical help ?
      ❑ not at all, or selected mainly random or inappropriate items ?

   B. Did {S} usually <u>pay</u> for items without supervision or physical help ?

Yes	No	Don't Know
❑	❑	❑
❑	❑	❑

17. In the past 4 weeks, did {S} <u>keep appointments</u> or meetings with other people,
   such as relatives, a doctor, the hairdresser, etc. ?
   If yes, which best describes his/her awareness of the meeting ahead of time:
      ❑ usually remembered, may have needed written reminders
         (e.g., notes, a diary, or calendar)
      ❑ only remembered the appointment after verbal reminders on the day
      ❑ usually did not remember, in spite of verbal reminders on the day

Yes	No	Don't Know
❑	❑	❑

Figure 8-9.   *continued*

ID Number: _____   Date: _____

18. In the past 4 weeks, was {S} ever <u>left on his/her own</u> ?

	Yes	No	Don't Know
	☐	☐	☐

If yes, ask all questions:
Was {S} left:
a) away from home, for 15 minutes or longer, during the day ?
b) at home, for an hour or longer, during the day ?
c) at home, for less than 1 hour, during the day ?

Yes	No	Don't Know
☐	☐	☐
☐	☐	☐
☐	☐	☐

19. In the past 4 weeks, did {S} <u>talk about **current** events</u> ?
(This means events or incidents that occurred during the past month)

	Yes	No	Don't Know
	☐	☐	☐

If yes, ask all questions:
Did {S} talk about events that…:
a) he/she heard or read about or saw on TV but did not take part in ?
b) {S} took part in <u>outside home</u> involving family, friends, or neighbors ?
c) events that occurred <u>at home</u> that he/she took part in or watched ?

Yes	No	Don't Know
☐	☐	☐
☐	☐	☐
☐	☐	☐

20. In the past 4 weeks, did {S} <u>read a magazine, newspaper or book</u> for more than 5 minutes at a time ?

If yes, ask all questions:
Did {S} usually:
a)   talk about details of what he/she read while or shortly
     (< than 1 hour) after reading ?
b)   talk about what he/she read 1 hour or longer after reading ?

Yes	No	Don't Know
☐	☐	☐
☐	☐	☐
☐	☐	☐

21. In the past 4 weeks, did {S} ever <u>write</u> things down ?
<u>Note</u>: *If {S} wrote things only after encouragement or with help, the response should still be 'yes'.*

If yes, which best describes the most complicated things that he/she wrote:

Yes	No	Don't Know
☐	☐	☐

❑ letters or long notes that other people understood
❑ short notes or messages that other people understood
❑ his/her signature or name

22. In the past 4 weeks, did {S} perform a <u>pastime, hobby or game</u> ?
If yes, which pastime <u>did</u> he/she perform:

Yes	No	Don't Know
☐	☐	☐

Ask about all of the following, check all that apply:
☐ card or board games (including bridge, chess, checkers)

☐ bingo	☐ reading
☐ crosswords	☐ gardening
☐ art	☐ golf
☐ musical instrument	☐ tennis
☐ knitting	☐ workshop
☐ sewing	☐ fishing
☐ other _____	

<u>Note</u>: *Walking does <u>NOT</u> count as a hobby/ pastime for this scale.*

❑ **If {S} performs hobbies/ pastimes only at day care, check here.**

If yes, how did {S} usually perform his/her most common pastimes:
❑ without supervision or help
❑ with supervision
❑ with help

Figure 8-9. *continued*

ID Number: _____   Date: _____

23. In the past 4 weeks, did {S} <u>use a household appliance</u> to do chores ?

Yes	No	Don't Know
☐	☐	☐

   Ask about all of the following, and check those that were used:

☐ washer	☐ dryer	☐ vacuum
☐ dishwasher	☐ toaster	☐ toaster oven
☐ range	☐ microwave	☐ food processor
☐ other _____		

   If yes, for <u>the most commonly used</u> appliances, which best describes how {S} usually used them:
   ❑ without help, operating more than on-off controls if needed
   ❑ without help, but operated only on-off controls
   ❑ with supervision, but no physical help
   ❑ with physical help

Figure 8-9.   *continued*

assessment of abilities in patients with AD. A shorter version of 23 items was published (Galasko et al., 1997). Scores on the 23-item version could range from 0–78, and this version was used in two recent clinical trials (Aisen et al., 2003; Tariot et al., 2000). Yes/no answers are provided to specific questions regarding aspects of each functional domain. Like the DAD and FAST, the specific questions describe functional tasks the patient might or might not be able to do but also address the need for supervision during performance of specific tasks.

Administration

The ADCS-ADLI score is derived from a caregiver interview.

Time

Administration of the ADCS-ADLI takes from 30 to 45 minutes.

Reliability and Validity

The ADCS-ADLI was developed by the Alzheimer's Disease Cooperative Studies Unit to meet the needs for a comprehensive and responsive scale to measure function in patients with AD. It has face validity as well as convergent validity with psychometric measures and other clinical measures, including the GDS. Some of the items on the complete scale were deemed likely to be nonresponsive. Kappa values assessing reliability of individual questions ranged

from a low of 0.41 for "makes conversation" to a high of 0.73 for bathing. Change over time and percent of subjects attempting individual items changes with the MMSE.

Special Considerations

By emphasizing functional elements in everyday performance, the ASCS-ADLI allows the clinician to identify areas of difficulty that may be related to caregiving. As noted in Advantages, the scale shows sensitivity to change in clinical trials, but long-range changes are not studied, as yet. It is anticipated that the scale would be sensitive to change throughout the course of dementia.

Advantages

This scale includes a range of functional abilities from basic to IADLs and, hence, may be useful across a range of dementia severity. Comprehensive information available for levels of cognitive severity might allow selection of items appropriate for stage of dementia. The scale has been used in two recent clinical trials, one that showed beneficial effects of an intervention (Tariot et al., 2000), and one that did not (Aisen et al., 2003). Thus, this scale can be feasibly applied to the clinical trials setting.

Disadvantages

Its application to non-AD dementia has not been studied. The relationship between the ADCS-ADLI and other specific cognitive or functional scales is not clear, but its comprehensive nature should make it useful for future studies of dementia.

Global Assessment Instruments

Global measures that give an overall idea of a patient's status are very useful both as a summary measure integrating cognitive and functional status, and as communication to families. Global measures have long been used to stage the severity of disease. Although global scales have been used when patients have already been diagnosed with dementia, they may also be useful in guiding the earliest steps in diagnosis by integrating all the available clinical information. Two such systems are the CDR and the GDS. They both span the range of severity from mildly to severely impaired. Moreover, both of these scales are responsive to disease progression, which is an essential feature for a scale to be used in grading severity of disease.

Clinical Dementia Rating

Description

The CDR consists of six domains (memory, orientation, judgment and problem solving, home and hobbies, community affairs, and personal care), each of which is graded on a scale of 0–3 (Hughes et al., 1982; Figure 8-10). Possible scores are: 0 = no impairment; 0.5 = questionable dementia; 1 = mild dementia; 2 = moderate dementia; or 3 = severe dementia. Although the memory domain is weighted above all others, it is not the sole determinant of the final score.

Administration

Ratings are obtained through a combination of caregiver interview and direct patient assessment. It is important to obtain examples of the patient's behavior in each of the domains while obtaining the functional history. Examples can be presented to the caregiver for facilitation of the grading if they can't provide them (see Table 8-4 for questions useful as probes for the CDR). The caregiver should be asked about autobiographic details of the patient and examples of recent activities or events attended by the patient to probe the patient's memory in a separate interview. The

patient interview is used to refine the gradation in the cognitive domains by mental status testing. Although a standard mental status examination, such as the MMSE, can be incorporated into the patient interview, additional assessment of memory (especially for recent and remote events), insight (e.g., into the memory disorder), problem solving, and abstract reasoning should be performed to grade these domains (see Table 8-5 for examples). An overall CDR score is obtained through a system that assigns a priority to the memory subscore.

The score is the same as the memory score unless at least three of the other items are higher or lower than the memory score, in which case the score is the same as the majority of the items. The exception to this scoring occurs when two items are to one side of the memory score and three items are on the other side. In that situation, the score is the same as the memory score (Morris, 1993). When the memory score is 0.5, a score of 0 cannot be obtained; the score must be 0.5 or 1, depending on the score on the other items. If the memory score is 0, but 2 other items are scored 1 or more, then the CDR score would be 0.5. The algorithm for scoring can be checked on the investigator's Web site (http://www.biostat.wustl.edu/~adrc/cdrpgm/index.html). The sum of all the scores has been examined as an outcome measure in clinical trials in mildly impaired patients (Homma et al., 2000) as well as in the nursing home setting (Tariot et al., 2001).

Time

An accurate assessment—interviewing the caregiver and the patient independently—takes a minimum of 30–45 minutes.

Reliability and Validity

Face validity of the scale follows from the fact that the scale was developed directly from established clinical criteria for the diagnosis of dementia. The scale has also been validated against pathologically verified cases of AD (Morris et al., 1988) and with prospectively assessed subjects with mild cognitive impairment (Morris et al., 1996). High inter-rater reliability was found in studies of physicians (Burke et al., 1988) and nonphysicians (McCulla et al., 1989) (weighted kappa = 0.87).

Special Considerations

The caregiver who has the most contact with the patient should be interviewed. Others may not be able

ID Number: _____   Date: _____

CLINICAL DEMENTIA RATING SCALE (CDR)

SCORE SHEET

Rater _____   Protocol _____

Instructions for assigning the CDR are as follows:
Use all information and make the best judgment. Score each category (M, O, JPS, CA, HH, PC) as independently as possible. Mark only one item in each category row, rating each according to subject's cognitive function. For determining the CDR, memory is considered the primary category; all others are secondary. If at least three secondary categories are given a score greater or less than the memory score, CDR = score of majority of secondary categories, unless three secondary categories are scored on one side of M and two secondary categories are scored on the other side of M. In this last circumstance, CDR = M.

When M = 0.5, CDR = 1 if at least three of certain others (O, JPS, CA, HH) are scored 1 or greater (PC not influential here). If M = 0.5, CDR cannot be 0; CDR can only be 0.5 or 1. If M = 0, CDR = 0 unless there is slight impairment in two or more secondary categories, in which case CDR = 0.5.

	Healthy CDR 0	Questionable Dementia CDR 0.5	Mild Dementia CDR 1	Moderate Dementia CDR 2	Severe Dementia CDR 3
Memory	No memory loss or slight inconsistent forgetfulness	Mild consistent forgetfulness; partial recollection of events; "benign" forgetfulness	Moderate memory loss, more marked for recent events; defect interferes with everyday activities	Severe memory loss; only highly learned material retained; new material rapidly lost	Severe memory loss; only fragments remain
Orientation	Fully oriented	Fully oriented	Some difficulty with time relationships; oriented for place and person at examination but may have geographic disorientation	Usually disoriented	Orientation to person only
Judgment and Problem Solving	Solves everyday problems well; judgment good in relation to past performance	Only doubtful impairment in solving problems, similarities, differences	Moderate difficulty in handling complex problems; social judgment usually maintained	Severely impaired in handling problems, similarities, differences; social judgment usually impaired	Unable to make judgments or solve problems
Community Affairs	Independent function at usual level in job, shopping, business and financial affairs, volunteer and social groups	Only doubtful mild impairment in these activities	Unable to function independently at these activities though may still be engaged in some; may still appear normal to casual inspection	No pretense of independent function outside the home Appears well enough to be taken to functions outside a family home	No pretense of independent function outside the home Appears too ill to be taken to functions outside a family home
Home and Hobbies	Life at home, hobbies, intellectual interests well maintained	Life at home, hobbies, intellectual interests slightly impaired	Mild but definite impairment of function at home: more difficult chores abandoned; more complicated hobbies and interests abandoned	Only simple chores preserved; very restricted interests, poorly sustained	No significant function in home or outside of own home
Personal Care	Fully capable of self care	Fully capable of self care	Needs occasional prompting	Requires assistance in dressing, hygiene, keeping of personal effects	Requires much help with personal care; often incontinent

CDR Score: _____

Figure 8-10. (From Morris JC. The Clinical Dementia Rating [CDR]: current version and scoring rules. *Neurology* 1993;43[11]:2412–2414, with permission.)

Table 8-4.   Probe Questions for Caregiver Portion of the Clinical Dementia Rating Interview

1. Memory

   Does the patient have problems with her or his thinking or memory? Is this consistent? Does it interfere with everyday activities now? Has it worsened in the last year? Give some examples.

   Can the patient recall a short shopping list?

   Does the patient recall recent events? What about remote events (e.g., birthdays, anniversaries, major holidays, place of work)?

   Does the patient recall details of events?

   Can you give an example of an event that the patient attended in the last week or month, or any unusual event from the last week or month? Provide some details so that I can ask the patient about them later.

   Where was the patient born? What is her or his birthday?

   Where did the patient go to school? What was the name of the school?

2. Orientation

   Does the patient get lost in the home? In the neighborhood? Beyond your neighborhood?

   Does the patient usually know where she or he is?

   Does the patient usually know the day, month, date, and year?

3. Judgment and problem solving

   How is the patient's problem solving? Can you give an example (examples include handling money [e.g., leaving a tip, using a checkbook] or household repairs)?

   How do you think the patient would handle a household emergency?

   How does the patient do in social situations? Does the patient ever interact inappropriately?

4. Home and hobbies

   Has the patient given up his or her job, or any chores or hobbies? Give examples of activities that he or she has given up (good examples include cooking, using appliances, yard work, games).

   What is the patient able to do?

5. Community affairs

   What was the patient's last employment?

   Why did she or he retire?

   Does the patient attend activities outside of the home? Examples of such activities include driving, group discussions, and shopping.

6. Self-care

   Is the patient able to take care of him- or herself in terms of everyday activities?

   Does the patient need prompting?

   Does the patient need assistance in dressing, hygiene, and personal care?

Adapted from unpublished materials provided by John Morris, M.D.

Table 8-5. Additional Questions for the Patient Portion of the Clinical Dementia Rating Interview

1. Memory

   Can you give an example of an event that you attended in the last week or month, or any unusual event from the last week or month?

   Provide some details (may prompt for the occasion, names of people who were there, and so on).

   What was your last employment?

   Why did you retire?

   Where did you go to school? What was the name of the school?

   Where did you grow up?

   Where were you born? What is your birthday?

   Use Mini-Mental State Examination, Blessed, or other standardized instrument.

2. Orientation

   Use Mini-Mental State Examination, Blessed, or other standardized instrument.

3. Judgment and problem solving

   I am going to ask you how some words are alike. For example, a pen and a pencil are alike because they're both used for writing.

   How are an apple and orange alike?

   How are a chair and a table alike?

   How are painting and music alike?

   What would you do if you arrived in a strange city and you wanted to find a friend who you knew lived in that city?

   How many nickels are there in a dollar?

   How many quarters are there in $6.75?

   Can you subtract 3 from 21 and keep subtracting from the answer you get?

Adapted from unpublished materials provided by John Morris, MD.

to give accurate information. Although the global score is not particularly sensitive to change, sensitivity can be improved by using the total score, which is easily generated by adding the domain scores.

Advantages

The CDR is clinically based. It rates domains beyond psychometric testing, thereby integrating cognitive and functional domains. It is valid and reliable. A sum of the scores gives an overall quantitative severity rating, which could potentially be used for following disease progression. The scale is multidimensional and can be used with people in the community and in institutions. The scale has been used in a number of clinical trials and has been shown to be reliable across centers (Morris, 1997; Morris et al., 1997).

Another advantage is that it formalizes clinically relevant history taking. This has been applied in a study that used the CDR to screen for dementia (Juva et al., 1995). These authors found the sensitivity of the CDR to be 0.95 with a specificity of 0.94. These data suggest that the CDR might make an excellent assessment tool for research studies and for clinical practice. The CDR was recently shown to be strongly correlated with the GDS, another widely used global rating scale (Choi et al., 2003).

Disadvantages

One disadvantage of this scale is its inability to make distinctions as severely impaired patients continue to deteriorate. Future versions of the CDR will include more gradation at the higher level of severity, but validation of the extended scale is not yet published.

Another potential issue is the lack of language, depression, and behavior domains. These items may not be reflected in the functional domains graded on the CDR. Moreover, changes in affect and problem behaviors occur at all stages of the disease and, therefore, do not represent features that can be used for staging. Subgroups of patients may have prominent behavioral problems, executive, language, visuospatial or motor dysfunction, which are a consequence of specific pathologic or neurochemical features. These features may have prognostic implications but can present early and may persist through the course of disease in individual patients, arguing against inclusion of these items in a staging system. One group of investigators has validated a scale, the Functional Rating Scale, adapted from the CDR, which includes language and behavior domains (Tuokko, 1993). The Functional Rating Scale has not been as widely used as the CDR in the longitudinal setting.

Global Deterioration Scale

The GDS was developed by Reisberg and colleagues for staging patients with dementia (Reisberg et al., 1982; Figure 8-11). It is a widely used scale that has been extensively studied (Eisdorfer et al., 1992). In the context of clinical trials it has generally been used to rate severity of disease at baseline.

Description

The GDS is a hierarchically organized, seven-level scale with a score of 1 representing the absence of cognitive decline and a score of 7 indicating very severe cognitive impairment. It has a parallel structure to the FAST, and it can be related to traditional global ratings based on cognitive status.

Administration

The scale is derived from a caregiver interview.

Time

An accurate assessment takes approximately 20 minutes.

Reliability and Validity

Concurrent validity was established for the GDS by Reisberg et al. (1994) by comparing scores on the GDS with performance on the MMSE. Reisberg et al. also showed that the GDS correlates significantly (p <.05) with psychometric tests ($r = 0.30$–0.60), the Inventory of Psychic and Somatic Complaints-Elderly ($r = 0.30$–0.70), CT scan measures ($r = 0.50$ for sulcal enlargement and 0.60 for ventricular dilatation), and cerebral blood flow ($r = 0.70$–0.80) (Reisberg et al., 1988). Longitudinal change can also be assessed (Reisberg et al., 1986). Inter-rater reliability for the GDS is quite high, ranging from 0.82 to 0.97 in different studies (Reisberg et al., 1994). Although the scale has generally been used to assess global severity for baseline staging of subjects, it has been used as an outcome measure in clinical trials (Scharf et al., 1999).

Special Considerations

The caregiver who has the most contact with the patient should be interviewed. Others may not be able to give accurate information. The scale is applicable to patients living in nursing facilities where the caregivers are the nursing staff. In this situation it may be difficult to find an individual who knows the patient well enough to apply the scale. In such circumstances, nursing notes may be relied on. It is generally useful to discuss individual items mentioned in the nursing notes with a caregiver who knows the patient.

Advantages

This scale remains one of the few validated, reliable staging systems for patients with dementia. It can easily be related to a simpler three-stage system: mild (GDS = 2–3); moderate (GDS = 4–5); severe (GDS = 6–7). Furthermore, it is relatively easy to apply (Reisberg et al., 1982). The available version of the GDS has been validated in patients with severe dementia, an advantage over other available scales.

Disadvantages

Unlike the CDR, in which the structure helps with documenting a dementia diagnosis, this scale is structured such that it presumes a diagnosis of dementia. This is not a major problem because, in practice, this is usually the case. The GDS has not been validated in pathologically verified cases of AD to our knowledge.

ID Number: _____   Date: _____

Global Deterioration Scale (GDS)

SCORE SHEET

Rater _____   Protocol _____

Informant's Name _____   Relationship with Subject _____

Rate the subject's level of cognitive functioning

1 **No cognitive decline**	* No subjective complaints of memory deficit. No memory deficit evident on clinical interview.
2 **Very mild cognitive decline**	* Subjective complaints of memory deficit, most frequently in following areas: a) forgetting where one has placed familiar objects; b) forgetting names one formerly knew well. No objective evidence of memory deficit on clinical interview. No objective deficits in employment or social situations. Appropriate concern with respect to symptomatology.
3 **Mild cognitive decline**	* Earliest clear-cut deficits. Manifestations in more than one of the following areas: a) patient may have gotten lost when travelling to an unfamiliar location; b) co-workers become aware of patient's relatively poor performance; c) word and name finding deficits become evident to intimates; d) patient may read a passage or book and retain relatively little material; e) patient may demonstrate decreased facility in remembering names upon introduction to new people; f) patient may have lost or misplaced an object of value; g) concentration deficit may be evident on clinical testing. * Objective evidence of memory deficits obtained only with intensive interview. * Decreased performance in demanding employment and social settings. Denial begins to become manifest in patient. Mild to moderate anxiety accompanies symptoms.
4 **Moderate cognitive decline**	* Clear-cut deficit on careful clinical interview. Deficit manifest in following areas: a) decreased knowledge of current and recent events; b) may exhibit some deficit in memory of one's personal history; c) concentration deficit elicited on serial subtractions; d) decreased ability to travel, handle finances, etc. * Frequently no deficit in following areas: a) orientation to time and person; b) recognition of familiar persons and faces; c) ability to travel to familiar locations. * Inability to perform complex tasks. Denial is dominant defense mechanism. Flattening of affect with withdrawal from challenging situations occur.

Figure 8-11. (From Reisberg B, Ferris SH, de Leon MJ, et al. The Global Deterioration Scale for assessment of primary degenerative dementia. *Am J Psychiatry* 1982;139[9]:1136–39, with permission. Copyright 1982, the American Psychiatric Association; http://ajp.psychiatryonline.org.)

ID Number: _____   Date: _____

5 **Moderately severe cognitive decline**	* Patient can no longer survive without some assistance. Patient is unable during interview to recall a major relevant aspect of their current life, e.g.: a) an address or telephone number of many years; b) the names of close members of their family (such as grandchildren); c) the name of the high school or college from which they graduated. * Frequently some disorientation to time (date, day of week, season, etc.) or to place. An educated person may have difficulty counting back from 40 by 4's or from 20 by 2's. * Persons at this stage retain knowledge of many major facts regarding themselves and others. They invariably know their own names and generally know their spouse's and children's names. They require no assistance with toileting and eating, but may have some difficulty choosing the proper clothing to wear.
6 **Severe cognitive decline**	* May occasionally forget the name of the spouse upon who they are entirely dependent for survival. Will be largely unaware of all recent events and experiences in their lives. Retain some knowledge of their past lives but this is very sketchy. Generally unaware of their surroundings, the year, the season, etc. May have difficulty counting from 10, both backward and sometimes, forward. Will require some assistance with activities of daily living, e.g.: may become incontinent; will require travel assistance but occasionally will display ability to be able to travel to familiar locations. Diurnal rhythm frequently disturbed. Almost always recall their own names. Frequently continue to be able to distinguish familiar from unfamiliar persons in their environment. * Personality and emotional changes occur. These are quite variable and include: a) delusional behavior, e.g., patients may accuse their spouse of being an imposter; may talk to imaginary figures in the environment, or to their own reflection in the mirror; b) obsessive symptoms, e.g., person may continually repeat simple cleaning activities; c) anxiety symptoms, agitation, and even previously non-existent violent behavior may occur; d) cognitive abulia, i.e., loss of willpower because an individual cannot carry a thought long enough to determine a purposeful course of action.
7 **Very severe cognitive decline**	* All verbal abilities are lost. Frequently there is no speech at all - only grunting. Incontinent of urine; requires assistance toileting and feeding. Loses basic psychomotor skills, e.g., ability to walk. The brain appears to no longer be able to tell the body what to do. * Generalized and cortical neurologic signs and symptoms are frequently present.

Rating: _____

Figure 8-11.   *continued*

Clinician Interview Based Impression of Change

The Clinician Interview Based Impression of Change (CIBIC-plus) is a formalized approach to form a global impression of change that incorporates caregiver input and assessment of patient function (Figure 8-12). It is a mandatory instrument for clinical dementia trials and should be performed independent of other rating scales, although reference to a baseline assessment is allowed.

Description

The CIBIC-plus is a rating of the impression of change from a baseline state in a clinical trial. The investigator assesses the patient and interviews a caregiver and rates the patient as unchanged (0), improved, or worsened, compared with a baseline assessment. Improvement or worsening are rated at three levels, mild (+/–1), moderate (+/–2) or marked (+/–3), giving a total range of 7 points.

Administration

The CIBIC-plus should be administered by the same assessor throughout a study. Assessors should be experienced in evaluating patients with dementia and can include physicians and others. In the study by Quinn, both neurologists and non-neurologists (who were also experienced in dementia assessment) rated patients with similar validity (Quinn et al., 2002).

Time

Thirty to 45 minutes are generally required to appropriately rate the subject's change.

Reliability and Validity

Although this scale and approach are widely used as key outcome measures in clinical trials, they are relatively insensitive to change. A recent study showed that the impression of change differed from that suggested by assessors' notes recorded as part of the procedure, suggesting a tendency among raters to assign patients to the "no change" level (Joffres et al., 2003). One study showed that validity (rating the direction of change appropriately) was good, ranging from 85% to 90% correct when videotapes were viewed in the true order in a study, and 53% to 63% when viewed in reverse order.

Advantages

The CIBIC-plus is a measure of global change that integrates all aspects of a patient's performance, including cognition, behavior, and function. It is widely used in clinical trials in which it has successfully been able to detect change.

Disadvantages

The poor reliability of the scale is a major concern. In a study in which raters viewed videotaped patient interviews, kappa of 0.18 was obtained using the full 7-point scale (Quinn et al., 2002). Collapsing the scale into unchanged, improved, or worsened improved reliability of kappa = 0.76 when videos of patients were presented in a true order, when improvement in a trial might be expected. This decreased to kappa = 0.12 when the order was reversed. Other global scales (the CDR and the GDS) show better reliability. Nevertheless, change of the CIBIC-plus correlates with change on other objective measures. Although it makes intuitive sense to include a global rating of function in clinical trials, the poor reliability of the CIBIC-plus, even when administered in a structured manner, raises concerns about its use. Nevertheless, considerable data exist regarding its use, and sample size calculations can be based on its properties. Any rated change likely represents a real change (Joffres et al., 2000; Knopman et al., 1994b; Oremus et al., 2000; Rockwood & Joffres, 2002b; Schneider et al., 1997; Spear et al., 2002).

Behavior/Psychopathology Assessment

Personality and behavior changes are well-documented features of the dementias. Both the American Psychiatry Association's criteria for dementia (American Psychiatric Association, 1994) and the diagnostic criteria for AD of the National Institute of Neurological and Communicative Diseases and Stroke/Alzheimer's Disease and Related Disorders Association (McKhann et al., 1984) state that changes in personality and behavior are supportive of the diagnosis of dementia. Many new instruments are available for assessment of various aspects of psychopathology in demented elderly. Some have been developed specifically for use with dementia patients whereas others have more general applications such as the Brief Psychiatric Rat-

ID Number: _____   Date: _____

Clinician Interview Based Impression of Change Plus (CIBIC+)

SCORE SHEET

Rater _____   Protocol _____

_____

Circle the response which best indicates the extent of change observed **SINCE** the **INITIAL BASELINE INTERVIEW:**

0 = Not assessed

1 = Marked Improvement

2 = Moderate Improvement

3 = Minimal Improvement

4 = No Change

5 = Minimal Worsening

6 = Moderate Worsening

7 = Marked Worsening

Figure 8-12. (From Schneider LS, Olin JT, Doody RS, et al. Validity and reliability of the Alzheimer's Disease Cooperative Study-Clinical Global Impression of Change. The Alzheimer's Disease Cooperative Study. *Alzheimer Dis Assoc Disord* 1997;11[Suppl 2]:S22–32, with permission.)

ing Scale (Devanand et al., 1998; Freedman et al., 1998). Articles have reviewed a broad range of behavioral and psychiatric assessment tools (Teri & Logsdon, 1995; Weiner et al., 1996).

Behavioral Pathology in Alzheimer's Disease Rating Scale

The Behavioral Pathology in Alzheimer's Disease Rating Scale (BEHAVE-AD) was developed to assess potentially remediable behaviors in patients with AD, independent of cognitive symptomatology (Reisberg et al., 1987; Figure 8-13). It was intended for use in prospective studies of pharmacologic interventions in the treatment of behavioral symptoms in AD. Items were selected based on chart reviews of outpatients with a diagnosis of AD. It continues to be a widely used instrument for the assessment of behavioral disturbance.

Description

The BEHAVE-AD is a 25-item scale covering the following domains: paranoid and delusional ideation, hallucinations, activity disturbances, aggressiveness, diurnal rhythm disturbances, affective disturbance, and anxieties and phobias. There is one additional item providing a global rating of behavioral disturbance. Items are rated on a 4-point scale based on a clinical interview with a reliable informant. Each item is rated as not present or by descriptive categories of increasing severity, which are specific to each item. Some items have fairly distinct categories whereas others are on a continuum of severity. For example, purposeless activities are rated in terms of the degree of restraint or physical harm resulting from the activity as indicators of severity of the behavior.

Administration

The caregiver is interviewed by a clinician either in person or by telephone. Some of the items, such as one related to delusions of infidelity, are more easily rated by spousal caregivers than by other family members or paid caregivers.

Time

The administration time has been estimated to be approximately 45 minutes (Weiner et al., 1996). Typically, the greater number of difficult behaviors, the longer the interview.

Reliability and Validity

In a comparison of the BEHAVE-AD, the Brief Psychiatric Rating Scale, and the Cornell Scale for Depression in Dementia (CSDD), the BEHAVE-AD was found to have the most items rated as occurring frequently in AD patients but not in control subjects (Mack & Patterson, 1994). Eighty-seven percent of those patients were reported to have at least one symptom. Content validity is based on derivation of items from chart review.

Inter-rater agreement ranged from 81% to 100% across the 25 items, with an overall agreement of 94% (Mack & Patterson, 1994). When corrected for chance agreement, kappa statistics ranged from 0.29 to 1.0, with a median of 0.70.

Special Considerations

Some items of the BEHAVE-AD make it more suitable for use with spouse caregivers. Similarly, some items assume that the patient lives at home, making this instrument inappropriate for use in nursing homes or assisted-living situations. Although it provides a good overview of most behavioral disturbances, it is less comprehensive in some domains than some other instruments.

Advantages

The items of the BEHAVE-AD address most of the behaviors reported to occur frequently in patients with AD. This scale has been shown to be a sensitive measure of change in behavioral pathology and has good reliability. It has been shown to be sensitive to behavioral effects in recent clinical trials assessing behavioral disturbance in dementia (Brodaty et al., 2003a; De Deyn et al., 1999; Katz et al., 1999; Sultzer et al., 2001). Some studies have been negative (Chan et al., 2001).

Disadvantages

The items of this scale do not assess frequency of behavior. Although caregiver distress or burden can be extrapolated from severity ratings, it is not directly evaluated. Of particular concern is the means of rating severity; for some items the behaviors used to describe severity may be indirectly related to the behavior in question. For example, anger or aggression is frequently used as a benchmark of severity for individual items, although aggressiveness is a separate domain within the

ID Number: _____   Date: _____

BEHAVE - AD

SCORE SHEET

Rater _____   Protocol _____

Assessment Interval: Specify _____weeks   Total Score: _____

PART I – SYMPTOMATOLOGY

A. Paranoid and Delusional Ideation

1. "People are Stealing Things" Delusion

> 0 = Not present.
> 1 = Delusion that people are hiding objects.
> 2 = Delusion that people are coming into the home and hiding objects or stealing objects.
> 3 = Talking and listening to people coming into the home.

2. "One's House Is Not One's Home" Delusion

> 0 = Not present.
> 1 = Conviction that the place in which one is residing is not one's home (e.g., packing to go home; complaints, while at home, of "take me home").
> 2 = Attempt to leave domiciliary to go home.
> 3 = Violence in response to attempts to forcibly restrict exit.

3. "Spouse (or Other Caregiver) is an Imposter" Delusion

> 0 = Not present.
> 1 = Conviction that spouse (or other caregiver) is an imposter.
> 2 = Anger toward spouse (or other caregiver) for being an imposter.
> 3 = Violence towards spouse (or other caregiver) for being an imposter.

4. "Delusion of Abandonment" (e.g., to an Institution)

> 0 = Not present.
> 1 = Suspicion of caregiver plotting abandonment or institutionalization (e.g., on telephone).
> 2 = Accusation of a conspiracy to abandon or institutionalize.
> 3 = Accusation of impending or immediate desertion or institutionalization.

5. "Delusion of Infidelity"

> 0 = Not present.
> 1 = Conviction that spouse and/or children and/or other caregivers are unfaithful.
> 2 = Anger toward spouse, relative, or other caregiver for infidelity.
> 3 = Violence toward spouse, relative, or other caregiver for supposed infidelity.

Figure 8-13.   BEHAVE-AD = Behavioral Pathology in Alzheimer's Disease Rating Scale. (Adapted from Reisberg B, Borenstein J, Salob SP, et al. Behavioral symptoms in Alzheimer's disease: phenomenology and treatment. *J Clin Psychiatry* 1987;48[Suppl]:9–15. Copyright 1987, Physicians Postgraduate Press.) (continued)

6. **"Suspiciousness/Paranoia" (other than above)**

    0 = Not present.
    1 = Suspicious (e.g., hiding objects that he/she later may be unable to locate).
    2 = Paranoid (i.e., fixed conviction with respect to suspicions and/or anger as a result of suspicions).
    3 = Violence as a result of suspicions.
    Unspecified? _____
    Describe _____
    _____

7. **Delusions (other than above)**

    0 = Not present.
    1 = Delusional.
    2 = Verbal or emotional manifestations as a result of delusions.
    3 = Physical actions or violence as a result of delusions.
    Unspecified? _____
    Describe _____
    _____

B. Hallucinations

8. **Visual Hallucinations**

    0 = Not present.
    1 = Vague: not clearly defined.
    2 = Clearly defined hallucinations of objects or persons (e.g., sees other people at the table).
    3 = Verbal or physical actions or emotional responses to the hallucinations.

9. **Auditory Hallucinations**

    0 = Not present.
    1 = Vague: not clearly defined.
    2 = Clearly defined hallucinations of words or phrases.
    3 = Verbal or physical actions or emotional response to the hallucinations.

10. **Olfactory Hallucinations**

    0 = Not present.
    1 = Vague: not clearly defined.
    2 = Clearly defined
    3 = Verbal or physical actions or emotional responses to the hallucinations.

11. **Haptic Hallucinations**

    0 = Not present.
    1 = Vague: not clearly defined.
    2 = Clearly defined.
    3 = Verbal or physical actions or emotional responses to the hallucinations.

12. **Other Hallucinations**

    0 = Not present.
    1 = Vague: not clearly defined.
    2 = Clearly defined.
    3 = Verbal or physical actions or emotional responses to the hallucinations.
    Unspecified? _____

Figure 8-13. *continued*

ID Number: _____   Date: _____

Describe_____
_____

C. Activity Disturbances

13. Wandering: Away From Home or Caregiver

    0 = Not present.
    1 = Somewhat, but not sufficient to necessitate restraint.
    2 = Sufficient to require restraint.
    3 = Verbal or physical actions or emotional responses to attempts to prevent wandering.

14. Purposeless Activity (Cognitive Abulia)

    0 = Not present.
    1 = Repetitive, purposeless activity (e.g., opening and closing pocketbook, packing and unpacking clothing, repeatedly putting on and removing clothing, opening and closing drawers, insistent repeating of demands or questions).
    2 = Pacing or other purposeless activity sufficient to require restraint.
    3 = Abrasions or physical harm resulting from purposeless activity.

15. Inappropriate Activity

    0 = Not present.
    1 = Inappropriate activities (e.g., storing and hiding objects in inappropriate places, such as throwing clothing in wastebasket or putting empty plates in the oven; inappropriate sexual behavior, such as inappropriate exposure.
    2 = Present and sufficient to require restraint.
    3 = Present, sufficient to require restraint, and accompanied by anger or violence when restraint is used.

D. Aggressiveness

16. Verbal Outbursts

    0 = Not present.
    1 = Present (including unaccustomed use of foul or abusive language).
    2 = Present and accompanied by anger.
    3 = Present, accompanied by anger, and clearly directed at other persons.

17. Physical Threats and/or Violence

    0 = Not present.
    1 = Threatening behavior.
    2 = Physical violence.
    3 = Physical violence accompanied by vehemence.

18. Agitation (other than above)

    0 = Not present.
    1 = Present.
    2 = Present with emotional component.
    3 = Present with emotional and physical component.
Unspecified? _____
Describe_____
_____

Figure 8-13. *continued*

ID Number: _____   Date: _____

E. Diurnal Rhythm Disturbances

19. Day/Night Disturbance

        0   = Not present.
        1   = Repetitive wakenings during night.
        2   = 50% to 75% of former sleep cycle at night.
        3   = Complete disturbance of diurnal rhythm (i.e., less than 50% of former sleep cycle at night).

F. Affective Disturbance

20. Tearfulness

        0   = Not present.
        1   = Present.
        2   = Present and accompanied by clear affective component.
        3   = Present and accompanied by affective and physical component (e.g., "wrings hands" or other gestures).

21. Depressed Mood: Other

        0   = Not present.
        1   = Present (e.g., occasional statement "I wish I were dead," without clear affective concomitants).
        2   = Present with clear concomitants (e.g., thoughts of death).
        3   = Present with emotional and physical component (e.g., suicide gestures).
Unspecified? _____
Describe_____
_____

G. Anxieties and Phobias

22. Anxiety Regarding Upcoming Events (Godot Syndrome)

        0   = Not present.
        1   = Present: Repeated queries and/or other activities regarding upcoming appointments and/or events.
        2   = Present and disturbing to caregivers.
        3   = Present and intolerable to caregivers.

23. Other Anxieties

        0   = Not present.
        1   = Present.
        2   = Present and disturbing to caregivers.
        3   = Present and intolerable to caregivers.
Unspecified? _____
Describe_____
_____

24. Fear of being Left Alone

        0   = Not present.
        1   = Present: Vocalized fear of being alone.
        2   = Vocalized and sufficient to require specific action on part of caregiver.
        3   = Vocalized and sufficient to require patient to be accompanied at all times.

Figure 8-13. *continued*

ID Number: _____   Date: _____

25. Other Phobias

        0   = Not present.
        1   = Present.
        2   = Present and of sufficient magnitude to require specific action on part of caregiver.
        3   = Present and sufficient to prevent patient activities.
        Unspecified? _____
        Describe_____

PART II – GLOBAL RATING

With respect to the above symptoms, they are of sufficient magnitude as to be:

        0   = Not at all troubling to the caregiver or dangerous to the patient.
        1   = Mildly troubling to the caregiver or dangerous to the patient.
        2   = Moderately troubling to the caregiver or dangerous to the patient.
        3   = Severely troubling or intolerable to the caregiver or dangerous to the patient.

TOTAL SCORE: _____

Figure 8-13. *continued*

scale. Other items indicate severity in terms of impact on caregiver (e.g., "disturbing to caregiver" versus "intolerable to caregiver").

Consortium to Establish a Registry for Alzheimer's Disease Behavior Rating Scale for Dementia

The Consortium to Establish a Registry for Alzheimer's Disease (CERAD) developed this scale to assess a wide range of psychopathology in patients with AD. The CERAD-B (Figure 8-14) is based on clinical experience and a review of existing instruments and literature to elicit information covering symptoms relevant to dementia (Tariot et al., 1995). It has been used to demonstrate the prevalence of behavioral problems in patients with AD (Tractenberg et al., 2003).

Description

The CERAD-B consists of 48 items, most of which are rated on a frequency scale ranging from 0 (has not occurred since illness began) to 4 (present 16 days or more in the past month). Ratings are also available for behaviors that have occurred since the illness began but not in the past month. Five items (e.g., changes in appetite and weight) are rated only as present, absent, or having occurred but not in the past month. At the completion of the interview, the clinician rates the validity of the informant's responses. Scores are not totaled, but rather number of items endorsed can be summed for a rough index of behavioral pathology.

Administration

The patient's informant is questioned by a trained examiner or clinician. Positive responses on certain items require further probing.

ID Number: _____   Date: _____

CERAD Behavior Rating Scale for Dementia (CERAD-B)

SCORE SHEET

Rater _____   Protocol _____

Circle one response for each item, using the following rating scale:

> **RATING SCALE**
> 0 = Has not occurred since illness began
> 1 = 1–2 days in past month
> 2 = 3–8 days in the past month (up to twice per week)
> 3 = 9–15 days in past month (up to half the day in the past month)
> 4 = 16 days or more in past month
> 8 = Occurred since illness began, but not in past month
> 9 = Unable to rate

Question	Rating Scale
1. Has [S] said that [S] feels anxious, worried, tense or fearful? (For example, has [S] expressed worry or fear about being left alone? Has [S] said [S] is anxious or afraid of certain situations?) *If so, describe.*	0 8 1 2 9 3 4
2. Has [S] shown physical signs of anxiety, worry, tension or fear? (For example, is [S] easily startled? Does [S] appear nervous? Does [S] have a tense or worried facial expression?) *If so, describe.*	0 8 1 2 9 3 4
3. Has [S] appeared sad or blue or depressed?	0 8 1 2 9 3 4
4. Has [S] expressed feelings of hopelessness or pessimism?	0 8 1 2 9 3 4
5. Has [S] cried within the past month?	0 8 1 2 9 3 4
6. Has [S] said that [S] feels guilty? (For example, has [S] blamed [S's] self for things [S] did in the past?) *If yes, describe nature and extent of guilt.*	0 8 1 2 9 3 4
7. Has [S] expressed feelings of poor self-esteem? For example, has [S] said that [S] feels like a failure or that [S] feels worthless? *This item is intended to reflect global loss of self-esteem rather than simply a concern over loss of, for example, a particular ability.*	0 8 1 2 9 3 4
8. Has [S] said [S] feels life is not worth living? Or has [S] expressed a wish to die or talked about committing suicide? *If yes, specify what subject said.*	0 8 1 2 9 3 4
9. Has [S] made any suicide attempts? *Include any suicidal gestures in rating this item.*	0 8 1 2 9 3 4
10. Have there been times when [S] doesn't enjoy the things [S] does as much as [S] used to? *This item refers to any specific loss of enjoyment so long as [S] actually engages in the activity in question. [S] need not be an active participant in this activity; [S] need only be present.*	0 = No 8 1 = Yes 9

Figure 8-14. CERAD = Consortium to Establish a Registry for Alzheimer's Disease. (From Patterson MB, Mack JL. CERAD behavior rating scale for dementia. *Alzheimer Dis Assoc Disord* 1997;11:S90–97, with permission.)

11. Do you find [S] sometimes can't seem to **get started** on things [S] used to do, even though [S] is **capable** of doing them? (For example, do you find [S] won't start a task or pastime on [S's] own, but with a little encouragement [S] goes ahead and carries it out?) *This item refers to any failure to initiate activities, so long as the activities are those which S is still capable of carrying out when given the opportunity.*	0 = No 8 1 = Yes 9
12. Has [S] seemed tired or lacking in energy?	0 8 1 2 9 3 4
13. Has [S] had physical complaints that seemed out of proportion to [S's] actual physical problems?	0 8 1 2 9 3 4
14. Was [S's] sleeping pattern in the past month different from the way it was before [S's] dementia began? (For example, does [S] sleep more or less than [S] used to? Does [S] sleep at a different time of day than [S] used to?) *If yes, describe changes.*	0 = No 8 1 = Yes 9
15. Has [S] had difficulty falling asleep or remaining asleep? *If yes, describe.*	0 8 1 2 9 3 4

16. Has [S's] appetite during the past month changed from the way it was before [S's] dementia began? (For example, at meal times does [S's] desire to eat seem different?) *"Appetite" refers to [S's] response to food when it is presented in the usual manner.*
 	
    If yes, circle either increased or decreased   1   Increased
    appetite according to informant's judgment.   2   Decreased
	0 = No 8
	
	1 = Yes 9

17. In the past month, has [S] gained or lost weight without intending to?
 	
                          Gained: 1   Up to 5 lbs
If yes, circle amount gained or lost: 2   More than 5 lbs
                       Lost: 1   Up to 5 lbs
                           2   More than 5 lbs
	0 = No 8
	
	1 = Yes 9

18. In the past month, has [S's] sexual interest been different from the way it was before [S's] dementia began? *If yes, describe.*	0 = No 8 1 = Yes 9
19. Has [S] shown sudden changes in [S's] emotions? (For example, does [S] go from laughter to tears quickly?)	0 8 1 2 9 3 4
20. Have there been times when [S] was agitated or upset? *This item refers to **observable** signs of emotional distress, such as verbal comments, facial expressions, or gestures. It is the **emotional component** that distinguishes this item from item 21.*	0 8 1 2 9 3 4
21. Has [S] seemed restless or overactive? (For example, does [S] fidget or pace? Does [S] finger things or seem unable to sit still?) *When the overactive behavior is associated with emotional agitation that is rated in item 20, it should not be rated here also.*	0 8 1 2 9 3 4

Figure 8-14. *continued*

22. Has [S] done things that seem to have no clear purpose or a confused purpose? (For example, does [S] open and close drawers? Does [S] put things in appropriate places? Does [S] hoard things or rummage through things?) *If [S's] behavior shows a high level of motor activity rather than confusion or lack of purpose, it should be rated under item 21.*	0 8 1 2 9 3 4
23. Does [S] tend to say the same things repeatedly? *This item refers to repetitive statements, including questions, phrases, demands, etc.*	0 8 1 2 9 3 4

24. Has there been a particular time of day during which [S] seemed more confused than at other times?
 	
              1 Daytime
              2 Evening – 6:00 pm to bedtime
   If yes, circle time of day. 3 Night
	0 = No 8
	
	1 = Yes 9

25. Has [S] done socially inappropriate things? (For example, does [S] make vulgar remarks? Does [S] talk excessively to strangers? Has [S] sexually exposed [S's] self or done other things such as making gestures or touching people inappropriately?) *This item is intended to reflect a loss of propriety, not simply confusion. If inappropriate behavior can be rated under a more specific item, such as abusive behavior (item 30) or aggressive behavior (item 31), it should not be rated here.*	0 8 1 2 9 3 4
26. Has [S] wandered or tried to wander for no apparent reason? *"Wandering" includes wandering away from one's residence or caregiver, as well as within the residence. If yes, describe incidents.*	0 8 1 2 9 3 4
27. Has [S] tried to leave home or get away from whoever was taking caring of [S] with an apparent purpose or destination in mind? *If yes, describe incidents.*	0 8 1 2 9 3 4
28. Have there been times when [S] was easily irritated or annoyed?	0 8 1 2 9 3 4
29. Has [S] been uncooperative? (For example, does [S] refuse to accept appropriate help? Does [S] insist on doing things [S's] own way?)	0 8 1 2 9 3 4
30. Has [S] been threatening or verbally abusive toward others?	0 8 1 2 9 3 4
31. Has [S] been physically aggressive toward people or things? (For example, has [S] shoved or physically attached people or thrown or broken objects?)	0 8 1 2 9 3 4
32. Has [S] harmed [S's] self in a way that was not an accident or suicide attempt? (For example, does [S] bang [S's] head or scratch [S's] self badly?) *If yes, describe. This item is intended to rate self-abusive behavior.*	0 8 1 2 9 3 4
33. Does [S] withdraw from social situations? (For example, does [S] avoid groups of people or prefer to be alone? Does [S] avoid participating in activities with others?)	0 8 1 2 9 3 4

Figure 8-14.   *continued*

34. Does [S] seek out more visual or physical contact with [S's] caregivers than before [S's] dementia began? (For example, has [S] seemed "clingy"? Does [S] follow you about or seem to want to be in the same room with you?)	0 = No 8 1 = Yes 9

35. Has [S] done or said anything that suggests [S] believes people are harming, threatening, or taking advantage of [S] in some way? (For example, with no good reason has [S] thought things have been given away or stolen; has [S] thought [S] was mischarged or overcharged for purchases; has [S] seemed suspicious or wary?)
 	
                                0 No
If yes, ask: If you try to correct [S], will [S] accept the truth?   1 Yes
                                  9 N/A
	0 8 1 2
	
	9 3 4

36. Has [S] done or said anything that suggests [S] thinks [S's spouse] is unfaithful?
 	
                                  0 No
If yes, ask: If you try to correct [S], will [S] accept the truth?   1 Yes
                                  9 N/A
	0 8 1 2
	9 3 4

37. Has [S] done or said anything that suggests [S] thinks [S's] spouse or caregiver] is plotting to abandon [S]?
 	
                                  0 No
If yes, ask: If you try to correct [S], will [S] accept the truth?   1 Yes
                                  9 N/A
	0 8 1 2
	9 3 4

38. Has [S] done or said anything that suggests [S] thinks [S's] spouse or caregiver] is an imposter?
                                  0 No
If yes, ask: If you try to correct [S], will [S] accept the truth?   1 Yes
                                  9 N/A
	0 8 1 2
	9 3 4

39. Has [S] done or said anything that suggests [S] thinks that characters on television are real? (For example, has [S] talked to them, acted as if they could hear or see [S], or said that they were friends or neighbors?)
 	
                                  0 No
If yes, ask: If you try to correct [S], will [S] accept the truth?   1 Yes
                                  9 N/A
	0 8 1 2
	9 3 4

40. Has [S] done or said anything that suggests [S] believes that there are people in or around the house beyond those who are actually there?
 	
                                  0 No
If yes, ask: If you try to correct [S], will [S] accept the truth?   1 Yes
                                  9 N/A
	0 8 1 2
	9 3 4

41. Has [S] done or said anything that suggests that [S] believes that a dead person is still alive even though [S] used to know they were dead? *Do not rate memory problems. If [S] simply cannot remember whether a particular person has died, it should not be rated as a mistaken belief.*
 	
                                  0 No
If yes, ask: If you try to correct [S], will [S] accept the truth?   1 Yes
                                  9 N/A
	0 8 1 2
	
	9 3 4

42. Has [S] done or said anything that suggests [S] thinks where [S] lives is not really [S's] home, even though [S] used to consider it home?
 	
                                  0 No
If yes, ask: If you try to correct [S], will [S] accept the truth?   1 Yes
                                  9 N/A
	0 8 1 2
	9 3 4

Figure 8-14. *continued*

ID Number: _____   Date: _____

43. Has [S] misidentified people? (For example, has [S] confused one familiar person with another, or has [S] thought that a familiar person was a stranger?) *"Misidentification" means an actual belief that one person was another, not simply a misnaming or failure to remember who someone is, and it refers to someone actually seen by [S].*	0 8 1 2 9 3 4
44. Has [S] looked at [S's] self in a mirror and not recognized [S's] self?	0 8 1 2 9 3 4
45. Has [S] misidentified things? Has [S] thought common things were something else? (For example, has [S] looked at a pillow and thought it was a person or said that a light bulb was a fire?) *If yes, describe.*	0 8 1 2 9 3 4
46. Has [S] heard voices or sounds when there was no sound? *If yes, describe.* *If yes, rate for clarity.* Vague 0 Clear 1	0 8 1 2 9 3 4
47. Has [S] seen things or people that were not there? *If yes, describe.* *If yes, rate for clarity.* Vague 0 Clear 1	0 8 1 2 9 3 4
48. Before we stop, I want to be sure we've covered all of [S's] problems, except, of course, for [S's] memory problems. Has [S] done anything else in the past month that has seemed strange or been a problem? Has [S] said anything that suggests [S] has some unusual ideas or beliefs that I haven't asked you about? *If response concerns behaviors that can be rated under other items, do so. Any behavior that is rated here should be described. Indicate the most frequently occurring problem and rate it.*	0 8 1 2 9 3 4

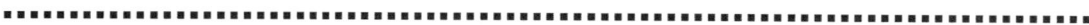

■■

QUALITY OF INTERVIEW (RATER'S JUDGMENT)
Rater should record the basis for judging the interview of 'questionable' or 'doubtful validity'.

Interview appeared valid.	0
Some questions about validity of interview, but it is probably acceptable.	1
Information from interview is of doubtful validity.	2
Comments:	

Figure 8-14. *continued*

Time

A thorough interview can take approximately 30–45 minutes.

Reliability and Validity

Validation of the scale has not yet been performed. However, in the original sample of 303 patients, the number of items endorsed grew with increasing dementia severity. Furthermore, global assessments of behavior or personality change were associated with a greater number of behavior problems on the CERAD-B. A factor analysis yielded eight clinically relevant domains: depressive features, psychotic features, defective self-regulation, irritability/agitation, vegetative features, apathy, aggression, and affective lability.

Inter-rater reliability was calculated for a subset of 104 patients for whom the CERAD-B was scored simultaneously by two raters. Agreement ranged from 91% to 100% across items.

On the basis of these analyses, the instrument has been modified. Some items have been discarded due to a very low rate of occurrence; others have been reworded to be more inclusive.

Advantages

This scale has been developed for use with AD patients. It has been administered to a large sample of carefully characterized subjects with probable AD. It covers a broad range of psychopathology in mildly to moderately impaired patients. Response choices are unambiguous and include the opportunity to report behaviors that have occurred since the illness began but not in the recent past.

Disadvantages

The length of the CERAD-B makes it impractical in some settings. Many patients will not manifest a large number of the behaviors described, yet the scale must be administered in its entirety. It has yet to be validated on the full range of dementia severity, notably those with very mild or very severe dementia. As a research instrument, it lacks an adequate scoring system.

Neuropsychiatric Inventory

The Neuropsychiatric Inventory (NPI, Cummings et al., 1994) was developed to assess behavioral disturbances in patients with dementia (Figure 8-15). Ten domains were selected for evaluation based on the frequency of their occurrence and their potential for distinguishing among the dementias. The NPI was reviewed by a panel of experts who rated the ability of the individual items to capture the important features of each behavioral domain.

Description

This instrument consists of 10 behavioral domains: delusions, hallucinations, dysphoria, anxiety, agitation/aggression, euphoria, disinhibition, irritability/lability, apathy, and aberrant motor behavior. Each domain includes a screening item and seven to eight subquestions. For example, if an informant responds in the affirmative to an initial question about hallucinations, seven additional items describing unusual sensory experiences are administered. If the respondent indicates that a behavior does not occur, the subsequent items in that domain are skipped. Each domain is rated in terms of frequency and severity, yielding a score based on the most aberrant or problematic behavior(s) within that domain. A maximum composite score of 120 is possible for the total NPI.

Administration

Information is obtained from an informed caregiver who is familiar with the patient's premorbid behavior. Daily contact with the patient is considered necessary to be able to respond adequately.

Time

The format of the NPI, whereby screening questions are sufficient for behaviors that are not present, makes it an efficient way to assess these domains. Administration time can take 30 minutes or less, depending on the number of behavioral domains probed.

Reliability and Validity

Content validity was based on ratings by a panel of experts on the adequacy of assessment within each domain. Concurrent validity was determined in a comparison of the NPI with comparable subscales of the BEHAVE-AD. Significant correlations demonstrated that the instruments are describing similar psychopathology. A comparison of AD patients with healthy controls yielded significant differences in scores on all 10 behavioral domains. Further, overall scores on the NPI were associated with dementia severity.

ADCO
Modified Neuropsychiatric Inventory
Adapted from the UCLA Neuropsychiatric Inventory

Page 1 of 4

Office Use Only

Clinic Site   Patient ID#   Patient Designation   Evaluation #

Patient Name _____

Evaluation Date ☐☐ ☐☐ ☐☐
                M   D   Y

Name of Informant _____

Name of Person Completing Form _____

Medical Record # _____

Evaluating Clinician _____

Relationship to patient _____

Date Completed _____

Instructions: SCORE behaviors present since onset of illness, NOT present throughout patient's life. If behavior *HAS occurred in the LAST MONTH*, check off all subquestions that apply and mark the overall frequency and severity of the behavior. *OTHERWISE* go to the next behavior.

A. IRRITABILITY/ LABILITY: Does (S) get irritated and easily disturbed? Are his/her moods very changeable? Is he/she abnormally impatient? We do not mean frustration over memory loss or inability to perform usual tasks; we are interested to know if (S) has abnormal irritability, impatience, or rapid emotional changes different from his/ her usual self.

☐ **N/A**, unable to assess, e.g., too impaired.
☐ **NO**, not since illness began.   } **Go directly to next behavior - Item B**
☐ **YES**, since illness began but not in the last month.

☐ **YES, has occurred in the last month**

☐ 1. Does (S) have a bad temper, flying "off the handle" easily over little things?
☐ 2. Does (S) rapidly change moods from one to another, being fine one minute and angry the next?
☐ 3. Does (S) have sudden flashes of anger?
☐ 4. Is (S) impatient, having trouble coping with delays or waiting for planned activities?
☐ 5. Is (S) cranky and irritable?
☐ 6. Is (S) argumentative and difficult to get along with?
☐ 7. Does (S) show any other signs of irritability?

Frequency:
☐ 1. **Occasionally** - less than once per week.
☐ 2. **Often** - about once per week.
☐ 3. **Frequently** - several times per week but less than every day.
☐ 4. **Very frequently** - essentially continuously present.

Severity:
☐ 1. **Mild** - irritability or lability is notable but usually responds to redirection and reassurance.
☐ 2. **Moderate** - irritability and lability are very evident and difficult to overcome by the caregiver.
☐ 3. **Marked** - irritability and lability are very evident, they usually fail to respond to any intervention by the caregiver, and they are a major source of distress.

Frequency x Severity Subscore ☐☐ (0-12)

B. AGITATION/ AGGRESSION: Does (S) have periods when he/she refuses to cooperate or won't let people help him/her? Is he/she hard to handle?

☐ **N/A**, unable to assess, e.g., too impaired.
☐ **NO**, not since illness began.   } **Go directly to next behavior - Item C**
☐ **YES**, since illness began but not in the last month.

☐ **YES, has occurred in the last month**

☐ 1. Does (S) get upset with those trying to care for him/her or resist activities such as bathing or changing clothes?
☐ 2. Is (S) stubborn, having to have things his/her way?
☐ 3. Is (S) uncooperative, resistive to help from others?
☐ 4. Does (S) have any other behaviors that make him/her hard to handle?
☐ 5. Does (S) shout or curse angrily?
☐ 6. Does (S) slam doors, kick furniture, throw things?
☐ 7. Does (S) attempt to hurt or hit others?
☐ 8. Does (S) have any other aggressive or agitated behaviors?

Frequency:
☐ 1. **Occasionally** - less than once per week.
☐ 2. **Often** - about once per week.
☐ 3. **Frequently** - several times per week but less than daily.
☐ 4. **Very frequently** - once or more per day.

Severity:
☐ 1. **Mild** - behavior is disruptive but can be managed with redirection or reassurance.
☐ 2. **Moderate** - behavior disruptive and difficult to redirect or control.
☐ 3. **Marked** - agitation is very disruptive and a major source of difficulty; there may be a threat of personal harm. Medications are often required.

Frequency x Severity Subscore ☐☐ (0-12)

C. ANXIETY: Is (S) very nervous, worried, or frightened for no apparent reason? Does he/she seem very tense or fidgety? Is the patient afraid to be apart from you?

☐ **N/A**, unable to assess, e.g., too impaired.
☐ **NO**, not since illness began.   } **Go directly to next behavior - Item D**
☐ **YES**, since illness began but not in the last month.

☐ **YES, has occurred in the last month**

☐ 1. Does (S) say that he/she is worried about planned events?
☐ 2. Does (S) have feelings of feeling shaky, unable to relax, or feeling excessively tense?
☐ 3. Does (S) have periods of [or complain of] shortness of breath, gasping, or sighing for no apparent reason other than nervous?
☐ 4. Does (S) complain of butterflies in his/her stomach, or of racing or pounding of the heart in association with nervousness? [Symptoms not explained by ill heath]
☐ 5. Does (S) avoid certain places or situations that make him/her more nervous such as riding in the car, meeting with friends, or being in crowds?
☐ 6. Does (S) become nervous and upset when separated from you [or his/her caregiver]? [Does he/she cling to you to keep you from being separated?]
☐ 7. Does (S) show any other signs of anxiety?

Frequency:
☐ 1. **Occasionally** - less than once per week.
☐ 2. **Often** - about once per week.
☐ 3. **Frequently** - several times per week but less than every day.
☐ 4. **Very frequently** - once or more per day.

Severity:
☐ 1. **Mild** - anxiety is distressing but usually responds to redirection or reassurance.
☐ 2. **Moderate** - anxiety is distressing, anxiety symptoms are spontaneously voiced by the patient and difficult to alleviate.
☐ 3. **Marked** - anxiety is very distressing and a major source of suffering for (S).

Frequency x Severity Subscore ☐☐ (0-12)

ADCONPInventory   2/9/96

Figure 8-15. (From Cummings JL, Mega M, Gray K, et al. The Neuropsychiatric Inventory: comprehensive assessment of psychopathology in dementia. *Neurology* 1994;44[12]:2308–14, with permission.)

Page 2 of 4

Office Use Only						
Patient's Name		Clinic Site	Patient ID#	Designation	Evaluation #	Evaluation Date

D. DEPRESSION/ DYSPHORIA: Does (S) seem sad or depressed? Does he/she say that he/she feels sad or depressed?

☐ **N/A**, unable to assess, e.g., too impaired.
☐ **NO**, not since illness began.   } **Go directly to next behavior - Item E**
☐ **YES**, since illness began but not in the last month.

☐ YES, has occurred in the last month

☐ 1. Does (S) have periods of tearfulness or sobbing that seem to indicate sadness?
☐ 2. Does (S) say or act as if he/she is sad or in low spirits?
☐ 3. Does (S) put him/herself down or say that he/she feels like a failure?
☐ 4. Does (S) say that he/she is a bad person or deserves to be punished?
☐ 5. Does (S) seem very discouraged or say that he/she has no future?
☐ 6. Does (S) say he/she is a burden to the family or that the family would be better off without him/her?
☐ 7. Does (S) express a wish for death or talk about killing him/herself?
☐ 8. Does (S) show any other signs of depression or sadness?

Frequency:
☐ 1. **Occasionally** - less than once per week.
☐ 2. **Often** - about once per week.
☐ 3. **Frequently** - several times per week but less than every day.
☐ 4. **Very frequently** - essentially continuously present.

Severity:
☐ 1. **Mild** - depression is distressing but usually responds to redirection or reassurance.
☐ 2. **Moderate** - depression is distressing, depressive symptoms are spontaneously voiced by (S) and difficult to alleviate.
☐ 3. **Marked** - depression is very distressing and a major source of suffering for (S).

Frequency x Severity Subscore ☐☐
(0-12)

E. ELATION/ EUPHORIA: Does (S) seem too cheerful or too happy for no reason? I don't mean the normal happiness that comes from seeing friends, receiving presents, or spending time with family members. I am asking if (S) has a persistent and <u>abnormally</u> good mood or finds humor where others do not.

☐ **N/A**, unable to assess, e.g., too impaired.
☐ **NO**, not since illness began.   } **Go directly to next behavior - Item F**
☐ **YES**, since illness began but not in the last month.

☐ YES, has occurred in the last month

☐ 1. Does (S) appear to feel too good or to be too happy, different from his/her usual self?
☐ 2. Does (S) find humor and laugh at things that others do not find funny?
☐ 3. Does (S) seem to have a childish sense of humor with a tendency to giggle or laugh inappropriately (such as when something unfortunate happens to others)?
☐ 4. Does (S) tell jokes or make remarks that have little humor for others but seem funny to him/her?
☐ 5. Does (S) play childish pranks such as pinching or playing "keep away" for the fun of it?
☐ 6. Does (S) "talk big" or claim to have more abilities or wealth than is true?
☐ 7. Does (S) show any other signs of feeling too good or being too happy?

Frequency:
☐ 1. **Occasionally** - less than once per week.
☐ 2. **Often** - about once per week.
☐ 3. **Frequently** - several times per week but less than every day.
☐ 4. **Very frequently** - essentially continuously present.

Severity:
☐ 1. **Mild** - elation is notable to friends and family but is not disruptive.
☐ 2. **Moderate** - elation is notably abnormal.
☐ 3. **Marked** - elation is very pronounced; (S) is euphoric and finds nearly everything to be humorous.

Frequency x Severity Subscore ☐☐
(0-12)

F. DISINHIBITION: Does (S) seem to act impulsively without thinking? Does he/she do or say things that are not usually done or said in public? Does he/she do things that are embarrassing to you or others?

☐ **N/A**, unable to assess, e.g., too impaired.
☐ **NO**, not since illness began.   } **Go directly to next behavior - Item G**
☐ **YES**, since illness began but not in the last month.

☐ YES, has occurred in the last month

☐ 1. Does (S) act impulsively without appearing to consider the consequences?
☐ 2. Does (S) talk to total strangers as if he/she knew them?
☐ 3. Does (S) say things to people that are insensitive or hurt their feelings?
☐ 4. Does (S) say crude things or make sexual remarks that they would not usually have said?
☐ 5. Does (S) talk openly about very personal or private matters not usually discussed in public?
☐ 6. Does (S) take liberties or touch or hug others in a way that is out of character?
☐ 7. Does (S) show any other signs of loss of control of his/her impulses?

Frequency:
☐ 1. **Occasionally** - less than once per week.
☐ 2. **Often** - about once per week.
☐ 3. **Frequently** - several times per week but less than every day.
☐ 4. **Very frequently** - essentially continuously present.

Severity:
☐ 1. **Mild** - disinhibition is notable but usually responds to redirection and guidance.
☐ 2. **Moderate** - disinhibition is very evident and difficult to overcome by the caregiver.
☐ 3. **Marked** - disinhibition usually fails to respond to any intervention by the caregiver, and is a source of embarrassment or social distress.

Frequency x Severity Subscore ☐☐
(0-12)

ADCONPInventory   2/9/96

Figure 8-15. *continued*

Office Use Only						
Patient's Name		Clinic Site	Patient ID#	Designation	Evaluation #	Evaluation Date

G. APATHY/ INDIFFERENCE:

Has (S) lost interest in the world around him/her? Has he/she lost interest in doing things or lack motivation for starting new activities? Is he/she more difficult to engage in conversation or in doing chores? Is the patient apathetic or indifferent?

☐ **N/A**, unable to assess, e.g., too impaired.
☐ **NO**, not since illness began.   } **Go directly to next behavior - Item H**
☐ **YES**, since illness began but not in the last month.

☐ YES, has occurred in the last month

1. Does (S) seem less spontaneous and less active than usual?
2. Is (S) less likely to initiate conversation?
3. Is (S) less affectionate or lacking in emotions when compared to his/her usual self?
4. Does (S) contribute less to household chores?
5. Does (S) seem less interested in the activities and plans of others?
6. Has (S) lost interest in friends and family members?
7. Is (S) less enthusiastic about his/her usual interests?
8. Does (S) show any other signs that he/she doesn't care about doing new things?

Frequency:
☐ 1. **Occasionally** - less than once per week.
☐ 2. **Often** - about once per week.
☐ 3. **Frequently** - several times per week but less than every day.
☐ 4. **Very frequently** - nearly always present.

Severity:
☐ 1. **Mild** - apathy is notable but produces little interference with daily routines; only mildly different from (S) usual behavior; (S) responds to suggestions to engage in activities.
☐ 2. **Moderate** - apathy is very evident; may be overcome by the caregiver with coaxing and encouragement; responds spontaneously only to powerful events such as visits from close relatives or family members.
☐ 3. **Marked** - apathy is very evident and usually fails to respond to any encouragement or external events.

Frequency x Severity Subscore ☐☐ (0-12)

H. ABERRANT MOTOR BEHAVIOR:

Does the patient pace, do things over and over such as opening closets or drawers, or repeatedly pick at things or wind string or threads?

☐ **N/A**, unable to assess, e.g., too impaired.
☐ **NO**, not since illness began.   } **Go directly to next behavior - Item I**
☐ **YES**, since illness began but not in the last month.

☐ YES, has occurred in the last month

1. Does (S) pace around the house without apparent purpose?
2. Does (S) rummage around opening and unpacking drawers or closets?
3. Does (S) repeatedly put on and take off clothing?
4. Does (S) have repetitive activities or "habits" that he/she performs over and over?
5. Does (S) engage in repetitive activities such as handling buttons, picking, wrapping string, etc.?
6. Does (S) fidget excessively, seem unable to sit still, or bounce his/her feet or tap his/her fingers a lot?
7. Does (S) do any other activities over and over?

Frequency:
☐ 1. **Occasionally** - less than once per week.
☐ 2. **Often** - about once per week.
☐ 3. **Frequently** - several times per week but less than every day.
☐ 4. **Very frequently** - essentially continuously present.

Severity:
☐ 1. **Mild** - abnormal motor activity is notable but produce little interference with daily routines.
☐ 2. **Moderate** - abnormal motor activity is very evident; can be overcome by the caregiver.
☐ 3. **Marked** - abnormal motor activity is very evident, it usually fails to respond to any intervention by the caregiver and is a major source of distress.

Frequency x Severity Subscore ☐☐ (0-12)

I. DELUSIONS:

Does (S) have beliefs that you know are not true? For example, insisting that people are trying to harm him/her or steal from him/her. Has he/she said that family members are not who they say they are or that the house is not their home? I'm not asking about mere suspiciousness; I am interested if (S) is <u>convinced</u> that these things are happening to him/her.

☐ **N/A**, unable to assess, e.g., too impaired.
☐ **NO**, not since illness began.   } **Go directly to next behavior - Item J**
☐ **YES**, since illness began but not in the last month.

☐ YES, has occurred in the last month

1. Does (S) believe that he/she is in danger - that others are planning to hurt him/her?
2. Does (S) believe that others are stealing from him/her?
3. Does (S) believe that his/her spouse is having an affair?
4. Does (S) believe that unwelcome guests are living in his/her house?
5. Does (S) believe that his/her spouse or others are not who they claim to be?
6. Does (S) believe that his/her house is not his/her home?
7. Does (S) believe that family members plan to abandon him/her?
8. Does (S) believe that television or magazine figures are actually present in the home? [Does he/she try to talk to them?]
9. Does (S) believe any other unusual things that I haven't asked about?

Frequency:
☐ 1. **Occasionally** - less than once per week.
☐ 2. **Often** - about once per week.
☐ 3. **Frequently** - several times per week but less than every day.
☐ 4. **Very frequently** - once or more per day.

Severity:
☐ 1. **Mild** - delusions present but seem harmless and produce little distress in the patient.
☐ 2. **Moderate** - delusions are distressing and disruptive.
☐ 3. **Marked** - delusions are very disruptive and are a major source of behavioral disruption. [If PRN medications are prescribed, their use signals that the delusions are of marked severity.]

Frequency x Severity Subscore ☐☐ (0-12)

ADCONPInventory   2/9/96

Figure 8-15. *continued*

Office Use Only						
Patient's Name			Clinic Site	Patient ID#	Designation	Evaluation #	Evaluation Date

J. HALLUCINATIONS:

Does (S) have hallucinations such as false visions or voices? Does he/she seem to see, hear or experience things that are not present? By this question we do not mean just mistaken beliefs such as stating that someone who has died is still alive; rather we are asking if the patient actually has abnormal experiences of sounds, or visions.

☐ **N/A**, unable to assess, e.g., too impaired.
☐ **NO**, not since illness began.   } **Go directly to next behavior - Item K**
☐ **YES**, since illness began but not in the last month.

☐ **YES, has occurred in the last month**

☐ 1. Does (S) describe hearing voices or act as if he/she hears voices?
☐ 2. Does (S) talk to people who are not there?
☐ 3. Does (S) describe seeing things not seen by others or behave as if he/she is seeing things not seen by others (people, animals, lights, etc.)?
☐ 4. Does (S) report smelling odors not smelled by others?
☐ 5. Does (S) describe feeling things on his/her skin or otherwise appear to be feeling things crawling or touching him/her?
☐ 6. Does (S) describe tastes that are without any known cause?
☐ 7. Does (S) describe any other unusual sensory experiences?

Frequency:
☐ 1. **Occasionally** - less than once per week.
☐ 2. **Often** - about once per week.
☐ 3. **Frequently** - several times per week but less than every day.
☐ 4. **Very frequently** - once or more per day

Severity:
☐ 1. **Mild** - hallucinations are present but harmless and cause little distress for the patient.
☐ 2. **Moderate** - hallucinations are distressing and are disruptive to the patient.
☐ 3. **Marked** - hallucinations are very disruptive and are a major source of behavioral disturbance. PRN medications may be required to control them.

Frequency x Severity Subscore ☐☐ (0-12)

K. SLEEP:

Does (S) have difficulty sleeping (do not count as present if (S) simply gets up once or twice per night only to go to the bathroom and falls back asleep immediately)? Is he/she up at night? Does he/she wander at night, get dressed, or disturb your sleep?

☐ **N/A**, unable to assess, e.g., too impaired.
☐ **NO**, not since illness began.   } **Go directly to next behavior - Item L**
☐ **YES**, since illness began but not in the last month.

☐ **YES, has occurred in the last month**

☐ 1. Does (S) have difficulty falling asleep?
☐ 2. Does (S) get up during the night (do not count if the patient gets up once or twice per night only to go to the bathroom and falls back asleep immediately)?
☐ 3. Does (S) wander, pace, or get involved in inappropriate activities at night?
☐ 4. Does (S) awaken you during the night?
☐ 5. Does (S) awaken at night, dress, and plan to go out thinking that it is morning and time to start the day?
☐ 6. Does (S) awaken too early in the morning (earlier than was his/her habit)?
☐ 7. Does (S) sleep excessively during the day?
☐ 8. Does (S) have any other night-time behaviors that bother you that we haven't talked about?

Frequency:
☐ 1. **Occasionally** - less than once per week.
☐ 2. **Often** - about once per week.
☐ 3. **Frequently** - several times per week but less than every day.
☐ 4. **Very frequently** - once or more per day (every night).

Severity:
☐ 1. **Mild** - night-time behaviors occur but they are not particularly disruptive.
☐ 2. **Moderate** - night-time behaviors occur and disturb the patient and the sleep of the caregiver; more than one type of night-time behavior may be present.
☐ 3. **Marked** - night-time behaviors occur; several types of night-time behavior may be present; (S) is very distressed during the night and the caregiver's sleep is markedly disturbed.

Frequency x Severity Subscore ☐☐ (0-12)

L. APPETITE AND EATING DISORDERS:

Has (S) had any change in appetite, weight, or eating habits (count as N/A if (S) is incapacitated and has to be fed)? Has there been any change in type of food he/she prefers?

☐ **N/A**, unable to assess, e.g., too impaired.
☐ **NO**, not since illness began.   } **End**
☐ **YES**, since illness began but not in the last month.

☐ **YES, has occurred in the last month**

☐ 1. Has (S) had a loss of appetite?
☐ 2. Has (S) had in an increase in appetite?
☐ 3. Has (S) had a loss of weight?
☐ 4. Has (S) gained weight?
☐ 5. Has (S) had a change in eating behavior such as putting too much food in his/her mouth at once?
☐ 6. Has (S) had a change in the kind of food he/she likes such as eating too many sweets or other specific types of food?
☐ 7. Has (S) developed eating behaviors such as eating exactly the same types of food each day or eating the food in exactly the same order?
☐ 8. Have there been any other changes in appetite or eating that I haven't asked about?

Frequency:
☐ 1. **Occasionally** - less than once per week.
☐ 2. **Often** - about once per week.
☐ 3. **Frequently** - several times per week but less than every day.
☐ 4. **Very frequently** - once or more per day or continuously.

Severity:
☐ 1. **Mild** - changes in appetite or eating are present but have not led to changes in weight and are not disturbing.
☐ 2. **Moderate** - changes in appetite or eating are present and cause minor fluctuations in weight.
☐ 3. **Marked** - obvious changes in appetite or eating are present and cause fluctuations in weight, are embarrassing, or otherwise disturb (S).

Frequency x Severity Subscore ☐☐ (0-12)

Total Neuropsychiatric Inventory Score ☐☐☐ (0-244)

ADCONPInventory   2/9/96

Figure 8-15.   *continued*

Inter-rater agreement ranged from 89% for apathy to 100% for several other subscale scores. Overall test-retest correlations were 0.79 for frequency and 0.86 for severity; all subscale test-retest reliabilities yielded significant correlations. Cronbach's coefficient alpha was 0.88, demonstrating good internal consistency among items of the NPI.

Advantages

The screening approach allows time for more detailed questioning of areas relevant to a particular patient while not belaboring areas that are less germane. This is one of the few scales that was developed with the intention of distinguishing among the dementias based on behavior changes, although, as yet, those studies have not been performed. The NPI is distinct from others in its assessment of a behavior's frequency, severity, and impact on a caregiver. The NPI has been used to measure behavioral problems in a number of recent clinical trials (Aisen et al., 2003; Brodaty et al., 2003b; Morris et al., 1998; Tariot et al., 2001; Tariot et al., 2000), including a study examining patients with dementia with Lewy bodies (McKeith et al., 2000a) in which rivastigmine was shown to significantly improve behavioral function. A nursing home version of the NPI was developed and has been used in clinical trials (Clark et al., 2001).

Disadvantages

It may occur that a caregiver denies problems based on the screening item but would respond in the affirmative to probe items within that domain. These would be missed by use of the screening approach. Despite its face validity, the NPI hasn't been as widely used in clinical trials of dementia other than AD, but it has been used to compare AD with frontotemporal dementia (Nyatsanza et al., 2003). As noted in Advantages earlier, it has been used in dementia with Lewy bodies in one trial, and it may well be of use in vascular dementia. But this needs further validation. Although the use of individual items from the scale (e.g., NPI-4, which specifically examines delusions, hallucinations, apathy, and depression) has been evaluated, this approach requires further validation.

Whereas the scales described thus far were developed to provide comprehensive assessments of behavioral disturbances in dementia patients, the remaining instruments have as their goal the quantification of particular domains of psychopathology. One scale provides a detailed assessment of agitated behaviors, whereas depressive symptomatology is the focus of several instruments, two of which will be described below.

Cohen-Mansfield Agitation Inventory

Agitation has been operationally defined by Jiska Cohen-Mansfield as "inappropriate verbal, vocal, or motor activity that is not judged by an outside observer to result directly from the needs or confusion of the agitated individual" (Figure 8-16; Cohen-Mansfield, 1986). The Cohen-Mansfield Agitation Inventory (CMAI; Cohen-Mansfield & Billig, 1986) was originally developed as a research instrument for use in nursing homes. Items were selected based on nurses' perceptions and a review of the literature. A community-based version added several items specific to that population.

Description

The current form of the CMAI consists of 29 items rated on a seven-point scale of frequency, from 1 = never to 7 = several times an hour (Cohen-Mansfield & Libin, 2004). Behaviors are rated on the basis of the prior 2 weeks. A factor analysis revealed three factors: aggressive behavior (e.g., hitting, grabbing, pushing), physically nonaggressive behavior (e.g., pacing, repetitious mannerisms, trying to get to a different place), and verbally agitated behavior (e.g., complaining, screaming, constant requests for attention). A 14-item short form has been developed, where behaviors are rated on a 5-point scale. Computation of total scores is not recommended; factor scores or analyses of individual items may provide more meaningful information. We reproduce all 36 behaviors from the original scale.

Administration

The CMAI may be self-administered by a caregiver or can be completed by interviewing the informant.

Time

It should take no longer than 15–20 minutes to administer the 29 items in an interview. Caregiver self-administration tends to take less time.

Reliability and Validity

Several studies have reported reliability and validity data for the CMAI. Concurrent validity has

ID Number: _____   Date: _____

Cohen-Mansfield Agitation Inventory (CMAI)

SCORE SHEET

Rater _____   Protocol _____

_____

Say to the Informant: "I would like to ask you about certain specific behaviors sometimes seen in older persons. Some are verbal. Some are physical. Some are quiet behaviors and others are disruptive. I do not expect that all of these behaviors will apply to your relative (patient). I will read you a description of the 36 behaviors on this list. I will want to know how often the behavior occurred in the past two weeks. I have given you a card with a list of the behaviors I will be asking you about. I would like you to indicate the frequency of each behavior on the card".

"The frequencies listed on the card are:"

- Never = 1
- Less than once a week but still occurring = 2
- Once or twice a week = 3
- Several times a week (3 or more) = 4
- Once or twice a day = 5
- Several times a day (3 or more) = 6
- Several times an hour (2 or more) = 7
- Not Applicable

QUESTIONS	Never	Less than once a week	Once or twice a week	Several times a week	Once or twice a day	Several times a day	Several times an hour	Not Applicable
1. During the past two weeks, how often did {S} repeat sentences or questions ? (was repetitive, whether or not addressed to any particular person)								
2. During the past two weeks, how often did {S} verbally interrupt or cut short others' interactions or conversations by saying something that was <u>relevant</u> to the conversation or ongoing activity ?								
3. During the past two weeks, how often did {S} verbally interrupt or cut short others' interactions or conversations by saying something that was <u>not relevant</u> to the conversation or ongoing activity ?								
4. During the past two weeks, how often did {S} make strange noises, including strange laughter, moaning, or crying ?								
5. During the past two weeks, how often did {S} scream, shout, or howl ?								
6. During the past two weeks, how often did {S} complain or whine ?								
7. During the past two weeks, how often did {S} make unwarranted requests for attention or help ? (includes nagging, pleading, calling out)								
8. During the past two weeks, how often was {S} negative, uncooperative or unwilling to participate in activities ? (bad attitude, doesn't like anything, nothing is right, includes social activities, eating, bathing)								

Figure 8-16. (From Cohen-Mansfield J. Alzheimer's disease cooperative study: a multicenter evaluation of new treatment efficacy instruments for AD clinical trials. *Alzheimer Dis Assoc Disord* 1997;11:S98–100, with permission.) (continued)

9. During the past two weeks, how often did {S} curse or was {S} verbally threatening or insulting ? (verbal aggression; score only if intelligible words were used; otherwise score under item 5)									
10. During the past two weeks, how often did {S} spit (including during meals) ? (does not include involuntary salivation or drooling)									
11. During the past two weeks, how often was {S} verbally bossy or pushy ?									
12. During the past two weeks, how often did {S} make verbal sexual advances (includes direct sexual propositioning or obvious sexual hints)									
13. During the past two weeks, how often did {S} make physical sexual advances or expose his/her sexual parts ? (includes inappropriate sexual touching of self or others)									
14. During the past two weeks, how often was {S} restless or fidgety, tended to move around when in a seat, or repeatedly get up and sit down (couldn't sit still)?									
15. During the past two weeks, how often did {S} pace, walk repeatedly back and forth, or wander aimlessly ? (includes wandering when done in a wheelchair)									
16. During the past two weeks, how often did {S} try to get out of doors inappropriately, sneak out, or inappropriately enter other places ?									
17. During the past two weeks, how often did {S} dress or undress inappropriately ? (such as undressing in public or repeatedly dressing and undressing; does not refer to inability to get dressed. If only sexual parts are exposed, rate on item 13)									
18. During the past two weeks, how often did {S} perform repetitious mannerisms ? (includes rocking, rubbing, tapping, picking at skin)									
19. During the past two weeks, how often did {S} handle things inappropriately ? (rummaging through drawers, picking up others' possessions or things that should not be touched)									
20. During the past two weeks, how often did {S} grab or snatch things from others ? (including food from others' plates)									
21. During the past two weeks, how often did {S} hoard or collect objects ?									
22. During the past two weeks, how often did {S} hide objects ?									
23. During the past two weeks, how often did {S} exhibit strange movements, such as making faces (frowning or grimacing) inappropriately, or moving arms and legs aimlessly ?									
24. During the past two weeks, how often did {S} have a temper outburst, including verbal or nonverbal expressions of anger ?									
25. During the past two weeks, how often did {S} hit people, self or objects ?									
26. During the past two weeks, how often did {S} kick people or objects?									
27. During the past two weeks, how often did {S} throw things (such as food) or knock objects off surfaces ?									
28. During the past two weeks, how often did {S} tear or destroy objects or property ?									
29. During the past two weeks, how often did {S} grab on to or cling to people physically ?									
30. During the past two weeks, how often did {S} push other people ?									
31. During the past two weeks, how often did {S} bite people or things ?									
32. During the past two weeks, how often did {S} scratch people, self or things ?									
33. During the past two weeks, how often did {S} hurt him/herself by									

Figure 8-16. *continued*

ID Number: _____   Date: _____

using a harmful object ? (cutting, burning or other means)									
34. During the past two weeks, how often did {S} hurt others by using a harmful object ? (cutting, burning or other means)									
35. During the past two weeks, how often did {S} appear to fall intentionally (includes from bed or wheelchair)									
36. During the past two weeks, how often did {S} attempt to or did {S} actually eat or drink nonfood substances ?									
37. During the past two weeks, how did {S} engage in any other inappropriate behavior ?									
If yes, please describe:									
38. Did agitated behavior(s) occur most often: ❑ Morning ❑ Afternoon ❑ Evening ❑ No time more than others ❑ Different times for different behaviors									
Total for each Rating									

TOTAL SCORE

Figure 8-16. *continued*

been demonstrated by significant correlations with scores on the Nursing Home Behavior Problems Scale (0.91; Ray et al., 1992) and the Behavioral and Emotional Activities Manifested in Dementia (0.91, 0.79, and 0.92 for three nursing home shifts; Miller et al., 1995). The three factors originally described have been confirmed in other nursing home populations (Miller et al., 1995).

The original manual provides reliability data based on nursing home assessments. Average inter-rater agreement across items ranged from 0.88 to 0.92 across three residential units.

Advantages

By referring to specific observable behaviors, the items of the CMAI do not rely on caregivers' interpretations of emotional states or causality of symptoms.

Each behavior is intended to include multiple, closely related behaviors, many of which are described in expanded items. For example, an item concerning the inappropriate handling of objects offers exemplars to assist the informant. Research has shown this to be a reliable measure of behavioral disturbance in nursing home patients. The scale continues to be used for overall assessment of agitation and has been recently used in clinical trials in AD (Ballard et al., 2002; Brodaty et al., 2003a; Sultzer et al., 2001).

Disadvantages

Although the CMAI offers a comprehensive assessment of a particular domain of behavioral disturbances, it does not address several other symptoms, including disturbances of mood, hallucinations, delusions, and problems of impulse control. Although the original form has been adapted for use with community-residing people, reliability data are not yet available with that population.

Cornell Scale for Depression in Dementia

Unlike other measures of depression that are more widely used, such as the Beck Depression Inventory (Beck et al., 1961) and the Hamilton Depression Rating Scale (Hamilton, 1960), the CSDD was developed specifically for use with dementia patients (Figure 8-17; Alexopoulos et al., 1988a). As the items of this scale are based primarily on observations, it excludes symptoms that cannot be reliably observed. This measure was designed not as a diagnostic tool but for assessment of mood disturbance in pharmacologic studies.

Description

This 19-item scale assesses five domains of mood disturbance: mood-related signs, behavioral disturbance, physical signs, cyclic functions, and ideational disturbance. Ratings are based on interviews with both the patient and informant, although primary emphasis is given to caregiver input. Items are rated on a 3-point scale based on observations in the prior week: absent, mild or intermittent, or severe. There is also an "unable to evaluate" response choice. The clinician is instructed to disregard responses based on physical disability or illness, for example, in rating weight loss or multiple physical complaints. Recommended cutoff scores are 8 or more for mild depression, 12 or more for moderate depression.

Administration

Following interviews with patient and caregiver, the clinicians provide ratings of each behavior. In instances of discrepancy between the two sources of information, greater weight is given to the caregiver's responses.

Time

Interview of both patient and caregiver should take no longer than 30 minutes.

Reliability and Validity

In a comparison of five depression measures, Logsdon and Teri (1995) found the CSDD to be the most sensitive measure in the detection of depression. Scores on the CSDD were able to distinguish between patients with diagnoses of major and minor depression regardless of the severity of their dementia. Alexopoulos et al. (1988b) validated the CSDD in a nondemented patient sample and found that scores discriminated among the diagnostic categories of major depression versus minor depression versus other psychiatric diagnoses.

Inter-rater reliability across items has been reported to range from 0.82 to 1.00, with overall reliability of 0.74 (Alexopoulos et al., 1988b). A Kuder-Richardson coefficient for internal consistency was 0.98. Mack and Patterson (1994) report inter-rater agreement across items to range from 78% to 100%. They caution, however, that the restricted range of choices inflates inter-rater agreement.

Advantages

As one of the few measures of depression in dementia, this scale is particularly suited for AD patients. It contains few items that focus on somatic signs and symptoms that occur commonly in elderly nondepressed patients. Unlike another widely used instrument, the Hamilton Dementia Rating Scale, it does not rely exclusively on patient self-reports, which are notably unreliable in patients with moderate to severe dementia. The scale and the Hamilton Depression Rating Scale have been shown to be sensitive to change in recent clinical trials in patients with AD (Brodaty et al., 2003b; Lyketsos et al., 2003; Lyketsos et al., 2000; Panisset et al., 2002; Teri et al., 2003).

Disadvantages

Ratings are based on behaviors in the week before the assessment, which may fail to capture behaviors that occur sporadically but are troublesome. The three-point frequency/severity scale is unlikely to detect subtle changes in behavior. In some instances it may be difficult to rate symptoms independent of other medical conditions and may make this scale less appropriate with dementia patients who have comorbidities. Like other measures of specific domains, the CSDD does not provide a comprehensive assessment of the range of behavioral disturbances frequently described in dementia patients.

Geriatric Depression Scale

The Geriatric Depression Scale was developed for use with nondemented elderly (Yesavage et al., 1982). It

ID Number: _____   Date: _____

Cornell Scale for Depression in Dementia

SCORE SHEET

Rater _____   Protocol _____

SCORING SCALE
a = unable to evaluate   0 = absent   1 = mild or intermittent   2 = severe

Rating should be based on symptoms and signs occurring during the week prior to interview. No score should be given if symptoms result from physical disability or illness.

A. Mood-Related Signs	Score			
1. Anxiety (anxious expression, ruminations, worrying)	a	0	1	2
2. Sadness (sad expression, sad voice, tearfulness)	a	0	1	2
3. Lack of reactivity to pleasant events	a	0	1	2
4. Irritability (easily annoyed, short tempered)	a	0	1	2
B. Behavioral Disturbances				
5. Agitation (restlessness, hand wringing, hair pulling)	a	0	1	2
6. Retardation (slow movements, slow speech, slow reactions)	a	0	1	2
7. Multiple physical complaints (score 0 if GI symptoms only)	a	0	1	2
8. Loss of interest (less involved in usual activities) (score only if change occurred acutely, i.e., in less than 1 month)	a	0	1	2
C. Physical Signs				
9. Appetite loss (eating les than usual)	a	0	1	2
10. Weight loss (score 2 if greater than 5 lbs in 1 month)	a	0	1	2
11. Lack of energy (fatigues easily, unable to sustain activities) (score only if change occurred acutely, i.e., in less than 1 month)	a	0	1	2
D. Cyclic Functions				
12. Diurnal variation of mood symptoms worse in the morning	a	0	1	2
13. Difficulty falling asleep (later than usual for this individual)	a	0	1	2
14. Multiple awakenings during sleep	a	0	1	2
15. Early morning awakening (earlier than usual for this individual)	a	0	1	2
E. Ideational Disturbance				
16. Suicide (feels life is not worth living, has suicidal wishes, or makes suicide attempt)	a	0	1	2
17. Poor self-esteem (self-blame, self-depreciation, feelings of failure)	a	0	1	2
18. Pessimism (anticipation of the worst)	a	0	1	2
19. Mood-congruent delusions (delusions of poverty, illness, or loss)	a	0	1	2
TOTAL SCORE (0 – 38) =				

Figure 8-17.   GI = gastrointestinal. (From Alexopoulos GS, Abrams RC, Young RC, et al. Cornell Scale for Depression in Dementia. *Biol Psychiatry* 1988;23[3]:271–84, with permission. Copyright 1988 Society of Biological Psychiatry.)

has been widely used in a variety of geriatric populations (Figure 8-18).

Description

This is a 30-item questionnaire with a yes/no response format. Items are worded to minimize a response bias so that both positive and negative responses can be indicative of depressive symptomatology. Suggested cutoff scores are 11 for mild depression and 14 for moderate depression.

Administration

This is a self-report inventory.

Time

It should take no longer than 10 minutes to read and respond to the 30 questions. Respondents with more severe dementia might need to have the test items read aloud. (See Reliability and Validity and Disadvantages later for a discussion of use of this instrument with severely impaired dementia patients.)

Reliability and Validity

When compared with other measures of depression, Geriatric Depression Scale scores correlated significantly with the Beck Depression Inventory (0.80), the Hamilton Depression Rating Scale (0.32), the CSDD (0.36), and the Center for Epidemiological Studies—Depression Scale (0.69) (Logsdon & Teri, 1995). In that study, caregiver surrogate ratings on the Geriatric Depression Scale were found to perform as well as the original self-report measure in describing depressive symptoms in demented elderly. A study of nursing home residents found the Geriatric Depression Scale to have lower sensitivity and specificity in patients with severe levels of dementia (McGivney et al., 1994). They report sensitivity and specificity values as follows: for residents with MMSE scores higher than 14, sensitivity (84%) and specificity (91%); for MMSE scores less than 14, sensitivity (27%) and specificity (69%). They conclude that first determining the level of dementia will greatly improve the utility of the Geriatric Depression Scale in detecting depression.

Advantages

The Geriatric Depression Scale has been shown to be a valid and reliable measure of depression in older adults. It is sensitive to both major and minor depression. As a self-report inventory it is able to assess mood and internal states that are not amenable to observation. A version that has been modified to be used as a caregiver report has been reported to be equally sensitive and reliable.

Disadvantages

This instrument was not developed for use with demented patients. As a self-report, it is of questionable use with more severely demented patients whose insight is impaired. Use of the Geriatric Depression Scale in an institutionalized population needs further validation given the high rate of dementia in nursing home residents. More demented patients may not reliably endorse symptoms on the Geriatric Depression Scale (Gilley & Wilson, 1997). The CSDD and the Hamilton Depression Rating Scale have been more commonly used in clinical trials. The CSDD may be more reliable in patients with advanced dementia.

Summary

We have discussed scales for the assessment of four aspects of dementia: cognition, functional abilities, global function, and behavior. For office use the MMSE and a brief assessment of functional abilities are most useful for initial assessment and follow-up. This could be supplemented by the CDR or the GDS for longitudinal assessment. Clinical trials, on the other hand, should use a cognitive scale, such as the Alzheimer's Disease Assessment Scale (ADAS-Cog), which may be more sensitive to clinical change. Early detection of dementia should include tests, such as expanded word lists, which are more sensitive to the earliest manifestations of degenerative dementias. Behavioral assessment is an essential part of the assessment of dementia. All patients should have an assessment of mood using one of the proposed instruments during the diagnostic evaluation. This should be repeated periodically and if the caregiver or patient expresses a complaint that could be explained on the basis of depression. The proposed scales can be used to track the response of a depressed patient to antidepressant medications. It is essential that instruments that grade mood are included in clinical trials. Abnormal behaviors should also be assessed. The NPI may find use in both the clinic and in clinical trials because it is relatively simple to use and may be sensitive enough to change to be useful in longitudinal follow-up. The physician need not perform all of the evaluations if adequately trained personnel are available to perform assessments. Clinical trials are usually designed to maximize the use of nonphysician personnel in the assessment of dementia. Recent trials

ID Number: _____   Date: _____

The Geriatric Depression Scale (GDS) - 30 item

SCORE SHEET

Rater _____   Protocol _____

Choose the best answer for how you felt over the past week

#	Question	Answer	Score
1	Are you basically satisfied with your life ?	Yes No	
2	Have you dropped many of your activities and interests ?	Yes No	
3	Do you feel that your life is empty ?	Yes No	
4	Do you often get bored ?	Yes No	
5	Are you hopeful about the future ?	Yes No	
6	Are you bothered by thoughts you can't get out of your head ?	Yes No	
7	Are you in good spirits most of the time ?	Yes No	
8	Are you afraid that something bad is going to happen to you ?	Yes No	
9	Do you feel happy most of the time ?	Yes No	
10	Do you often feel helpless ?	Yes No	
11	Do you often get restless and fidgety ?	Yes No	
12	Do you prefer to stay at home, rather than going out and doing new things ?	Yes No	
13	Do you frequently worry about the future ?	Yes No	
14	Do you feel you have more problems with memory than most ?	Yes No	
15	Do you think it is wonderful to be alive now ?	Yes No	
16	Do you often feel downhearted and blue ?	Yes No	
17	Do you feel pretty worthless the way you are now ?	Yes No	
18	Do you worry a lot about the past ?	Yes No	
19	Do you find life very exciting ?	Yes No	
20	Is it hard for you to get started on new projects ?	Yes No	
21	Do you feel full of energy ?	Yes No	
22	Do you feel that your situation is hopeless ?	Yes No	
23	Do you think that most people are better off than you are ?	Yes No	
24	Do you frequently get upset over little things ?	Yes No	
25	Do you frequently feel like crying ?	Yes No	
26	Do you have trouble concentrating ?	Yes No	
27	Do you enjoy getting up in the mornings ?	Yes No	
28	Do you prefer to avoid social gatherings ?	Yes No	
29	Is it easy for you to make decisions ?	Yes No	
30	Is your mind as clear as it used to be ?	Yes No	
		TOTAL SCORE =	

Score 1 for "NO" on questions: 1, 5, 7, 9, 15, 19, 21, 27, 29, 30
Score 0 for all other questions

Figure 8-18.   (From Yesavage JA, Brink TL, Rose TL, et al. Development and validation of a geriatric depression screening scale: a preliminary report. *J Psychiatr Res* 1982;17[1]:37–49, with permission. Copyright 1983, with permission from Elsevier.)

have incorporated assessments of quality of life (Aisen et al., 2003; Spector et al., 2003). This is likely to become more common, as it is highly relevant to patient outcomes. In addition, tailoring treatment goals for individual patients may be complementary to current approaches that are often based on clinical scales (Rockwood et al., 2002a). In conclusion, clinical scales are an important complement to the routine history and physical examination in the assessment of patients with dementia. These can readily be incorporated into clinical practice, and they are an essential part of clinical trials.

Acknowledgments

Supported by grants from the Department of Veterans' Affairs and the Oregon Alzheimer's Disease Center of Oregon Health Sciences University (NIA grant #AG08017) and the University of Alberta. Sheri Foster assisted in preparing the manuscript.

References

Aisen PS, Schafer KA, Grundman M, et al. Effects of rofecoxib or naproxen vs placebo on Alzheimer disease progression: a randomized controlled trial. *JAMA* 2003; 289(21):2819–26.

Albert M, Cohen C. The Test for Severe Impairment: an instrument for the assessment of patients with severe cognitive dysfunction. *J Am Geriatr Soc* 1992;40(5):449–53.

Alexopoulos GS, Abrams RC, Young RC, et al. Cornell Scale for Depression in Dementia. *Biol Psychiatry* 1988a; 23(3): 271–84.

Alexopoulos GS, Abrams RC, Young RC, et al. Use of the Cornell scale in nondemented patients. *J Am Geriatr Soc* 1988b;36(3):230–36.

American Psychiatric Association. *Diagnostic and statistical manual of mental disorders: DSM-IV-TR* (4th ed., text revision). Washington: American Psychiatric Association, 2000.

Ballard CG, O'Brien JT, Reichelt K, et al. Aromatherapy as a safe and effective treatment for the management of agitation in severe dementia: the results of a double-blind, placebo-controlled trial with Melissa. *J Clin Psychiatry* 2002;63(7):553–58.

Barberger-Gateau P, Commenges D, Gagnon M, et al. Instrumental activities of daily living as a screening tool for cognitive impairment and dementia in elderly community dwellers. *J Am Geriatr Soc* 1992;40(11): 1129–34.

Barberger-Gateau P, Dartigues JF, Letenneur L. Four instrumental activities of daily living scores as a predictor of one-year incident dementia. *Age Ageing* 1993;22(6): 457–63.

Beck AT, Ward CH, Mendelson M, et al. An inventory for measuring depression. *Arch Gen Psychiatry* 1961;4:561–71.

Blesa R, Davidson M, Kurz A, et al. Galantamine provides sustained benefits in patients with "advanced moderate" Alzheimer's disease for at least 12 months. *Dement Geriatr Cogn Disord* 2003;15(2):79–87.

Blessed G, Tomlinson BE, Roth M. The association between quantitative measures of dementia and of senile change in the cerebral grey matter of elderly subjects. *Br J Psychiatry* 1968;114(512):797–811.

Boller F, Verny M, Hugonot-Diener L, et al. Clinical features and assessment of severe dementia. A review. *Eur J Neurol* 2002;9(2):125–36.

Braekhus A, Laake K, Engedal K. A low, "normal" score on the Mini-Mental State Examination predicts development of dementia after three years. *J Am Geriatr Soc* 1995;43(6):656–61.

Brodaty H, Ames D, Snowdon J, et al., A randomized placebo-controlled trial of risperidone for the treatment of aggression, agitation, and psychosis of dementia. *J Clin Psychiatry* 2003a;64(2):134–43.

Brodaty H, Draper BM, Millar J, et al. Randomized controlled trial of different models of care for nursing home residents with dementia complicated by depression or psychosis. *J Clin Psychiatry* 2003b;64(1):63–72.

Brodaty H, Howarth GC, Mant A, et al. General practice and dementia. A national survey of Australian GPs. *Med J Aust* 1994;160(1):10–14.

Bucks RS, Ashworth DL, Wilcock GK, et al. Assessment of activities of daily living in dementia: development of the Bristol Activities of Daily Living Scale. *Age Ageing* 1996;25(2):113–20.

Burke WJ, Miller JP, Rubin EH, et al. Reliability of the Washington University Clinical Dementia Rating. *Arch Neurol* 1988;45(1):31–32.

Burns A, Lawlor B, Craig S. *Assessment scales in old age psychiatry*. London: Martin Dunitz Ltd., 1999.

Byrne LM, Wilson PM, Bucks RS, et al. The sensitivity to change over time of the Bristol Activities of Daily Living Scale in Alzheimer's disease. *Int J Geriatr Psychiatry* 2000;15(7):656–61.

Chan WC, Lam LC, Choy CN, et al. A double-blind randomised comparison of risperidone and haloperidol in the treatment of behavioural and psychological symptoms in Chinese dementia patients. *Int J Geriatr Psychiatry* 2001;16(12):1156–62.

Choi SH, Lee BH, Kim S, et al. Interchanging scores between clinical dementia rating scale and global deterioration scale. *Alzheimer Dis Assoc Disord* 2003; 17(2):98–105.

Chui HC, Victoroff JI, Margolin D, et al. Criteria for the diagnosis of ischemic vascular dementia proposed by the State of California Alzheimer's Disease Diagnostic and Treatment Centers. *Neurology* 1992;42(3 Pt 1):473–80.

Clarfield AM. The reversible dementias: do they reverse? *Ann Intern Med* 1988;109(6):476–86.

Clark WS, Street JS, Feldman PD, et al. The effects of olanzapine in reducing the emergence of psychosis among nursing home patients with Alzheimer's disease. *J Clin Psychiatry* 2001;62(1):34–40.

Cohen-Mansfield J. Agitated behaviors in the elderly. II. Preliminary results in the cognitively deteriorated. *J Am Geriatr Soc* 1986;34(10):722–27.

Cohen-Mansfield J, Billig N. Agitated behaviors in the elderly. I. A conceptual review. *J Am Geriatr Soc* 1986; 34(10):711–21.

Cohen-Mansfield J, Libin A. Assessment of agitation in elderly patients with dementia: correlations between informant rating and direct observation. *Int J Geriatr Psychiatry* 2004;19:881–91.

Cole MG, Dastoor DP. A new hierarchic approach to the measurement of dementia. Accurate results within 15 to 30 minutes. *Psychosomatics* 1987;28(6):298–301,304.

Cooper B, Bickel H, Schaufele M. The ability of general practitioners to detect dementia and cognitive impairment in their elderly patients: a study in Mannheim. *Int J Geriatr Psychiatry* 1992;7:591–98.

Crum RM, Anthony JC, Bassett SS, et al. Population-based norms for the Mini-Mental State Examination by age and educational level. *JAMA* 1993;269(18):2386–91.

Cullum S, Huppert FA, McGee M, et al. Decline across different domains of cognitive function in normal ageing: results of a longitudinal population-based study using CAMCOG. *Int J Geriatr Psychiatry* 2000;15(9):853–62.

Cummings JL, Benson DF. *Dementia: a clinical approach* (2nd ed.). Boston: Butterworth-Heinemann, 1992.

Cummings JL, Mega M, Gray K, et al. The Neuropsychiatric Inventory: comprehensive assessment of psychopathology in dementia. *Neurology* 1994;44(12):2308–14.

Davis PB, Morris JC, Grant E. Brief screening tests versus clinical staging in senile dementia of the Alzheimer type. *J Am Geriatr Soc* 1990;38(2):129–35.

De Deyn PP, Rabheru K, Rasmussen A, et al. A randomized trial of risperidone, placebo, and haloperidol for behavioral symptoms of dementia. *Neurology* 1999;53(5):946–55.

Devanand DP, Marder K, Michaels KS, et al. A randomized, placebo-controlled dose-comparison trial of haloperidol for psychosis and disruptive behaviors in Alzheimer's disease. *Am J Psychiatry* 1998;155(11): 1512–20.

Doody RS, Stevens JC, Beck C, et al. Practice parameter: management of dementia (an evidence-based review). Report of the Quality Standards Subcommittee of the American Academy of Neurology. *Neurology* 2001; 56(9):1154–66.

Doraiswamy PM, Bieber F, Kaiser L, et al. The Alzheimer's Disease Assessment Scale: patterns and predictors of baseline cognitive performance in multicenter Alzheimer's disease trials. *Neurology* 1997;48(6):1511–17.

Dubois B, Slachevsky A, Litvan I, et al. The FAB: a frontal assessment battery at bedside. *Neurology* 2000;55(11): 1621–26.

Eisdorfer C, Cohen D, Paveza GJ, et al. An empirical evaluation of the Global Deterioration Scale for staging Alzheimer's disease. *Am J Psychiatry* 1992;149(2):190–94.

Erkinjuntti T, Kurz A, Gauthier S, et al. Efficacy of galantamine in probable vascular dementia and Alzheimer's disease combined with cerebrovascular disease: a randomised trial. *Lancet* 2002;359(9314):1283–90.

Eslinger P, Damasio A, Benton A. *The Iowa screening battery for mental decline.* Iowa City: University of Iowa Press, 1984.

Feldman H, Gabathuler R, Kennard M, et al. Serum p97 levels as an aid to identifying Alzheimer's disease. *J Alzheimer's Dis* 2001a;3(5):507–16.

Feldman H, Gauthier S, Hecker J, et al. Efficacy of donepezil on maintenance of activities of daily living in patients with moderate to severe Alzheimer's disease and the effect on caregiver burden. *J Am Geriatr Soc* 2003; 51(6):737–44.

Feldman H, Gauthier S, Hecker J, et al. A 24-week, randomized, double-blind study of donepezil in moderate to severe Alzheimer's disease. *Neurology* 2001b;57(4): 613–20.

Fillenbaum GG. Screening the elderly. A brief instrumental activities of daily living measure. *J Am Geriatr Soc* 1985; 33(10):698–706.

Fillenbaum GG, Duke University. Center for the Study of Aging and Human Development. *Multidimensional functional assessment of older adults: the Duke Older Americans Resources and Services procedures.* Hillsdale, NJ: L. Erlbaum Associates, 1988.

Folstein MF, Folstein SE, McHugh PR. "Mini-Mental State." A practical method for grading the cognitive state of patients for the clinician. *J Psychiatr Res* 1975;12(3):189–98.

Fratiglioni L, Grut M, Forsell Y, et al. Clinical diagnosis of Alzheimer's disease and other dementias in a population survey. Agreement and causes of disagreement in applying Diagnostic and Statistical Manual of Mental Disorders, Revised Third Edition, Criteria. *Arch Neurol* 1992;49(9):927–32.

Freedman M, Rewilak D, Xerri T, et al. L-deprenyl in Alzheimer's disease: cognitive and behavioral effects. *Neurology* 1998;50(3):660–68.

Fuld PA. Psychological testing in the differential diagnosis of the dementias. In: Bick KL (ed.). *Alzheimer's disease:*

senile dementia and related disorders (aging). Vol. 7. New York: Raven Press, 1978;185–93.

Galasko D, Abramson I, Corey-Bloom J, et al. Repeated exposure to the Mini-Mental State Examination and the Information-Memory-Concentration Test results in a practice effect in Alzheimer's disease. *Neurology* 1993;43(8):1559–63.

Galasko D, Bennett D, Sano M, et al. An inventory to assess activities of daily living for clinical trials in Alzheimer's disease. The Alzheimer's Disease Cooperative Study. *Alzheimer Dis Assoc Disord* 1997;11(Suppl 2):S33–39.

Galasko D, Corey-Bloom J, Thal LJ. Monitoring progression in Alzheimer's disease. *J Am Geriatr Soc* 1991;39(9): 932–41.

Ganguli M, Belle S, Ratcliff G, et al. Sensitivity and specificity for dementia of population-based criteria for cognitive impairment: the MoVIES project. *J Gerontol* 1993;48(4): M152–61.

Gelinas I, Gauthier L, McIntyre M, et al. Development of a functional measure for persons with Alzheimer's disease: the Disability Assessment for Dementia. *Am J Occup Ther* 1999;53(5):471–81.

Gelinas I, Gauthier S, Cyrus PA. Metrifonate enhances the ability of Alzheimer's disease patients to initiate, organize, and execute instrumental and basic activities of daily living. *J Geriatr Psychiatry Neurol* 2000;13(1):9–16.

Gilley DW, Wilson RS. Criterion-related validity of the Geriatric Depression Scale in Alzheimer's disease. *J Clin Exp Neuropsychol* 1997;19(4):489–99.

Grace J, Nadler JD, White DA, et al. Folstein vs modified Mini-Mental State Examination in geriatric stroke. Stability, validity, and screening utility. *Arch Neurol* 1995; 52(5):477–84.

Grigoletto F, Zappala G, Anderson DW, et al. Norms for the Mini-Mental State Examination in a healthy population. *Neurology* 1999;53(2):315–20.

Hamilton M. A rating scale for depression. *Neurol Neurosurg Psychiat* 1960;23:56–62.

Hejl A, Hogh P, Waldemar G. Potentially reversible conditions in 1000 consecutive memory clinic patients. *J Neurol Neurosurg Psychiatry* 2002;73(4):390–94.

Hogan DB, Ebly EM. Predicting who will develop dementia in a cohort of Canadian seniors. *Can J Neurol Sci* 2000;27(1):18–24.

Homma A, Takeda M, Imai Y, et al. Clinical efficacy and safety of donepezil on cognitive and global function in patients with Alzheimer's disease. A 24-week, multicenter, double-blind, placebo-controlled study in Japan. E2020 Study Group. *Dement Geriatr Cogn Disord* 2000;11(6): 299–313.

Hughes CP, Berg L, Danziger WL, et al. A new clinical scale for the staging of dementia. *Br J Psychiatry* 1982; 140: 566–72.

Inzitari D, Rossi R, Lamassa M, et al. Validity of different linguistic versions of the Alzheimer's Disease Assessment Scale in an international multicentre Alzheimer's disease trial. *Dement Geriatr Cogn Disord* 1999;10(4):269–77.

Joffres C, Bucks RS, Haworth J, et al. Patterns of clinically detectable treatment effects with galantamine: a qualitative analysis. *Dement Geriatr Cogn Disord* 2003;15(1): 26–33.

Joffres C, Graham J, Rockwood K. Qualitative analysis of the clinician interview-based impression of change (plus): methodological issues and implications for clinical research. *Int Psychogeriatr* 2000;12(3):403–13.

Juva K, Sulkava R, Erkinjuntti T, et al. Usefulness of the Clinical Dementia Rating scale in screening for dementia. *Int Psychogeriatr* 1995;7(1):17–24.

Kahn RL, Goldfarb AI, Pollak M, et al. Brief objective measures for the determination of mental status in the aged. *Am J Psychiatry* 1960:326–28.

Katz IR, Jeste DV, Mintzer JE, et al. Comparison of risperidone and placebo for psychosis and behavioral disturbances associated with dementia: a randomized, double-blind trial. Risperidone Study Group. *J Clin Psychiatry* 1999;60(2):107–15.

Katzman R, Brown T, Fuld P, et al. Validation of a short Orientation-Memory-Concentration Test of cognitive impairment. *Am J Psychiatry* 1983;140(6):734–39.

Katzman R, Brown T, Thal LJ, et al. Comparison of rate of annual change of mental status score in four independent studies of patients with Alzheimer's disease. *Ann Neurol* 1988;24(3):384–89.

Katzman R, Rowe JW. *Principles of geriatric neurology*. Philadelphia: Davis, 1992.

Kawas C, Karagiozis H, Resau L, et al. Reliability of the Blessed Telephone Information-Memory-Concentration Test. *J Geriatr Psychiatry Neurol* 1995;8(4):238–42.

Kiernan RJ, Mueller J, Langston JW, et al. The Neurobehavioral Cognitive Status Examination: a brief but quantitative approach to cognitive assessment. *Ann Intern Med* 1987;107(4):481–85.

Kiyak HA, Teri L, Borson S. Physical and functional health assessment in normal aging and in Alzheimer's disease: self-reports vs family reports. *Gerontologist* 1994; 34(3):324–30.

Knopman D, Gracon S. Observations on the short-term "natural history" of probable Alzheimer's disease in a controlled clinical trial. *Neurology* 1994a;44(2):260–65.

Knopman DS, DeKosky ST, Cummings JL, et al. Practice parameter: diagnosis of dementia (an evidence-based review). Report of the Quality Standards Subcommittee of the American Academy of Neurology. *Neurology* 2001;56(9):1143–53.

Knopman DS, Knapp MJ, Gracon SI, et al. The Clinician Interview-Based Impression (CIBI): a clinician's global change rating scale in Alzheimer's disease. *Neurology* 1994b;44(12):2315–21.

Knopman DS, Parisi JE, Boeve BF, et al. Vascular dementia in a population-based autopsy study. *Arch Neurol* 2003;60(4):569–75.

Knopman DS, Ryberg S. A verbal memory test with high predictive accuracy for dementia of the Alzheimer type. *Arch Neurol* 1989;46(2):141–45.

Kokmen E, Smith GE, Petersen RC, et al. The short test of mental status. Correlations with standardized psychometric testing. *Arch Neurol* 1991;48(7):725–28.

Lawton MP, Brody EM. Assessment of older people: self-maintaining and instrumental activities of daily living. *Gerontologist* 1969;9(3):179–86.

Lezak MD. *Neuropsychological assessment* (3rd ed.). New York: Oxford University Press, 1995.

Linn MW, Linn BS. The rapid disability rating scale-2. *J Am Geriatr Soc* 1982;30(6):378–82.

Liu HC, Teng EL, Chuang YY, et al. The Alzheimer's Disease Assessment Scale: findings from a low-education population. *Dement Geriatr Cogn Disord* 2002;13(1):21–26.

Liu HC, Teng EL, Lin KN, et al. Performance on a dementia screening test in relation to demographic variables. Study of 5297 community residents in Taiwan. *Arch Neurol* 1994;51(9):910–15.

Locascio JJ, Growdon JH, Corkin S. Cognitive test performance in detecting, staging, and tracking Alzheimer's disease. *Arch Neurol* 1995;52(11):1087–99.

Loewenstein DA, Amigo E, Duara R, et al. A new scale for the assessment of functional status in Alzheimer's disease and related disorders. *J Gerontol* 1989;44(4):P114–21.

Logsdon RG, Teri L. Depression in Alzheimer's disease patients: caregivers as surrogate reporters. *J Am Geriatr Soc* 1995;43(2):150–55.

Lyketsos CG, DelCampo L, Steinberg M, et al. Treating depression in Alzheimer disease: efficacy and safety of sertraline therapy, and the benefits of depression reduction: the DIADS. *Arch Gen Psychiatry* 2003;60(7):737–46.

Lyketsos CG, Sheppard JM, Steele CD, et al. Randomized, placebo-controlled, double-blind clinical trial of sertraline in the treatment of depression complicating Alzheimer's disease: initial results from the Depression in Alzheimer's Disease study. *Am J Psychiatry* 2000;157(10):1686–89.

Mace NL, Whitehouse PJ, Smyth KA. Management of patients with dementia. In: Whitehouse PJ (ed.). *Dementia* (40th ed.). Philadelphia: F.A. Davis, 1993:400–16.

Mack JL, Patterson MB. The evaluation of behavioral disturbances in Alzheimer's disease: the utility of three rating scales. *J Geriatr Psychiatry Neurol* 1994;7(2):99–115.

Mahurin RK, DeBettignies BH, Pirozzolo FJ. Structured assessment of independent living skills: preliminary report of a performance measure of functional abilities in dementia. *J Gerontol* 1991;46(2):P58–66.

Massoud F, Devi G, Moroney JT, et al. The role of routine laboratory studies and neuroimaging in the diagnosis of dementia: a clinicopathological study. *J Am Geriatr Soc* 2000;48(10):1204–10.

Mathuranath PS, Nestor PJ, Berrios GE, et al. A brief cognitive test battery to differentiate Alzheimer's disease and frontotemporal dementia. *Neurology* 2000;55(11):1613–20.

Mattis S. Mental status examination for organic mental syndrome in the elderly patient. In: Birenbaum C (ed.). *Geriatric psychiatry : a handbook for psychiatrists and primary care physicians.* New York: Grune & Stratton, 1976:77–121.

Mayeux R, Stern Y, Rosen J, et al. Depression, intellectual impairment, and Parkinson disease. *Neurology* 1981;31(6):645–50.

McCulla MM, Coats M, Van Fleet N, et al. Reliability of clinical nurse specialists in the staging of dementia. *Arch Neurol* 1989;46(11):1210–11.

McGivney SA, Mulvihill M, Taylor B. Validating the GDS depression screen in the nursing home. *J Am Geriatr Soc* 1994;42(5):490–92.

McKeith I, Del Ser T, Spano P, et al. Efficacy of rivastigmine in dementia with Lewy bodies: a randomised, double-blind, placebo-controlled international study. *Lancet* 2000a;356(9247):2031–36.

McKeith IG, Ballard CG, Perry RH, et al. Prospective validation of consensus criteria for the diagnosis of dementia with Lewy bodies. *Neurology* 2000b;54(5):1050–58.

McKeith IG, Cumming JL, Lovestone S, et al. *Outcome measures in Alzheimer's disease.* London: Martin Dunitz Ltd., 1999.

McKhann G, Drachman D, Folstein M, et al. Clinical diagnosis of Alzheimer's disease: report of the NINCDS-ADRDA Work Group under the auspices of Department of Health and Human Services Task Force on Alzheimer's Disease. *Neurology* 1984;34(7):939–44.

McKhann GM, Albert MS, Grossman M, et al. Clinical and pathological diagnosis of frontotemporal dementia: report of the Work Group on Frontotemporal Dementia and Pick's Disease. *Arch Neurol* 2001;58(11):1803–09.

Mendez MF, Ala T, Underwood KL. Development of scoring criteria for the clock drawing task in Alzheimer's disease. *J Am Geriatr Soc* 1992;40(11):1095–99.

Miller RJ, Snowdon J, Vaughan R. The use of the Cohen-Mansfield Agitation Inventory in the assessment of behavioral disorders in nursing homes. *J Am Geriatr Soc* 1995;43(5):546–49.

Mohs RC, Knopman D, Petersen RC, et al. Development of cognitive instruments for use in clinical trials of antidementia drugs: additions to the Alzheimer's Disease Assessment Scale that broaden its scope. The Alzheimer's Disease Cooperative Study. *Alzheimer Dis Assoc Disord* 1997;11(Suppl 2):S13–21.

Molloy DW. *Standardized Mini-Mental State Examination (SMMSE)*. Troy, Canada: New Grange Press, 1999.

Molloy DW, Alemayehu E, Roberts R. Reliability of a Standardized Mini-Mental State Examination compared with the traditional Mini-Mental State Examination. *Am J Psychiatry* 1991;148(1):102–05.

Molloy DW, Standish TI. A guide to the standardized Mini-Mental State Examination. *Int Psychogeriatr* 1997; 9(Suppl 1):87–94; discussion 143–50.

Morris JC. The Clinical Dementia Rating (CDR): current version and scoring rules. *Neurology* 1993;43(11): 2412–14.

Morris JC. Clinical dementia rating: a reliable and valid diagnostic and staging measure for dementia of the Alzheimer type. *Int Psychogeriatr* 1997;9(Suppl 1):173–76; discussion 177–78.

Morris JC, Cyrus PA, Orazem J, et al. Metrifonate benefits cognitive, behavioral, and global function in patients with Alzheimer's disease. *Neurology* 1998;50(5):1222–30.

Morris JC, Ernesto C, Schafer K, et al. Clinical dementia rating training and reliability in multicenter studies: the Alzheimer's Disease Cooperative Study experience. *Neurology* 1997;48(6):1508–10.

Morris JC, Heyman A, Mohs RC, et al. The Consortium to Establish a Registry for Alzheimer's Disease (CERAD). Part I. Clinical and neuropsychological assessment of Alzheimer's disease. *Neurology* 1989;39(9):1159–65.

Morris JC, McKeel DW Jr., Fulling K, et al. Validation of clinical diagnostic criteria for Alzheimer's disease. *Ann Neurol* 1988;24(1):17–22.

Morris JC, Storandt M, McKeel DW Jr., et al. Cerebral amyloid deposition and diffuse plaques in "normal" aging: evidence for presymptomatic and very mild Alzheimer's disease. *Neurology* 1996;46(3):707–19.

Mungas D, Marshall SC, Weldon M, et al. Age and education correction of Mini-Mental State Examination for English and Spanish-speaking elderly. *Neurology* 1996; 46(3):700–6.

Murden RA, McRae TD, Kaner S, et al. Mini-Mental State exam scores vary with education in blacks and whites. *J Am Geriatr Soc* 1991;39(2):149–55.

Nyatsanza S, Shetty T, Gregory C, et al. A study of stereotypic behaviours in Alzheimer's disease and frontal and temporal variant frontotemporal dementia. *J Neurol Neurosurg Psychiatry* 2003;74(10):1398–402.

Oremus M, Perrault A, Demers L, et al. Review of outcome measurement instruments in Alzheimer's disease drug trials: psychometric properties of global scales. *J Geriatr Psychiatry Neurol* 2000;13(4):197–205.

Orgogozo JM, Rigaud AS, Stoffler A, et al. Efficacy and safety of memantine in patients with mild to moderate vascular dementia: a randomized, placebo-controlled trial (MMM 300). *Stroke* 2002;33(7):1834–39.

Panisset M, Gauthier S, Moessler H, et al. Cerebrolysin in Alzheimer's disease: a randomized, double-blind, placebo-controlled trial with a neurotrophic agent. *J Neural Transm* 2002;109(7–8):1089–104.

Parks RW, Zec RF, Wilson RS. *Neuropsychology of Alzheimer's disease and other dementias*. New York: Oxford University Press, 1993.

Patterson MB, Mack JL, Neundorfer MM, et al. Assessment of functional ability in Alzheimer disease: a review and a preliminary report on the Cleveland Scale for Activities of Daily Living. *Alzheimer Dis Assoc Disord* 1992; 6(3):145–63.

Paykel ES, Brayne C, Huppert FA, et al. Incidence of dementia in a population older than 75 years in the United Kingdom. *Arch Gen Psychiatry* 1994;51(4):325–32.

Pfeffer RI, Kurosaki TT, Harrah CH Jr., et al. Measurement of functional activities in older adults in the community. *J Gerontol* 1982;37(3):323–29.

Pfeiffer E. A short portable mental status questionnaire for the assessment of organic brain deficit in elderly patients. *J Am Geriatr Soc* 1975;23(10):433–41.

Quinn J, Moore M, Benson DF, et al. A videotaped CIBIC for dementia patients: validity and reliability in a simulated clinical trial. *Neurology* 2002;58(3):433–37.

Randolph C, Tierney MC, Mohr E, et al. The Repeatable Battery for the Assessment of Neuropsychological Status (RBANS): preliminary clinical validity. *J Clin Exp Neuropsychol* 1998;20(3):310–19.

Raskind MA, Peskind ER, Wessel T, et al. Galantamine in AD: a 6-month randomized, placebo-controlled trial with a 6-month extension. The Galantamine USA-1 Study Group. *Neurology* 2000;54(12):2261–68.

Ray WA, Taylor JA, Lichtenstein MJ, et al. The Nursing Home Behavior Problem Scale. *J Gerontol* 1992;47(1): M9–16.

Reed BR, Jagust WJ, Seab JP. Mental status as a predictor of daily function in progressive dementia. *Gerontologist* 1989;29(6):804–07.

Reisberg B, Borenstein J, Salob SP, et al. Behavioral symptoms in Alzheimer's disease: phenomenology and treatment. *J Clin Psychiatry* 1987;48(Suppl):9–15.

Reisberg B, Ferris SH, de Leon MJ, et al. The Global Deterioration Scale for assessment of primary degenerative dementia. *Am J Psychiatry* 1982;139(9):1136–39.

Reisberg B, Ferris SH, de Leon MJ, et al. Global Deterioration Scale (GDS). *Psychopharmacol Bull* 1988;24(4):661–63.

Reisberg B, Ferris SH, Shulman E, et al. Longitudinal course of normal aging and progressive dementia of the Alzheimer's type: a prospective study of 106 subjects over a 3.6 year mean interval. *Prog Neuropsychopharmacol Biol Psychiatry* 1986;10(3–5):571–78.

Reisberg B, Ferris SH, Torossian C, et al. Pharmacologic treatment of Alzheimer's disease: a methodologic critique based upon current knowledge of symptomatology and relevance for drug trials. *Int Psychogeriatr* 1992;4(Suppl 1):9–42.

Reisberg B, Sclan SG, Franssen E, et al. Dementia staging in chronic care populations. *Alzheimer Dis Assoc Disord* 1994;8(Suppl 1):S188–205.

Roccaforte WH, Burke WJ, Bayer BL, Wengel SP. Validation of a telephone version of the Mini-Mental State Examination. *J Am Geriatr Soc* 1992;40(7):697–702.

Rockwood K, Graham JE, Fay S. Goal setting and attainment in Alzheimer's disease patients treated with donepezil. *J Neurol Neurosurg Psychiatry* 2002a;73(5):500–07.

Rockwood K, Joffres C. Improving clinical descriptions to understand the effects of dementia treatment: consensus recommendations. *Int J Geriatr Psychiatry* 2002b;17(11):1006–11.

Roman GC, Tatemichi TK, Erkinjuntti T, et al. Vascular dementia: diagnostic criteria for research studies. Report of the NINDS-AIREN International Workshop. *Neurology* 1993;43(2):250–60.

Rosen WG, Mohs RC, Davis KL. A new rating scale for Alzheimer's disease. *Am J Psychiatry* 1984;141(11):1356–64.

Rothlind JC, Brandt J. A brief assessment of frontal and subcortical functions in dementia. *J Neuropsychiatry Clin Neurosci* 1993;5(1):73–77.

Royall DR. Precis of executive dyscontrol as a cause of problem behavior in dementia. *Exp Aging Res* 1994;20(2):73–94.

Saxton J, McGonigle-Gibson KL, Swihart AA, et al. Assessment of the severely impaired patient: description and validation of a new neuropsychological test battery. *Psychological Assessment* 1990;2(3):298–303.

Scharf S, Mander A, Ugoni A, et al. A double-blind, placebo-controlled trial of diclofenac/misoprostol in Alzheimer's disease. *Neurology* 1999;53(1):197–201.

Schneider LS, Olin JT, Doody RS, et al. Validity and reliability of the Alzheimer's Disease Cooperative Study-Clinical Global Impression of Change. The Alzheimer's Disease Cooperative Study. *Alzheimer Dis Assoc Disord* 1997;11(Suppl 2):S22–32.

Schwartz GE. Development and validation of the geriatric evaluation by relatives rating instrument (GERRI). *Psychol Rep* 1983;53(2):479–88.

Sclan SG, Reisberg B. Functional assessment staging (FAST) in Alzheimer's disease: reliability, validity, and ordinality. *Int Psychogeriatr* 1992;4(Suppl 1):55–69.

Spear J, Chawla S, O'Reilly M, et al. Does the HoNOS 65+ meet the criteria for a clinical outcome indicator for mental health services for older people? *Int J Geriatr Psychiatry* 2002;17(3):226–30.

Spector A, Thorgrimsen L, Woods B, et al. Efficacy of an evidence-based cognitive stimulation therapy programme for people with dementia: randomised controlled trial. *Br J Psychiatry* 2003;183:248–54.

Spreen O, Strauss E. *A compendium of neuropsychological tests: administration, norms, and commentary.* New York: Oxford University Press, 1991.

Standish TI, Molloy DW, Bedard M, et al. Improved reliability of the Standardized Alzheimer's Disease Assessment Scale (SADAS) compared with the Alzheimer's Disease Assessment Scale (ADAS). *J Am Geriatr Soc* 1996;44(6):712–16.

Stern RG, Mohs RC, Bierer LM, et al. Deterioration on the Blessed test in Alzheimer's disease: longitudinal data and their implications for clinical trials and identification of subtypes. *Psychiatry Res* 1992;42(2):101–10.

Stern RG, Mohs RC, Davidson M, et al. A longitudinal study of Alzheimer's disease: measurement, rate, and predictors of cognitive deterioration. *Am J Psychiatry* 1994;151(3):390–96.

Stevens T, Livingston G, Kitchen G, et al. Islington study of dementia subtypes in the community. *Br J Psychiatry* 2002;180:270–76.

Sultzer DL, Gray KF, Gunay I, et al. Does behavioral improvement with haloperidol or trazodone treatment depend on psychosis or mood symptoms in patients with dementia? *J Am Geriatr Soc* 2001;49(10):1294–300.

Swirsky-Sacchetti T, Field HL, Mitchell DR, et al. The sensitivity of the Mini-Mental State Exam in the white matter dementia of multiple sclerosis. *J Clin Psychol* 1992;48(6):779–86.

Tariot PN, Cummings JL, Katz IR, et al. A randomized, double-blind, placebo-controlled study of the efficacy and safety of donepezil in patients with Alzheimer's disease in the nursing home setting. *J Am Geriatr Soc* 2001;49(12):1590–99.

Tariot PN, Mack JL, Patterson MB, et al. The Behavior Rating Scale for Dementia of the Consortium to Establish a Registry for Alzheimer's Disease. The Behavioral Pathology Committee of the Consortium to Establish a Registry for Alzheimer's Disease. *Am J Psychiatry* 1995;152(9):1349–57.

Tariot PN, Solomon PR, Morris JC, et al. A 5-month, randomized, placebo-controlled trial of galantamine in AD. The Galantamine USA-10 Study Group. *Neurology* 2000;54(12):2269–76.

Teng EL, Chui HC. The Modified Mini-Mental State (3MS) examination. *J Clin Psychiatry* 1987;48(8):314–18.

Teng EL, Wimer C, Roberts E, et al. Alzheimer's dementia: performance on parallel forms of the dementia assessment battery. *J Clin Exp Neuropsychol* 1989;11(6):899–912.

Teri L, Gibbons LE, McCurry SM, et al. Exercise plus behavioral management in patients with Alzheimer disease: a randomized controlled trial. *JAMA* 2003;290(15):2015–22.

Teri L, Logsdon RG. Methodologic issues regarding outcome measures for clinical drug trials of psychiatric complications in dementia. *J Geriatr Psychiatry Neurol* 1995;8(Suppl 1):S8–17.

Terry RD, Masliah E, Salmon DP, et al. Physical basis of cognitive alterations in Alzheimer's disease: synapse loss is the major correlate of cognitive impairment. *Ann Neurol* 1991;30(4):572–80.

Tombaugh TN, McIntyre NJ. The Mini-Mental State Examination: a comprehensive review. *J Am Geriatr Soc* 1992;40(9):922–35.

Tractenberg RE, Weiner MF, Patterson MB, et al. Comorbidity of psychopathological domains in community-dwelling persons with Alzheimer's disease. *J Geriatr Psychiatry Neurol* 2003;16(2):94–99.

Tuokko H. Psychosocial evaluation and management of the Alzheimer's patient. In: Wilson RS (ed.). *Neuropsychology of Alzheimer's disease and other dementias*. New York: Oxford University Press, 1993:565–88.

Tuokko H, Hadjistavropoulos T, Miller JA, et al. The Clock Test: a sensitive measure to differentiate normal elderly from those with Alzheimer disease. *J Am Geriatr Soc* 1992;40(6):579–84.

Uhlmann RF, Larson EB. Effect of education on the Mini-Mental State Examination as a screening test for dementia. *J Am Geriatr Soc* 1991;39(9):876–80.

Wade DT. *Measurement in neurological rehabilitation.* Oxford: Oxford University Press, 1992.

Weiner MF, Koss E, Wild KV, et al. Measures of psychiatric symptoms in Alzheimer patients: a review. *Alzheimer Dis Assoc Disord* 1996;10(1):20–30.

Wilcock G, Mobius HJ, Stoffler A. A double-blind, placebo-controlled multicentre study of memantine in mild to moderate vascular dementia (MMM500). *Int Clin Psychopharmacol* 2002;17(6):297–305.

Wilcock GK, Lilienfeld S, Gaens E. Efficacy and safety of galantamine in patients with mild to moderate Alzheimer's disease: multicentre randomised controlled trial. Galantamine International-1 Study Group. *BMJ* 2000; 321(7274):1445–49.

Wilkinson D, Doody R, Helme R, et al. Donepezil in vascular dementia: A randomized, placebo-controlled study. *Neurology* 2003;61(4):479–86.

Wind AW, Van Staveren G, Schellevis FG, et al. The validity of the judgment of general practitioners on dementia. *Int J Geriatr Psychiatry* 1994;9:543–49.

Yesavage JA, Brink TL, Rose TL, et al. Development and validation of a geriatric depression screening scale: a preliminary report. *J Psychiatr Res* 1982;17(1):37–49.

Zanetti O, Frisoni GB, Rozzini L, et al. Validity of direct assessment of functional status as a tool for measuring Alzheimer's disease severity. *Age Ageing* 1998;27(5):615–22.

9

Clinical Stroke Scales

Wayne M. Clark, M.D., and J. Maurice Hourihane, M.B., M.R.C.P.I.

T he ideal method of assessing a patient's deficit following a stroke has not yet been determined. Early clinical stroke therapy trials relied heavily on detailed neurologic scales, such as the National Institutes of Health Stroke Scale (NIHSS), to quantify a patient's deficits. Arbitrary levels of improvement (e.g., 4 points in the total scale score) were set as primary efficacy endpoints and were used to test whether a drug was therapeutically beneficial. It soon became clear that such arbitrary endpoints may not be clinically meaningful in terms of the patient's recovery. For example, a severe stroke patient could have a 4-point improvement on the NIHSS and yet remain confined to bed. Furthermore, the various numeric ratings for each subset of the scales are arbitrary and may not accurately reflect the impact such deficits have on the patient. For instance, a moderate aphasia is given 2 points on the NIHSS, the same as a hemisensory numbness. For these reasons, beginning in the early 1990s, there has been a general trend toward assessing a patient's level of function using a variety of functional outcome assessments as opposed to relying solely on detailed neurologic examination

scores. This change is illustrated by the NIH tissue plasminogen activator (tPA) stroke treatment study results (National Institute of Neurological Disorders and Stroke [NINDS] rt-PA Stroke Study Group, 1995). In part 1 of the study, primary efficacy was assessed using a 4-point improvement on the NIHSS, whereas, in part 2, various functional outcome measures were used to determine the final efficacy for the tPA-treated patients.

Functional outcome testing measures are generally much easier to administer and have far fewer gradations than scales based on neurologic examination. Taking this simplified outcome assessment to an extreme, the most reliable efficacy endpoint would be to determine if the patient is normal or abnormal. This 2-point functional outcome assessment has been advocated by some investigators (Zivin & Waud, 1992). A problem with the simplified outcome assessments is that patients can achieve a fairly normal score and still have significant cognitive deficits. A patient may be able to perform all activities of daily living (ADLs) and still have problems with cortical functioning and be unable to return to his or her prior level of employment. A combination of these two techniques, with weighting given to functional outcome as well as more detailed neurologic evaluations, would be the ideal method of determining outcome. To date, such a method has not been validated.

This chapter reviews both the detailed neurologic deficit stroke scales and the commonly used functional outcome scales that are currently employed in stroke therapeutic efficacy trials.

Neurologic Deficit Stroke Scales

National Institutes of Health Stroke Scale

The NIHSS (Table 9-1) was developed by investigators at the University of Cincinnati Stroke Center to quantify neurologic status in stroke patients. This scale is in widespread use in a variety of stroke therapy efficacy trials.

Description

The NIHSS was developed to quantify neurologic deficit status in stroke patients based on a scale originally devised at the University of Cincinnati Stroke Center (Brott et al., 1989a; Goldstein et al., 1989). It was revised in 1994 to measure both affected and nonaffected sides (Lyden et al., 1994). Its primary use is to determine drug efficacy comparing initial evaluations at baseline in acute stroke patients with 3-month follow-up assessments performed by the same examiner. The NIHSS is a 24-point scale (11 items), with zero being a normal score. Patients receive points depending on different areas of deficit. They are scored on their initial actual performance, not on what the evaluator thinks they should be able to do. In general, patients are also given the worst possible score if they are unable to perform a task. A patient who is completely mute from severe aphasia also receives 2 points for severe dysarthria even though he or she cannot actually speak at all. In general, patients who score higher than 15 points are assumed to have had a major stroke; a score of 4–15 points is indicative of a moderate stroke, and less than 4 points is considered a mild stroke. The less than 4-point criterion is frequently used by stroke studies to exclude patients with minimal deficit. In several studies an additional assessment of distal motor function has been added.

Validation

The NIHSS has high inter-rater reliability among neurologists, emergency room physicians, house officers, and stroke research nurses (Goldstein et al., 1989). It has also been shown to have high criterion validity by predicting stroke lesion size on brain computed tomography (Brott et al., 1989a, 1989b). This scale has been clinically validated in several drug therapy stroke trials (Brott et al., 1992; Haley et al., 1992, 1993).

Administration

The NIHSS is performed during the bedside neurologic evaluation. Although the examination could be performed by anyone with neurologic examination experience, it is now recommended that it be administered only by individuals who have passed a certification tape examination. Although many stroke studies require a board-certified neurologist to perform the test, it can actually be performed by neurologists, emergency room physicians, or neurologic nurses, provided that they have passed the certification examination. This certification process improves intra-rater reliability.

The test takes approximately 5 minutes to administer and another 5 minutes to record the proper scores.

Special Considerations

One of the main advantages of the NIHSS is that there is an associated training tape and certification examination. The tape consists of six patient examples for which a neurologist points out the proper scoring of the case (Lyden et al., 1994). After the viewing of this training tape, the individual sees six new cases and scores them appropriately. The scoring sheets are sent to a certification center, and the individual is notified whether he or she passed the examination. The use of this certification examination greatly increases the reliability of the scale. Individuals interested in obtaining the training and certification tape are directed to contact the National Institute of Neurological Disorders and Stroke or the National Stroke Association.

Advantages/Disadvantages

The advantage of the NIHSS is that it can be rapidly performed in the acute stroke setting. It has been well validated in a large number of studies. The training tape, along with the certification examination, is an added feature that ensures high reliability between raters. The scale is easy to learn. With the aid of the training tape, people can become highly competent in its use following a single afternoon training session.

Table 9-1. Modified National Institutes of Health Stroke Scale

Item	Name	Response
1A	Level of consciousness	0 = Alert
		1 = Not alert, but arousable easily
		2 = Not alert, obtunded
		3 = Unresponsive
1B	Questions	0 = Answers both correctly
		1 = Answers one correctly
		2 = Answers neither correctly
1C	Commands	0 = Performs both tasks correctly
		1 = Performs one task correctly
		2 = Performs neither task correctly
2	Gaze	0 = Normal
		1 = Partial gaze palsy
		2 = Total gaze palsy
3	Visual fields	0 = No vision loss
		1 = Partial hemianopsia
		2 = Complete hemianopsia
		3 = Bilateral hemianopsia
4	Facial palsy	0 = Normal
		1 = Minor paralysis
		2 = Partial paralysis
		3 = Complete paralysis
5	Motor arm	0 = No drift
	Left	1 = Drifts before 10 sec
	Right	2 = Falls before 10 sec
		3 = No effort against gravity
		4 = No movement
6	Motor leg	0 = No drift
	Left	1 = Drifts before 5 sec
	Right	2 = Falls before 5 sec
		3 = No effort against gravity
		4 = No movement
7	Ataxia	0 = Absent
		1 = One limb
		2 = Two limbs

(continued)

Table 9-1. *(continued)*

Item	Name	Response
8	Sensory	0 = Normal
		1 = Mild loss
		2 = Severe loss
9	Language	0 = Normal
		1 = Mild aphasia
		2 = Severe aphasia
		3 = Mute or global aphasia
10	Dysarthria	0 = Normal
		1 = Mild
		2 = Severe
11	Extinction/inattention	0 = Normal
		1 = Mild
		2 = Severe

Note: There are 15 items in this version of the National Institutes of Health Stroke Scale. Complete scale with instructions can be obtained from the National Institute of Neurological Disorders and Stroke (Lyden P, Brott T, Tilley B, et al. Improved reliability of the NIH stroke scale using video training. *Stroke* 1994;25:2220–26).

A disadvantage of the NIHSS scale is that it is not good for posterior circulation strokes. The scale is weighted toward language-related functions and, as such, individuals who have mainly brainstem features may receive scores that are less severe despite significant deficits.

Summary

The NIHSS is the most commonly used clinical rating score for acute stroke patients. This scale has been well validated in stroke patients and provides an additional advantage of having a training tape available. Its ease of use and associated training tape make it the most widely recommended scale for evaluating acute stroke patients in the United States. It shows the weakness of all neurologic scores in that changes in the examination may not accurately reflect meaningful changes in the patient's status.

Scandinavian Stroke Scale

The Scandinavian Stroke Scale (SSS) was developed to test therapeutic efficacy of hemodilution treatment in acute middle cerebral artery stroke (Scandinavian Stroke Study Group, 1985; Scandinavian Stroke Study Group, 1987; Lindenstrøm et al., 1991). The scale is currently in widespread use to determine therapeutic efficacy of a variety of potential stroke treatments in Europe.

Description

The SSS is a nine-item scale consisting of both a prognostic score and a long-term score. The prognostic score includes measures of consciousness, gaze palsy, and limb weakness. It is designed to stratify patients into several groups, depending on their prognosis for survival. The long-term score is meant for repeated evaluations of the patient during follow-up. The long-term score does not include consciousness or gaze palsy but does include limb strength, aphasia, facial palsy, orientation, and gait (Table 9-2). Limb strength is rated only on the symptomatic side. Unlike the NIH score, visual fields, ocular motor function, and sensation are not included. A score of 48 indicates normal performance on the long-term examination. The SSS is most suitable for assessing deficits in the carotid artery.

Table 9-2.   Unified Neurological Stroke Scale (Combination of the Scandinavian Stroke Scale and the Orgogozo Scale)

Item		SSS	Orgogozo
Consciousness	Normal/fully conscious	6	15
	Somnolent/drowsy	4	10
	Reacts to verbal command	2	10
	Stupor (reacts to pain only)	0	5
	Coma	0	0
Orientation	Correct for time, place, person	6	—
	Two of these	4	—
	One of these	2	—
	Completely disoriented	0	—
Speech/verbal communication	Normal/no aphasia	10	10
	Limited vocabulary or incoherent speech/difficult	6	5
	More than yes-no but not longer sentences/difficult	3	5
	Only yes-no or less/extremely difficult or impossible	0	0
Eye movements/eyes and head shift	No gaze palsy/none	4	10
	Gaze palsy/gaze failure	2	5
	Conjugate eye deviation/forced	0	0
Facial palsy	None/dubious/slight paresis	2	5
	Present/paralysis or marked paresis	0	0
Gait	Walks at least 5 m without aids	12	—
	Walks with aids	9	—
	Walks with help of another person	6	—
	Sits without support	3	—
	Bedridden/wheelchair	0	—
Arm: motor power/raising	Raises with normal strength/normal	6	10
	Raises with reduced strength/possible	5	10
	Raises with flexion in elbow/incomplete	4	5
	Can move but not against gravity/impossible	2	0
	Paralysis	0	0
Hand: motor power/movements	Normal strength/normal	6	15
	Reduced strength/skilled	4	10
	Fingertips do not reach palm/useful	2	5
	Paralysis/useless	0	0

(continued)

Table 9-2. *(continued)*

Item		SSS	Orgogozo
Leg: motor power/raising	Normal strength	6	15
	Raises with reduced strength/against resistance	5	10
	Raises with flexion of knee/against gravity	4	5
	Can move, but not against gravity/impossible	2	0
	Paralysis	0	0
Foot dorsiflexion	Against resistance/normal	—	15
	Against gravity	—	5
	Footdrop	—	0
Upper limb tone	Normal (even if brisk reflexes)	—	5
	Overtly spastic or flaccid	—	0
Lower limb tone	Normal (even if brisk reflexes)	—	5
	Overtly spastic or flaccid	—	0

SSS = Scandinavian Stroke Scale.

Validation

The SSS has been shown to have high inter-rater and intra-rater reliability (Lindenstrøm et al., 1991). It has been clinically validated in several stroke studies (Scandinavian Stroke Study Group, 1985; Scandinavian Stroke Study Group, 1987; Lindenstrøm et al., 1991).

Administration

The score is calculated during the bedside neurologic examination. Anyone with neurologic examination experience could administer it, although it has only been validated for neurologists. It takes approximately 5 minutes to administer.

Special Considerations

Acute stroke patients with scores of 40 or greater on the SSS long-term have a high likelihood of spontaneous recovery. Scores of less than 40 resulted in incomplete recovery. Therefore, the 40-point cutoff is frequently used as an inclusion criterion for acute stroke trials.

Advantages/Disadvantages

The SSS is easy to administer and can be performed with minimal prior training as part of the neu-

rologic evaluation. It is one of the few scales that includes gait as one of the items to be tested. Gait evaluation is an important component of the patient's outcome. One of the main disadvantages is that the scale is weighted heavily toward middle cerebral artery stroke, so a patient with a substantial brainstem infarction may not be adequately assessed.

Summary

The SSS is an easily administered neurologic scoring scale for acute middle cerebral artery stroke patients. It has been well validated and is in widespread use in several European stroke studies.

Orgogozo Scale

The Orgogozo Scale, also called the Neurological Scale for Middle Cerebral Artery Infarction, is a neurologic deficit scale designed to test the degree of deficit in middle cerebral artery infarction patients.

Description

The scale is rated from 0 to 100, with 100 being normal (Orgogozo et al., 1983; Orgogozo & Dartigues, 1986; see Table 9-2). The scale is weighted heavily to measure hemiplegia due to middle cerebral artery infarction. As such, patients receive scores for both upper and lower extremity weakness and abnormalities of tone. Facial abnormalities are given minimal weighting, and there are no assessments of confusion, visual fields, or sensory deficits. Consciousness is rated on a 3-point scale.

Validation

Inter-rater reliability is very high even when the scale is used by less trained personnel (Orgogozo & Dartigues, 1991). The items have good construct validity and have been shown to be a powerful predictor of neurologic outcome (Orgogozo & Dartigues, 1986). The scale has been changed from its original form to improve interrater reliability (Orgogozo & Dartigues, 1986).

Administration

Due to the additional tone and detailed motor assessments for this scale, some expertise with a general neurologic evaluation is required of the examiner. This scale can be performed in approximately 10 minutes.

Advantages/Disadvantages

The main advantage of the Orgogozo scale is the detailed assessment of the patient's motor weakness. A disadvantage is the minimal assessment of neurologic items outside of motor weakness. An additional disadvantage is that it has not been used in any large clinical drug trials.

Summary

Although it is a potentially important method of determining motor outcome of a patient, the Orgogozo scale is not in widespread use. Several of the other stroke scales are easier to learn and have greater clinical validation.

Canadian Neurologic Scale

The Canadian Neurologic Scale (Table 9-3) was designed as a simple clinical instrument to be used by neurologists and nonphysicians alike to evaluate and monitor the neurologic status of acute stroke patients (Côté et al., 1989; Côté et al., 1986).

Description

The eight-item scale measures level of consciousness, orientation, speech, motor function, and facial weakness for a maximum score of 10 points in the normal patient. A separate section measuring motor response is used for patients who have comprehension deficits.

Validation

Validation and reliability have been measured extensively by Côté (Côté et al., 1988). Criterion validity was shown in that the test was able to accurately predict morbidity and mortality; patients with low total scores had higher mortality at 6 months, along with a greater incidence of recurrent strokes (Côté et al., 1989). Inter-observer agreement levels of 0.92 have been reported with this scale (Côté et al., 1989). The scale has been used in several clinical trials evaluating neuroprotective efficacy.

Advantages/Disadvantages

The advantages of the Canadian Neurologic Scale include its ease of administration, which enables even nonphysicians to administer the test with high reproducibility. A disadvantage is that the scale is weighted toward anterior circulation strokes.

Summary

The Canadian Neurologic Scale is simple to administer and a highly reliable method of assessing neurologic deficit. It appears to have inter-observer reliability and has good construct validity.

Toronto Stroke Scale

The Toronto Stroke Scale (Table 9-4) was developed to assess neurologic deficit in acute stroke patients as part of a steroid therapy efficacy trial (Norris, 1976).

Description

The Toronto stroke scale is a 317-point (11 categories) assessment measuring consciousness, motor weakness, sensory impairment, visual field deficit, aphasia, higher cortical functions, confusion, gaze function, incoordination, dysarthria, and dysphagia. Each item is measured from 0 to 4, reflecting the amount of deficit.

Validation

The Toronto Stroke Scale has not been extensively validated. It did appear to accurately reflect neu-

Table 9-3. Canadian Neurologic Scale

Mentation	Level of consciousness	Alert	3.0
		Drowsy	1.5
	Orientation	Oriented	1.0
		Disoriented/nonapplicable	0.0
	Speech	Normal	1.0
		Expressive deficit	0.5
		Receptive deficit	0.0
Section A1	Motor functions	Weakness	
No comprehension deficit	Face	None	0.5
		Present	0
	Arm: proximal	None	1.5
		Mild	1.0
		Significant	0.5
		Total	0.0
	Arm: distal	None	1.5
		Mild	1.0
		Significant	0.5
		Total	0.0
	Leg: proximal	None	1.5
		Mild	1.0
		Significant	0.5
		Total	0.0
	Leg: distal	None	1.5
		Mild	1.0
		Significant	0.5
		Total	0.0
Section A2	Motor response		
Comprehension deficit	Face	Symmetrical	0.5
		Asymmetrical	0.0
	Arms	Equal	1.5
		Unequal	0.0
	Legs	Equal	1.5
		Unequal	0.0

Table 9-4. Toronto Stroke Scale

1. Consciousness	Alert	0	×	25	0
	Drowsy	1	×	25	0–25
	Stupor	2	×	25	0–50
	Light coma	3	×	25	0–75
	Deep coma	4	×	25	0–100
2. Paresis	Face	0–3	×	1	0–3
	Arm	0–4	×	3.5	0–14
	Leg	0–4	×	2.5	0–10
3. Sensory loss	Face	0–2	×	1.5	0–3
	Arm	0–2	×	6	0–12
	Leg	0–2	×	4.5	0–9
4. Hemianopia		0–2	×	3	0–6
5. Aphasia	Mild, moderate, severe, total	0–4	×	10	0–40
6. Higher cortical function	Frontal	0–2	×	12	0–48
	Parietal	0–2	×	12	0–48
7. Dementia		0–3	×	3	0–9
8. Forced gaze		0–2	×	2	0–4
9. Incoordination		0–3	×	3	0–9
10. Dysarthria		0–3	×	2	0–6
11. Dysphagia		0–2	×	4	0–8

rologic impairments as part of the original therapy trial. It also has been compared with several other stroke studies and has high correlation (Brown et al., 1990).

Administration

Due to the complexity of the Toronto Stroke Scale, it probably needs to be administered by a neurologist trained in cerebrovascular disease. The time of administration ranges from 10 to 20 minutes, depending on the severity of the case.

Special Considerations

The Toronto Stroke Scale is one of the more comprehensive neurologic scales. As such, strokes of any vascular territory appear to be assessed as part of this scale.

Advantages/Disadvantages

The main advantage of the Toronto Stroke Scale is that it can be used outside of the middle cerebral artery territory. Disadvantages include the fact that it is relatively difficult to learn to administer and has had little validation in terms of testing in clinical trials.

Summary

The Toronto Stroke Scale is a comprehensive neurologic deficit assessment scale. It is relatively difficult to learn and there is little reported experience with its use.

Hemispheric Stroke Scale

The Hemispheric Stroke Scale was designed to test neurologic deficit as part of an acute stroke therapy trial using hemodilution (Adams et al., 1987).

Description

The Hemispheric Stroke Scale is a 100-point (19 items) neurologic assessment scale. This comprehensive scale measures level of consciousness, language, cortical function, motor function, and sensory capacity, with higher scores reflecting more deficits. Due to the length and complexity of the scale, it is not included here. Readers are referred to the original paper by Adams and colleagues (1987). The Hemispheric Stroke Scale actually includes the Glasgow Coma Scale.

Validation

The Hemispheric Stroke Scale has been shown to have good construct validity in comparison with the Glasgow Coma Scale ($r = 0.89$), as well as both the Toronto Stroke Scale and the Mathew Scale (Adams et al., 1987; Brown et al., 1990). Intra-observer reliability has not been reported.

Administration

The Hemispheric Stroke Scale should take 15–30 minutes to administer. Due to the complexity of the neurologic evaluation, a neurologist with cerebrovascular training is probably required.

Special Considerations

Due to testing at least some higher cortical functions, the Hemispheric Stroke Scale may be more sensitive for nondominant cortical infarctions.

Advantages/Disadvantages

Due to the relative large amount of neurologic information obtained, the Hemispheric Stroke Scale can be used to measure strokes in a variety of vascular territories. Its disadvantages are similar to those of the Toronto scale in that it is relatively difficult to administer and time-consuming, and several of the scores appear to test redundant information.

Summary

The Hemispheric Stroke Scale is a comprehensive neurologic deficit assessment scale. Although it appears to have fairly high construct validity, it has not been validated in recorded therapeutic stroke trials.

Mathew Stroke Scale

The Mathew Stroke Scale (Table 9-5) was originally designed to test neurologic deficit as part of an acute stroke study testing the therapeutic efficacy of glycerol.

Description

The Mathew Stroke Scale is a comprehensive neurologic scale measuring cognition, cranial nerve function, motor power, global disability status, reflexes, and sensation. It is a 100-point scale (10 items), with lower scores reflecting more severe deficit (Mathew et al., 1972). A modified Mathew scale has been used in studies of nimodipine or hemodilution for acute stroke (Gelmers et al., 1988a; Koller et al., 1990).

Validation

The Mathew Stroke Scale has high construct validity in that it has been shown to be highly correlated with several other stroke scales. It has also been shown to be predictive of long-term outcome (Frithz & Werner, 1976). It appears to have fairly poor inter-observer reliability, with several of the items in the scale having only "slight" inter-observer agreement (Gelmers et al., 1988b). The scale has also been shown to have low internal consistency compared with other measures (Brown et al., 1990). It has had fairly extensive validation in several clinical studies (Gelmers et al., 1988a; Koller et al., 1990).

Administration

Due to the neurologic complexity of the Mathew Stroke Scale, a neurologist with cerebrovascular training is required. The test takes approximately 15 minutes to administer.

Advantages/Disadvantages

An advantage of the Mathew Stroke Scale is that it should be able to detect strokes in many vascular territories due to its relatively comprehensive nature. Disadvantages include the relatively poor inter-observer agreement on several of the items, the time required to administer the test, and the need for specialized neurologic training to properly perform the test.

Table 9-5. Mathew Stroke Scale

Factor	Score	Factor	Score
Mentation		**Motor power***	
Level of consciousness		Normal strength	5
Fully conscious	8	Contracts against resistance	4
Lethargic but mentally intact	6	Elevates against gravity	3
Obtunded	4	Flicker	2
Stuporous	2	No movements	0
Comatose	0		
Orientation		**Performance or disability status scale**	
Oriented × 3	6	Normal	28
Oriented × 2	4	Mild impairment	21
Oriented × 1	2	Moderate impairment	14
Disoriented	0	Severe impairment	7
		Death	0
Speech		**Reflexes**	
Normal	23	Normal	3
Incoherent words	15	Asymmetrical or pathological reflexes	2
Expressive or impressive words	10	Clonus	1
Speechless	0	No reflexes elicited	0
Cranial nerves			
Homonymous hemianopsia		**Sensation**	
Intact	3	Normal	3
Mild	2	Mild sensory abnormality	2
Moderate	1	Severe sensory abnormality	1
Severe	0	No response to pain	0
Conjugate/deviation of eyes			
Intact	3		
Mild	2		
Moderate	1		
Severe	0		
Facial weakness			
Intact	3		
Mild	2		
Moderate	1		
Severe	0		

*Each limb separately.

Summary

The Mathew Stroke Scale is a comprehensive neurologic deficit assessment scale. It has good construct validation in several clinical therapeutic trials, but it appears to have poor intra-observer reliability and requires specialized neurologic training to administer.

European Stroke Scale

The European stroke scale (Table 9-6) is a test designed to detect therapeutic effects in acute stroke treatment trials. The scale is intended to test only middle cerebral artery stroke and is heavily weighted toward motor items (Hantson et al., 1994).

Description

The European Stroke Scale was designed for clinical stroke trials in patients with middle cerebral artery stroke. The scale can be used both for matching patients into severity groups and for long-term efficacy evaluations similar to the SSS. It consists of 14 items selected on the basis of prognostic value: level of consciousness, comprehension, speech, visual field, gaze, facial movement, maintenance of arm position, arm raising, wrist extension, finger strength, maintenance of leg position, leg flexing, foot dorsal flexion, and gait. A normal individual will score 106 on this scale. The scale is similar to the NIHSS except that there are more levels for consciousness evaluation, and there is an inclusion of a gait assessment (Hantson et al., 1994).

Validation

The European Stroke Scale has high construct validity, showing correlations with the other neurologic stroke scales ranging between 0.93 and 0.95. The scale also correlated well with long-term functional recovery measured by the Barthel Index. There was high inter-rater and intra-rater reliability in a development study (Hantson et al., 1994). This scale has not been validated in published clinical therapeutic trials to date.

Administration

Given its similarity to the NIHSS, it appears that both physicians and nurses could learn to administer the European Stroke Scale. The average time of administration is 8 minutes.

Advantages/Disadvantages

Advantages include ease of administration and the ability of non-neurologists to learn the scale. Disadvantages include the fact that it is not in widespread use, so results obtained with the scale may not be directly comparable with those from other scales.

Summary

The European Stroke Scale is a scale designed to test therapeutic effects in acute stroke therapy trials. It appears to have good validity and good prognostic ability, but further experience in clinical trials is needed before widespread use can be recommended.

Unified Neurological Stroke Scale

The Unified Neurological stroke scale is a newly developed "composite" scale for the assessment of acute stroke patients.

Description

The Unified Neurological Stroke Scale is a combination of the Orgogozo Scale and the SSS (see Table 9-2). An alternate way of looking at it is that it is the SSS with the addition of assessments of foot dorsal flexion and extremity tone.

Validation

Both construct and predictive validity were determined in a study by Edwards and colleagues (Edwards et al., 1995; Orgogozo et al., 1992; Brown et al., 1990). Not surprisingly, there was high construct validity as assessed by correlations with the SSS and the Orgogozo Scale. The Unified Neurological Stroke Scale was also shown to be a good predictor of functional outcome for both ischemic stroke and hemorrhagic stroke. In this study, the investigators also looked at the use of this scale for subarachnoid hemorrhage and traumatic brain injury and found it to be a less reliable predictor of outcome than it is in stroke. The scale has also been shown to have high inter-rater agreement (Treves et al., 1994).

Administration

The Unified Neurological Stroke Scale probably needs to be administered by a neurologist because of the inclusion of the tone assessments. The time of

Table 9-6. European Stroke Scale

Level of consciousness		
Alert, keenly responsive		10
Drowsy, but can be aroused by minor stimulation to obey, answer, or respond		8
Requires repeated stimulation to attend, or is lethargic or obtunded, requiring stroke or painful stimulation to make movements		6
Cannot be roused by any stimulation, does react purposefully to painful stimuli		4
Cannot be roused by any stimulation, does react with decerebration to painful stimuli		2
Cannot be roused by any stimulation, does not react to painful stimuli		0
Comprehension		
Verbally give the patient the following commands (IMPORTANT: DO NOT DEMONSTRATE):		
1. Stick out your tongue	Patient performs 3 commands	8
2. Put your finger (of the unaffected side) on your nose	Patient performs 2 or 1 commands	4
3. Close your eyes	Patient does not perform any commands	0
Speech		
The examiner makes a conversation with the patient (how is the patient feeling, did he/she sleep well, for how long has the patient been in the hospital...).	Normal speech	8
	Slight word-finding difficulties, conversation is possible	6
	Severe word-finding difficulties, conversation is difficult	4
	Only yes or no	2
	Mute	0
Visual field		
The examiner stands at arm's length and compares the patient's field of vision by advancing a moving finger from the periphery inwards. The patient must fixate on the examiner's pupil (first with one eye and then with the other eye closed).	Normal	8
	Deficit	0
Gaze		
The examiner steadies the patient's head and asks him/her to follow his/her finger. The examiner observes the resting eye position and, subsequently, the full range of movements by moving the index finger from the left to the right and vice versa.	Normal	8
	Median eye position, deviation to one side impossible	4
	Lateral eye position, return to midline possible	2
	Lateral eye position, return to midline impossible	0
Facial movement		
The examiner observes the patient as he/she talks and smiles, noting any asymmetrical elevation of one corner of mouth, flattening of nasolabial fold. Only the muscles in the lower half of the face are assessed.	Normal	8
	Paresis	4
	Paralysis	0

(continued)

Table 9-6.   *(continued)*

Arm (maintain outstretched position)		
The examiner asks the patient to close the eyes and actively lifts the patient's arms into position so that they are outstretched at 45 degrees in relation to the horizontal plane with both hands in mid-position so that the palms face each other. The patient is asked to maintain this position for 5 sec after the examiner withdraws the arms. Only the affected side is evaluated.	Arm maintains position for 5 sec	4
	Arm maintains position for 5 sec, but affected arm pronates	3
	Arm drifts before 5 sec pass and maintains a lower position	2
	Arm can't maintain position, but attempts to oppose gravity	1
	Arm falls	0

Arm (raising)		
The patient's arm is rested next to the leg with the hand in the mid-position. The examiner asks the patient to raise the arm outstretched to 90 degrees.	Normal	4
	Straight arm, movement not full	3
	Flexed arm	2
	Trace movements	1
	No movement	0

Extension of the wrist		
The patient is tested with the forearm supported and the hand unsupported, relaxed in pronation. The patient is asked to extend the hand.	Normal (full isolated movement, no decrease in strength)	8
	Full isolated movement, reduced strength	6
	Movement not isolated and/or full	4
	Trace movements	2
	No movement	0

Fingers		
The examiner asks the patient to form with both hands and as strongly as possible a pinch grip with the thumb and forefinger and to try to resist a weak pull. The examiner checks the strength of this grip by pulling the pinch with one finger.	Equal strength	8
	Reduced strength on affected side	4
	Pinch grip impossible on affected side	0

Leg (maintain position)		
The examiner actively lifts the patient's affected leg into position so that the thigh forms an angle of 90 degrees with the bed, with the shin parallel with the bed. The examiner asks the patient to close the eyes and to maintain this position for 5 sec without support.	Leg maintains position for 5 sec	4
	Leg drifts to intermediate position by the end of 5 sec	2
	Leg drifts to bed within 5 sec, but not immediately	1
	Leg falls to bed immediately	0

Leg (flexing)		
The patient is in the supine position with the legs outstretched. The examiner asks the patient to flex the hip and knee.	Normal	4
	Movement against resistance, reduced strength	3
	Movement against gravity	2
	Trace movements	1
	No movement	0

Table 9-6.   *(continued)*

Dorsiflexion of the foot		
The patient is tested with the leg outstretched. The examiner asks the patient to dorsiflex the foot.	Normal (leg outstretched, full movement, full strength)	8
	Leg outstretched, full movement, reduced strength	6
	Leg outstretched, movement not full or knee flexed or foot in supination	4
	Trace movements	2
	No movements	0
Gait		
	Normal	10
	Gait has abnormal aspect and/or distance/speed limited	8
	Patient can walk with aid	6
	Patient can walk with the physical assistance of person(s)	4
	Patient cannot walk, but can stand supported	2
	Patient cannot walk or stand	0

administration would only require 1 minute additional to that required by the SSS (i.e., it should be done in less than 15 minutes).

Advantages/Disadvantages

The Unified Neurological Stroke Scale appears to have good reliability and good construct validity. It appears to be an improvement over the SSS alone, with only minimal additional time being required to administer it compared to the SSS. An additional advantage of the Unified Neurological Stroke Scale is that it is the only scale that has been validated in terms of assessing patients with intracerebral hemorrhage. Disadvantages include the fact that it is not in widespread use and, therefore, has not been validated in published therapeutic efficacy trials.

Summary

The Unified Neurological Stroke Scale is a newly developed composite scale that appears to be valid in both ischemic stroke and intracerebral hemorrhage. Further work is needed to determine if it will prove useful in therapeutic efficacy trials.

Conclusion

A large number of stroke scales have been developed to assess neurologic deficits following acute stroke. These scales range from relatively simple and rapid measurements—the Canadian Neurologic Scale—to much more detailed time-consuming assessments, such as the Toronto Stroke Scale and the Hemispheric Stroke Scale. Many of these scales are designed primarily to assess middle cerebral artery strokes and almost all are heavily weighted toward motor function. All of the scales appear to have fairly high construct validity and many of them have shown good predictive validity. The NIHSS and the Canadian Neurologic Scale have had the largest amount of work done assessing inter- and intra-observer reliability, both of which have been found to be very good. The NIHSS and the SSS appear to be the most frequently used for current stroke clinical trials.

Although each neurologic deficit stroke scale has its proponents and merit, overall we think that the NIHSS is currently the preferred scale, given its widespread use, high reliability, and the availability of a training tape. If a simpler scale is desired, the Canadian Neurologic Scale would be the choice, whereas, if a more comprehensive scale is desired, the Unified Neurological Stroke Scale appears to offer a good balance between detailed assessment and ease of use.

Functional Outcome Scales

As opposed to the previously discussed stroke scales, which attempt to define a patient's neurologic examination, the various functional outcome scales attempt to quantify the patient's functional status as measured by ability to perform tasks of daily living. There are two general categories of outcome scales. The first is global assessment. Such scales give broad-based gestalt assessments of the overall functional status of a patient. The second type of outcome scale involves more detailed testing of either routine ADLs or more detailed instrumental ADLs. ADL scales measure performance of functions that are used for independent living. One of the advantages of such scales is that they can be administered by any health care professional and can actually be done through conversation with family or patient over the telephone. A general disadvantage is that they are impractical in the acute stroke setting, where it is inappropriate to test several of the activities.

Overall, functional outcome scales have been receiving more attention in several ongoing clinical trials. As is evidenced in the tPA NIH study (NINDS rt-PA Stroke Study Group, 1995), several companies have abandoned neurologic stroke scales as their primary endpoint and have gone on to functional outcome assessments. The driving force behind this trend is the belief that while a drug may improve a finding on a neurologic examination, e.g., improve a patient by 4 points on the NIHSS, the patient may have no meaningful improvement in terms of ability to function. It is the patient's ability to resume his or her prior ADLs that patients, providers, and insurance companies measure as the *gold standard* for measuring the effectiveness of a drug.

Global Outcome Scales

Glasgow Outcome Scale

The Glasgow Outcome Scale is a 5-point global outcome scale (Table 9-7) that was originally designed as a companion to the Glasgow Coma Scale (Jennett et al.,

Table 9-7. Glasgow Outcome Scale

Score	Circle the Appropriate Score
1	Dead.
2	Persistent vegetative state: patient exhibits no obvious cortical function.
3	Severe disability (conscious but disabled): patient depends on others for daily support due to mental or physical disability or both.
4	Moderate disability (disabled but independent): patient is independent as far as daily life is concerned. The disabilities found include varying degrees of dysphasia, hemiparesis, or ataxia, as well as intellectual and memory deficits and personality changes.
5	Good recovery: resumption of normal activities even though there may be minor neurological or psychological deficits.

1979; Jennett & Bond, 1975). The scale has been extensively used in studies of head injury and nontraumatic coma (Jennett et al., 1979; Levy et al., 1991). It is in widespread use in many clinical therapeutic stroke trials.

Description

The Glasgow Outcome Scale is a 5-point scale with 1 = dead and 5 = good recovery. Although the scale is simple to administer—having only five scores—there is sometimes confusion in that there is no clear demarcation between some of the levels. This is particularly true in some cases between the severe disability and moderate disability scores.

Administration

The Glasgow Outcome Scale can be administered by any trained health care worker. It takes only seconds to complete.

Validation

The Glasgow Outcome Scale has high reliability in several studies of head injury, but reliability assessments in stroke population have not been extensively published. Of interest, it has actually been used as a *gold standard* to measure whether several of the clinical stroke scales previously discussed in Neurologic Deficit Stroke Scales had good construct validity (Côté et al., 1989).

Advantages/Disadvantages

Advantages include ease of use and the ability of nonstroke neurologists to fill out the form. Disadvantages include the relative lack of proven construct validity in stroke, along with the problem of poor demarcation between several of the categories.

Summary

The Glasgow Outcome Scale is in widespread use in clinical stroke trials. It is easy to administer and appears to provide a good overview of a patient's functional outcome.

Modified Rankin Scale

The Modified Rankin Scale (Table 9-8) is a 5-point global assessment categorization of a patient's function based on the ability to perform ADLs.

Description

Groups are ranked from 0 = no symptoms to 5 = severe disability (Rankin, 1957; van Swieten et al., 1988). Ratings are given as to how much assistance the patient requires to achieve various levels of function. Some clinical stroke trials also add a grade 6 for

Table 9-8. Modified Rankin Scale

Grade	Description
0	No symptoms at all
1	No significant disability despite symptoms: able to carry out all usual duties and activities
2	Slight disability: unable to carry out all previous activities but able to look after own affairs without assistance
3	Moderate disability: requiring some help, but able to walk without assistance
4	Moderately severe disability: unable to walk without assistance and unable to attend to own bodily needs without assistance
5	Severe disability: bedridden, incontinent, and requiring constant nursing care and attention

patients who have expired. Similar to the Glasgow Outcome Scale, the Modified Rankin Scale sometimes suffers from poor demarcation between various levels. As an example, a patient with a middle cerebral artery stroke could have severe disability in many categories yet still be scored as only moderate in that he or she frequently is able to ambulate without assistance.

Administration

The Modified Rankin Scale can be administered by a neurologist or other health care professional.

Validation

The Modified Rankin Scale has been reported to have moderate inter-observer reliability. It has had significant use in several stroke therapeutic outcome trials (Tomasello et al., 1982; Bonita & Beaglehole, 1988).

Activities of Daily Living Scales

Barthel Index

The Barthel Index (Table 9-9) is a widely used measure of functional outcome that has been used not only in stroke but also in a multitude of neurologic disorders (Mahoney & Barthel, 1965; Gresham et al., 1980; Brown et al., 1990; Wade & Hewer, 1987).

Description

The Barthel Index comprises 10 weighted items measuring feeding, bathing, grooming, dressing, bowel control, bladder control, toileting, chair transfer, ambulation, and stair climbing. A maximum score of 100 is normal.

Administration

The Barthel Index can be administered by any health care professional. It takes approximately 5 minutes to administer. The score can be obtained from discussing the questions with the patient, family, or rehabilitation facility nurses.

Validation

The Barthel Index has been extensively studied and has had high construct validation (Brown et al.,

Table 9-9.   Barthel Index

1. Feeding	10 =	Independent. Able to apply any necessary device. Feeds in reasonable time.
	5 =	Needs help (i.e., for cutting).
	0 =	Inferior performance.
2. Bathing	5 =	Performs without assistance.
	0 =	Inferior performance.
3. Personal toilet (grooming)	5 =	Washes face, combs hair, brushes teeth, shaves (manages plug if electric razor).
	0 =	Inferior performance.
4. Dressing	10 =	Independent. Ties shoes, fastens fasteners, applies braces.
	5 =	Needs help but does at least half of task within reasonable time.
	0 =	Inferior performance.
5. Bowel control	10 =	No accidents. Able to use enema or suppository if needed.
	5 =	Occasional accidents or needs help with enema or suppository.
	0 =	Inferior performance.
6. Bladder control	10 =	No accidents. Able to care for collecting device if used.
	5 =	Occasional accidents or needs help with device.
	0 =	Inferior performance.
7. Toilet transfers	10 =	Independent with toilet or bedpan. Handles clothes, wipes, flushes, or cleans pan.
	5 =	Needs help for balance, handling clothes or toilet paper.
	0 =	Inferior performance.
8. Chair/bed transfers	15 =	Independent, including locks of wheelchair and lifting footrests.
	10 =	Minimum assistance or supervision.
	5 =	Able to sit, but needs maximum assistance to transfer.
	0 =	Inferior performance.
9. Ambulation	15 =	Independent for 50 yd. May use assistive devices, except for rolling walker.
	10 =	With help for 50 yd.
	5 =	Independent with wheelchair for 50 yd, only if unable to walk.
	0 =	Inferior performance.
10. Stair climbing	10 =	Independent. May use assistive devices.
	5 =	Needs help or supervision.
	0 =	Inferior performance.

1990; Wade & Hewer, 1987). The scale has also been shown to predict length of hospital stay as well as the odds of independent living (Granger et al., 1979, 1989). Barthel Index scores obtained from telephone interviews have been shown to correlate highly with those obtained from direct examinations (Shinar et al., 1987). It has also been shown to have high inter-rater reliability (Shinar et al., 1987).

Advantages/Disadvantages

Advantages include ease of use and the ability to conduct interviews by telephone follow-up. Disadvantages include the fact that the scale only measures very basic functions. Patients can have significant cognitive impairment and still score 100 on the Barthel Index.

Summary

The Barthel Index is a widely used ADL scale with high reliability and construct validation. It is in widespread use as the primary endpoint in many ongoing clinical therapeutic trials.

Activity Index

The Activity Index (Table 9-10) was originally developed using components of other ADL scales to measure the functional outcome of acute stroke patients.

Description

The Activity Index includes four mental capacity items, six measures of motor function, and five measures of ADL. There is a strong correlation between the Activity Index and the Barthel Index (Lindmark, 1988).

Administration

The Activity Index can be administered by any health care professional. No evaluation of whether it can be administered by telephone has been reported.

Validation

The Activity Index has shown excellent construct validity in that it correlates highly with the Barthel Index ($r = 0.94$; Hamrin & Wohlin, 1989). This scale has also been shown to have a good predictive validity in that initial scores on the scale are highly predictive of 3-week functional outcome (Hamrin & Wohlin, 1989). The scale has been shown to have high internal consistency (Lindmark, 1988).

Advantages/Disadvantages

Advantages include ease of use and the ability of any health care professional to administer it. Disadvantages include the fact that the scale is not in widespread use in clinical stroke trials.

Summary

Although it is a potential improvement over the Barthel Index, the Activity Index has not received widespread acceptance.

Functional Independence Measure

The Functional Independence Measure (FIM) is a measure of disability. Widely used in the United States, it was originally developed by Uniform Data Systems in Buffalo, New York, based on a large database of patients discharged from rehabilitation facilities (Dodds et al., 1993; Heinemann et al., 1993).

Description

The 18 items of the FIM are organized into six subscales and assess two dimensions:

1. Physical: eating, grooming, bathing, dressing, toiletry, bowel and bladder control, transferring, and ambulation.
2. Cognitive: communication, social interaction, problem-solving, and memory.

Each of the 18 items is assessed on a 7-point scale ranging from 1 (requiring complete dependence) to 7 (being completely independent). The scale is under copyright protection. Copies can be obtained from the Research Foundation—State University of New York.

Validation

The FIM has been extensively validated in patients who have had either neurologic or orthopedic disabilities (Kidd et al., 1995). It has been shown to have high inter-rater agreement even when administered by telephone (Ottenbacher et al., 1994). The FIM was validated in several stroke outcome studies and was found to be a predictor of long-term stroke outcome (Owen et al., 1995; Segal & Schall, 1994).

Administration

The FIM is usually administered by a rehabilitation physician or nurse. This scale comes with a 24-page instruction manual and is time-consuming to learn. The ratings can be determined through either patient interview or family/provider interview.

Advantages/Disadvantages

Advantages include the fact that it provides a more detailed assessment of the various functional abilities of the patient compared to the Barthel Index. However, it is difficult to learn, and the gradations between the 7-point assistance scale for each item are relatively poorly defined. The FIM is available from the Uniform System

Table 9-10. Activity Index

Variable	Score	Variable	Score
Mental capacity		Left hand	
Degree of consciousness		Normal or nearly normal activity, isolated gripping and finger movements	4
Completely awake	8	Simple functional grips	3
Somnolent	6	Activity without functional value	2
Precomatose	4	No activity	1
Comatose	1	Left leg	
Orientation in time, space, and person (identity)		Normal or nearly normal activity	4
Orientation in all three dimensions	6	Activity of some functional value	3
Orientation in two dimensions	4	Activity without functional value	2
Orientation in one dimension	3	No activity	1
Disoriented	1		
Ability to communicate verbally		ADL function	
Normal verbal communication	12	Ambulation	
Slight difficulties in communication	8	Able to walk	6
Severe difficulties in communication	4	Walks if supported by somebody, able to move her-/himself about in a wheelchair	4
No verbal communication	1	Confined to a wheelchair, able to stand with support of somebody	3
Psychological activities		Confined to bed or wheelchair, cannot stand even with the support of somebody	1
Takes initiative him-/herself, wants information, etc.	6	Personal hygiene	
Takes some initiative, talks to people around	4	Manages personal hygiene by him-/herself	6
Takes no initiative, apathetic	3	Help needed only for her/his lower toilet	4
No noticeable psychological activity	1	Assists when washing her-/himself but needs help both for upper and lower toilet	3
		Does not assist in her/his personal hygiene at all	1
Motor activity		Dressing	
Right arm		Dresses her-/himself	6
Normal or nearly normal activity	4	Dresses her-/himself on the whole, needs help only with stockings/socks, for example	4
Activity of some functional value	3	Can assist in certain minor elements of the dressing procedure	3
Activity without functional value	2	Must be dressed completely by somebody else	1
No activity	1	Feeding	
Right hand		Eats completely by her-/himself	6
Normal or nearly normal activity, isolated gripping and finger movements	4	Eats with some assistance	4
Simple functional grips	3	Is fed	3
Activity without functional value	2	Fed by tube or intravenous infusion	1
No activity	1	Emptying/function of bladder	
Right leg		Continent	6
Normal or nearly normal activity	4	Occasional failures	4
Activity of some functional value	3	Uridome and/or assistance with toilet and bedpan	3
Activity without functional value	2	Incontinent	1
No activity	1	Maximum score	92
Left arm			
Normal or nearly normal activity	4		
Activity of some functional value	3		
Activity without functional value	2		
No activity	1		

ADL = activities of daily living.

for Rehabilitation Project Office, Buffalo General Hospital, 100 High Street, Buffalo, NY 14203.

Summary

The FIM is a comprehensive disability evaluation scale. Although it is in widespread use in the rehabilitation literature, it is not frequently used in clinical stroke research.

Several other ADL scales are in use in other neurologic diseases. These include the Kennedy self-care evaluation scale (Schoening et al., 1965; Gresham et al., 1980) and the Katz index of ADLs (Katz et al., 1963; Katz & Akpom, 1976). These scales have been shown to be highly correlative with the Barthel Index (Wade & Hewer, 1987; Gresham et al., 1980). Both scales use performance in ambulation, dressing, personal hygiene, feeding activities, and continence. Because they are not in widespread use in clinical stroke studies, the reader is referred to the original description of the scales for more details.

The previous scales measure routine ADLs. As such, they measure whether a patient can perform basic activities that are required for them to be independent. One of the weaknesses of the ADL scales is that they neglect all aspects of higher cortical function, including such activities as the ability to read, manage money, perform hobbies, drive, and perform general house maintenance functions. In an effort to measure these more complex functions of daily life, measurements of instrumental ADLs have been developed. Four such scales have been applied to acute stroke patients. These include the Rivermead ADL Assessment Scale (Whiting & Lincoln, 1980), the Hamrin Activity Index (Holbrook & Skilbeck, 1983), the Frenchay Activities Index (Lincoln & Edmans, 1990), and the Nottingham Extended ADL scale (Nouri & Lincoln, 1987) (Table 9-11). Although they offer a theoretical advantage over the ADL scales previously discussed in Activities of Daily Living Scales, they have not received widespread acceptance in the stroke community. To our knowledge, they are not used in any acute stroke therapeutic trial. For this reason, we do not undertake a detailed discussion of each scale in this chapter. Interested readers are referred to a paper by Chong (1995) for an in-depth discussion of these scales as well as a discussion of their validity and reliability.

Functional outcome scales are receiving more attention as primary outcome for various therapeutic trials. Of the scales currently in use, the Modified Rankin Scale, the Glasgow Outcome Scale, and the Barthel Index all appear to have good construct validity and reliability. These three scales are in widespread use in many acute stroke trials. They are easily administered by any health care professional. A potential weakness is the fact that they do not measure activities that require significant cognitive abilities, so patients who still have major impairments may attain good scores on these scales.

Conclusion

In this chapter we have reviewed both the neurologic deficit scales and the functional outcome scales that are in widespread use in clinical stroke studies. Brief discussions of the validity and reliability of the various scales have been included. For readers interested in a more detailed review of these areas, we recommend the excellent article by Lyden and Lau (1991), in which they critically review many of the stroke scales that are discussed in this chapter. Many ongoing therapeutic trials use a combination of several of the neurologic and outcome scales. Both types of scales have their apparent advantages, with the neurologic scales being able to detect smaller changes in the patient's neurologic examination, whereas the functional outcome scales appear to have more relevance to the patient's ability to function independently. Clearly, both types of scales have their weaknesses and, to date, there is no agreement on a single method of determining either an individual patient's outcome or a *gold standard* for measuring a drug's therapeutic efficacy.

The results from the NIH tPA trial found that all of the endpoints, including the Modified Rankin Scale, Glasgow Outcome Scale, Barthel Index, and NIHSS, showed therapeutic benefit (NINDS rt-PA Stroke Study Group, 1995). This suggests that if the effect of a drug is real, any of these scales appear capable of detecting this. Currently, the most widely accepted tests are the Modified Rankin Scale and the NIHSS. It is hoped that additional outcome assessments will be used in the future. These may include measurements of infarct size reduction based on magnetic resonance imaging diffusion weighted imaging technology. Finally, several clinical therapeutic trials are now also using pharmacoeconomic assessments as secondary endpoints to assess therapeutic efficacy. In the managed health care environment, such pharmacoeconomic endpoints may actually prove to be the most powerful indicator of a drug's benefit.

Acknowledgment

The authors thank Sandi Hungerford for her excellent assistance in the preparation of this chapter.

Table 9-11. Instrumental Activities of Daily Living Scales

Rivermead Scale	Hamrin Scale	Frenchay Scale	Nottingham Scale
Household 1	Household work	Preparing meals	Mobility
Preparation of hot drink	Make coffee/tea	Washing dishes	Walk outside
Preparation of snack	Simple cooking	Washing clothes	Climb stairs
Cope with money	Dishwashing	Dusting/vacuum cleaning	Get in/out of car
Get in/out of car	Make bed	Cleaning	Walk over uneven ground
Prepare meal	Vacuum cleaning, wash floors	Local shopping	Cross roads
Carry shopping	Easy laundry (by hand or machine)	Social activities	Public transport
Crossing roads	Locomotion	Walks	Kitchen
Transport self to shop	Move from bed to chair	Hobby/sport	Feed self
Public transport	Move about in home	Car/bus travel	Make hot drink
Household 2	Manage stairs	Gardening	Take hot drinks from one room to another
Washing	Walk outdoors	Books	
Ironing	Unlock and close entrance door	Outings	Washing up
Light cleaning	Psychosocial functions	House/car maintenance	Make hot snack
Hang out washing	Write letters	Employment	Domestic tasks
Bed-making	Telephone	Manage own money	Wash small items of clothing
Heavy cleaning	Visit someone	Housework	Wash full load of clothes
	Use municipal means of transport	Shopping	Leisure activities
	Go to public premises		Read newspapers or books
	Shopping		Telephone
	Intellectual activities		Write letters
	Read daily newspapers		Go out socially
	Listen to news on radio or TV		Manage own garden
	Read books		Drive a car
	Keep own accounts		

References

Adams RJ, Meador KJ, Sethi KD, et al. Graded neurologic scale for use in acute hemispheric stroke treatment protocols. *Stroke* 1987;18:655–69.

Bonita R, Beaglehole R. Recovery of motor function after stroke. *Stroke* 1988;19:1497–1500.

Brott TG, Adams HP, Olinger CP, et al. Measurements of acute cerebral infarction: a clinical examination scale. *Stroke* 1989a;20:864–70.

Brott T, Haley EC Jr., Levy DE, et al. Urgent therapy for stroke. Part 1: pilot study of tissue plasminogen activator administered within 90 minutes. *Stroke* 1992;23:632–40.

Brott T, Marler JR, Olinger CO, et al. Measurements of acute cerebral infarction: lesion size by computerized tomography. *Stroke* 1989b;20:871–75.

Brown EB, Tietjen GE, Deveshwar RK, et al. Clinical stroke scales: an intra- and interscale evaluation. *Neurology* 1990;40S1:352–55.

Chong DKH. Measurement of instrumental activities of daily living in stroke. *Stroke* 1995;26:1119–22.

Côté R, Battista RN, Wolfson CM. Stroke assessment scales: guidelines for development, validation, and reliability assessment. *Can J Neurol Sci* 1988;115:261–65.

Côté R, Battista RN, Wolfson CM, et al. The Canadian neurological scale: validation and reliability assessment. *Neurology* 1989;39:638–43.

Côté R, Hachinski V, Shurvell BL, et al. The Canadian neurological scale: a preliminary study in acute stroke. *Stroke* 1986;17:731–37.

Dodds TA, Martin DP, Stolov WC, et al. A validation of the functional independence measure and its performance among rehabilitation inpatients. *Arch Phys Med Rehabil* 1993;74:531–36.

Edwards DF, Chen YW, Diringer MN. Unified neurological stroke scale is valid in ischemic and hemorrhagic stroke. *Stroke* 1995;26:1852–58.

Frithz G, Werner I. Clinical findings and short-term prognosis in a stroke material. *Acta Med Scand* 1976;199:133–40.

Gelmers HJ, Gorter K, de Weerdt CJ, et al. A controlled trial of nimodipine in acute ischemic stroke. *N Engl J Med* 1988a;318:203–7.

Gelmers HJ, Gorter K, de Weerdt CJ, et al. Assessment of interobserver variability in a Dutch multicenter study on acute ischemic stroke. *Stroke* 1988b;19:709–11.

Goldstein LB, Bartels C, Davis JN. Interrater reliability of the NIH stroke scale. *Arch Neurol* 1989;46:660–62.

Granger CV, Dewis LS, Peters NC, et al. Stroke rehabilitation: analysis of repeated Barthel Index measures. *Arch Phys Med Rehabil* 1979;60:14–17.

Granger CV, Hamilton BB, Gresham GE, et al. The stroke rehabilitation outcome study: part II. Relative merit of the total Barthel Index score and a four-item subscore in predicting patient outcomes. *Arch Phys Med Rehabil* 1989;70:100–3.

Gresham GE, Phillips TF, Labi MLC. ADL status in stroke: relative merits of three standard indexes. *Arch Phys Med Rehabil* 1980;61:355–58.

Haley EC Jr., Brott TG, Sheppard GL, et al. Pilot randomized trial of tissue plasminogen activator in acute ischemic stroke. *Stroke* 1993;24:1000–4.

Haley EC Jr., Levy DE, Brott TG, et al. Urgent therapy for stroke. Part 2: pilot study of tissue plasminogen activator administered 91–180 minutes from onset. *Stroke* 1992;23:641–45.

Hamrin E, Wohlin A. Evaluation of the functional capacity of stroke patients through an activity index. *J Clin Physiol* 1989;14:93–100.

Hantson L, de Weerdt W, de Keyser J, et al. The European stroke scale. *Stroke* 1994;25:2215–19.

Heinemann AW, Linacre JM, Wright BD, et al. Prediction of rehabilitation outcomes with disability measures. *Arch Phys Med Rehabil* 1993;74:566–73.

Holbrook M, Skilbeck C. An activities index for use with stroke patients. *Age Ageing* 1983;12:166–70.

Jennett B, Bond M. Assessment of outcome after severe brain damage: a practical scale. *Lancet* 1975;5:480–84.

Jennett B, Teasdale G, Braakman R, et al. Prognosis of patients with severe head injury. *Neurosurgery* 1979;4:283–89.

Katz S, Akpom CA. A measure of primary sociobiological functions. *Intl J Health Serv* 1976;6:493–507.

Katz S, Ford AB, Moskowitz RW, et al. The index of ADL: a standardized measure of biological and psychosocial function. *JAMA* 1963;185:913–19.

Kidd D, Steward G, Baldry J, et al. The functional independence measure: a comparative validity and reliability study. *Disabil Rehabil* 1995;17:10–14.

Koller M, Haenny P, Hess K. et al. Adjusted hypervolemic hemodilution in acute ischemic stroke. *Stroke* 1990;21:1429–34.

Levy DE, Bates D, Garonna JJ, et al. Prognosis in nontraumatic coma. *Ann Int Med* 1991;94:293–301.

Lincoln NB, Edmans JA. A re-validation of the Rivermead ADL scale for elderly patients with stroke. *Age Ageing* 1990;19:19–24.

Lindenstrøm E, Boysen G, Christiansen LW, et al. Reliability of Scandinavian neurological stroke scale. *Cerebrovasc Dis* 1991;1:103–7.

Lindmark B. Evaluation of functional capacity after stroke with special emphasis on motor function and ADL. *Scand J Rehab Med* 1988;21S:1–40.

Lyden P, Brott T, Tilley B, et al. Improved reliability of the NIH stroke scale using video training. *Stroke* 1994;25:2220–26.

Lyden PD, Lau GT. A critical appraisal of stroke evaluation and rating scales. *Stroke* 1991;22:1345–52.

Mahoney FT, Barthel DW. Functional evaluation: Barthel Index. *Md State Med J* 1965;14:61–65.

Mathew NT, Rivera VM, Meyer JS, et al. Double-blind evaluation of glycerol therapy in acute cerebral infarction. *Lancet* 1972;2:1327–29.

National Institute of Neurological Disorders and Stroke rt-PA Stroke Study Group. Tissue plasminogen activator for acute ischemic stroke. *N Engl J Med* 1995;333:1581–87.

Norris JW. Steroid therapy in acute cerebral infarction. *Arch Neurol* 1976;33:69–71.

Nouri FM, Lincoln NB. An extended activities of daily living scale for stroke patients. *Clin Rehab* 1987;1:301–5.

Orgogozo JM, Asplund K, Boysen J. A unified form for neurologic scoring of hemispheric stroke with motor impairment. *Stroke* 1992;23:1678–79.

Orgogozo JM, Calpideo R, Anagnostou CN. Mise au point d'un score neurologique pour revaluation clinique des infarctus sylviens. *Presse Med* 1983;12:3039–44.

Orgogozo JM, Dartigues JF. Clinical trials in brain infarction. The question of assessment criteria. In: Battistini N (ed.). *Acute brain ischemia. Medical and surgical therapy.* New York: Raven, 1986:201–8.

Orgogozo JM, Dartigues JF. Methodology of clinical trials in acute cerebral ischemia: survival, functional and neurological outcome measures. *Cerebrovasc Dis* 1991;1(Suppl 1):100–11.

Ottenbacher KJ, Mann WC, Granger CV, et al. Inter-rater agreement and stability of functional assessment in the community-based elderly. *Arch Phys Med Rehabil* 1994; 75:1297–1301.

Owen DC, Getz PA, Bulla S. A comparison of characteristics of patients with completed stroke: those who achieve continence and those who do not. *Rehabil Nurs* 1995; 20:197–203.

Rankin J. Cerebral vascular accidents in patients over the age of 60: prognosis. *Scott Med J* 1957;2:200–15.

Scandinavian Stroke Study Group. Multicenter trial of hemodilution in ischemic stroke. Background and study protocol. *Stroke* 1985;16:885–90.

Scandinavian Stroke Study Group. Multicenter trial of hemodilution in ischemic stroke. *Stroke* 1987;18:691–99.

Schoening HA, Anderegg L, Bergstrom D, et al. Numerical scoring of self-care status of patients. *Arch Phys Med Rehabil* 1965;46:689–97.

Segal ME, Schall RR. Determining function/health status and its relation to disability in stroke survivors. *Stroke* 1994;25:2391–97.

Shinar D, Gross CR, Bronstein KS, et al. Reliability of the activities of daily living scale and its use in the telephone interview. *Arch Phys Med Rehabil* 1987;68:723–28.

Tomasello F, Mariani F, Fieschi C, et al. Assessment of interobserver differences in the Italian multicenter study on reversible cerebral ischemia. *Stroke* 1982;13:32–34.

Treves TA, Karepov VG, Aronovich BD, et al. Interrater agreement in evaluation of stroke patients with the unified neurological stroke scale. *Stroke* 1994;25:1263–64.

van Swieten JC, Koudstall PJ, Visser MC, et al. Interobserver agreement for the assessment of handicap in stroke patients. *Stroke* 1988;19:604–7.

Wade DT, Hewer RL. Functional abilities after stroke: measurement, natural history, and prognosis. *J Neurol Neurosurg Psychiatry* 1987;50:177–82.

Whiting S, Lincoln N. An ADL assessment for stroke patients. *Br J Occup Ther* 1980;43:44–6.

Zivin JA, Waud DR. Quantal bioassay and stroke. *Stroke* 1992;23:767–73.

10 Peripheral Neuropathy and Pain Scales

Robert M. Herndon, M.D.

H istorically, the findings in peripheral neuropathy were simply
recorded as part of the neurologic examination with little
attempt at quantitation. However, over the past three
decades, methods and scales have been developed to
assess neuropathic signs and symptoms and pain in a
more systematic manner. Methods of assessing peripheral neuropathy and pain are many and varied. They
range from simple visual/analogue and symptom scales
to quantitative sensory and motor testing to electrophys-
iologic measurement of motor and sensory nerve conduction and electromyography.

Scales for the study of neuropathies range from
disease specific, such as the neurologic symptom score
and neurologic disability score for diabetes (Dyck et
al., 1980), to that of Merkies and the Inflammatory
Neuropathy Cause and Treatment Group for assessing
sensory neuropathic symptoms (Merkies et al., 2000).

Recently, the American Academy of Neurology,
the American Association of Neuromuscular & Electrodiagnostic Medicine, and the American Academy of
Physical Medicine and Rehabilitation have published a
definition of *distal symmetric polyneuropathy* for research
purposes. The diagnostic algorithm is fairly complex,

and those planning research in this area should refer to
the original article (England et al., 2005).

Assessment of pain is complicated by its variability and subjective nature. Different individuals have
differing pain thresholds and respond to pain differently. Descriptions of pain quality are also complicated
by subjectivity and by the differences in the way individuals experience pain. A number of attempts have
been made to categorize pain, the best known being
the McGill Pain Questionnaire (Melzack, 1975). We
here discuss several questionnaires and scales used for
assessment of neuropathies and neuropathic pain.

McGill Pain Questionnaire

Description

The McGill Pain Questionnaire, developed at the
McGill Pain Center, consists of three major classes of
word descriptors—sensory (the quality of the pain),
affective (that describe emotional and anxiety responses
to pain), and evaluative (that describe overall intensity)—
which are used by patients to describe their pain experience. The words were ranked on a severity scale, and it

was found that the ranking was consistent both for doctors and patients. Using these descriptors, the investigators developed three major measures, a pain rating index, the number of words chosen, and the present pain intensity. These form a semiquantitative method for assessing pain. Administration and scoring are somewhat complicated. Subsequent studies have shown that different types of pain are characterized by different descriptors, so the questionnaire can distinguish between pain due to different causes (Dubuisson & Melzack, 1976).

Validation

The system was tested in 297 patients suffering various types of pain and then used in an experimental study. The scales are based on the idea that, despite the subjective nature of the pain experience, individuals rate the terms used similarly. Correlation coefficients between rank and scale values for the 20 subclasses of the pain questionnaire were quite high with most above 0.85. The scales also proved sensitive to change in the clinical trial.

Administration

Administration is by a physician or trained technician and requires 10–20 minutes. Self-administration was not found to be satisfactory.

Forms for the McGill Pain Questionnaire can be found in Melzack (1975). Those interested in using this scale should refer to the original article to understand its development and appreciate its uses and capabilities.

Advantages/Disadvantages

This is one of the best general pain scales and is useful for all types of pain. It has a modest length and provides a good, reproducible description of the pain quality and intensity. Scale result cannot be reduced to a single number but rather reduces to descriptors and intensities. Aside from the time required to administer it, it has no substantial disadvantages.

Short-Form McGill Pain Questionnaire

Description

This is a shorter version of the McGill Pain Questionnaire derived by selecting a small representative set of descriptors from the sensory and affective terms of the standard McGill form along with the present pain intensity scale and the visual analog scale (Table 10-1). The investigators selected the descriptors used by more than one-third of a set of patients with varied pain disorders, with the addition of a key descriptor for dental pain. The intensity of the sensation is then assessed for each of the terms and recorded and the visual analog scale and present pain intensity recorded (Melzack, 1987; Melzack & Wall, 2004).

Validation

The scale was validated relative to the full McGill Pain Scale and correlation values were highly significant.

Administration

Like the full pain scale, this is administered by a health professional. Administration should require less than 5 minutes.

Advantages

This is a well-validated, brief pain questionnaire that appears sensitive to change and is suitable for pharmacologic trials. Although the result cannot be reduced to a single number, the effect of analgesics on different aspects of the pain can be elucidated by both this and the full McGill questionnaire.

Disadvantages

The short form provides somewhat less information than the full McGill Pain Questionnaire.

Polyneuropathies

In January 2005 (England et al., 2005), a committee composed of members of the American Academy of Neurology, the American Association of Neuromuscular & Electrodiagnostic Medicine, and the American Academy of Physical Medicine and Rehabilitation published a clinical research definition of distal symmetrical polyneuropathy. This is a consensus document that ranks probability of the disease based on various characteristics based on a review of the literature (Table 10-2).

Neurological Symptom Score

Description

The Neurological Symptom Score was developed by Dr. Peter Dyck and the Rochester Diabetes Neuropathy Study group (Dyck & Thomas, 1975; Dyck et al., 1980) to assess change in diabetic polyneuropathy. It is a straightforward assessment of the presence or absence of a list of motor, sensory, and autonomic

Table 10-1. Short-Form McGill Pain Questionnaire

Patient's Name: _____   Date: _____

	None	Mild	Moderate	Severe
1. Throbbing	0)_____	1)_____	2)_____	3)_____
2. Shooting	0)_____	1)_____	2)_____	3)_____
3. Stabbing	0)_____	1)_____	2)_____	3)_____
4. Sharp	0)_____	1)_____	2)_____	3)_____
5. Cramping	0)_____	1)_____	2)_____	3)_____
6. Gnawing	0)_____	1)_____	2)_____	3)_____
7. Hot-burning	0)_____	1)_____	2)_____	3)_____
8. Aching	0)_____	1)_____	2)_____	3)_____
9. Heavy	0)_____	1)_____	2)_____	3)_____
10. Tender	0)_____	1)_____	2)_____	3)_____
11. Splitting	0)_____	1)_____	2)_____	3)_____
12. Tiring-exhausting	0)_____	1)_____	2)_____	3)_____
13. Sickening	0)_____	1)_____	2)_____	3)_____
14. Fearful	0)_____	1)_____	2)_____	3)_____
15. Punishing-cruel	0)_____	1)_____	2)_____	3)_____

Visual analog scale

No pain_____Worst possible pain

Present pain intensity

0	No pain	_____
1	Mild	_____
2	Discomforting	_____
3	Distressing	_____
4	Horrible	_____
5	Excruciating	_____

Note: Descriptors 1–11 represent the sensory dimension of pain experience, and 12–15 represent the affective dimension. Each descriptor is ranked on an intensity scale of 0 = none; 1 = mild; 2 = moderate; or 3 = severe. The present pain intensity of the standard long-form McGill Pain Questionnaire and the visual analog scale are included to provide overall intensity scores. Reprinted with the kind permission of Ronald Melzack, Ph.D.

symptoms, which are simply scored as present or absent (Table 10-3).

Validation

As a simple list of common symptoms of peripheral neuropathy, it has face validity. It has good construct validity and good criterion-related validity in that its scores correlated significantly with other measures of the presence of diabetic neuropathy.

Administration

The scale is administered by a physician who records volunteered symptoms and elicits symptoms using non-leading questions relative to neuropathic symptoms.

Table 10-2. Estimated Likelihood of Distal Symmetric Polyneuropathy for Case Definitions That Include Symptoms, Signs, and Nerve Conduction Studies: Recommendations for Clinical Research Studies

Neuropathic Symptoms	Decreased or Absent Ankle Reflexes[1]	Decreased Distal Sensation	Distal Muscle Weakness or Atrophy	NCSs[2]	Ordinal Likelihood
Present	Present	Present	Present	Abnormal	++++
Absent	Present	Present	Present	Abnormal	++++
Present	Present	Present	Absent	Abnormal	++++
Present	Present	Absent	Absent	Abnormal	++++
Present	Absent	Present	Absent	Abnormal	++++
Absent	Present	Absent	Present	Abnormal	+++
Present	Absent	Absent	Absent	Abnormal	+++
Absent	Absent	Absent	Absent	Abnormal	++
Absent	Present	Absent	Absent	Abnormal	++
Present	Present	Present	Absent	Normal	++
Present[3]	Absent	Present[3]	Absent	Normal[3]	+
Present[4]	Present[4]	Present[4]	Present[4]	Normal[4]	−

NCSs = nerve conduction studies.
Note: Neuropathic symptoms: numbness, altered sensation, or pain in the feet. For clinical research studies enrollment should be limited to cases above the bold horizontal line (i.e., ++++).
[1]Ankle reflexes may be decreased in normal individuals older than 65–70 years.
[2]Abnormal NCSs are defined in the body of the article.
[3]This phenotype is common in "small-fiber" sensory polyneuropathy. Determination of intraepithelial nerve fiber density in skin biopsy may be useful to confirm the diagnosis (see text).
[4]This phenotype in the presence of normal NCSs is not a distal symmetric polyneuropathy. This situation is given a negative (−) ordinal likelihood because the condition cannot be classified as a distal symmetric polyneuropathy. It is included here to emphasize the importance of including NCSs as part of the case definition for clinical research studies.
Comment: This is a definition developed for research on polyneuropathies. It has not been available for a long enough period to determine its usefulness or accuracy. It is based on the opinion of experts, and its role in research on neuropathies remains to be determined.

Time to Administer

Elicitation and recording of the symptoms should ordinarily take 3–6 minutes.

Advantages

It is a simple, straightforward, and valid elicitation of symptoms. It is a systematic compilation of the presence or absence of symptoms related to neuropathy.

Disadvantages

It is entirely subjective and may vary depending on the sophistication of the patient or the ability of the examiner to elicit specific symptoms in a nonleading fashion. It is an ordinal scale and requires nonparametric statistics.

Summary

This is a useful, systematic approach to recording symptoms of diabetic neuropathy probably best used in conjunction with the Neurological Disability Score.

Neurological Disability Score

Description

The Neurological Disability Score is a systematic neurologic examination with scoring of papilledema, motor function in the cranial nerves, 16 muscles or muscle groups on each side of the body, and reflexes and sensations in each extremity (Table 10-4). These

Table 10-3. Neurological Symptom Score

Score 1 point for the presence of a symptom.	Left	Right
Symptoms of muscle weakness		
Bulbar		
Extraocular	___	___
Facial	___	___
Tongue	___	___
Throat	___	___
Limbs		
Shoulder girdle and upper arm	___	___
Hand	___	___
Glutei and thigh	___	___
Legs	___	___
Sensory disturbances		
Negative symptoms		
Difficulty identifying objects in mouth	___	___
Difficulty identifying objects in hands	___	___
Unsteadiness walking	___	___
Positive symptoms		
Numbness, asleep feeling, like Novocain, prickling at any site	___	___
Pain—burning, deep aching, tenderness at any location	___	___
Autonomic symptoms		
Postural fainting	___	___
Impotence in male	___	___
Loss of urinary control	___	___
Night diarrhea	___	___
Sum	___	___

are scored on a 0–4 scale ranging from no deficit to severest deficit.

Validation

This scale has reasonable face validity and correlates fairly well with other measures of diabetic neuropathy.

Table 10-4. Neurological (Neuropathy) Disability Score

Scoring—Enter 0 for no deficit, 1 for mild deficit, 2 for moderate deficit, 3 for severe deficit, and 4 for complete absence of function or severest deficit.	Right	Left
Cranial nerves		
Papilledema	___	___
EOM weakness cranial nerve III	___	___
EOM weakness cranial nerve IV	___	___
Face weakness	___	___
Palate weakness	___	___
Tongue weakness	___	___
Muscle weakness		
Respiratory	___	___
Shoulder abduction	___	___
Biceps brachii	___	___
Brachioradialis	___	___
Extension at elbow	___	___
Extension at wrist	___	___
Flexion at wrist	___	___
Flexion of fingers	___	___
Intrinsic hand	___	___
Iliopsoas	___	___
Glutei	___	___
Quadriceps	___	___
Hamstrings	___	___
Dorsiflexors	___	___
Plantar flexors	___	___
Reflexes		
Biceps brachii	___	___
Triceps brachii	___	___
Brachioradialis	___	___
Quadriceps femoris	___	___
Triceps surae	___	___
Sensation		
Index finger (below base of nail)		
Touch-pressure	___	___
Pricking pain	___	___
Vibration	___	___
Joint position	___	___
Great toe		
Touch-pressure	___	___
Pricking pain	___	___
Vibration	___	___
Joint position	___	___
Sum	___	___

EOM = extraocular movement.

Administration

This scale is administered by a neurologist as part of the neurologic examination that is administered and recorded in a somewhat more detailed manner than the standard neurologic examination. It should add no more than 5–10 minutes to a standard neurologic examination to perform and record the results.

Advantages

This is a simple, systematic recording of the parts of the neurologic examination that may be affected by diabetic neuropathies, with scoring based on the unweighted sum of the various noncommensurate deficits.

Disadvantages

Because scoring is based on the unweighted sum of the grading of multiple signs and symptoms based on a 5-point scale, inter-rater reliability is likely to be fair, at best. It does not distinguish between symptoms that are due to diabetic peripheral polyneuropathy and mononeuritis multiplex secondary to diabetes, which are probably caused by different mechanisms.

Neuropathic Pain Scale

Description

The Neuropathic Pain Scale (Galer & Jensen, 1997) uses 10 descriptors of pain quality (sharp, dull, deep, itchy, etc.) and severity, each with a 0–10 scale of intensity to describe the qualities of neuropathic pain. It is not intended to discriminate between types of neuropathic pain but can be used to look at the aspects of pain that respond to particular treatments. The individual item scores are used rather than being summed (Figure 10-1).

Validation

The scale items have fairly good discriminant validity with relatively little overlap between the various qualities. It has some predictive validity in that the quality of post-herpetic pain is distinct from that of complex regional pain syndromes, diabetic neuropathy, and nerve injury.

Administration

This is a self-report scale. It normally would require 1–3 minutes to fill out the questionnaire.

Advantages

To the author's knowledge, this is the only neuropathic pain scale. It differs somewhat from the McGill Pain Questionnaire.

Disadvantages

Like all pain scales, it is subjective.

Summary

This scale appears useful for the study of neuropathic pain and its treatment. It is relatively simple to use and has the potential to differentiate the effects of different treatments on different aspects of pain. It can be used as a profile showing the type(s) of pain sensations or as a tool to follow changes in different aspects of pain.

Neuropathy Total Symptom Score

Description

This is a brief, six-question scale involving severity and frequency of various neuropathic symptoms designed for use in diabetic neuropathy. It is novel in that it uses frequency × intensity to estimate overall severity (Table 10-5).

Validation

This is a well-validated symptom inventory that appears reasonably responsive to symptom change.

Administration

The score is administered by a trained health professional and typically would require 4–8 minutes.

Advantages

This is a brief symptom inventory with good reliability and reproducibility. A similar but shorter version with only four questions has also been used (Ziegler et al., 1995).

Disadvantages

The score is based entirely on the subject's report of symptoms. Patients may differ significantly in pain threshold so comparison between patients with similar disease severity may differ considerably.

1. Please use the scale below to tell us how **intense** your pain is. Place an "X" through the number that best describes the intensity of your pain.

No Pain   The most **intense** pain
                                                                                   sensation imaginable

0	1	2	3	4	5	6	7	8	9	10

2. Please use the scale below to tell how **sharp** your pain feels. Words used to describe "sharp" feelings include "like a knife," "like a spike," "jabbing" or "like jolts."

                                                                                   The most **sharp** sensation imaginable
Not sharp   ("like a knife")

0	1	2	3	4	5	6	7	8	9	10

3. Please use the scale below to tell us how **hot** your pain feels. Words used to describe very hot pain include "burning" and "on fire."

                                                                                   The most **hot** sensation
Not hot   imaginable ("on fire")

0	1	2	3	4	5	6	7	8	9	10

4. Please use the scale below to tell us how **dull** your pain feels. Words used to describe very dull pain include "like a dull toothache," "dull pain," "aching" and "like a bruise."

                                                                                   The most **dull**
Not dull   sensation imaginable

0	1	2	3	4	5	6	7	8	9	10

5. Please use the scale below to tell us how **cold** your pain feels. Words used to describe very cold pain include "like ice" and "freezing."

                                                                                   The most **cold**
                                                                                   sensation imaginable
Not cold   ("freezing")

0	1	2	3	4	5	6	7	8	9	10

Figure 10-1.   Neuropathic Pain Scale.

Instructions: There are several different aspects of pain that we are interested in measuring: pain **sharpness, heat/cold, dullness, intensity,** overall **unpleasantness**, and **surface vs. deep** pain.

The distinction between these aspects of pain might be clearer if you think of taste. For example, people might agree on how *sweet* a piece of pie might be (the *intensity* of the sweetness), but some might enjoy it more if it were sweeter, whereas others might prefer it to be less sweet. Similarly, people can judge the loudness of music and agree on what is quieter and what is louder but disagree on how it makes them feel. Some prefer quiet music, and some prefer it loud. In short, the *intensity* of a sensation is not the same as how it makes you feel. A sound might be unpleasant and still be quiet (think of someone grating his or her fingernails along a chalkboard). A sound can be quiet and *dull* or loud and *dull*.

Pain is the same. Many people are able to tell the difference between many aspects of their pain, for example, *how much* it hurts and *how unpleasant* or annoying it is. Although often the intensity of pain has a strong influence on how unpleasant the experience of pain is, some people are able to experience more pain than others before they feel very bad about it.

There are scales for measuring different aspects of pain. For one patient, a pain might feel extremely hot but not at all dull, whereas another patient may not experience any heat, but feel like the pain is very dull. We expect you to rate very high on some of the scales and very low on others. We want you to use the measures to tell us exactly what you experience.

(continued)

6. Please use the scale below to tell us how **sensitive** your skin is to light touch or clothing. Words used to describe sensitive skin include "like sunburned skin" and "raw skin."

Not sensitive

The most **sensitive** sensation imaginable ("raw skin")

0	1	2	3	4	5	6	7	8	9	10

7. Please use the scale below to tell us how **itchy** your pain feels. Words used to describe itchy pain include "like poison oak" and "like a mosquito bite."

Not itchy

The most **itchy** sensation imaginable ("like poison oak")

0	1	2	3	4	5	6	7	8	9	10

8. Which of the following best describes the **time** quality of your pain? Please check only one answer.

( ) I feel a background pain <u>all of the time</u> **and** occasional flare-ups (break-through pain) <u>some of the time.</u>

Describe the background pain: _____

Describe the flare-up (break-through) pain: _____

( ) I feel a single type of pain <u>all the time</u>. Describe this pain: _____

( ) I feel a single type of pain only <u>sometimes</u>. Other times, I am pain free.

Describe this occasional pain: _____

9. Now that you have told us the different physical aspects of your pain, the different types of sensations, we want you to tell us overall how **unpleasant** your pain is to you. Words used to describe very unpleasant pain include "miserable" and "intolerable." Remember, pain can have a low intensity, but still feel extremely unpleasant, and some kinds of pain can have a high intensity but be very tolerable. With this scale, please tell us how **unpleasant** your patient feels.

The most **unpleasant** sensation imaginable ("intolerable")

Not unpleasant

0	1	2	3	4	5	6	7	8	9	10

10. Lastly, we want you to give us an estimate of the severity of your <u>deep</u> versus <u>surface</u> pain. We want you to rate each location of pain separately. We realize that it can be difficult to make these estimates, and most likely it will be a "best guess," but please give us your best estimate.

HOW INTENSE IS YOUR DEEP PAIN?

No **Deep** Pain

The most **intense deep** pain sensation imaginable

0	1	2	3	4	5	6	7	8	9	10

HOW INTENSE IS YOUR SURFACE PAIN?

No **Surface** Pain

The most **intense surface** pain sensation imaginable

0	1	2	3	4	5	6	7	8	9	10

Figure 10-1. *continued*

Table 10-5. Total Symptom Score Worksheet

The evaluating health care professional will complete a score of frequency × intensity by asking patients about their symptoms of deep aching pain, burning pain, and prickling sensation, as well as numbness in their lower extremities. The questionnaire is modified from a previously published symptom scale* with the addition of two questions on lancinating pain and allodynia. A copy of the questionnaire is included.

A symptom score for frequency × intensity is estimated separately for each deep aching, superficial burning, prickling, or lancinating pain, as well as for numbness. *Tight, compressing, boring, squeezing* descriptions of pain are to be included with deep aching pain. Grading of pain is to be for the feet and legs. Allodynia is also graded. It is graded on intensity (mild, moderate, or severe) and on frequency (never or occasional [not beyond normal], occasional but abnormal [<33% of the time], often [>33% to <66%], or most continuous [≥66%]). The results of the intensity and frequency are scored as below. The total score possible for each symptom is 3.66.

Symptom Score of Frequency × Intensity

Symptom	Not Present	Mild	Moderate	Severe
Never or occasional (normal amount)	0.00	0.00	0.00	0.00
Occasional, but abnormal (<33% of time)	0.00	1.00	2.00	3.00
Often (≥33% to <66%)	0.00	1.33	2.33	3.33
Almost continuous (≥66%)	0.00	1.66	2.66	3.66

1. Do you experience a deep, aching, tightening, boring, pulling, or squeezing pain in your feet or legs? Please mark an *X* over the number in the most appropriate box. Record this number on the case report form.

Aching Pain	Not Present	Mild	Moderate	Severe
Never or occasional (normal amount)	0.00	0.00	0.00	0.00
Occasional, but abnormal (<33% of time)	0.00	1.00	2.00	3.00
Often (≥33% to <66%)	0.00	1.33	2.33	3.33
Almost continuous (≥66%)	0.00	1.66	2.66	3.66

2. Do you experience burning pain in your feet or legs? Please mark an *X* over the number in the most appropriate box. Record this number on the Case Report Form.

Burning Pain	Not Present	Mild	Moderate	Severe
Never or occasional (normal amount)	0.00	0.00	0.00	0.00
Occasional, but abnormal (<33% of time)	0.00	1.00	2.00	3.00
Often (≥33% to <66%)	0.00	1.33	2.33	3.33
Almost continuous (≥66%)	0.00	1.66	2.66	3.66

3. Do you experience a *prickling* or *tingling* feeling with or without an asleep feeling in your feet or legs? Please mark an *X* over the number in the most appropriate box. Record this number on the case report form.

Prickling Sensation	Not Present	Mild	Moderate	Severe
Never or occasional (normal amount)	0.00	0.00	0.00	0.00
Occasional, but abnormal (<33% of time)	0.00	1.00	2.00	3.00
Often (≥33% to <66%)	0.00	1.33	2.33	3.33
Almost continuous (≥66%)	0.00	1.66	2.66	3.66

(continued)

Table 10-5. *(continued)*

4. Do you experience asleep numbness, lost sensation, *dead feeling* like an anesthetic without prickling in your feet or legs? Please mark an *X* over the number in the most appropriate box. Record this number on the case report form.

Numbness	Not Present	Mild	Moderate	Severe
Never or occasional (normal amount)	0.00	0.00	0.00	0.00
Occasional, but abnormal (<33% of time)	0.00	1.00	2.00	3.00
Often (≥33% to <66%)	0.00	1.33	2.33	3.33
Almost continuous (≥66%)	0.00	1.66	2.66	3.66

Additional questions:

5. Do you experience sharp, stabbing, or shooting pain, electrical shock-like pain, or surges of pain that lasts seconds to minutes in your feet or legs? Please mark an *X* over the number in the most appropriate box. Record this number on the case report form.

Lancinating Pain	Not Present	Mild	Moderate	Severe
Never or occasional (normal amount)	0.00	0.00	0.00	0.00
Occasional, but abnormal (<33% of time)	0.00	1.00	2.00	3.00
Often (≥33% to <66%)	0.00	1.33	2.33	3.33
Almost continuous (≥66%)	0.00	1.66	2.66	3.66

6. Do you experience unusual sensitivity or tenderness when your feet are touched or are used in activities such as walking? Please mark an *X* over the number in the most appropriate box. Record this number on the case report form.

Allodynia	Not Present	Mild	Moderate	Severe
Never or occasional (normal amount)	0.00	0.00	0.00	0.00
Occasional, but abnormal (<33% of time)	0.00	1.00	2.00	3.00
Often (≥33% to <66%)	0.00	1.33	2.33	3.33
Almost continuous (≥66%)	0.00	1.66	2.66	3.66

Summary

The Neuropathy Total Symptom Score is a useful, brief symptom inventory for diabetic neuropathy.

Inflammatory Neuropathy Cause and Treatment Group Sensory Sum Score

Description

This is a sensory scale developed by the Inflammatory Neuropathy Cause and Treatment Group (Merkies et al., 2000) to assess sensory symptoms in polyneuropathy (Table 10-6). It assesses the normality of sensory sensations at various levels from distal to proximal in the upper and lower extremities.

Validation

There was general agreement among the 13 members of the development group that the scale has good face and construct validity. Inter-observer agreement was good with an *r* value of 0.89 and intra-observer agreement had an *r* value of 0.85. The sensory score also correlated with the Nine-Hole Peg Test score. Patient follow-up during treatment demonstrated good agreement between the patients' subjective estimate of

Table 10-6. Sensory Sum Score

Pinprick Sensation, Sites of Examination, and Corresponding Grades			
Arms		Legs	
Normal at index finger	0	Normal at hallux	0
Abnormal at:		Abnormal at:	
Index finger	1	Hallux	1
Wrist	2	Ankle	2
Elbow	3	Knee	3
Shoulder	4	Groin	4

Vibration Sensation, Sites of Examination, and Corresponding Grades			
Arms		Legs	
Normal at index finger	0	Normal at hallux	0
Abnormal at:		Abnormal at:	
Index finger	1	Hallux	1
Wrist	2	Ankle	2
Elbow	3	Knee	3
Shoulder	4	Groin	4

2-Point Discrimination	
Normal (<4 mm)	0
Abnormal:	
5–9 mm	1
10–14 mm	2
15–19 mm	3
>20 mm	4

improvement or worsening and changes in the sensory sum score.

Administration

Testing is generally done by a neurologist and requires a mean of 3.5 minutes.

Advantages/Disadvantages

This is a relatively simple, responsive measure that can be performed in a relatively short time and has good inter- and intra-observer reliability. Like all sensory scales, it is subjective.

Summary

Scales for pain and neuropathy have been developing steadily for the past three decades with new scales appearing at frequent intervals. Validation of these scales has improved steadily but, given the subjective nature of many of the symptoms, quantitative measures are difficult to develop. In this chapter we have covered a few of the more commonly used scales. Those with a particular interest in measuring pain would do well to study Melzack's classic article on development and validation of the McGill Pain Questionnaire (Melzack, 1975).

References

Dyck PJ, Sherman WE, Hallcher L, et al. Human diabetic endoneurial sorbitol, fructose, and myo-inositol related to sural nerve morphometry. *Ann Neurol* 1980;8:590–96.

Dyck PJ, Thomas PK, Lambert EH (eds.). *Peripheral neuropathy*. Philadelphia: Saunders, 1975.

Dubuisson D, Melzack R. Classification of clinical pain descriptions by multiple group discriminant analysis. *Exp Neurol* 1976;51:480–87.

England JD, Gronseth GS, Franklin G, et al. Distal symmetric polyneuropathy: a definition for clinical research. *Neurology* 2005;64:199–207.

Galer BS, Jensen MP. Development and preliminary validation of a pain measure specific to neuropathic pain: the neuropathic pain scale. *Neurology* 1997;48:332–38.

Melzack R. The McGill pain questionnaire: major properties and scoring methods. *Pain* 1975;1:277–99.

Melzack R. The short-form McGill pain questionnaire. *Pain* 1987;30:191–97.

Melzack R, Wall PD (eds.). *Textbook of pain*. Edinburgh: Churchill Livingston, 2004.

Merkies IS, Schmitz PI, van der Meché FG, et al. Psychometric evaluation of a new sensory scale in immune-mediated polyneuropathies. Inflammatory Neuropathy Cause and treatment (INCAT) group. *Neurology* 2000; 54:943–49.

Ziegler D, Hanefeld M, Ruhnau KJ, et al. The ALADIN Study Group: treatment of symptomatic diabetic peripheral neuropathy with the anti-oxidant alpha-lipoic acid: a 3-week randomized controlled trial (ALADIN Study). *Diabetologia* 1995;38:1425–33.

11 Diagnostic Headache Criteria and Instruments

Elcio J. Piovesan, M.D., and Stephen D. Silberstein, M.D.

Headache is one of the most common medical complaints of humankind, accounting for more than 18 million outpatient visits per year in the United States (Ries, 1986). More than 1% of physician's office visits and emergency department visits are primarily for headache (Silberstein & Silberstein, 1990). Because pain and associated symptoms are subjective and must be described by the patient, history is the key to diagnosing headache, and because patients are not always good historians, taking a precise history takes time (Silberstein et al., 2001).

In 1988, the International Headache Society (IHS) introduced new diagnostic criteria for headache disorders (Headache Classification Committee of the International Headache Society, 1988). Like the first edition, the second edition of the International Headache Classification (IHC-2003) is intended to be used both for research and clinical practice. The IHS divides headaches into two broad categories: the primary headache disorders (categories 1–4), which include migraine, tension-type headache, trigeminal-autonomic cephalalgias, and other primary headaches, and headache attributed to secondary disorders (categories 5–14) (Table 11-1). The IHS

classification represents an enormous step forward in the codification of headache. Systematic scientific classification of primary headaches is inexact because the disorders lack diagnostic markers; on clinical features, however, the IHS classification has created relatively homogeneous clinical groups for pathophysiologic and therapeutic studies. The IHS criteria have been translated into many languages and have been the basis for clinical trials and epidemiologic research since 1990.

How to Use the International Headache Classification

The IHC-2003 has suggested some steps to use this classification.

1. This classification is hierarchical, and one must decide how detailed the diagnosis needs to be. In general practice, the diagnosis is usually coded only to the first or second digit; in specialty practices and specialized centers, it is appropriate to diagnose to the third or fourth digit.

Table 11-1. Second Edition of the International Headache Classification (IHC-2003)

A. Primary headache disorders
  1. Migraine
    1.1 Migraine without aura
    1.2 Migraine with aura
      1.2.1 Typical aura with migraine headache
      1.2.2 Typical aura with nonmigraine headache
      1.2.3 Typical aura without headache
      1.2.4 Familial hemiplegic migraine
      1.2.5 Sporadic hemiplegic migraine
      1.2.6 Basilar type migraine
    1.3 Childhood periodic syndromes that are commonly precursors of migraine
      1.3.1 Cyclical vomiting
      1.3.2 Abdominal migraine
      1.3.3 Benign paroxysmal vertigo of childhood
    1.4 Retinal migraine
    1.5 Complications of migraine
      1.5.1 Chronic migraine
      1.5.2 Status migrainosus
      1.5.3 Persistent aura without infarction
      1.5.4 Migrainous infarction
      1.5.5 Migraine-triggered seizures
    1.6 Probable migraine
      1.6.1 Probable migraine without aura
      1.6.2 Probable migraine with aura
  2. Tension-type headache
    2.1 Infrequent episodic tension-type headache
      2.1.1 Associated with disorder of pericranial tenderness
      2.1.2 Not associated with disorder of pericranial tenderness
    2.2 Frequent episodic tension-type headache
      2.2.1 Associated with pericranial tenderness
      2.2.2 Not associated with pericranial tenderness
    2.3 Chronic tension-type headache
      2.3.1 Associated with pericranial tenderness
      2.3.2 Not associated with pericranial tenderness
  3. Cluster headache and other trigeminal-autonomic cephalalgias
    3.1 Cluster headache
      3.1.1 Episodic cluster headache
      3.1.2 Chronic cluster headache
    3.2 Paroxysmal hemicrania
      3.2.1 Episodic paroxysmal hemicrania
      3.2.2 Chronic paroxysmal hemicrania

    3.3 Short-lasting unilateral neuralgiform headache with conjunctival injection and tearing
    3.4 Probable trigeminal autonomic cephalalgia
  4. Other primary headaches
    4.1 Primary stabbing headache
    4.2 Primary cough headache
    4.3 Primary exertional headache
    4.4 Primary headache associated with sexual activity
      4.4.1 Preorgasmic headache
      4.4.2 Orgasmic headache
    4.5 Hypnic headache
    4.6 Primary thunderclap headache
    4.7 Hemicrania continua
    4.8 New daily persistent headache
B. Secondary headache disorders
  5. Headache attributed to head and/or neck trauma
    5.1 Acute posttraumatic headache
      5.1.1 Acute posttraumatic headache with moderate or severe head injury
      5.1.2 Acute posttraumatic headache with mild head injury
    5.2 Chronic posttraumatic headache
      5.2.1 Chronic posttraumatic headache with moderate or severe head injury
      5.2.2 Chronic posttraumatic headache with mild head injury
    5.3 Acute postwhiplash injury headache
    5.4 Chronic postwhiplash injury headache
    5.5 Headache attributed to traumatic intracranial hematoma
      5.5.1 Epidural hematoma
      5.5.2 Chronic subdural hematoma
    5.6 Headache attributed to other head and neck trauma
    5.7 Postcraniotomy headache
      5.7.1 Acute postcraniotomy headache
      5.7.2 Chronic postcraniotomy headache
  6. Headache attributed to cranial or cervical vascular disorders
    6.1 Ischemic stroke and transient ischemic attacks
      6.1.1 Ischemic stroke (cerebral infarction)
      6.1.2 Transient ischemic attacks
    6.2 Nontraumatic intracranial hemorrhage
      6.2.1 Intracerebral hemorrhage
      6.2.2 Subarachnoid hemorrhage
    6.3 Unruptured vascular malformations
      6.3.1 Saccular aneurysm
      6.3.2 Arteriovenous malformation

Table 11-1. *(continued)*

6.3.3 Dural arteriovenous fistula

6.3.4 Cavernous angiomas

6.3.5 Encephalotrigeminal or leptomen-
ingeal angiomatosis (Sturge-Weber
syndrome)

6.4 Arteritis

6.4.1 Giant cell arteritis

6.4.2 Primary central nervous system
(CNS) angiitis (isolated CNS angiitis, granulomatous CNS angiitis)

6.4.3 Secondary central nervous system
angiitis

6.5 Carotid or vertebral artery pain

6.5.1 Arterial dissection

6.5.2 Postendarterectomy headache

6.5.3 Carotid angioplasty headache

6.5.4 Headache associated with intracranial endovascular procedures

6.5.5 Angiography headache

6.6 Cerebral venous thrombosis

6.7 Other intracranial vascular disorders

6.7.1 Cerebral autosomal dominant arte-
riopathy with subcortical infarcts
and leukoencephalopathy

6.7.2 Mitochondrial encephalopathy, lac-
tic acidosis, and strokelike episodes

6.7.3 Benign angiopathy of the central
nervous system

6.7.4 Pituitary apoplexy

7. Headache attributed to nonvascular intracranial
disorder

7.1 High cerebrospinal fluid pressure

7.1.1 Idiopathic intracranial hypertension

7.1.2 Intracerebral hemorrhage secondary to metabolic, toxic, or hor-
monal causes

7.1.3 Intracerebral hemorrhage secondary to hydrocephalus

7.2 Low cerebrospinal fluid pressure

7.2.1 Postdural puncture headache

7.2.2 Cerebrospinal fluid fistula headache

7.2.3 Spontaneous (or idiopathic) low
cerebrospinal fluid pressure

7.3 Noninfectious inflammatory diseases

7.3.1 Neurosarcoidosis

7.3.2 Aseptic (noninfectious) meningitis

7.3.3 Other noninfectious inflammatory
disease

7.3.4 Lymphocytic hypophysitis

7.4 Intracranial neoplasm

7.4.1 Headache attributed to increased
intracranial pressure or hydrocephalus caused by neoplasm

7.4.2 Headache attributed directly to
neoplasm

7.4.3 Headache attributed to carcinoma-
tous meningitis

7.4.4 Headache attributed to colloid cyst
of the third ventricle

7.4.5 Headache attributed to pituitary
hypersecretion or hyposecretion

7.5 Headache related to intrathecal injections

7.6 Postseizure headache

7.7 Chiari malformation type I

7.8 Syndrome of transient headache and neurologic deficits with cerebrospinal fluid lym-
phocytosis

7.9 Headache attributed to other non-vascular
intracranial disorder

8. Headache attributed to a substance or its withdrawal

8.1 Headache induced by acute substance use
or exposure

8.1.1 Nitric oxide (NO) donor–induced
headache

8.1.1.1 Immediate NO donor–
induced headache

8.1.1.2 Delayed NO donor–
induced headache

8.1.2 Phosphodiesterase inhibitor–
induced headache

8.1.3 Carbon monoxide–induced headache

8.1.4 Alcohol-induced headache

8.1.4.1 Immediate alcohol-
induced headache

8.1.4.2 Delayed alcohol-induced
headache

8.1.5 Headache induced by food components and additives

8.1.5.1 Monosodium glutamate–
induced headache

8.1.6 Cocaine

8.1.7 Cannabis

8.1.8 Headache attributed to other acute
substance use (specify)

8.2 Medication-overuse headache

8.2.1 Ergotamine-overuse headache

8.2.2 Triptan-overuse headache

(continued)

Table 11-1. *(continued)*

8.2.3 Analgesic-overuse headache
8.2.4 Opioid-overuse headache
8.2.5 Combination drug–overuse headache
8.2.6 Other substance overuse
8.2.7 Headache as a side effect of drugs used for other indications
8.3 Headache as an adverse event of chronic exposure
8.4 Headache attributed to dependent substance withdrawal
  8.4.1 Caffeine-withdrawal headache
  8.4.2 Opioids
  8.4.3 Estrogen-withdrawal headache
  8.4.4 Headache attributed to withdrawal from chronic use of other substances
8.5 Exogenous hormone–induced headache
9. Headache attributed to infections
9.1 Intracranial infection
  9.1.1 Bacterial meningitis
  9.1.2 Lymphocytic meningitis
  9.1.3 Encephalitis
  9.1.4 Brain abscess
  9.1.5 Subdural empyema
  9.1.6 Acquired immunodeficiency syndrome
9.2 Extracranial infection
  9.2.1 Bacterial infection
  9.2.2 Viral infection
  9.2.3 Other infection
9.3 Human immunodeficiency virus/acquired immunodeficiency syndrome
9.4 Chronic postinfectious headache
10. Headache attributed to disorder of homeostasis
10.1 Headache attributed to hypoxia and/or hypercapnia
  10.1.1 High-altitude headache
  10.1.2 Diving headache
  10.1.3 Sleep apnea
10.2 Dialysis
10.3 Arterial hypertension
  10.3.1 Headache attributed to pheochromocytoma
  10.3.2 Headache attributed to hypertensive crisis without hypertensive encephalopathy
  10.3.3 Headache attributed to hypertensive encephalopathy
  10.3.4 Headache attributed to pre-eclampsia
  10.3.5 Headache attributed to eclampsia
  10.3.6 Headache attributed to acute pressor response to exogenous agents

10.4 Headache attributed to hypothyroidism
10.5 Headache attributed to fasting
10.6 Cardiac cephalgia
10.7 Headache attributed to other disturbance of homeostasis
11. Headache or facial pain attributed to disorder of cranium, neck, eyes, ears, nose, sinuses, teeth, mouth, or other facial or cranial structures
11.1 Cranial bone
11.2 Neck
  11.2.1 Cervicogenic headache
  11.2.2 Retropharyngeal tendinitis
  11.2.3 Craniocervical dystonia
11.3 Eyes
  11.3.1 Acute glaucoma
  11.3.2 Refractive errors
  11.3.3 Heterophoria or heterotropia (latent or manifest squint)
  11.3.4 Ocular inflammatory disorders
11.4 Ears
  11.4.1 Primary otalgia
  11.4.2 Referred otalgia
11.5 Rhinosinusitis
11.6 Teeth, jaws, and related structures
11.7 Temporomandibular joint disease
11.8 Headache attributed to other disorder of cranium, neck, eyes, ears, nose, sinuses, teeth, mouth, or other cranial facial or cervical structures
12. Headache attributed to psychiatric disorders
12.1 Headache attributed to somatization disorder
12.2 Headache attributed to a psychotic disorder
13. Cranial neuralgias and central causes of facial pain
13.1 Trigeminal neuralgia
  13.1.1 Classical trigeminal neuralgia
  13.1.2 Symptomatic trigeminal neuralgia
13.2 Glossopharyngeal neuralgia
  13.2.1 Classical glossopharyngeal neuralgia
  13.2.2 Symptomatic glossopharyngeal neuralgia
13.3 Nervus intermedius neuralgia
13.4 Superior laryngeal neuralgia
13.5 Nasociliary neuralgia (Charlin's neuralgia)
13.6 Supraorbital neuralgia
13.7 Other terminal branch neuralgias
13.8 Occipital neuralgia
13.9 Neck-tongue syndrome

Table 11-1. *(continued)*

13.10 External compression headache	13.17 Ophthalmoplegic migraine
13.11 Cold stimulus headache	13.18 Central causes of head and facial pain
13.11.1 External application of a cold stimulus	13.18.1 Anesthesia dolorosa
13.11.2 Ingestion of a cold stimulus	13.18.2 Central poststroke pain
13.12 Constant pain caused by compression, irritation, or distortion of cranial nerves or upper cervical roots by structural lesions	13.18.3 Multiple sclerosis
	13.18.4 Persistent idiopathic facial pain
	13.18.5 Burning mouth syndrome
13.13 Optic neuritis	13.18.6 Other cranial neuralgia or other centrally mediated facial pain
13.14 Ocular diabetic neuropathy	14. Other headache, cranial neuralgia, central or primary facial pain
13.15 Herpes zoster	14.1 Headache not elsewhere classified
13.15.1 Acute herpes zoster	14.2 Headache unspecified
13.15.2 Postherpetic neuralgia	
13.16 Tolosa-Hunt syndrome	

2. If more than one diagnosis is made, the diagnoses should be listed in the order of importance indicated by the patient.

3. If one type of headache fits the diagnostic criteria for two different sets of explicit diagnostic criteria, then all information that is not part of explicit diagnostic criteria should be used.

4. If a new type of headache occurs for the first time in close temporal relation to a known cause of headache, the new headache is coded as a secondary headache.

5. If a patient has a headache disorder that fulfills one set of diagnostic criteria, there may also be episodes that do not quite satisfy the criteria. This can be due to treatment, the patient's lack of ability to remember symptoms exactly, or other factors.

6. If headache persists more than 3 months after remission or cure of a secondary cause of headache, the diagnosis is "chronic headache attributed to . . . ."

Diagnostic Criteria for Headache

Migraine

Migraine (see Table 11-1) is a common episodic headache disorder characterized by attacks that consist of various combinations of headache and neurologic, gastrointestinal, and autonomic symptoms. Migraine is divided into different types according to clinical characteristics (see Table 11-1). Migraine may be preceded by an aura. The aura is the complex of neurologic symptoms; it may include visual (Queiroz et al., 1997), sensory, or motor phenomena and may involve language or brainstem disturbances (Table 11-2) (Silberstein et al., 2001). Most patients have attacks without aura exclusively (Table 11-3), but others have attacks both with (Table 11-4) and without aura. The typical aura develops gradually over 5–20 minutes and lasts less than 60 minutes. The aura can accompany the typical migraine, accompany a nonmigraine headache, or occur without headache. Familial hemiplegic migraine is migraine with an aura of motor weakness and at least one first- or second-degree relative having a migraine with an aura of motor weakness; when no first- or second-degree relative has aura (including motor weakness), the disorder is sporadic hemiplegic migraine. Basilar-type migraine is migraine with aura symptoms that clearly originate from the brainstem (dysarthria, vertigo, tinnitus, decreased hearing, double vision, ataxia, decreased level of consciousness, simultaneous bilateral visual symptoms in both the temporal and nasal field of both eyes, or simultaneous bilateral paresthesias) or from both hemispheres simultaneously with no motor weakness (see Table 11-4). Retinal migraine is repeated attacks of monocular visual phenomena, including scintillations, scotoma, or blindness associated with migraine headache (Table 11-5). The most common complication of migraine is chronic migraine, a type of daily headache that used to be called *transformed migraine* (Table 11-6). Medication overuse is often the cause of daily

Table 11-2. Types of Aura in Migraine, Basilar Migraine, and Headache Cluster

Migraine with Aura	Basilar Migraine	Cluster
1. Visual		
1.1 Positive visual phenomena	No	1.1 Visual hallucinations
1.1.1 Small bright dots ("stars")		
1.1.2 White spots/flashes of light (photopsias)		
1.1.3 Fortification spectra (teichopsia)		
1.1.4 Other zigzag lines		
1.1.5 Colored spots of light		
1.1.6 Other lines (curves, straight)		
1.2 Negative visual phenomena		
1.2.1 "Blind spots" (scotomata)	1.2.1 Defects of nasal and temporal fields	
1.2.2 Black dots/spots		
1.2.3 Hemianopsia		
1.3 Disturbances of visual perception		
1.3.1 "Foggy"/blurred vision	1.3.1 Diplopia	1.3.1 Achromatopsia (loss of color vision)
1.3.2 "As looking through heat waves/water"		1.3.2 Shooting lights
1.3.3 "Tunnel vision"		1.3.3 Black-and-white flashing lights
1.3.4 "Mosaic"/fractured vision		
1.3.5 Micropsia/macropsia/teleopsia		
1.3.6 Corona phenomena		
1.3.7 Complex hallucination		
1.3.8 "Slanted vision"		
1.3.9 "Like a negative of a film"		
2. Sensory		
2.1 Paresthesia, often migrating in different parts of the body	2.1 Bilateral paresthesia	2.1 Olfactory hallucinations
2.2 Olfactory hallucinations	2.2 Cerebellovestibular ataxia	
2.3 Allodynia	2.3 Dizziness	
2.4 Burning sensation		
3. Motor		
3.1 Weakness in different parts of body	3.1 Bilateral weakness	
3.2 Ataxia		
4. Language		
4.1 Dysarthria	4.1 Dysarthria	
4.2 Aphasia		
5. Auditory		
5.1 Auditory hallucinations	5.1 Tinnitus	
5.2 Oscillocusis	5.2 Decreased hearing	
5.3 Tinnitus		
5.4 Fluctuating low-frequency and hearing loss		
5.5 Sudden deafness		
6. Delusions and disturbed consciousness		
6.1 Déjà vu	6.1 Decreased consciousness	
6.2 Multiple conscious trancelike states	6.2 Confusion	

Table 11-3. Migraine without Aura (1.1)

Diagnostic criteria

A. At least five attacks fulfilling B–D

B. Headache attacks lasting 4–72 hr and occur <15 days/mo (untreated or unsuccessfully treated)

C. Headache has at least two of the following characteristics:

1. Unilateral location

2. Pulsating quality

3. Moderate or severe intensity

4. Aggravation by or causing avoidance from routine physical activity (e.g., walking or climbing stairs)

D. During headache at least one of the following:

1. Nausea and/or vomiting

2. Photophobia and phonophobia

E. Not attributed to another disorder

headache. This is coded as *migraine associated with medication overuse.* If chronicity persists after drug withdrawal, the disorder is called *chronic migraine* rather than *headache attributed to drug overuse* (Table 11-7). Other complications of migraine include status migrainosus, persistent aura without infarction, migrainous infarction, and migraine-triggered seizure (see Table 11-6).

Tension-Type Headache and New Daily Persistent Headache

Epidemiologic studies of the general population have shown that tension-type headache (see Table 11-1) is the most common type of headache, with a lifetime prevalence of 78% and a yearly prevalence of 38% (Rasmussen et al., 1991; Schwartz et al., 1998). The diagnostic criteria are based on IHS classification (Table 11-8).

Cluster Headache and Other Trigeminal-Autonomic Cephalgias

The short-lasting primary headache syndrome may be conveniently divided into those that exhibit marked autonomic activation and those without autonomic activation. This group includes cluster headache (episodic or chronic) (see Tables 11-1 and 11-9), paroxysmal hemicrania (episodic or chronic) (Table 11-10), and short-lasting unilateral neuralgiform headache with conjunctival injection and tearing (Table 11-11).

Other Primary Headaches

The last group of primary headaches is heterogeneous (see Table 11-1). These headaches can mimic organic disorders and need to be carefully evaluated (Table 11-12). This group includes primary stabbing headache, primary cough headache, primary exertional headache, primary headache associated with sexual activity, hypnic headache, and primary thunderclap headache. Hemicrania continua (Table 11-13) and new daily persistent headache are subsets of chronic daily headache. New daily persistent headache is characterized by the relatively abrupt onset of an unremitting primary chronic daily headache (see Table 11-13) (Silberstein et al., 1994). The daily headache develops abruptly, over less than 3 days. Patients are generally younger than those with chronic migraine (Vanast, 1986).

Primary headaches can be associated with the overuse of analgesics or other substances and their withdrawal. This disorder consists of a new form of headache (including migraine, tension-type headache, or cluster headache) that develops in close temporal relation to substance use or substance withdrawal as specified in special groups (see Table 11-7). Doses and temporal relationships have not yet been determined for most substances.

Instruments and Scales in Headache

Headaches can severely interfere with daily functioning and productivity (Lipton & Stewart, 1993; Osterhaus et al., 1992). Research has demonstrated that improvement in symptoms and quality of life (QOL) are not perfectly correlated; symptoms may improve, but function may not (Deyo, 1984). Consequently, it is important to include instruments that measure QOL. Instruments that assess migraine disability can improve headache care by facilitating physician–patient communication and guiding treatment decisions. Various headache scales are in use. The scales can be divided into two main groups: scales that measure the impact of a single migraine attack (with or without therapy) over 24 hours and scales that measure the impact of migraine over weeks or months. The first group of scales were used in randomized, placebo-controlled trials and are highly sensitive to acute treatment effects (Santanello et al., 1997). The second group of scales has been chosen to compare results in randomized trials (Block et al., 1998).

Table 11-4. Migraine with Aura (1.2)

1.2.1 Typical aura with migraine headache

Diagnostic criteria

    A. At least two attacks fulfilling B–E

    B. Fully reversible visual and/or sensory and/or speech symptoms but no motor weakness

    C. Homonymous or bilateral visual symptoms, including positive features (e.g., flickering lights, spots, lines) or negative features (i.e., loss of vision), and/or unilateral sensory symptoms, including positive features (i.e., vision loss, pins and needles) and/or negative features (e.g., numbness)

    D. At least one of two:

        1. At least one symptom develops gradually over ≥5 min and/or different symptoms occur in succession

        2. Each symptom lasts ≥5 min and ≤60 min

    E. Headache that meets criteria B–D for migraine without aura (1.1) begins during the aura or follows the aura within 60 min

    F. Not attributed to another disorder

1.2.2 Typical aura with nonmigraine headache

Diagnostic criteria

    A. At least two attacks fulfilling criteria B–E

    B. Fully reversible visual and/or sensory and/or speech symptoms but no motor weakness

    C. Homonymous or bilateral visual symptoms, including positive features (e.g., flickering lights, spots, lines) or negative features (e.g., loss of vision), and/or unilateral sensory symptoms, including positive features (e.g., vision loss, pins and needles) and/or negative features (e.g., numbness)

    D. At least one of two:

        1. At least one symptom develops gradually over ≥5 min and/or different symptoms occur in succession

        2. Each symptom lasts ≥5 min and ≤60 min

    E. Headache that does not meet criteria B–D for migraine without aura (1.1) begins during the aura or follows aura within 60 min

    F. Not attributed to another disorder

1.2.3 Typical aura without headache

Diagnostic criteria

    A. At least two attacks fulfilling criteria B–E

    B. Fully reversible visual and/or sensory and/or speech symptoms but no motor weakness

    C. Homonymous or bilateral visual symptoms, including positive features (e.g., flickering lights, spots, lines) or negative features (e.g., loss of vision), and/or unilateral sensory symptoms, including positive features (e.g., vision loss, pins and needles) and/or negative features (e.g., numbness)

    D. At least one of two:

        1. At least one symptom develops gradually over ≥5 min and/or different symptoms occur in succession

        2. Each symptom lasts ≥5 min and ≤60 min

    E. No headache begins during the aura or follows the aura within 60 min

    F. Not attributed to another disorder

1.2.4 Familial hemiplegic migraine

Diagnostic criteria

    A. At least two attacks fulfilling B–E

Table 11-4. *(continued)*

B. Fully reversible motor weakness and at least one of the following other aura symptoms: visual, sensory, or speech disturbance

C. At least two of the following:

  1. At least one aura symptom develops gradually over ≥5 min and/or different symptoms occur in succession

  2. Each aura symptom lasts <24 hr

  3. Headache that meets criteria B–D for migraine without aura (1.1) begins during the aura or follows aura within 60 min

D. At least one first- or second-degree relative has attacks with aura, including motor weakness (fulfill 1.2.1 criteria A, B, C, and E).

E. Not attributed to another disorder

1.2.5   Sporadic hemiplegic migraine

Diagnostic criteria

A. At least two attacks fulfilling B–D

B. Fully reversible motor weakness and at least one of the following other aura symptoms: visual, sensory, or speech disturbance

C. At least two of the following:

  1. At least one aura symptom develops gradually over ≥5 min and/or different symptoms occur in succession

  2. Each aura symptom lasts <24 hr

  3. Headache that meets criteria B–D for migraine without aura (1.1) begins during the aura or follows the aura within 60 min

D. No first- or second-degree relative has migraine attacks with aura, including motor weakness

E. Not attributed to another disorder

1.2.6   Basilar type migraine

Diagnostic criteria

A. At least two attacks fulfilling criteria B–E

B. Fully reversible visual and/or sensory and/or speech symptoms but no motor weakness

C. Two or more fully reversible aura symptoms of the following types:

Dysarthria

Vertigo

Tinnitus

Decreased hearing

Double vision

Ataxia

Decreased level of consciousness

Simultaneous bilateral visual symptoms in both the temporal and nasal field of both eyes

Simultaneous bilateral paresthesias

D. Headache that meets criteria B–D for migraine without aura (1.1) begins during the aura or follows the aura within 60 min

E. Not attributed to another disorder

Table 11-5. Retinal Migraine

1.4 Retinal migraine

Diagnostic criteria

A. At least two attacks fulfilling B–C.

B. Fully reversible monocular positive visual phenomena, scotomata, or blindness confirmed by examination during attack or (after proper instruction) by patient's drawing of monocular field defect during an attack.

C. Headache fulfilling criteria for 1.1 migraine without aura is associated with the visual symptoms.

D. Normal ophthalmologic examination outside of attack. Appropriate investigations exclude other causes of transient monocular blindness.

The scales that measure the impact of an acute attack include (1) QOL (24-Hour Migraine Quality of Life Questionnaire [MQoLQ] and Migraine-Specific Quality of Life Questionnaire [MSQ version 2.1]) and (2) headache impact and disability (Headache Needs Assessment [HANA] survey). The scales that measure long-term impact are (1) QOL (Migraine-Specific Quality of Life [MSQOL]), (2) headache impact (Headache Impact Test [HIT], Headache Impact Questionnaire [HImQ], Henry Ford Hospital Headache Disability Inventory [Headache Disability Inventory, or HDI]), and (3) migraine disability (Migraine Disability Assessment [MIDAS] scale).

Scales That Assess Quality of Life

QOL is influenced by environmental, economic, social, health-related, spiritual, and political factors. The fundamental domains of instruments to measure QOL include physical, psychological, and social areas. Both generic and disease-specific measures have been used to measure QOL. The most commonly used generic measure is the Medical Outcomes Study Instrument, which includes the Short Form 20 (SF-20) (Stewart et al., 1988), the Short Form 36 (SF-36) (McHorney et al., 1993), and the Short Form 12 (SF-12) (Ware et al., 1996). Other generic QOL scales used in headache studies include the Sickness Impact Profile (Damiano, 1996), the Nottingham Health Profile (McEwen et al., 1996), and the Psychological General Well-Being index (Dahlof & Dimenas, 1995). The spe-

cific QOL scales for migraine fall into two broadly defined categories: those that measure QOL in a single migraine attack (MQoLQ and MSQ version 2.1) and those that measure the QOL over a period of weeks or months (MSQOL).

Generic Scales That Assess Quality of Life in Headache

Medical Outcomes Study 36-Item Short-Form Health Survey

The SF-36 (Figure 11-1) was designed for use in clinical practice and research, health policy evaluations, and general population surveys (Ware & Sherbourne, 1992). This instrument facilitates comparisons across patient populations and disease states, but it is less sensitive to changes in QOL in headache within the context of a clinical intervention. The SF-36 includes one multi-item scale that assesses eight health concepts: (1) limitations in physical activities; (2) limitations in social activities because of physical or emotional problems; (3) limitations in usual role activities because of physical health problems; (4) bodily pain; (5) general mental health (psychological distress and well-being); (6) limitations in usual role activities because of emotional problems; (7) vitality (energy and fatigue); and (8) general health perceptions. This scale was constructed for self-administration by persons 14 years of age and older and for administration by a trained interviewer in person or by telephone. The SF-36 emphasizes both kinds of tests: psychometric tests, which are the foundation of scale construction and scoring, and applied tests of relevance and usefulness that approximate a particular use of the measure (McHorney et al., 1993). The SF-36 has been used for chronic diseases such as diabetes, hypertension, depression, osteoarthritis, low back pain, and migraine headaches (Chatterton et al., 2002; Jhingran et al., 1996; Mushet et al., 1996; Osterhaus & Townsend, 1991; Osterhaus et al., 1994; Solomon, 1994; Solomon et al., 1995; Terwindt et al., 2000), chronic daily headache (Guitera et al., 2002; Monzon et al., 1998; Wang et al., 2001), and chronic tension-type headaches (Mannix et al., 1999). Depression accounts for the low scores on most SF-36 scales (McHorney et al., 1993) and therefore may confound the comparisons of SF-36 scales among patients with different headache diagnoses (Wang et al., 2001).

Table 11-6. Complications of Migraine (1.5) and Probable Migraine (1.6)

1.5.1 Chronic migraine

Diagnostic criteria

A. Average migraine frequency ≥15 days/mo for ≥3 mo fulfilling B–D

B. Some attacks fulfill criteria for 1.1 (migraine without aura)

C. No overuse of acute medication

D. Not attributed to another disorder

1.5.2 Status migrainosus

Diagnostic criteria

A. Previous attacks fulfill criteria for 1.1 migraine without aura

B. The present attack fulfills criteria for migraine without aura except for duration

C. Headache lasts >72 hr, is continuous, is severe, and prevents normal activities

D. Not attributed to another disorder

1.5.3 Persistent aura without infarction

Diagnostic criteria

A. Previous attacks fulfill criteria for 1.2

B. The present attack is typical of previous attacks, but one or more aura symptoms persist for >2 wks

C. Not attributed to another disorder

1.5.4 Migrainous infarction

Diagnostic criteria

A. Previous attacks fulfill criteria for 1.2

B. The present attack is typical of previous attacks, but one or more aura symptoms last >60 min

C. Neuroimaging demonstrates ischemic infarction in a relevant area

D. Not attributed to another disorder

1.5.5 Migraine-triggered seizure

Diagnostic criteria

A. Migraine fulfilling 1.3

B. A seizure fulfilling diagnostic criteria for one type of epileptic attack occurs during or within 1 hr after a migraine aura

1.6.1 Probable migraine without aura

Diagnostic criteria

A. Fulfills all but one of criteria A–D for 1.1 migraine without aura

B. Not attributed to another disorder

1.6.2 Probable migraine with aura

Diagnostic criteria

A. Fulfills all criteria but one for one of the types of migraines with aura (1.2.1–1.2.6)

B. Headache that meets criteria B–D for migraine without aura (1.1) begins during the aura or follows the aura within 60 min

C. Not attributed to another disorder

Table 11-7. Headache Induced by Acute Substance Use or Exposure (8.1)

8.1.4   Alcohol-induced headache

    8.1.4.1   Immediate alcohol-induced headache

        Diagnostic criteria

        A.   Headache has at least one of the following characteristics: bilateral, frontotemporal, pulsating, aggravated by physical activity

        B.   Ingestion of beverage containing alcohol; effective dose has not been determined

        C.   Headache occurs within 3 hr after ingestion of alcoholic beverage

        D.   Headache lasts <72 hr

    8.1.4.2   Delayed alcohol-induced headache

        Diagnostic criteria

        A.   Headache has at least one of the following characteristics: bilateral, frontotemporal, pulsating, aggravated by physical activity

        B.   Ingestion of a modest amount of alcoholic beverage in migraine sufferers or intoxicating amounts in nonheadache sufferers

        C.   Headache occurs after the effects of alcohol have disappeared

        D.   Headache lasts <72 hr

8.1.5   Food component and additives

    Diagnostic criteria

    A.   Headache has at least one of the following characteristics: bilateral, frontotemporal, pulsating, aggravated by physical activity

    B.   Follows ingestion of a minimum dose of food or component

    C.   Onset within 12 hr of substance intake

    D.   Headache lasts <72 hr after single intake

    8.1.5.1   Monosodium glutamate–induced headache

        Diagnostic criteria

        A.   Headache has at least one of the following characteristics: bilateral, frontotemporal, pulsating, aggravated by physical activity

        B.   Follows ingestion of monosodium glutamate

        C.   Occurs within 1 hr of monosodium glutamate ingestion

        D.   Headache lasts <72 hr after single intake

8.1.6   Cocaine

    Diagnostic criteria

    A.   Headache has at least one of the following characteristics: bilateral, frontotemporal, pulsating, aggravated by physical activity

    B.   Exposure to cocaine

    C.   Onset within 12 hr of exposure

    D.   Headache lasts <72 hr after single use

8.2   Medication-overuse headache

    8.2.1   Ergotamine-overuse headache

        Diagnostic criteria

        A.   Headache has at least one of the following characteristics: chronic (≥15 days/mo), pressing/tightening quality, frequency ≥15 days/mo, mild or moderate intensity (may inhibit but does not prohibit activities), bilateral location

Table 11-7.   *(continued)*

B. Ergotamine intake >10 days/mo on a regular basis for ≥3 mo

C. Headache worsening has occurred during ergotamine overuse

D. Headache reverts back to previous pattern within 2 mo after discontinuation of ergotamine

8.2.2 Triptan-overuse headache

Diagnostic criteria

A. Headache has at least one of the following characteristics:

1. Chronic headaches (≥15 days/mo)

2. Predominantly unilateral location

3. Pulsating quality

4. Moderate or severe pain intensity

5. Aggravation by or causing avoidance of routine physical activity (e.g., walking or climbing stairs)

6. During headache at least one of the following:

a. Nausea and/or vomiting

b. Photophobia and phonophobia

B. ≥10 days/mo with intake of triptan (any formulation) on a regular basis for >3 mo

C. Migraine frequency has increased during triptan overuse

D. Headache reverts back to previous pattern within 2 mo after discontinuation of triptan

8.2.3 Analgesic/opioid-overuse headache

Diagnostic criteria

A. Headache has at least one of the following characteristics:

1. Chronic headaches (≥15 days/mo)

2. Pressing/tightening (nonpulsating) quality

3. Mild or moderate intensity (may inhibit but does not prohibit activities)

4. Bilateral location

B. ≥15 days with intake for >3 mo

C. Headache worsening has occurred during analgesic overuse

D. Headache reverts back to previous pattern within 2 mo after discontinuation of analgesics

8.2.4 Opioid-overuse headache

Diagnostic criteria

A. Headache has at least one of the following characteristics: chronic headache (≥15 days/month)

B. ≥15 days with intake for >3 mo

C. Headache worsening occurs during opioid overuse

D. Headache reverts back to previous pattern within 2 mo after discontinuation of opioid

8.2.5 Combination drug–overuse headache

Diagnostic criteria

A. Headache has at least one of the following characteristics:

1. Chronic headache (>15 days/mo)

2. Pressing/tightening (nonpulsating) quality

3. Mild or moderate intensity (may inhibit but does not prohibit activities)

4. Bilateral location

(continued)

Table 11-7. *(continued)*

        B. ≥15 days with intake for >3 mo

        C. Headache worsening has occurred during combination analgesic overuse

        D. Headache reverts back to previous pattern within 2 mo after discontinuation of combination analgesics

8.3   Headache as an adverse event of chronic exposure

    Diagnostic criteria

    A. Headache has at least one of the following characteristics: chronic headaches (≥15 days/mo)

    B. Minimum exposure to agent required for minimum time

    C. Headache worsening has occurred during overuse

    D. Headache reverts back to previous pattern within 2 mo after discontinuation of overuse

8.4   Headache secondary to dependent substance withdrawal

    8.4.1 Caffeine-withdrawal headache

        Diagnostic criteria

        A. Headache has at least one of the following characteristics: bilateral, throbbing

        B. Patient has consumed ≥200 mg caffeine/day for ≥2 wk

        C. Occurs within 24 hr after last caffeine intake and is relieved within 1 hr by 100 mg of caffeine

        D. Headache lasts <7 days after caffeine withdrawal

    8.4.2 Opioid-withdrawal headache

        Diagnostic criteria

        A. Headache has at least one of the following characteristics: bilateral, throbbing

        B. Patient has taken opioids for >3 mo on a daily basis

        C. Occurs within 24 hr of opioid withdrawal

        D. Headache lasts <7 days after opioid withdrawal

    8.4.3 Estrogen-withdrawal headache

        Diagnostic criteria

        A. Headache or migraine

        B. Daily use of exogenous estrogen

        C. Onset of headache within 5 days of estrogen cessation

        D. Headache lasts <3 mo after estrogen withdrawal

    8.4.4 Headache attributed to withdrawal from chronic use of other substances

        Diagnostic criteria

        A. Headache has at least one of the following characteristics: bilateral, throbbing

        B. Daily intake of a substance not mentioned in this classification for >3 mo

        C. Headache occurs in close temporal relation to withdrawal of the substance

        D. Headache lasts <3 mo after substance withdrawal

8.5   Exogenous hormone–induced headache

    Diagnostic criteria

    A. New onset or increased frequency of headache or migraine

    B. Use of exogenous hormones

    C. Onset within 3 mo of commencing exogenous hormones

    D. Headache greatly improves or disappears <3 mo after discontinuation of exogenous hormones

Table 11-8. Tension-Type Headache (2)

2.1 Infrequent episodic tension-type headache

Diagnostic criteria

A. At least 10 episodes fulfilling criteria B–E; number of days with such headache <1 day/mo (<12 days/yr)

B. Headache lasting from 30 min to 7 days

C. At least two of the following pain characteristics:

    1. Pressing/tightening (nonpulsating) quality

    2. Mild or moderate intensity (may inhibit, but does not prohibit activities)

    3. Bilateral location

    4. No aggravation by walking stairs or similar routine physical activity

D. Both of the following:

    1. No nausea or vomiting (anorexia may occur)

    2. Photophobia and phonophobia are absent, or one but not the other may be present

E. Not attributed to another disorder

  2.1.1 Associated with pericranial tenderness

    Diagnostic criteria

    A. Fulfills criteria for 2.1

    B. Increased tenderness on pericranial manual palpation

  2.1.2 Not associated with pericranial tenderness

    Diagnostic criteria

    A. Fulfills criteria for 2.1

    B. Not associated with increased pericranial tenderness

2.2 Frequent episodic tension-type headache

Diagnostic criteria

A. At least 10 episodes fulfilling criteria B–E; number of days with such headache ≥1 day/mo and <15 days/mo for at least 3 mo (≥12 days and <180 days/yr)

B. Headache lasting from 30 min to 7 days

C. At least two of the following pain characteristics:

    1. Pressing/tightening (nonpulsating) quality

    2. Mild or moderate intensity (may inhibit but does not prohibit activities)

    3. Bilateral location

    4. No aggravation by walking stairs or similar routine physical activity

D. Both of the following:

    1. No nausea or vomiting (anorexia may occur)

    2. Photophobia and phonophobia are absent, or one but not the other may be present

E. Not attributed to another disorder

  2.2.1 Associated with pericranial tenderness

    Diagnostic criteria

    A. Fulfills criteria for 2.2

    B. Increased tenderness on pericranial manual palpation

(continued)

Table 11-8. *(continued)*

    2.2.2 Not associated with pericranial tenderness

        Diagnostic criteria

        A. Fulfills criteria for 2.2

        B. Not associated with increased pericranial tenderness

2.3 Chronic tension-type headache

  Diagnostic criteria

  A. At least 10 episodes fulfilling criteria B–F; number of days with such headache ≥15 days/mo for at least a 3-mo period (≥180 days/yr)

  B. Headache lasts hours or may be continuous

  C. At least two of the following pain characteristics:

    1. Pressing/tightening (nonpulsating) quality

    2. Mild or moderate intensity (may inhibit but does not prohibit activities)

    3. Bilateral location

    4. No aggravation by walking stairs or similar routine physical activity

  D. Both of the following:

    1. No more than one of the following: photophobia, phonophobia, or mild nausea

    2. No moderate or severe nausea and no vomiting

  E. Use of analgesics or other acute medication on ≤10 days/mo

  F. Not attributed to another disorder

    2.3.1 Associated with pericranial tenderness

        Diagnostic criteria

        A. Fulfills criteria for 2.3

        B. Increased tenderness on pericranial manual palpation

    2.3.2 Not associated with pericranial tenderness

        Diagnostic criteria

        A. Fulfills criteria for 2.3

        B. Not associated with increased pericranial tenderness

2.4   Probable tension-type headache

  Diagnostic criteria

  A. Fulfills all but one criterion for one of the types of tension-type headaches given above

  B. Does not fulfill criteria for migraine without aura (1.1)

Table 11-9. Cluster Headache (3.1)

Diagnostic criteria

A. At least five attacks fulfilling B–D

B. Severe or very severe unilateral orbital, supraorbital, and/or temporal pain lasting 15–180 min untreated for more than half of the period (or time if chronic)

C. Headache accompanied by least one of the following signs, which have to be present on the side of the pain:

    1. Conjunctival injection, lacrimation, or both

    2. Nasal congestion, rhinorrhea, or both

    3. Forehead and facial sweating

    4. Miosis, ptosis, or both

    5. Eyelid edema

    6. Headache is associated with a sense of restlessness or agitation

D. Frequency of attacks: from one every other day to eight per day, for more than half of the period/or time if chronic

E. Not attributed to another disorder

3.1.1 Episodic cluster headache

    Diagnostic criteria

    A. All alphabetical headings of 3.1

    B. At least two periods of headaches (cluster periods) lasting (untreated patients) from 7 days to 1 yr and separated by remissions of at least 1 mo

3.1.2 Chronic cluster headache

    Diagnostic criteria

    A. All alphabetical headings of 3.1

    B. Absence of remission phases for 1 yr or more or with remissions lasting <1 mo

Table 11-10. Paroxysmal Hemicrania (3.2)

Diagnostic criteria

A. At least 20 attacks fulfilling B–D

B. Attacks of severe unilateral orbital, supraorbital, or temporal pain lasting 2–30 min

C. Attack frequency above five a day for more than half of the time, although periods with lower frequency may occur

D. Pain associated with at least one of the following signs/symptoms on the pain side:

    1. Conjunctival injection, lacrimation, or both

    2. Nasal congestion, rhinorrhea, or both

    3. Eyelid edema

    4. Forehead and facial sweating

    5. Miosis, ptosis, or both

E. Headache stopped completely by indomethacin

F. Not attributed to another disorder

3.2.1 Episodic paroxysmal hemicrania

    Diagnostic criteria

    A. All alphabetical headings of 3.2

    B. At least two periods of headaches lasting (untreated patients) from 7 days to 1 yr and separated by remissions of at least 1 mo

3.2.2 Chronic paroxysmal hemicrania

    Diagnostic criteria

    A. All alphabetical headings of 3.2

    B. Absence of remission phases for 1 yr or more or with remissions lasting <1 mo

Table 11-11. Short-Lasting Unilateral Neuralgiform Headache with Conjunctival Injection and Tearing (3.3)

Diagnostic criteria

A. At least 20 attacks fulfilling B–E

B. Attacks of unilateral orbital, supraorbital, or temporal, stabbing, or throbbing pain lasting from 5 to 240 sec

C. Attack frequency from 3 to 200/day

D. Pain is associated with conjunctival injection and lacrimation

E. Not attributed to another disorder

Medical Outcomes Study 20-Item Short-Form General Health Survey (Downsized Version of SF-36)

The SF-20 consists of 20 items that measure six health concepts (Stewart et al., 1988; Tarlov et al., 1989). These include physical functioning, role functioning, social functioning, mental health, health perceptions, and pain. This scale has been used in hypertension, diabetes, heart disease, depression, health perceptions, and back problems (Stewart et al., 1989). The SF-20 was validated in headache populations in two different studies (Osterhaus & Townsend, 1991; Solomon et al., 1993). The SF-20 has been used to examine two components of psychological well-being: life satisfaction and affective well-being in community-dwelling elderly with and without chronic headaches (Jelicic et al., 1998). The scale is easy to complete, and patients can administer it in approximately 10 minutes (Figure 11-2).

Medical Outcomes Study 12-Item Short-Form Health Survey

The SF-12 health survey represents another step in the "downsizing" of measures from the Medical Outcomes Study. The SF-12 is designed to accomplish three objectives: reproduction of more than 90% of the variance in SF-36; accurate reproduction of average scores for both SF-36 summary measures (but less accurately for the eight-scale profile); and reduction in length to allow the form to be printed on one to two pages and to allow the patient to self-administer the survey in 2 minutes or less. In choosing between forms, it is important to consider that the SF-36 defines more levels of health and better represents the content of

health measures than does the SF-12. SF-36 summary measures, particularly the eight-scale SF-36 profile, yield more reliable estimates of individual levels of health, giving the SF-36 a decided advantage over the SF-12 in smaller studies. Therefore, the choice of the SF-12 over the SF-36 is justified in large sample size studies that have severe constraints on questionnaire length and in studies focusing on patient-based assessment of physical and mental health (Ware et al., 1996). Twenty cross-sectional and longitudinal tests of empirical validity previously published for the 36-item short-form scales and summary measures were replicated for the 12-item Physical Component Summary and the 12-item Mental Component Summary, including comparisons between patient groups known to differ or to change in terms of the presence and seriousness of physical and mental conditions, acute symptoms, age and aging, self-reported 1-year changes in health, and recovery from depression (Ware et al., 1996). The SF-12 has been used to assess the influence of migraine and comorbid depression on health-related QOL in a population with migraine and nonmigraine controls (Figure 11-3) (Lipton et al., 2000a).

Specific Scales That Assess Quality of Life in Headache

Migraine-Specific Quality of Life Questionnaire

MQoLQ is a questionnaire to assess the short-term QOL decrements associated with acute migraine headache attacks (Hartmaier et al., 1995). This questionnaire evaluates the impairment of QOL in the 24-hour period after the onset of a migraine headache in adult migraine headache patients. The questionnaire is self-administered and completed quickly and easily (Figure 11-4). The questionnaire consists of 15 items with five domains: (1) work functioning, (2) social functioning, (3) energy/vitality, (4) migraine headache symptoms, and (5) feelings and concerns. There are three items within each domain. Response options for each of the items are on a 7-point scale in which 1 indicates maximum impairment of QOL and 7 indicates no impairment. Each domain has a maximum score of 21 and a minimum score of 3. The scores are compared between migraine-free and migraine periods. The construct validity of the questionnaire has been established by showing that there are significant relationships between subjects' 24-hour MQoLQ scores and other indices of clinical migraine headache, such as headache severity,

Table 11-12. Primary Stabbing Headache, Primary Cough Headache, Primary Exertional Headache, Primary Headache Associated with Sexual Activity, Hypnic Headache, Primary Thunderclap Headache

4.1 Primary stabbing headache

Diagnostic criteria

A. Pain occurring as a single stab or a series of stabs confined to the head and exclusively or predominantly felt in the distribution of the first division of the trigeminal nerve (orbit, temple, and parietal area)

B. Stabs last for up to a few seconds and recur with irregular frequency, ranging from one to many per day

C. No accompanying symptoms

D. Not attributed to another disorder

4.2 Primary cough headache

Diagnostic criteria

A. Headache of sudden onset, lasts from 1 sec to 30 min

B. Headache brought on by coughing, straining, and/or Valsalva's maneuver

C. The same headache does not occur without coughing or straining

D. Not attributed to another disorder

4.3 Primary exertional headache

Diagnostic criteria

A. Throbbing headache lasting from 5 min to 48 hr

B. Headache occurs during physical exertion

C. The same headache does not occur without exertion

D. Not attributed to another disorder

4.4 Primary headache associated with sexual activity

4.4.1 Preorgasmic headache

Diagnostic criteria

A. A dull ache in the head and neck usually bilateral and associated with awareness of neck and/or jaw muscle contraction

B. Occurs during sexual activity and increases with excitement

C. Not attributed to another disorder

4.4.2 Orgasmic headache

Diagnostic criteria

A. Sudden severe ("explosive") headache

B. Headache occurs at orgasm

C. Not attributed to another disorder

4.5 Hypnic headache

Diagnostic criteria

A. Headache has onset during and awakens patient from sleep and does not occur at other times

B. Headache has at least two of the following characteristics:

1. Occurs >15 times/mo

2. Lasts at least 15 min after waking

3. Onset after age 50 yr

C. No autonomic symptoms

(continued)

Table 11-12. *(continued)*

D. No more than one of the following:

1. Nausea

2. Photophobia

3. Phonophobia

E. Not attributed to another disorder

4.6 Primary thunderclap headache

Diagnostic criteria

A. Head pain is very severe and of sudden onset, reaching maximum intensity in <1 min

B. Pain lasts 1 hr to 10 days

C. Headache may recur within the first week after onset but does not recur regularly over subsequent weeks or months

D. Not attributed to another disorder: normal cerebrospinal fluid and normal brain imaging required

Table 11-13. Hemicrania Continua (4.7) and New Daily Persistent Headache (4.8)

4.7 Hemicrania continua

Diagnostic criteria

A. Headache present for at least 2 mo fulfilling criteria B–E

B. Unilateral headache without side shift

C. Pain has the following qualities:

1. Daily and without pain-free periods

2. Moderate severity but with exacerbations when it becomes severe

D. Complete response to indomethacin

E. At least one of the following autonomic features in association with exacerbations of pain on the affected side:

1. Conjunctival injection and/or lacrimation

2. Nasal congestion and/or rhinorrhea

3. Ptosis and/or miosis

F. Not attributed to another disorder

4.8 New daily persistent headache (4.8)

Diagnostic criteria

A. Headache with acute onset (within 24 hr) fulfilling criteria B–F

B. The headache is present ≥15 days/mo for at least 3 mo

C. At least two of the following pain characteristics:

1. Pressing/tightening (nonpulsating) quality

2. Mild or moderate intensity (may inhibit but does not prohibit activities)

3. Bilateral location

4. No aggravation by walking stairs or similar routine physical activity

D. Both of the following:

1. No more than one of the following: photophobia, phonophobia, or mild nausea

2. No moderate or severe nausea and no vomiting

E. Use of analgesics or other acute medication on ≤10 days/mo

F. Not attributed to another disorder

1. In general, would you say your health is:

☐ [1] Excellent   ☐ [2] Very Good   ☐ [3] Good   ☐ [4] Fair   ☐ [5] Poor

---

2. Compared to one year ago, how would you rate your health in general now?

☐ [1] Much better now than one year ago   ☐ [2] Somewhat better now than one year ago

☐ [3] About the same as one year ago   ☐ [4] Somewhat worse now than one year ago

☐ [5] Much worse than one year ago

---

3. The following items are about activities you might do during a typical day. Does your health now limit you in these activities? If so, how much?

	Yes	Limited a lot	Limited a little	No	Not limited at all
a. Vigorous activities, such as running, lifting heavy objects, participating in strenuous sports	[1] ☐	[2] ☐	[3] ☐	[4] ☐	[5] ☐
b. Moderate activities, such as moving a table, pushing a vacuum cleaner, bowling, or playing golf	[1] ☐	[2] ☐	[3] ☐	[4] ☐	[5] ☐
c. Lifting or carrying groceries	[1] ☐	[2] ☐	[3] ☐	[4] ☐	[5] ☐
d. Climbing several flights of stairs	[1] ☐	[2] ☐	[3] ☐	[4] ☐	[5] ☐
e. Climbing one flight of stairs	[1] ☐	[2] ☐	[3] ☐	[4] ☐	[5] ☐
f. Bending, kneeling, or stooping	[1] ☐	[2] ☐	[3] ☐	[4] ☐	[5] ☐
g. Walking more than a mile	[1] ☐	[2] ☐	[3] ☐	[4] ☐	[5] ☐
h. Walking several blocks	[1] ☐	[2] ☐	[3] ☐	[4] ☐	[5] ☐
i. Walking one block	[1] ☐	[2] ☐	[3] ☐	[4] ☐	[5] ☐
j. Bathing or dressing yourself	[1] ☐	[2] ☐	[3] ☐	[4] ☐	[5] ☐

---

4. During the past 4 weeks, have you had any of the following problems with your work or other regular daily activities as a result of your physical health?

a. Cut down the amount of time you spent on work or other activities   [1] ☐ Yes   [0] ☐ No

b. Accomplished less than you would like   [1] ☐ Yes   [0] ☐ No

c. Were limited in the kind of work or other activities   [1] ☐ Yes   [0] ☐ No

d. Had difficulty performing the work or other activities (e.g., it took extra effort)   [1] ☐ Yes   [0] ☐ No

Figure 11-1.   Medical Outcomes Study 36-Item Short-Form General Health Survey (SF-36). (From Ware JE Jr., Sherbourne CD. The MOS 36-Item Short-Form heath survey [SF-36]. I. Conceptual framework and item selection. *Med Care* 1992; 30:473–83, with permission.) (continued)

5. During the past 4 weeks, have you had any of the following problems with your work or other regular daily activities as a result of any emotional problems (such as feeling depressed or anxious)?

a. Cut down the amount of time you spent on work or other activities   1 ☐ Yes   0 ☐ No

b. Accomplished less than you would like   1 ☐ Yes   0 ☐ No

c. Didn't do work or other activities as carefully as usual   1 ☐ Yes   0 ☐ No

6. During the past 4 weeks, to what extent has your physical health or emotional problems interfered with your normal social activities with family, friends, neighbors, or groups?

☐ 1 Not at all   ☐ 2 Slightly   ☐ 3 Moderately   ☐ 4 Quite a bit   ☐ 5 Extremely

7. How much bodily pain have you had during the past 4 weeks?

☐ 1 None   ☐ 2 Very mild   ☐ 3 Mild   ☐ 4 Moderate   ☐ 5 Severe   ☐ 6 Very severe

8. During the past 4 weeks, how much did pain interfere with your normal work (including both work outside the home and housework)?

☐ 1 Not at all   ☐ 2 A little bit   ☐ 3 Moderately   ☐ 4 Quite a bit   ☐ 5 Extremely

9. These questions are about how you feel and how things have been with you during the past 4 weeks. For each question, please give the one answer that comes closest to the way you have been feeling. How much of the time during the past 4 weeks

a. Did you feel full of pep?   1 All of the time ☐   2 Most of the time ☐   3 A good bit of the time ☐   4 Some of the time ☐   5 A little of the time ☐   6 None of the time ☐

b. Have you been a very nervous person?   1 All of the time ☐   2 Most of the time ☐   3 A good bit of the time ☐   4 Some of the time ☐   5 A little of the time ☐   6 None of the time ☐

c. Have you felt so down in the dumps that nothing could cheer you up?   1 All of the time ☐   2 Most of the time ☐   3 A good bit of the time ☐   4 Some of the time ☐   5 A little of the time ☐   6 None of the time ☐

d. Have you felt calm and peaceful?   1 All of the time ☐   2 Most of the time ☐   3 A good bit of the time ☐   4 Some of the time ☐   5 A little of the time ☐   6 None of the time ☐

e. Did you have a lot or energy?   1 All of the time ☐   2 Most of the time ☐   3 A good bit of the time ☐   4 Some of the time ☐   5 A little of the time ☐   6 None of the time ☐

f. Have you felt downhearted and blue?   1 All of the time ☐   2 Most of the time ☐   3 A good bit of the time ☐   4 Some of the time ☐   5 A little of the time ☐   6 None of the time ☐

Figure 11-1. *continued*

g. Did you feel worn out?

¹ All of the time ☐ ² Most of the time ☐ ³ A good bit of the time ☐
⁴ Some of the time ☐ ⁵ A little of the time ☐ ⁶ None of the time ☐

h. Have you been a happy person?

¹ All of the time ☐ ² Most of the time ☐ ³ A good bit of the time ☐
⁴ Some of the time ⁵ A little of the time ☐ ⁶ None of the time ☐

i. Did you feel tired?

¹ All of the time ☐ ² Most of the time ☐ ³ A good bit of the time ☐
⁴ Some of the time ☐ ⁵ A little of the time ☐ ⁶ None of the time ☐

10. During the past 4 weeks, how much of the time has your physical health or emotional problems interfered with your social activities (like visiting with friends, relatives, etc.)?

☐ ¹ All the time   ☐ ² Most of the time

☐ ³ Some of the time   ☐ ⁴ A little of the time

☐ ⁵ None of the time

11. How TRUE or FALSE is each of the following statements for you?

a. I seem to get sick a little easier than other people
☐ ¹ Definitely true ☐ ² Mostly True ☐ ³ Don't Know
☐ ⁴ Mostly false ☐ ⁵ Definitely false

b. I am as healthy as anybody I know
☐ ¹ Definitely true ☐ ² Mostly True ☐ ³ Don't Know
☐ ⁴ Mostly false ☐ ⁵ Definitely false

c. I expect my health to get worse
☐ ¹ Definitely true ☐ ² Mostly True ☐ ³ Don't Know
☐ ⁴ Mostly false ☐ ⁵ Definitely false

d. My health is excellent
☐ ¹ Definitely true ☐ ² Mostly True ☐ ³ Don't Know
☐ ⁴ Mostly false ☐ ⁵ Definitely false

Figure 11-1. *continued*

Instructions: Answer every question by checking the appropriate box, 1,2,3, etc.... If you are unsure about how to answer a question, please give the best answer you can and make a comment in the left margin.

1. In general, would you say your health is: (check one box)

    [ ] ¹ Excellent   [ ] ² Very good   [ ] ³ Good   [ ] ⁴ Fair   [ ] ⁵ Poor

2. Compared to one year ago, how would you rate your health in general now? (check one box)

    [ ] ¹ Much better now than one year ago   [ ] ⁴ Somewhat worse now than one year ago

    [ ] ² Somewhat better now than one year ago   [ ] ⁵ Much worse now than one year ago

    [ ] ³ About the same

3. The following questions are about activities you might do during a typical day. During the past 8 weeks, has your health limited you in these activities? If so, how much? (check one box on each line)

	Yes, limited a lot	Yes, limited a little	No, not limited at all
a. Vigorous activities, such as running, lifting heavy objects, participating in strenuous sports	[ ] ¹	[ ] ¹	[ ] ¹
b. Moderate activities, such as moving a table, pushing a vacuum cleaner, bowling, or playing golf	[ ] ¹	[ ] ¹	[ ] ¹
c. Lifting or carrying groceries	[ ] ¹	[ ] ¹	[ ] ¹
d. Climbing several flights of stairs	[ ] ¹	[ ] ¹	[ ] ¹
e. Climbing one flight of stairs	[ ] ¹	[ ] ¹	[ ] ¹
f. Bending, kneeling, or stooping	[ ] ¹	[ ] ¹	[ ] ¹
g. Walking more than a mile	[ ] ¹	[ ] ¹	[ ] ¹
h. Walking several blocks	[ ] ¹	[ ] ¹	[ ] ¹
i. Walking one block	[ ] ¹	[ ] ¹	[ ] ¹
j. Bathing and dressing yourself	[ ] ¹	[ ] ¹	[ ] ¹

4. During the past 8 weeks, have you had any of the following problems with your work or other regular daily activities as a result of your physical health? (please answer yes or no by checking the appropriate box)

    a. Cut down on the amount of time you spent on work or other activities   [ ] ¹ Yes   [ ] ⁰ No

    b. Accomplished less than you would like   [ ] ¹ Yes   [ ] ⁰ No

    c. Were limited in the kind of work or other activities   [ ] ¹ Yes   [ ] ⁰ No

    d. Had difficulty performing the work or other activities (for example, it took extra effort)   [ ] ¹ Yes   [ ] ⁰ No

Figure 11-2.   Medical Outcomes Study 20-Item Short-Form General Health Survey (SF-20). (From Stewart A, Hays R, Ware JE Jr. The MOS short form general health survey. Reliability and validity in a patient population. *Med Care* 1988;26:724–35, with permission.)

5. During the past 8 weeks, have you had any of the following problems with your work or other regular daily activities as a result of any emotional problems (such as feeling depressed or anxious)? (Please answer yes or no by checking the appropriate box).

    a. Cut down on the amount of time spent on work or other activities   yes ^{1} ☐   no ^{0} ☐

    b. Accomplished less than you would like   yes ^{1} ☐   no ^{0} ☐

    c. Didn't do work or other activities as carefully as usual   yes ^{1} ☐   no ^{0} ☐

6. During the past 8 weeks, to what extent has your physical health or emotional problems interfered with your normal social activities with family, friends, neighbors, or groups? (Check one box)

☐ ^{1} Not at all   ☐ ^{2} Slightly   ☐ ^{3} Moderately   ☐ ^{4} Quite a bit   ☐ ^{5} Extremely

7. How much bodily pain have you had during the past 8 weeks? (Check one box).

☐ ^{1} None   ☐ ^{2} Very Mild   ☐ ^{3} Mild   ☐ ^{4} Moderate   ☐ ^{5} Severe   ☐ ^{6} Very Severe

8. During the past 8 weeks, how much did pain interfere with your normal work (including work both outside the home and housework)? (Check one box)

☐ ^{1} Not at all   ☐ ^{2} Slightly   ☐ ^{3} Moderately   ☐ ^{4} Quite a bit   ☐ ^{5} Extremely

9. These questions are about how you feel and how things have been with you during the past 8 weeks. For each question, please indicate the one answer that comes closest to the way you have been feeling. (Check one box on each line)

How much of the time during the past 8 weeks	All of the Time	Most of the Time	A Good bit of the Time	Some of the Time	A Little of the Time	None of the Time
a. did you feel full of pep?	☐ 1	☐ 2	☐ 3	☐ 4	☐ 5	☐ 6
b. have you been a very nervous person?	☐ 1	☐ 2	☐ 3	☐ 4	☐ 5	☐ 6
c. have you felt so down in the dumps nothing could cheer you up?	☐ 1	☐ 2	☐ 3	☐ 4	☐ 5	☐ 6
d. have you felt calm and peaceful?	☐ 1	☐ 2	☐ 3	☐ 4	☐ 5	☐ 6
e. did you have a lot of energy?	☐ 1	☐ 2	☐ 3	☐ 4	☐ 5	☐ 6
f. have you felt downhearted and blue?	☐ 1	☐ 2	☐ 3	☐ 4	☐ 5	☐ 6
g. did you feel worn out?	☐ 1	☐ 2	☐ 3	☐ 4	☐ 5	☐ 6
h. have you been a happy person?	☐ 1	☐ 2	☐ 3	☐ 4	☐ 5	☐ 6
i. did you feel tired?	☐ 1	☐ 2	☐ 3	☐ 4	☐ 5	☐ 6
j. has your health limited your social activities (like visiting with friends or close relatives)	☐ 1	☐ 2	☐ 3	☐ 4	☐ 5	☐ 6

Figure 11-2. *continued*

10. Please choose the answer that best describes how true or false each of the following statements is for you. (Check one box on each line)

	Definitely True	Mostly True	Not Sure	Mostly False	Definitely False
a. I seem to get sick a little easier than other people	☐ 1	☐ 2	☐ 3	☐ 4	☐ 5
b. I am as healthy as anybody I know	☐ 1	☐ 2	☐ 3	☐ 4	☐ 5
c. I expect my health to get worse	☐ 1	☐ 2	☐ 3	☐ 4	☐ 5
d. My health is excellent	☐ 1	☐ 2	☐ 3	☐ 4	☐ 5

Figure 11-2. *continued*

activity limitation, number of associated migraine symptoms, global change in migraine symptoms, and migraine duration (Hartmaier et al., 1995; Santanello et al., 1995). The ability of the MQoLQ to capture within-subject change in QOL was evaluated by comparing QOL scores during a "migraine-free" period to MQoLQ scores 24 hours after migraine onset (see Figure 11-4) (Santanello et al., 1997). The MQoLQ should be applicable to all adults suffering from episodic migraine headache. It was designed primarily for use in clinical trials to assess migraine management and to be responsive to subject changes in QOL in the 24 hours after the onset of a migraine headache. The MQoLQ assesses subjective well-being and daily ability to function, in addition to measuring the typical associated symptoms of migraine such as nausea, photophobia/phonophobia, and head pain. The 24-hour MQoLQ should not be used to measure global QOL between headache episodes.

Migraine-Specific Quality of Life Questionnaire (MSQ Version 2.1)

The MSQ is a disease-specific QOL instrument with three hypothesized scales. It has been developed, tested, and revised (Martin et al., 2000). The MSQ (version 2.1) was structured secondary to older versions of the MSQ (version 1.0 and 2.0). The revised 14-item MSQ (version 2.1) consists of seven items in the role-restrictive dimension that measure the degree to which performance of normal activities is limited by migraines; four items in the role-preventive dimen-

sions that measure the degree to which performance of normal activities is interrupted by migraines; and three items in the emotional function that measure the emotional effects of migraine (Martin et al., 2000). The MSQ dimensions had low to modest correlations with the two component scores of the SF-36 and were modestly to moderately correlated with migraine symptoms (Table 11-14). The validation was structured in three separate analyses applied in 267 subjects (Martin et al., 2000). The MSQ provides clinicians, researchers, and those who fund health care with a measurement tool to assess health-related QOL. The questionnaire was designed to be completed quickly and easily in a self-administered form (see Table 11-14). This study suggested the mean MSQ (version 2.1) scores 6–12 points higher (indicating better QOL).

Migraine-Specific Quality of Life

MSQOL is used to assess migraine patients' QOL over a long period (average 3 weeks). The MSQOL is a valid and reliable self-administered measure and a useful tool in clinical migraine research (Table 11-15) (Wagner et al., 1996). The information it provides can add important information about migraine's impact on QOL and the potential benefits of therapeutic interventions. This questionnaire has 25 items, each question having four answers. The general format and scoring are as follows: 1, very much; 2, quite a lot; 3, a little; 4, not at all. The total score is then transferred to a scale of 0–100, a higher number representing a better

INSTRUCTIONS: This survey asks for your views about your health. This information will help keep track of how you feel and how well you are able to do your usual activities.

Please answer every question by marking one box. If you are unsure about how to answer, please give the best answer you can.

1. In general, would you say your health is:

☐ Excellent   ☐ Very good   ☐ Good   ☐ Fair   ☐ Poor

The following items are about activities you might do during a typical day. Does your health now limit you in these activities? If so, how much?

	Yes, Limited A Lot	Yes, Limited A Little	No, Not Limited At All
2. Moderate activities, such as moving a table, pushing a vacuum cleaner, bowling, or playing golf	☐	☐	☐
3. Climbing several flights of stairs	☐	☐	☐

During the past 4 weeks, have you had any of the following problems with your work or other regular daily activities as a result of your physical health?

	YES	NO
4. Accomplished less than you would like	☐	☐
5. Were limited in the kind of work or other activities	☐	☐

During the past 4 weeks, have you had any of the following problems with your work or other regular daily activities as a result of any emotional problems (such as feeling depressed or anxious)?

	YES	NO
6. Accomplished less than you would like	☐	☐
7. Don't do work or other activities as carefully as usual	☐	☐

8. During the past 4 weeks how much did pain interfere with your normal work (including both work outside the home and housework)?

☐ Not at all   ☐ A little bit   ☐ Moderately   ☐ Quite a bit   ☐ Extremely

Figure 11-3. Medical Outcomes Study 12-Item Short-Form General Health Survey (SF-12). (From Ware J, Kosinski M, Keller SD. A 12-item short form health survey: construction of scales and preliminary tests of reliability and validity. *Med Care* 1996;34:220–33, with permission.) (continued)

These questions are about how you feel and how things have been with you during the past four weeks. For each question, please give the one answer that comes closest to the way you have been feeling. How much of the time during the past four weeks

	All of the Time	Most of the Time	A good bit of the Time	Some of the Time	A little of the Time	None of the Time
9. Have you felt calm and peaceful?	☐	☐	☐	☐	☐	☐
10. Did you have a lot energy?	☐	☐	☐	☐	☐	☐
11. Have you felt downhearted and blue?	☐	☐	☐	☐	☐	☐

12. During the past four weeks, how much of the time has your physical   health or emotional problems interfered with your social activities (like visiting with friends, relatives, etc.)?

☐ All of the time   ☐ Most of the time   ☐ Some of the time

☐ A little of the time   ☐ None of the time

Figure 11-3.   *continued*

QOL. For the MSQOL, Cronbach's alpha was 0.92, suggesting that the items are tapping into a single concept. The MSQOL has the potential to provide valuable information on a migraineur's QOL and be a useful adjuvant measure when assessing long-term treatment outcomes (see Table 11-15).

Scales That Assess Headache Impact and Disability

Headache impairs physical, social, and emotional functioning, but a diagnosis is not always made despite the availability of helpful tools. One reason for this is poor patient–physician communication. If the impact that headaches are having on a person's life can be communicated adequately to the physician, the likelihood of appropriate management increases (Pryse-Phillips, 2002). Impact and disability instruments are scored differently and have different interpretations. Generally, the impact is scaled in a positive direction, with higher scores reflecting better QOL (i.e., lower impact). For disability measures, higher scores reflect greater activity limitation (i.e., higher impact). Measuring headache-related disability, together with assessments of pain intensity, head-

ache frequency, tiredness, mood alterations and cognition, can be used to assess the impact of migraine on sufferers' lives and on society (Dowson, 2001). The tools currently used for assessing headache impact are *HIT* and *HIT-6*, *HImQ*, *HANA*, and *HDI* (Henry Ford questionnaire). These scales, when adequately used, can improve communication between patients and physicians, assess migraine severity, and act as outcome measures to monitor treatment efficacy. Impact tools are also used to produce an individualized treatment plan for each patient along with other clinical assessments (Dowson, 2001). Disability measures assess impairment in role functioning—that is, reduced ability to function in defined roles, such as paid work (Lipton et al., 2001a). The disability instruments used are the *HDI* (or Henry Ford Hospital Headache Disability Inventory) and the *MIDAS*.

Headache Impact Test

HIT is a tool that measures headache's impact on a person's ability to function on the job, at home, and in social situations (Figure 11-5). The HIT was developed by the psychometricians who developed the SF-36 health assessment. HIT was designed for greater accessibility

The following questions are to be completed 24 HOURS after your take your first dose of medication for your migraine headache, and ask how your quality of life was affected.

In the past 24 HOURS after you took your first dose of medication for your migraine headache, how much of the time did you: (*Please check one box for each question*)

	(1) All of the time	(2) Most of the time	(3) A good bit of the time	(4) Some of the time	(5) A little of the time	(6) Hardly any of the time	(7) None of the time
1 have increased sensitivity to light and/or noise...............	☐	☐	☐	☐	☐	☐	☐
2 have nausea...........................	☐	☐	☐	☐	☐	☐	☐
3 have throbbing head pain............	☐	☐	☐	☐	☐	☐	☐
4 feel upset about having migraine headaches	☐	☐	☐	☐	☐	☐	☐
5 feel physically uncomfortable........	☐	☐	☐	☐	☐	☐	☐
6 feel concerned that your migraine medication wouldn't relieve your migraine headache symptoms.......	☐	☐	☐	☐	☐	☐	☐

In the past 24 HOURS after you took your first dose of migraine medication, how much of the time did your migraine headache and accompanying symptoms limit your ability to: (*Please check one box for each question*)

	(1) All of the time	(2) Most of the time	(3) A good bit of the time	(4) Some of the time	(5) A little of the time	(6) Hardly any of the time	(7) None of the time
7 do normal everyday work (job outside the home, schoolwork, housework).............	☐	☐	☐	☐	☐	☐	☐
8 stay alert................................	☐	☐	☐	☐	☐	☐	☐
9 operate machinery or a motor vehicle (including home appliances and office equipment)..............	☐	☐	☐	☐	☐	☐	☐
10 enjoy life............................	☐	☐	☐	☐	☐	☐	☐

Figure 11-4. Migraine Quality of Life Questionnaire—24 hours (MQoLQ). (From Hartmaier SL, Santanello NC, Epstein RS, et al. Development of a brief 24-hour migraine-specific quality of life questionnaire. *Headache* 1995;35:320–29, with permission.) (continued)

In the past 24 hours after you took your first dose of migraine medication, how much did your migraine headache and accompanying symptoms <u>negatively</u> affect your: *(Please check <u>one</u> box for each question)*

	(1) All of the time	(2) Most of the time	(3) A good bit of the time	(4) Some of the time	(5) A little of the time	(6) Hardly any of the time	(7) None of the time
11 interactions with people who are close to you................	☐	☐	☐	☐	☐	☐	☐
12 interactions with other people................................	☐	☐	☐	☐	☐	☐	☐
13 energy level............................	☐	☐	☐	☐	☐	☐	☐
14 ability to have a good night's sleep...................................	☐	☐	☐	☐	☐	☐	☐
15 mood.......................................	☐	☐	☐	☐	☐	☐	☐

Figure 11-4. *continued*

Table 11-14. Migraine-Specific Quality of Life Questionnaire (MSQ Version 2.1)

Dimension	Item	Variable	Abbreviated Item Content
Role function restrictive	1	FAMILY	… interfered with how well you dealt with family, friends, and others
	2	LEISURE	… interfered with your leisure time activities such as reading or exercising
	3	ACTIVITY	… had difficulty in performing work or daily activities
	4	WORK	… kept you from getting as much done at work or at home
	5	CONCTRAT	… limited your ability to concentrate on work or daily activities
	6	TIRED	… left you too tired to do work or daily activities
	7	ENERGY	… limited the number of days you felt energetic
Role preventive	8	CANCEL	… canceled work or daily activities
	9	HELP	… needed help in handling routine tasks
	10	STOP	… stopped work or daily activities
	11	SOCIAL	… not able to go to social activities
Emotional function	12	FRUSTRAT	… felt fed up or frustrated
	13	BURDEN	… felt like a burden on others
	14	AFRAID	… afraid of letting others down

From Martin BC, Pathak DS, Sharfman MI, et al. Validity and reliability of the migraine-specific quality of life questionnaire (MSQ Version 2.1). *Headache* 2000;40:204–15, with permission.

Table 11-15. Migraine-Specific Quality of Life

Migraine affects people's lives in different ways. Please circle the number of the statement that best describes how you feel in between your migraines.

1. It is important to avoid changes in the pace of my life because of my migraines. (*Please circle the number of your answer.*)

    1—Yes, it is very important.

    2—Yes, it is quite important.

    3—No, it is not very important.

    4—No, it is not important at all.

2. I try to avoid getting too tired because of my migraines. (*Please circle the number of your answer.*)

    1—Yes, I try very hard.

    2—Yes, I try quite hard.

    3—No, I do not try very hard.

    4—No, I do not try at all.

3. It is important for me to stay in familiar surroundings because of my migraines. (*Please circle the number of your answer.*)

    1—Yes, it is very important.

    2—Yes, it is quite important.

    3—No, it is not very important.

    4—No, it is not important at all.

4. I feel helpless when a migraine starts. (*Please circle the number of your answer.*)

    1—Yes, very much.

    2—Yes, quite a lot.

    3—Yes, a little.

    4—No, not at all.

5. I worry about my migraines disrupting other people's lives. (*Please circle the number of your answer.*)

    1—Yes, I worry about it very much.

    2—Yes, I worry about it quite a lot.

    3—Yes, I worry about it a little.

    4—No, I don't worry about it at all.

6. My life revolves around my migraines. (*Please circle the number of your answer.*)

    1—Yes, very much.

    2—Yes, quite a lot.

    3—No, not very much.

    4—No, not at all.

7. It is important for me to eat regularly because of my migraines. (*Please circle the number of your answer.*)

    1—Yes, it is very important.

    2—Yes, it is quite important.

    3—No, it is not very important.

    4—No, it is not important at all.

8. I worry that I neglect people close to me because of my migraines. (*Please circle the number of your answer.*)

    1—Yes, I worry about it very much.

    2—Yes, I worry about it quite a lot.

    3—Yes, I worry about it a little.

    4—No, I don't worry about it at all.

(continued)

Table 11-15.   *(continued)*

9. I resent losing time because of my migraines. (*Please circle the number of your answer.*)

    1—Yes, I resent it very much.

    2—Yes, I resent it quite a lot.

    3—Yes, I resent it a little.

    4—No, I do not resent it at all.

10. I dislike having to rely on other people because of my migraines. (*Please circle the number of your answer.*)

    1—Yes, very much.

    2—Yes, quite a lot.

    3—No, not very much.

    4—No, not at all.

11. I am reluctant to make plans because of my migraines. (*Please circle the number of your answer.*)

    1—Yes, I am very reluctant.

    2—Yes, I am quite reluctant.

    3—No, I am not very reluctant.

    4—No, I am not reluctant at all.

12. I try to avoid too much activity for fear of bringing on a migraine. (*Please circle the number of your answer.*)

    1—Yes, I try very hard.

    2—Yes, I try quite hard.

    3—No, I do not try very hard.

    4—No, I do not try at all.

13. I worry about getting a migraine if I have to travel long distances. (*Please circle the number of your answer.*)

    1—Yes, I worry about it very much.

    2—Yes, I worry about it quite a lot.

    3—Yes, I worry about it a little.

    4—No, I don't worry about it at all.

14. My migraines put a strain on my close relationships. (*Please circle the number of your answer.*)

    1—Yes, very much so.

    2—Yes, quite a lot.

    3—No, not very much.

    4—No, not at all.

15. I try to avoid places that might bring on a migraine (e.g., bright, noisy, or smoky places). (*Please circle the number of your answer.*)

    1—Yes, I try very hard.

    2—Yes, I try quite hard.

    3—No, I do not try very hard.

    4—No, I do not try at all.

16. I worry about the future because of my migraines. (*Please circle the number of your answer.*)

    1—Yes, I worry about it very much.

    2—Yes, I worry about it quite a lot.

    3—Yes, I worry about it a little.

    4—No, I don't worry about it at all.

17. I try to avoid pushing myself too hard because of my migraines. (*Please circle the number of your answer.*)

    1—Yes, very much.

    2—Yes, quite a lot.

Table 11-15. *(continued)*

3—No, not very much.

4—No, not at all.

18. I get nervous if I think I am going to get a migraine. (*Please circle the number of your answer.*)

    1—Yes, I get very nervous.

    2—Yes, I get quite nervous.

    3—Yes, I get a little nervous.

    4—No, I don't get nervous at all.

19. I feel depressed about having migraines. (*Please circle the number of your answer.*)

    1—Yes, I feel very depressed.

    2—Yes, I feel quite depressed.

    3—Yes, I feel a little depressed.

    4—No, I don't feel depressed at all.

20. I worry about letting people down because of my migraines. (*Please circle the number of your answer.*)

    1—Yes, I worry about it very much.

    2—Yes, I worry about it quite a lot.

    3—Yes, I worry about it a little.

    4—No, I don't worry about it at all.

21. I doubt my ability to do a good job because of my migraines. (*Please circle the number of your answer.*)

    1—Yes, very much.

    2—Yes, quite a lot.

    3—No, not very much.

    4—No, not at all.

22. It is important for me to keep to a routine because of my migraines. (*Please circle the number of your answer.*)

    1—Yes, it is very important.

    2—Yes, it is quite important.

    3—No, it is not very important.

    4—No, it is not important at all.

23. I find my migraines frightening. (*Please circle the number of your answer.*)

    1—Yes, very much.

    2—Yes, quite a lot.

    3—No, not very much.

    4—No, not at all.

24. I feel angry that nothing can stop a migraine. (*Please circle the number of your answer.*)

    1—Yes, I feel very angry.

    2—Yes, I feel quite angry.

    3—Yes, I feel a little angry.

    4—No, I don't feel angry at all.

25. I worry that people think I use my migraines as an excuse. (*Please circle the number of your answer.*)

    1—Yes, I worry about it very much.

    2—Yes, I worry about it quite a lot.

    3—Yes, I worry about it a little.

    4—No, I don't worry about it at all.

From Wagner TH, Patrick DL, Galer BS, et al. A new instrument to assess the long-term quality of life effects from migraine: Development and psychometric testing of the MSQOL. *Headache* 1996;36:484–92, with permission.

This questionnaire was designed to help you describe and communicate the way you feel and what you cannot do because of headaches.
To complete, please circle one answer for each question.

1 When you have headaches, how often is the pain severe?
Never   Rarely   Sometimes   Very Often   Always

2 How often do headaches limit your ability to do usual daily activities including household work, work, school, or social activities?
Never   Rarely   Sometimes   Very Often   Always

3 When you have a headache, how often do you wish you could lie down?
Never   Rarely   Sometimes   Very Often   Always

4 In the past 4 weeks, how often have you felt too tired to do work or daily activities because of your headaches?
Never   Rarely   Sometimes   Very Often   Always

5 In the past 4 weeks, how often have you felt fed up or irritated because of your headaches?
Never   Rarely   Sometimes   Very Often   Always

6 In the past 4 weeks, how often did headaches limit your ability to concentrate on work or daily activities?
Never   Rarely   Sometimes   Very Often   Always

Column 1	Column 2	Column 3	Column 4	Column 5
(6 points each)	(8 points each)	(10 points each)	(11 points each)	(13 points each)

To score, add points for answers in each column.   **Total Score**

Figure 11-5. Headache Impact Test (HIT-6). (From Ware JE, Bjorner JB, Kosinski M. Practical implications of item response theory and computerized adaptive testing: A brief summary of ongoing studies of widely used headache impact scales. *Med Care* 2000;38[Suppl 2]:S73–82, with permission.)

(on the Internet at http://www.headachetest.com and http://www.amihealthy.com and as a paper-based form known as *HIT-6*). The HIT-6 is a practical test with six questions. The patient can complete the test in less than 2 minutes. The HIT-6 assesses disability over a 4-week period. The score range is 36–78. Higher scores indicate greater disability impact. A score of 60 or above indicates a severe impact (headache stops family, work, school, or social activities), a score between 56 and 59 a substantial impact, a score between 50 and 55 some impact, and a score below 49 no impact (Pryse-Phillips, 2002; Ware et al., 2000; Bjorner et al., 2003). The availability of this test on the Internet, with feedback provided, makes this a useful tool to help headache sufferers to understand the burden of their migraines and seek appropriate management.

Headache Impact Questionnaire

The HImQ measures pain and activity limitations over a 3-month period. This instrument was the precursor to the MIDAS instrument (see Instruments and Scales in Headache). The HImQ score is derived from four frequency-based questions (i.e., number of headaches, missed days of work, missed days of chores, or missed days of nonwork activity) and four summary measures of average experience across headaches (i.e., average pain intensity and average reduced effectiveness when having a headache at work, during household chores, and in nonwork activity) (Figure 11-6). This scale was validated after assessing the pain and activity limitations in a population-based sample of 132 migraine headache sufferers enrolled in a 90-day daily diary study who completed the HImQ at the end of the study. Previous studies of the validity of retrospective pain and disability reporting were mixed (Basilicato et al., 1992; Hunter et al., 1979; Kent, 1985; Linton & Melin, 1982; Linton & Gotestam, 1983; Means et al., 1989; Roche & Gijsbers, 1986; Solovey et al., 1992; Stewart et al., 1998). Study participants completed the HImQ in person and then completed daily diaries for 90 days. The HImQ was developed to identify headache sufferers who have the greatest need for medical care. Self-administered questionnaires can adequately capture information to rate pain severity.

Headache Needs Assessment Survey

The HANA questionnaire was designed to assess two dimensions (frequency and bothersomeness) of migraine's impact (Cramer et al., 2001). Seven issues related to living with migraine were used as ratings of frequency and bothersomeness. Validation studies were performed in a Web-based survey, a clinical trial responsiveness population, and a retest reliability population. Headache characteristics (e.g., frequency, severity, and treatment), demographic information, and the HDI were used for external validation. The HANA can be used in medical practice groups (e.g., headache centers, managed care groups) as a screening tool to detect potential problems. The scores from the scale were compared before and after treatment to determine the impact of the headache. Primary care physicians could use the HANA to screen patients with migraine for further evaluation. Once identified, those with severe migraine may be candidates for further evaluation and immediate treatment. The HANA has several advantages: (1) It can select who should be treated; (2) it can increase productivity by adequately treating headaches; and (3) it can identify the need for aggressive treatment without the usual slow advancement through stepped-care algorithms. This brief, self-applied questionnaire may be a useful screening tool to evaluate the impact of migraines. The two-dimensional approach to patient-reported QOL allows individuals to weigh the impact of both frequency and bothersomeness of chronic migraines on multiple aspects of daily life (Figure 11-7).

Henry Ford Hospital Headache Disability Inventory

The HDI is useful in assessing the impact of headache, and its treatment, on daily living (Figure 11-8) (Bauer et al., 1999; Jacobson et al., 1994, 1995; Mannix et al., 1999). It is a paper and pencil instrument that probes the functional and emotional effects of headache on everyday life. The HDI is a 25-item headache disability inventory, each item requiring a "yes" (4 points), "sometimes" (2 points), or "no" (0 points) response. Thus, a maximum score of 100 points reflects severe self-perceived headache disability. The scale is easy to complete and simple to score and interpret (see Figure 11-8). The HDI has high internal consistency, reliability, and good content validity; the long-term (2 months) test-retest stability of the HDI was robust (Jacobson et al., 1994, 1995). The test-retest reliability for the beta-HDI was acceptable for the total score and functional and emotional subscale scores (Jacobson et al., 1994). Scales of this nature help investigators understand the

Diary – First Part.

Note the actual day and date you completed:

_____   _____/_____/_____
Day of Week   Month   Day   Year

1. Did you go to work today?   ☐ Yes   ☐ No/ Not Applicable (Skip to 3)

2. Compared to your usual ability to work (100%) what was your effectiveness at work today?
Mark an "X" on the line,

0   10%   20%   30%   40%   50%   60%   70%   80%   90%   100%

Not able   Usual
to work   ability

3. Did you do chores today?   ☐ Yes   ☐ No (Skip to 5)

4. Compared to your usual ability to do housework or chores, what was your effectiveness in doing these activities today? Mark an "X" on the line.

0   10%   20%   30%   40%   50%   60%   70%   80%   90%   100%

Not able   Usual
to work   ability

5. Record any medication you took today for any reason EXCEPT medications to relieve headache pain, or to prevent a headache. Do not include any medication you take daily, such as birth control pills, blood pressure medication, etc.

Name of Medication	Dosage	Reason for taking it

Figure 11-6.   Headache Impact Questionnaire (HImQ). (From Stewart WF, Lipton RB, Simon D, et al. Validity of an illness severity measure for headache in a population sample of migraine sufferers. *Pain* 1999;79:291–301, with permission.)

6. Overall Mood

Please describe your overall sense of well-being today. Mark an "X" on the line at the point which best describes your mood today, on average.

Today you felt...

Least Relaxed	_____	Most Relaxed
Least Sociable	_____	Most Sociable
Extremely Depressed	_____	Not at all Depressed
Extremely Stressed	_____	No at all Stressed

Your overall mood today is....

Worst	_____	Best

7. Did you have a headache today?

☐ NO, STOP – You have completed today's diary. Thank you.

☐ YES, Please continue.

If you had more than one headache today, answer all the following questions ONLY for your WORST headache.

A. Your headache today began at: ____:____   ☐ AM   ☐ PM

B. Do you still have the headache?   ☐ Yes   ☐ No

C. Your headache today ended at: ____:____   ☐ AM   ☐ PM

Please complete a new Symptom Checklist (in the back of this diary) for each headache you have this week.

Figure 11-6.   *continued*

Diary – Second Part.

Today's Data ___/_____/_____

ABOUT MY HEADACHE TODAY...

Please complete the following checklist to describe today's headache. If you had more than one headache today, please describe the worst headache. If you don't know an answer, please check ( ) "DK".

With this headache.

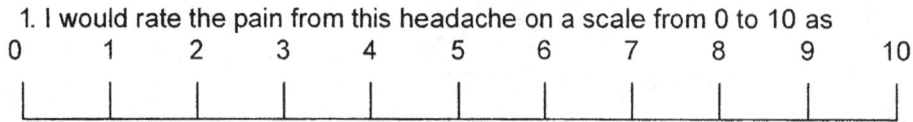

1. I would rate the pain from this headache on a scale from 0 to 10 as

```
0   1   2   3   4   5   6   7   8   9   10
```

▲ No pain at all   ▲ Pain as bad as it can be

2. I had to lie down and rest   no ☐   yes ☐   DK ☐
   If YES how many hours did you lie down ? ____hr(s)

3. I had pain that was worse on one side of the head   no ☐   yes ☐   DK ☐

4. I had pain that was worse around only one eye   no ☐   yes ☐   DK ☐
   or temple.

5. I had pain on both sides of the head   no ☐   yes ☐   DK ☐

6. I had pressing/tightening pain   no ☐   yes ☐   DK ☐

7. I had pounding/pulsating pain   no ☐   yes ☐   DK ☐

8. I was especially bothered by light   no ☐   yes ☐   DK ☐

   If YES, how bad was it   mild ☐   moderate ☐   severe ☐

9. I was especially bothered by sound   no ☐   yes ☐   DK ☐

   If YES, how bad was it   mild ☐   moderate ☐   severe ☐

10. I felt nauseous or sick to my stomach   no ☐   yes ☐   DK ☐

   If YES, how bad was it?   mild ☐   moderate ☐   severe ☐
                                       vomited ☐

11. I had changes in my vision before or   no ☐   yes ☐   DK ☐
    during my headache

   If YES, check all that apply   zigzag ☐   spots ☐   heat waves ☐
                                   flashes ☐
                                   Complete or partial visual loss ☐

Figure 11-6. *continued*

12. I missed work or school for all or   no ☐ part of day ☐ all of the day ☐
                                                 NA (go to 14) ☐

13. How much was your ability to work reduced today because of this headache? Make an "X" on the line.

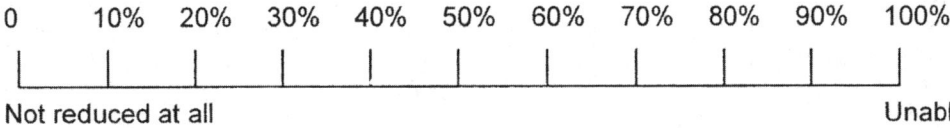

0   10%   20%   30%   40%   50%   60%   70%   80%   90%   100%

Not reduced at all   Unable to work

14. I was unable to do housework or chores for at   No ☐   Yes ☐   NA ☐
    least half of the day*   (go to 16)

15. How much was your ability to do housework or chores reduced today because of this headache? Make an "X" on the line.

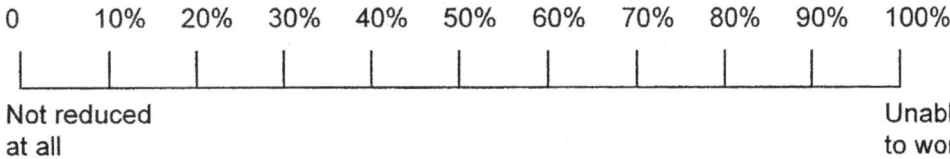

0   10%   20%   30%   40%   50%   60%   70%   80%   90%   100%

Not reduced   Unable
at all   to work

16. I was unable to do non-work activities (family,   No ☐   Yes ☐   NA ☐
    social, or recreational) for at least half of the day*

17. How much was your ability to engage in non-work activities (family, social, recreational) reduced today because of this headache? Make an "X" on the line.

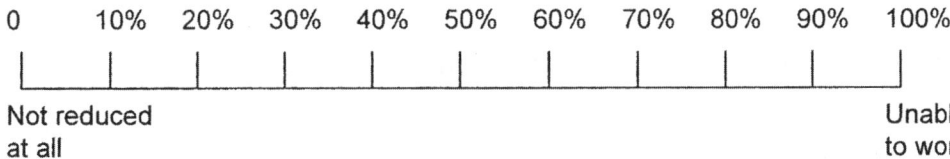

0   10%   20%   30%   40%   50%   60%   70%   80%   90%   100%

Not reduced   Unable
at all   to work

18. Did you take my medication to treat this headache?   No ☐   Yes ☐
If Yes answer questions 19 & 20.

19. How long did the headache last before took the medication?   _____ hours.

20. What medication(s) did you take for this headache?

Name of Medication	# Pills Taken	Dosage of Each Pill

*If you <u>did not plan</u> to go to work, do housework, or engage in non-work activities today answer this as "NA".

Figure 11-6.   *continued*

We are interested in knowing how you feel about having migraine headaches and the problems caused by your headaches in usual daily activities. This information wil help us to understand the problems you face related to having frequent and severe migraine headaches. Please answer questions A and B for each problem listed (1–7) describing how migraine headaches affected your life in the past 4 weeks.

	Problem area:	Question A	Question B
		How often has this problem occurred?	How much has this problem bothered you?
		1= never,	1= not at all,
		2= rarely,	2= a little,
		3= sometimes,	3= some,
		4= often,	4= a lot,
	In the past month,…	5= all the time	5= a great deal

	A	B

Problem 1. I have felt **anxious or worried** (tense, wound-up, frightened) about having another severe headache.

Problem 2. I have felt **depressed, discouraged** about my headaches.

Problem 3. I have felt that I am not in **control** of myself because of my headaches.

Problem 4. I have had less **energy**; I am more **tired** than I should have been because of my headaches.

Problem 5. I **functioned** and **worked** (attention, concentration, etc.) at a lower level than I should have because of my headaches.

Problem 6. I have felt that my **family and social activities** were limited because of my headaches.

Problem 7. I have felt that my **life centered or revolved** around my headaches.

Figure 11-7.   Headache Needs Assessment Questionnaire. (From Cramer JA, Silberstein SD, Winner P. Development and validation of the Headache Needs Assessment [HANA] survey. *Headache* 2001;41:402–9, with permission.)

E= emotional subscale, F= functional subscale. A "yes" response is scored as 4 points, a "sometimes" response is scored as 2 points, and a "no" response is scored as zero points. The maximum score is 100 points, reflecting severe spouse-perceived headache disability.

INSTRUCTIONS – PLEASE READ CAREFULLY

The purpose of this scale is to evaluate your perceptions of your spouse's headaches. Please answer "yes", "sometimes", or "no" to each item (mark one only per item). Answer each question as it pertains to your spouse's headache only.

		Yes	Sometimes	No
E1:	Because of headaches, my spouse feels handicapped	___	___	__
F2:	Because of headaches, my spouse feels restricted in performing his/her routine daily activities	___	___	__
E3:	No one understands the effect that my spouse's headaches have on his/her life	___	___	__
F4:	My spouse restricts his/her recreational activities (eg, sports, hobbies) because of his/her headaches	___	___	__
E5:	My spouse's headaches make him/her angry	___	___	__
E6:	Sometimes my spouse feels that he/she is going to lose control because of his/her headaches	___	___	__
F7:	What I am going through because of my spouse's headaches is not understood by family, friends, or even my spouse himself/herself	___	___	__
E8:	My spouse, family, and friends have no idea what I am going through because of his/her headaches	___	___	__
E9:	My spouse's headaches are so bad that he/she feels he/she is going to go insane	___	___	__
E10:	My spouse's outlook on the world is affected by his/her headaches	___	___	__
E11:	My spouse is afraid to go outside when he/she feels that a headache is starting	___	___	__
E12:	My spouse feels desperate because of his/her headaches	___	___	__
F13:	My spouse is concerned that he/she is paying penalties at work or at home because of headaches	___	___	__
E14:	My spouse's headaches place stress on his/her relationships with family or friends	___	___	__
F15:	My spouse avoids being around people when he/she has a headache	___	___	__

Figure 11-8.   Headache Disability Inventory. (From Jacobson GP, Ramadan NM, Aggarwal SK, et al. The Henry Ford Hospital Headache Disability Inventory [HDI]. *Neurology* 1994;44:837–42, with permission.) (continued)

F16:   My spouse believes his/her headaches are making it difficult
       for him/her to achieve goals in life   ———   ————   ——

F17:   My spouse is unable to think clearly because of his/her headaches   ———   ————   ——

F18:   My spouse gets tense (eg, muscle tension) because of his/her
       headaches   ———   ————   ——

F19:   My spouse does not enjoy social gatherings because of his/her
       headaches   ———   ————   ——

E20:   My spouse feels irritable because of his/her headaches   ———   ————   ——

F21:   My spouse avoids traveling because of his/her headaches   ———   ————   ——

E22:   My spouse's headaches make him/her feel confused   ———   ————   ——

E23:   My spouse's headaches make him/her feel frustrated   ———   ————   ——

F24:   My spouse finds it difficult to read because of his/her
       headaches   ———   ————   ——

F25:   My spouse finds it difficult to focus his/her attention away
       from headaches and on other things   ———   ————   ——

Figure 11-8.   *continued*

impact of headache on everyday life. Thus, the HDI can be used to (1) assess the impact of headache on the patient's daily living; (2) monitor the effect of therapeutic intervention; and (3) plan for a global approach to coping with headache, involving the patient.

Migraine Disability Assessment Scale

The MIDAS was developed to measure headache-related disability and improve doctor–patient communication about the functional consequences of migraine. The MIDAS questionnaire was based on five disability questions that focus on lost time in three domains: school work or work for pay; household work or chores; and family, social, and leisure activities (Stewart et al., 2001). This scale can be used by physicians, nurses, pharmacists, and alternative practitioners. The questionnaire is easy to complete and takes only a few minutes. The MIDAS questionnaire has demonstrated reliability (Stewart et al., 1999b), as reported in two separate population-based studies in the United States and United Kingdom, and validity, using a 3-month daily diary study as the gold standard (Stewart et al., 2000).

Scores on the MIDAS are highly correlated with physician judgments about the severity of illness and need for treatment (Holmes et al., 2001; Lipton et al., 2000b). The score of this instrument is as follows: little or no disability, 5–10; moderate disability, 10–20; and severe disability, more than 20. The MIDAS questionnaire is an important part of a package of educational, investigative, and therapeutic measures and could play a major role in improving the care of patients with migraine and other types of headaches (Chatterton et al., 2002; D'Amico et al., 2001; Dowson, 2001; Edmeads et al., 2001; Fragoso, 2002; Henry et al., 2002; Lipton et al., 2001b; Mathew et al., 2002; Stewart & Lipton, 2002). A randomized, placebo-controlled trial showed that the MIDAS grade provides a basis for selecting initial treatment in stratified care (Figure 11-9) (Lipton et al., 2000c; Sculpher et al., 2002).

Pediatric Migraine Disability Assessment Scale

The PedMIDAS scale is a pediatric version of the MIDAS that assesses disability in school-aged chil-

INSTRUCTIONS: Please answer the following questions about ALL your headaches you have had over the last 3 months. Write your answer in the box next to each question. Write zero if you did not do the activity in the last 3 months.

1 On how many days in the last 3 months did you miss work or school because of your headache?   ☐ days

2 How many days in the last 3 months was your productivity at work or school reduced by half or more because of your headaches? (Do not include days you counted in question 1 where you missed work or school).   ☐ days

3 On how many days in the last 3 months did you not do household work because of your headache?   ☐ days

4 How many days in the last 3 months was your productivity in household worked reduced by half or more because of your headaches? (Do not include days you counted in question 3 where you did not do household work).   ☐ days

5 On how many days in the last 3 months did you miss family, social or leisure activities because of your headaches?   ☐ days

TOTAL   ☐ days

A On how many days in the last 3 months did you have a headache? (If a headache lasted more than 1 day, count each day).   ☐ days

B On a scale of 0–10, on average how painful were these headaches? (where 0 = no pain at all, and 10 = pain as bad as it can be).   ☐ days

Once you have filled in the questionnaire, add up the total number of days from questions 1–5 (ignore A and B).

Grading system for the MIDAS Questionnaire:

Grade	Definition	Score
I	Little or no disability	0–5
II	Mild disability	6–10
III	Moderate disability	11–20
IV	Severe disability	21+

Figure 11-9. Migraine Disability Assessment (MIDAS) questionnaire. (From Stewart WF, Lipton RB, Dowson AJ, et al. Development and testing of the Migraine Disability Assessment [MIDAS] Questionnaire to assess headache-related disability. *Neurology* 2001;56[Suppl 1]:S20–28, with permission.)

dren and adolescents. The PedMIDAS questionnaire was administered to 441 patients for a total of 724 trials (Hershey et al., 2001). The validity was assessed by correlating scores with headache frequency, severity, and duration. Internal consistency and test-retest reliability were assessed. The PedMIDAS proved to be a sensitive, reliable, and valid assessment of the disability of childhood and adolescent headaches (Hershey et al., 2001). It can be used by physicians, nurses, or others involved in the care of children and adolescents. It is a tool to assess the impact of migraines in school-aged children and to monitor response to treatment (Figure 11-10).

Miscellaneous

Other instruments have been used in different studies to assess the quality, impact, or disability of headaches and the influence of treatment [Migraine Background Questionnaire (Lambert et al., 2002)]. Migraine Therapy Assessment Questionnaire (Chatterton et al., 2002) is a reliable and valid questionnaire to identify migraineurs whose migraine management may be suboptimal in a primary care setting. This tool is a brief, self-administered, reliable, valid instrument that may be used to help clinicians identify a migraine population who may have received inappropriate management (Figure 11-11).

Scales That Measure Pain

Verbal Descriptor Scales

Scales consisting of verbal descriptors have been used for simple reporting of subjective pain. These require only the choice of the best word descriptor from the patient. This scale can use words, numbers, letters, facial expression pictures, and colors.

Four-Level Categorical Scale

Headache pain intensity in clinical trials is usually measured using a four-level categorical scale (0 = none, 1 = mild, 2 = moderate, and 3 = severe). A score of "0" indicates that the patient has not felt pain; "1" indicates that the pain does not prohibit activities and

does not negatively influence the patient's job performance. At level "2," the pain influences the patient's job performance, but the patient does not miss work. At level "3," the pain influences work, school, and social situations, and the patient loses time from activities. This is the scale used in the IHS criteria to assess disability.

Numeric Rating Scale

Patients are asked to indicate how strong their pain is on a scale from 0 to 10 on which *0* represents *no pain at all* and *10* is *the worst pain imaginable.* This scale is easily understood by most patients and can be administered either orally or in written form (Chapman & Syrjala, 1990).

Visual Analog Scale

An equally simple and efficient alternative is the visual analog scale, which usually consists of a 10-cm line anchored at one end by a label such as "no pain" and at the other end by a label such as "the worst pain imaginable." The measurement can be marked on either a 1- to 10-cm or 1- to 100-mm scale (Figure 11-12). This scale has been validated in acute pain (Ohnhaus & Adler, 1975). Older patients have more difficulty with visual analog scale instruction. Examples using common pain problems can be helpful for patients who do not understand how to use the scale. Carlsson critically evaluated the visual analog scale as an indicator of pain state or pain relief in chronic pain patients, comparing different forms of the scale (Carlsson, 1983). Other research, however, has supported the reliability and validity of the visual analog scale as a sensitive measure of pain and change in pain (Ohnhaus & Adler, 1975).

Tactile Analog Scale

The tactile analog scale assesses the pain during migraine or other types of headaches in blind patients and those who cannot use vision during clinical tests. This scale was compared with the visual analog scale and validated in patients with normal vision (Piovesan et al., 2000).

INSTRUCTIONS: The following questions try to assess how much the headaches are affecting day-to-day activity. Your answers should be based on the last three months. There are no "right" or "wrong" answers so please put down your best guess.

1   How many full days of school were missed in the last 3 months due to headaches?   ☐☐ days

2   How many partial days of school were missed in the last 3 months due to headaches (do not include full days counted in the first question)?   ☐☐ days

3   How many days in the last 3 months did you function at less than half your ability in school because of a headache (do not include days counted in the first two questions)?   ☐☐ days

4   How many days were you not able to do things at home (i.e., chores, homework, etc.)?   ☐☐ days

5   How many days did you not participate in other activities due to headaches (i.e., play, go out, sports, etc.)?   ☐☐ days

How many days did you participate in these activities, but functioned at less than half your ability (do not include days counted in the 5th question)?   ☐☐ days

Total PedMIDAS Score   ☐☐

A   On how many days in the last 3 months did you have a headache? (If a headache lasted more than 1 day, count each day).   ☐☐ days

B   On a scale of 0–10, on average how painful were these headaches? (where 0 = no pain at all, and 10 = pain as bad as it can be).   ☐☐ days

Figure 11-10.   Pediatric Migraine Disability Assessment Scale (PedMIDAS) questionnaire. (From Hershey AD, Powers SW, Vockell AL, et al. PedMIDAS: Development of a questionnaire to assess disability of migraines in children. *Neurology* 2001;57:2034–39, with permission.)

YES   NO

☐   ☐   Most times, I get relief from my migraine symptoms within 2 hours after I take my migraine medicine.

☐   ☐   Most times, I can get back to what I was doing within 2 hours after I take my migraine medicine.

☐   ☐   Most months, I get 3 or more migraines.

☐   ☐   I take daily medicine to reduce how often I get migraines.

☐   ☐   I know what may bring on my migraines.

☐   ☐   Most times, I try not to use my migraine medicines right away.

☐   ☐   In the past month, I missed some school, work, or other activity because of a migraine.

☐   ☐   In the past 6 months, I had to go to an emergency or urgent care center for a migraine.

☐   ☐   I am satisfied with my migraine treatment.

Figure 11-11.   Migraine Therapy Assessment Questionnaire. (From Chatterton ML, Lofland JH, Shechter A, et al. Reliability and validity of the Migraine Therapy Assessment Questionnaire. *Headache* 2002;42:1006–15, with permission.)

INSTRUCTIONS: Mark on the lines below how strong your pain are right during the days.

Day

_____   No pain
               at all   ———————————————————————————— The worst
                                                         pain
                                                         imaginable

_____   ————————————————————————————

_____   ————————————————————————————

_____   ————————————————————————————

_____   ————————————————————————————

_____   ————————————————————————————

Figure 11-12.   Visual analog scale. (From Ohnhaus EE, Adler R. Methodological problems in the measurement of pain: a comparison between the verbal rating scale and the visual analogue scale. *Pain* 1975;1:379, with permission.)

References

Basilicato S, Groves M, Nisbet L, et al. Effect of concurrent chest pain assessment on retrospective reports by cardiac patients. *J Cardiovasc Nurs* 1992;7:56–67.

Bauer B, Evers S, Gralow I, et al. Psychosocial handicap due to chronic headaches. Evaluation of the inventory of disabilities caused by headache. *Nervenarzt* 1999;70:522–29.

Bjorner JB, Kosinsk M, Ware JE. Using item response theory to calibrate the Headache Impact Test (HIT) to the metric of traditional headache scales. *Qual Life Res* 2003;12:981–1002.

Block GA, Goldstein J, Polis A, et al. Efficacy and safety of rizatriptan versus standard care during long-term treatment for migraine. Rizatriptan Multicenter Study Group. *Headache* 1998;38:764–71.

Carlsson AM. Assessment of chronic pain. I. Aspects of the reliability and validity of the visual analog scale. *Pain* 1983;16:87–101.

Chapman CR, Syrjala KL. Measurement of pain. In: Bonica JJ, Loeser JD, Chapman CR, et al. *The management of pain*, 2nd ed., vol 1. Philadelphia: Lea & Febiger, 1990:581–94.

Chatterton ML, Lofland JH, Shechter A, et al. Reliability and validity of the Migraine Therapy Assessment Questionnaire. *Headache* 2002;42:1006–15.

Cramer JA, Silberstein SD, Winner P. Development and validation of the Headache Needs Assessment (HANA) survey. *Headache* 2001;41:402–9.

Dahlof C, Dimenas E. Migraine patients experience poorer subjective well-being quality of life even between attacks. *Cephalalgia* 1995;15:31–36.

D'Amico D, Mosconi P, Genco S, et al. The Migraine Disability Assessment (MIDAS) questionnaire: translation and reliability of the Italian version. *Cephalalgia* 2001;21:947–52.

Damiano A. The sickness impact profile. In: Spilker B (ed.). *Quality of life and pharmacoeconomics in clinical trials*. Philadelphia: Lippincott–Raven, 1996:347–54.

Deyo RA. Measuring functional outcomes in therapeutic trials for chronic disease. *Control Clin Trials* 1984;5:223–40.

Dowson AJ. Assessing the impact of migraine. *Curr Med Res Opin* 2001;17:298–309.

Edmeads J, Lainez JM, Brandes JL, et al. Potential of the Migraine Disability Assessment (MIDAS) questionnaire as a public health initiative and in clinical practice. *Neurology* 2001;56(Suppl 1):S29–34.

Fragoso YD. MIDAS (Migraine Disability Assessment): a valuable tool for work-site identification of migraine in workers in Brazil. *Sao Paulo Med J* 2002;120:118–21.

Guitera V, Munoz P, Castillo J, et al. Quality of life in chronic daily headache: a study in a general population. *Neurology* 2002;58:1062–65.

Hartmaier SL, Santanello NC, Epstein RS, et al. Development of a brief 24-hour migraine-specific quality of life questionnaire. *Headache* 1995;35:320–29.

Headache Classification Committee of the International Headache Society. Classification and diagnostic criteria for headache disorders, cranial neuralgias, and facial pain. *Cephalalgia* 1988;8(Suppl 7):1–96.

Henry P, Auray JP, Gaudin AF, et al. Prevalence and clinical characteristics of migraine in France. *Neurology* 2002;59:232–37.

Hershey AD, Powers SW, Vockell AL, et al. PedMIDAS: Development of a questionnaire to assess disability of migraines in children. *Neurology* 2001;57:2034–39.

Holmes WF, MacGregor EA, Sawyer JP, et al. Information about migraine disability influences physicians' perceptions of illness severity and treatment needs. *Headache* 2001;41:343–50.

Hunter M, Philips C, Rachman S. Memory for pain. *Pain* 1979;6:35–46.

Jacobson GP, Ramadam NM, Norris L, et al. Headache disability inventory (HDI): short-term test-retest reliability and spouse perceptions. *Headache* 1995;35:534–39.

Jacobson GP, Ramadan NM, Aggarwal SK, et al. The Henry Ford Hospital Headache Disability Inventory (HDI). *Neurology* 1994;44:837–42.

Jelicic M, Kempen GI, Passchier J. Psychological well-being in older adults suffering from chronic headache. *Headache* 1998;38:292–94.

Jhingran P, Cady RK, Rubino J, et al. Improvements in health-related quality of life with sumatriptan treatment for migraine. *J Fam Pract* 1996;42:36–42.

Kent G. Memory for dental pain. *Pain* 1985;21:187–94.

Lambert J, Carides GW, Meloche JP, et al. Impact of migraine symptoms on health care use and work loss in Canada in patients randomly assigned in a phase III clinical trial. *Can J Clin Pharmacol* 2002;9:158–64.

Linton SJ, Gotestam KG. A clinical comparison of two pain scales: correlation, remembering chronic pain, and a measure of compliance. *Pain* 1983;17:57–65.

Linton SJ, Melin L. The accuracy of remembering chronic pain. *Pain* 1982;13:281–85.

Lipton RB, Stewart WF. Migraine in the United States: a review of epidemiology and health care use. *Neurology* 1993;43(Suppl 3):S6–10.

Lipton RB, Hamelsky SW, Stewart WF. Epidemiology and impact of headache. In: Silberstein SD, Lipton RB, Dalessio DJ (eds.). *Wolff's headache and other head pain* (7th ed.). New York: Oxford University Press, 2001a:88–107.

Lipton RB, Stewart WF, Sawyer J, et al. Clinical utility of an instrument assessing migraine disability: the Migraine Disability Assessment (MIDAS) questionnaire. *Headache* 2001b;41:854–61.

Lipton RB, Hamelsky SW, Kolodner KB, et al. Migraine, quality of life, and depression: a population-based case-control study. *Neurology* 2000a;55:629–35.

Lipton RB, Goadsby PJ, Sawyer JP, et al. Migraine: diagnosis and assessment of disability. *Rev Contemp Pharmacother* 2000b;11:63–73.

Lipton RB, Stewart WF, Stone AM, et al. Stratified care vs step care strategies for migraine: the Disability in Strategies of Care (DISC) study: a randomized trial. *JAMA* 2000c;284:2599–605.

Mannix LK, Chandurkar RS, Rybicki LA, et al. Effect of guided imagery on quality of life for patients with chronic tension-type headache. *Headache* 1999;39:326–34.

Martin BC, Pathak DS, Sharfman MI, et al. Validity and reliability of the migraine-specific quality of life questionnaire (MSQ Version 2.1). *Headache* 2000;40:204–15.

Mathew NT, Kailasam J, Meadors L. Prophylaxis of migraine, transformed migraine, and cluster headache with topiramate. *Headache* 2002;42:796–803.

McEwen J, McKenna S. Nottingham health profile. In: Spilker B (ed.). *Quality of life and pharmacoeconomics in clinical trials*. Philadelphia: Lippincott–Raven, 1996:281–86.

McHorney C, Ware J, Raczek AE. The MOS 36-item short form health survey (SF-36): II. Psychometric and clinical tests of validity in measuring physical and mental health constructs. *Med Care* 1993;31:247–63.

Means F, Nigam A, Zarrow M. Autobiographical memory for health related events. National Center for Health Statistics. *Vital Health Stat* 1989;6:1–37.

Monzon MJ, Lainez MJ. Quality of life in migraine and chronic daily headache patients. *Cephalalgia* 1998; 18:638–43.

Mushet GR, Miller D, Clements B, et al. Impact of sumatriptan on workplace productivity, nonwork activities, and health-related quality of life among hospital employees with migraine. *Headache* 1996;36:137–43.

Ohnhaus EE, Adler R. Methodological problems in the measurement of pain: a comparison between the verbal rating scale and the visual analogue scale. *Pain* 1975; 1:379.

Osterhaus JT, Townsend RJ. The quality of life of migraineurs: a cross sectional profile. *Cephalalgia* 1991; 11(Suppl 11):103–4.

Osterhaus JT, Townsend RJ, Gandek B, et al. Measuring the functional status and well-being of patients with migraine headache. *Headache* 1994;34:337–43.

Osterhaus JT, Gutterman DL, Plachetka JR. Healthcare resource and lost labour costs of migraine headache in the U.S. *Pharmacoeconomics* 1992;2:67–76.

Piovesan EJ, Lange MC, Werneck LC, et al. Comparison study between visual analogue scale (VAS) and tactile analogue scale (TAS), a new scale. *Cephalalgia* 2000; 20(P-140):323.

Pryse-Phillips W. Evaluating migraine disability: the Headache Impact Test instrument in context. *Can J Neurol Sci* 2002;29(Suppl 2):S11–15.

Queiroz LP, Rapaport AM, Weeks RE, et al. Characteristics of migraine visual aura. *Headache* 1997;37:137–41.

Rasmussen BK, Jensen R, Schroll M, et al. Epidemiology of headache in a general population: a prevalence study. *J Clin Epidemiol* 1991;44:1147–57.

Ries PW. Current estimates from the national health interview survey, United States, 1984. National Center for Health Statistics: 1986 Vital and Health Statistics, Series 10, No. 156. Department of Health and Human Services Publication (PHS) 86-1584.

Roche PA, Gijsbers K. A comparison of memory for induced ischemic pain and chronic rheumatoid pain. *Pain* 1986;25:337–43.

Santanello N, Polis A, Hartmaier SL, et al. Improvement in migraine-specific quality of life in a clinical trial of rizatriptan. *Cephalalgia* 1997;17:867–72.

Santanello NC, Hartmaier SL, Epstein RS, et al. Validation of a new quality of life questionnaire for acute migraine headache. *Headache* 1995;35:330–37.

Schwartz BS, Stewart WF, Simon D, et al. Epidemiology of tension-type headache. *JAMA* 1998;279:381–83.

Sculpher SD, Millson D, Meddis D, et al. Cost-effectiveness analysis of stratified versus stepped care strategies for acute treatment of migraine: the Disability in Strategies for Care (DISC) study. *Pharmacoeconomics* 2002; 20:91–100.

Silberstein SD, Silberstein MM. New concepts in the pathogenesis of headache. Part II. *Pain Manage* 1990;3:334–42.

Silberstein SD, Lipton RB, Dalessio DJ. Overview, diagnosis, and classification of headache. In: Silberstein SD, Lipton RB, Dalessio DJ (eds.). *Wolff's headache and other head pain* (7th ed.). New York: Oxford University Press, 2001:6–26.

Silberstein SD, Lipton RB, Solomon S, et al. Classification of daily and near-daily headaches: proposed revisions to the IHS criteria. *Headache* 1994;34:1–7.

Solomon GD. Quality of life assessment in patients with headache. *Pharmacoeconomics* 1994;6:34–41.

Solomon GD, Skobieranda FG, Genzen JR. Quality of life assessment among migraine patients treated with sumatriptan. *Headache* 1995;35:449–54.

Solomon GD, Skobieranda FG, Gragg LA. Quality of life and well-being of headache patients: measurement by the Medical Outcomes Study instrument. *Headache* 1993; 33:351–58.

Solovey P, Sieber WJ, Smith AF, et al. Reporting chronic pain episodes in health surveys. National Center for Health Statistics. *Vital Health Stat* 1992;6:6.

Stewart W, Lipton R. Need for care and perceptions of MIDAS among headache sufferers study. *CNS Drugs* 2002;16(Suppl 1):5–11.

Stewart WF, Lipton RB, Dowson AJ, et al. Development and testing of the Migraine Disability Assessment (MIDAS) questionnaire to assess headache-related disability. *Neurology* 2001;56(Suppl 1):S20–28.

Stewart WF, Lipton RB, Kolodner KB, et al. Validity of the Migraine Disability Assessment (MIDAS) score in comparison to a diary-based measure in a population sample of migraine sufferers. *Pain* 2000;88:41–52.

Stewart WF, Lipton RB, Simon D, et al. Validity of an illness severity measure for headache in a population sample of migraine sufferers. *Pain* 1999a;79:291–301.

Stewart WF, Lipton RB, Whyte J, et al. An international study to assess reliability of the Migraine Disability Assessment (MIDAS) score. *Neurology* 1999b;53:988–94.

Stewart WF, Lipton RB, Simon D, et al. Reliability of an illness severity measure for headache in a population sample of migraine sufferers. *Cephalalgia* 1998;18:44–51.

Stewart AL, Greenfield S, Hays RD, et al. Functional status and well-being of patients with chronic conditions. Results from the Medical Outcomes Study. *JAMA* 1989;262:907–13.

Stewart A, Hays R, Ware JE Jr. The MOS short form general health survey. Reliability and validity in a patient population. *Med Care* 1988;26:724–35.

Tarlov AR, Ware JE Jr., Greenfeld S, et al. The Medical Outcomes Study. An application of methods for monitoring the results of medical care. *JAMA* 1989;262:925–30.

Terwindt GM, Ferrari MD, Tijhuis M, et al. The impact of migraine on quality of life in the general population: the GEM study. *Neurology* 2000;55:624–29.

Vanast WJ. New daily persistent headaches: definition of a benign syndrome. *Headache* 1986;26:317.

Wagner TH, Patrick DL, Galer BS, et al. A new instrument to assess the long-term quality of life effects from migraine: development and psychometric testing of the MSQOL. *Headache* 1996;36:484–92.

Wang SJ, Fuh JL, Lu SR, et al. Quality of life differs among headache diagnoses: analysis of SF-36 survey in 901 headache patients. *Pain* 2001;89:285–92.

Ware JE Jr., Sherbourne CD. The MOS 36-item short-form health survey (SF-36). I. Conceptual framework and item selection. *Med Care* 1992;30:473–83.

Ware JE, Bjorner JB, Kosinski M. Practical implications of item response theory and computerized adaptive testing: a brief summary of ongoing studies of widely used headache impact scales. *Med Care* 2000a;38(Suppl 2):S73–82.

Ware J, Kosinski M, Keller SD. A 12-item short form health survey: construction of scales and preliminary tests of reliability and validity. *Med Care* 1996;34:220–33.

12 Scales for Assessment of Ataxia

Robert M. Herndon, M.D.

T he spinocerebellar degenerations are a heterogeneous set of disorders with overlapping phenotypes. There are now some 26 genetically defined dominantly inherited spinocerebellar atrophies and several recessively inherited spinocerebellar diseases, the most common being Friedreich's ataxia. Clinical diagnostic criteria have been published for Friedreich's ataxia; however, they lack sensitivity (Filla et al., 2000), and molecular diagnosis is essential. Formal diagnostic criteria have not been found for the recessive spinocerebellar ataxias, for which genetic testing appears necessary for diagnosis given the extensive overlap in clinical syndromes. There are good clinical descriptions of these disorders, but given their variability, it is unlikely that satisfactory clinical diagnostic criteria can be developed. Genetic testing remains the gold standard for all of the hereditary ataxias. In addition to the hereditary ataxias, there are a substantial number of patients with progressive ataxia of unknown cause. Two rating scales for ataxia are discussed, the International Cooperative Ataxia Rating Scale (Storey et al., 2004) and one specifically for Friedreich's ataxia (Subramony et al., 2005). These are relatively new scales designed primarily for clinical trials.

International Cooperative Ataxia Rating Scale

Description

The International Cooperative Ataxia Rating Scale was developed by the Ataxia Neuropharmacology Committee of the World Federation of Neurology for the purpose of planning and developing clinical trials in the hereditary ataxias (Table 12-1) (Trouillas et al., 1997). It is a 100-point scale, with 0 being normal and the theoretical maximum being 100.

Administration

The scale is typically done by a physician but could be done by a trained technician.

Time to Administer

The estimated time to administer is 10–15 minutes.

Table 12-1.   International Cooperative Ataxia Rating Scale (World Federation of Neurology)

I. Posture and gait disturbances

  1. Walking capacities

     (Observed during a 10-m test, including a half turn, near a wall, at approximately 1.5 m)

     0 = Normal

     1 = Almost normal naturally but unable to walk with feet in tandem position

     2 = Walking without support but clearly abnormal and irregular

     3 = Walking without support but with considerable staggering; difficulties in half turn

     4 = Walking with autonomous support no longer possible; the patient uses the episodic support of the wall for a 10-m test

     5 = Walking only possible with one stick

     6 = Walking only possible with two special sticks or with a stroller

     7 = Walking only with accompanying person

     8 = Walking impossible, even with accompanying person (wheelchair)

     Score:

  2. Gait speed

     (Observed in patients with preceding scores 1–3; preceding score 4 and up automatically gives score 4 in this test)

     0 = Normal

     1 = Slightly reduced

     2 = Markedly reduced

     3 = Extremely slow

     4 = Walking with autonomous support no longer possible

     Score:

  3. Standing capacities, eyes open

     (The patient is asked first to try to stand on one foot; if impossible, to stand with feet in tandem position; if impossible, to stand feet together; for the natural position, the patient is asked to find a comfortable standing position.)

     0 = Normal: able to stand on one foot >10 sec

     2 = Able to stand with feet together but no longer able to stand with feet in tandem position

     3 = No longer able to stand with feet together but able to stand in natural position without support, with no or moderate sway

     4 = Standing in natural position without support, with considerable sway and considerable corrections

     5 = Unable to stand in natural position without strong support of one arm

     6 = Unable to stand at all, even with strong support of two arms

     Score:

  4. Spread of feet in natural position without support, eyes open

     (The patient is asked to find a comfortable position and then the distance between medial malleoli is measured.)

     0 = Normal (<10 cm)

     1 = Slightly enlarged (>10 cm)

     2 = Clearly enlarged (25 cm < spread <35 cm)

Table 12-1. *(continued)*

3 = Severely enlarged (>35 cm)

4 = Standing in natural position impossible

Score:

5. Body sway with feet together, eyes open

   0 = Normal

   1 = Slight oscillations

   2 = Moderate oscillations (<10 cm at the level of head)

   3 = Severe oscillations (>10 cm at the level of head), threatening the upright position

   4 = Immediate falling

   Score:

6. Body sway with feet together, eyes closed

   0 = Normal

   1 = Slight oscillations

   2 = Moderate oscillations (<10 cm at the level of head)

   3 = Severe oscillations (>10 cm at the level of head), threatening the upright position

   4 = Immediate falling

   Score:

7. Quality of sitting position

   (Thighs together, on a hard surface, arms folded)

   0 = Normal

   1 = With slight oscillations of the trunk

   2 = With moderate oscillations of the trunk and legs

   3 = With severe dysequilibrium

   4 = Impossible

   Score: Posture and gait score (static score): _____/34

II. Kinetic functions

8. Knee-tibia test (decomposition of movement and intention tremor)

   (The test is performed in the supine position, but the head is tilted so that visual control is possible. The patient is requested to raise one leg and place the heel on the knee, and then slide the heel down the anterior tibial surface of the resting leg toward the ankle. On reaching the ankle joint, the leg is again raised in the air to a height of approximately 40 cm, and the action is repeated. At least three movements of each limb must be performed for proper assessment.)

   0 = Normal

   1 = Lowering of heel in continuous axis, but the movement is decomposed in several phases, without real jerks, or abnormally slow

   2 = Lowering jerkily in the axis

   3 = Lowering jerkily with lateral movements

   4 = Lowering jerkily with extremely strong lateral movements or test impossible

   Score right: Score left:

(continued)

Table 12-1. *(continued)*

9. Action tremor in the heel-to-knee test

   (Same test as preceding one: The action tremor of the heel on the knee is specifically observed when the patient holds the heel on the knee for a few seconds before sliding down the anterior tibial surface; visual control is required.)

   0 = No trouble

   1 = Tremor stopping immediately when the heel reaches the knee

   2 = Tremor stopping in <10 sec after reaching the knee

   3 = Tremor continuing for >10 sec after reaching the knee

   4 = Uninterrupted tremor or test impossible

   Score right: Score left:

10. Finger-to-nose test: decomposition and dysmetria

    (The subject sits on a chair; the hand is resting on the knee before the beginning of the movement; visual control is required. Three movements of each limb must be performed for proper assessment.)

    0 = No trouble

    1 = Oscillating movement without decomposition of the movement

    2 = Segmented movement in two phases and/or moderate dysmetria in reaching nose

    3 = Segmented movement in more than two phases and/or considerable dysmetria in reaching nose

    4 = Dysmetria preventing the patient from reaching nose

    Score right: Score left:

11. Finger-to-nose test: intention tremor of the finger

    (The studied tremor is that appearing during the ballistic phase of the movement; the patient is sitting comfortably, with his or her hand resting on his or her thigh; visual control is required; three movements of each limb must be performed for proper assessment.)

    0 = No trouble

    1 = Simple swerve of the movement

    2 = Moderate tremor with estimated amplitude <10 cm

    3 = Tremor with estimated amplitude between 10 and 40 cm

    4 = Severe tremor with estimated amplitude >40 cm

    Score right: Score left:

12. Finger-finger test (action tremor and/or instability)

    (The sitting patient is asked to maintain medially his or her two index fingers pointing at each other for approximately 10 sec, at a distance of approximately 1 cm, at the level of the thorax, under visual control.)

    0 = Normal

    1 = Mild instability

    2 = Moderate oscillations of finger with estimated amplitude <10 cm

    3 = Considerable oscillations of finger with estimated amplitude between 10 and 40 cm

    4 = Jerky movements >40 cm of amplitude

    Score right: Score left:

Table 12-1. *(continued)*

13. Pronation-supination alternating movements

(The subject, comfortably sitting on a chair, is asked to raise his or her forearm vertically and to make alternative movements of the hand. Each hand is moved and assessed separately.)

0 = Normal

1 = Slightly irregular and slowed

2 = Clearly irregular and slowed but without sway of the elbow

3 = Extremely irregular and slowed movement, with sway of the elbow

4 = Movement completely disorganized or impossible

Score right: Score left:

14. Drawing of the Archimedes' spiral on a predrawn pattern

(The subject is comfortably settled in front of a table, the sheet of paper being fixed to avoid artifacts. The subject is asked to perform the task without timing requirements. The same conditions of examination must be used at each examination: same table, same pen. The dominant hand is examined.)

0 = Normal

1 = Impairment and decomposition, the line quitting the pattern slightly, but without hypermetric swerve

2 = Line completely out of the pattern with recrossings and/or hypermetric swerves

3 = Major disturbance due to hypermetria and decomposition

4 = Drawing completely disorganized or impossible

Score: Kinetic score (limb coordination):_____/52

III. Speech disorders

15. Dysarthria: fluency of speech

(The patient is asked to repeat several times a standard sentence, always the same, for instance, "A mischievous spectacle in Czechoslovakia.")

0 = Normal

1 = Mild modification of fluency

2 = Moderate modification of fluency

3 = Considerably slow and dysarthric speech

4 = No speech

Score:

16. Dysarthria: clarity of speech

0 = Normal

1 = Suggestion of slurring

2 = Definite slurring, most words understandable

3 = Severe slurring, speech not understandable

4 = No speech

Score: Dysarthria score:_____/8

(continued)

Table 12-1. *(continued)*

IV. Oculomotor disorders

17. Gaze-evoked nystagmus

(The subject is asked to look laterally at the finger of the examiner; the movements assessed are mainly horizontal, but they may be oblique, rotatory, or vertical.)

0 = Normal

1 = Transient

2 = Persistent but moderate

3 = Persistent and severe

Score:

18. Abnormalities of the ocular pursuit

(The subject is asked to follow the slow lateral movement performed by the finger of the examiner.)

0 = Normal

1 = Slightly saccadic

2 = Clearly saccadic

Score:

19. Dysmetria of the saccade

(The two index fingers of the examiner are placed in each temporal visual field of the patient, whose eyes are in the primary position; the patient is then asked to look laterally at the finger, on the right and on the left; the average overshoot or undershoot of the two sides is then estimated.)

0 = Absent

1 = Bilateral clear overshoot or undershoot of the saccade

Score: Oculomotor movement score:_____/6

Total ataxia score:_____/100

Validation

Storey et al. (2004) looked at inter-rater reliability in a group of patients that included 11 patients with spinocerebellar ataxia type I, one with spinocerebellar ataxia type II, and 10 with genetically confirmed Friedreich's ataxia. Videotapes were made of International Cooperative Ataxia Rating Scale assessment by neurologists not specifically trained in movement disorders. Excellent inter-observer reliability was obtained by two movement disorder specialists observing the videotapes, with a Kendall's ω ranging from 0.791 to 0.994 for various subscales. Further work is needed to assess sensitivity to change and reliability in larger populations and other ataxias.

Summary

This scale requires considerably more evaluation and use by the medical community before its characteristics will be fully understood. Work needs to be done to establish its sensitivity to change and its reliability in larger populations.

Friedreich's Ataxia Rating Scale

Description

Friedreich's Ataxia Rating Scale is a new scale developed by the cooperative ataxia group for assessing impairment in Friedreich's ataxia, with a view to initiating a clinical treatment trial (Table 12-2).

Table 12-2.   Friedreich's Ataxia Scale

I. Functional staging for ataxia (Increments of 0.5 may be used if the status is approximately the middle between two stages.)

Stage ☐ ☐

Stage 0	Normal.
Stage 1.0	Minimal signs detected by physician during screening. Can run or jump without loss of balance. No disability.
Stage 2.0	Symptoms present, recognized by patient, but still mild. Cannot run or jump without losing balance. The patient is physically capable of leading an independent life, but daily activities may be somewhat restricted. Minimal disability.
Stage 3.0	Symptoms are overt and significant. Requires regular or periodic holding onto wall/furniture or use of a cane for stability and walking. Mild disability. (Note: Many patients postpone obtaining a cane by avoiding open spaces and walking with the aid of walls/people, etc. These patients are graded as stage 3.0.)
Stage 4.0	Walking requires a walker, Canadian crutches, or two canes (or other aids such as walking dogs). Can perform several activities of daily living. Moderate disability.
Stage 5.0	Confined but can navigate a wheelchair. Can perform some activities of daily living that do not require standing or walking. Severe disability.
Stage 6.0	Confined to wheelchair or bed with total dependency for all activities of daily living. Total disability.

II. Activities of daily living (Increments of 0.5 may be used if strongly felt that a task falls between 2 scores.)

1. Speech   ☐

    0—Normal.

    1—Mildly affected. No difficulty being understood.

    2—Moderately affected. Sometimes asked to repeat statements.

    3—Severely affected. Frequently asked to repeat statements.

    4—Unintelligible most of the time.

2. Swallowing   ☐

    0—Normal.

    1—Rare choking (less than once a month).

    2—Frequent choking (less than once a week, more than once a month).

    3—Requires modified food or chokes multiple times a week, or patient avoids certain foods.

    4—Requires nasogastric tube or gastrostomy feedings.

3. Cutting food and handling utensils   ☐

    0—Normal.

    1—Somewhat slow and clumsy but no help needed.

    2—Clumsy and slow but can cut most foods with some help needed, or needs assistance when in a hurry.

    3—Food must be cut by someone but can still feed self slowly.

    4—Needs to be fed.

(continued)

Table 12-2. *(continued)*

4. Dressing

    0—Normal.

    1—Somewhat slow but no help needed.

    2—Occasional assistance with buttoning, getting arms in sleeves, etc., or has to modify activity in some way (e.g., having to sit to get dressed; use Velcro for shoes, stop wearing ties).

    3—Considerable help required but can do some things alone.

    4—Helpless.

5. Personal hygiene

    0—Normal.

    1—Somewhat slow but no help needed.

    2—Very slow hygienic care or has need for devices such as special grab bars, tub bench, shower chair, etc.

    3—Requires personal help with washing, brushing teeth, combing hair, or using toilet.

    4—Fully dependent.

6. Falling (assistive device = score 3)

    0—Normal.

    1—Rare falling (less than once a month).

    2—Occasional falls (once a week to once a month).

    3—Falls multiple times a week or requires device to prevent falls.

    4—Unable to stand or walk.

7. Walking (assistive device = score 3)

    0—Normal.

    1—Mild difficulty, perception of imbalance.

    2—Moderate difficulty but requires little or no assistance.

    3—Severe disturbance of walking, requires assistance or walking aids.

    4—Cannot walk at all even with assistance (wheelchair-bound).

8. Quality of sitting position

    0—Normal.

    1—Slight imbalance of the trunk but needs no back support.

    2—Unable to sit without back support.

    3—Can sit only with extensive support (geriatric chair, posy, etc.).

    4—Unable to sit.

9. Bladder function (if using drugs for bladder, automatic score of 3)

    0—Normal.

    1—Mild urinary hesitance, urgency, or retention (less than once a month).

    2—Moderate hesitance, urgency, rare retention/incontinence (more than once a month but less than once a week).

    3—Frequent urinary incontinence (more than once a week).

    4—Loss of bladder function requiring intermittent catheterization/indwelling catheter.

Total activities of daily living score:

Table 12-2. *(continued)*

III. Neurologic examination (Rate each item on the basis of the patient status during examination. To the extent possible, sequential patient examinations should be carried out at the same time of the day. If the patient is taking any medication, the examination should be carried out before dosing or at a fixed time after the dosing based on the maximum expected therapeutic response. Increments of 0.5 may be used if examiner believes an item falls between two defined severities.)

A. Bulbar

1. Facial atrophy, fasciculation, action myoclonus, and weakness

   0—None.

   1—Fasciculations or action myoclonus, but no atrophy.

   2—Atrophy present but not profound or complete.

   3—Profound atrophy and weakness.

2. Tongue atrophy, fasciculation, action myoclonus, and weakness

   0—None.

   1—Fasciculations or action myoclonus, but no atrophy.

   2—Atrophy present but not profound or complete.

   3—Profound atrophy and weakness.

3. Cough (patient asked to cough forcefully three times)

   0—Normal.

   1—Depressed.

   2—Totally or nearly absent.

4. Spontaneous speech (Ask the patient to read or repeat the sentences "The president lives in the White House" or "The traffic is heavy today.")

   0—Normal.

   1—Mild (all or most words understandable).

   2—Moderate (most words not understandable).

   3—Severe (no or almost no useful speech).

Total bulbar score:

B. Upper limb coordination

1. Finger-to-finger test (The index fingers are placed in front of each other, with flexion at the elbow approximately 25 cm from the sternum. Observe for 10 sec. Score amplitude of oscillations.)

   0—Normal.   Right   Left

   1—Mild oscillations of finger (<2 cm).

   2—Moderate oscillations of finger (2–6 cm).

   3—Severe oscillations of finger (>6 cm).

2. Nose-finger test (Assess kinetic or intention tremor during and toward the end of movement: examiner holds index finger at 90% reach of patient; test at least three nose-finger-nose trials; movement slow >3 sec.)

   0—None.   Right   Left

   1—Mild (<2 cm amplitude).

   2—Moderate (2–4 cm amplitude or persisting through movement).

   3—Severe (>6 cm and persisting through movement).

   4—Too poorly coordinated to perform task.

(continued)

Table 12-2. *(continued)*

3. Dysmetria (fast nose-finger) test (Assess dysmetria: The patient touches tip of examiner's finger eight times as rapidly as possible while the examiner moves his or her finger and stops at different locations at approximately 90% reach of the patient. Assess dysmetria—i.e., inaccuracy of reaching the target—at examiner's finger.)

    0—None.
    1—Mild (misses two or fewer times).
    2—Moderate (misses three to five times).
    3—Severe (misses six to eight times).
    4—Too poorly coordinated to perform task.

                Right   Left

4. Rapid alternating movements of hands (forearm pronation/supination 15 cm above thigh; 10 full cycles as fast as possible; assess rate, rhythm, accuracy; practice 10 cycles before rating, if time >7 sec, add 1 to score; use stopwatch)

    0—Normal.
    1—Mild (slightly irregular or slowed).
    2—Moderate (irregular and slowed).
    3—Too poorly coordinated to perform task.

                Right   Left

5. Finger taps (index fingertip-to-thumb crease; 15 repetitions as fast as possible; practice 15 repetitions once before rating; if time >6 sec, add 1 to rating; use stopwatch)

    0—Normal.
    1—Mild (misses one to three times).
    2—Moderate (misses four to nine times).
    3—Severe (misses 10–15 times).
    4—Cannot perform the task.

                Right   Left

Total upper limb coordination score:

C. Lower limb coordination

1. Heel-along-shin slide (Under visual control, slide heel on the contralateral tibia from the patella to the ankle up and down, three cycles at moderate speed, 2-sec cycle, one at a time. May be seated with contralateral leg extended or supine but perform same way each time. Circle which: supine   seated)

    0—Normal (stay on shin).
    1—Mild (abnormally slow, tremulous but contact maintained).
    2—Moderate (goes off shin a total of three or fewer times during three cycles).
    3—Severe (goes off shin four or more times during three cycles).
    4—Too poorly coordinated to attempt the task.

                Right   Left

2. Heel-to-shin tap (Patient taps heel on midpoint of contralateral shin eight times on each side from approximately 6–10 in., one at a time. May be seated with contralateral leg extended or supine, but perform the same way each time. Circle which: supine   seated)

    0—Normal (stays on target).
    1—Mild (misses shin two or more times).
    2—Moderate (misses shin three to five times).
    3—Severe (misses shin more than four times).
    4—Too poorly coordinated to perform task.

                Right   Left

Total lower limb coordination score:

Table 12-2. *(continued)*

D. Peripheral nervous system

1. Muscle atrophy (score most severe atrophy in either upper or lower limb)

   0—None.
   1—Present—mild/moderate.
   2—Severe/total wasting.

   Right   Left

2. Muscle weakness (Test deltoids, interossei, iliopsoas, and tibialis anterior. Score most severe weakness in either upper or lower limb.)

   0—Normal (5/5).
   1—Mild (movement against resistance but not full power 4/5).
   2—Moderate (movement against gravity but not with added resistance 3/5).
   3—Severe (movement of joint but not against gravity 2/5).
   4—Near paralysis (muscular activity without movement 1/5).
   5—Total paralysis (0/5).

   Right   Left

3. Vibratory sense (Educate patient regarding the sensation. Tested with 128 cps tuning fork set to near full vibration, eyes closed, test over index finger and great toe. Abnormal <15 sec for toes and <25 sec for hands.)

                        Right   Left
   Time felt for toes: _____   _____
   Time felt for fingers: _____   _____

   0—Normal.
   1—Impaired at toes.
   2—Impaired at toes or fingers.

   Right   Left

4. Position sense (Test using minimal random movement of distal interphalangeal joints of index finger and big toe.)

   0—Normal.
   1—Impaired at toes and/or fingers.
   2—Impaired at toes and fingers.

   Right   Left

5. Deep tendon reflexes (0—absent; 1—hyporeflexia; 2—normal; 3—hyperreflexia; 4—pathologic hyperreflexia)

   Right:
   Biceps jerk (BJ)_____   Brachioradialis jerk (BrJ)_____   Knee jerk (KJ)_____   Ankle jerk (AJ)_____

   Left:
   BJ_____   BrJ_____   KJ_____   AJ_____

   0—No areflexia.
   1—Areflexia in either upper or lower limbs.
   2—Generalized areflexia.

   Right   Left

Total peripheral nervous system score:

(continued)

Table 12-2.   *(continued)*

E. Upright stability (For sitting posture, patient can sit in a chair or on an examination table. For standing and walking assessment, instruct patient to wear best walking shoes, and record below if barefoot, footwear, or ankle-foot orthosis used. Stance assessment begins with feet 20 cm apart. Place marker tapes in the examination room 20 cm apart; the insides of the feet are lined up against these. Subsequent stance tests are more difficult. For feet together, the entire inside of the feet should be close together as much as possible. For tandem stance, the dominant foot is in the back, and the heel of the other foot is lined with the toes of the dominant foot but not in front of the toes [because this makes it even more difficult]. For one-foot stance, the patient is asked to stand on dominant foot, and the other leg is elevated by bringing it forward, with knee extended; this gives some advantage to the patient. If a patient can stand in a particular position for 1 min or longer in trial 1, then trials 2 and 3 are abandoned. Otherwise, each of three trials is timed and then averaged. Grading scores are then given as noted. Tandem walk and gait are performed in a hallway, preferably with no carpet, but at least serial examinations should be on the same surface. For gait, place markers 25 ft apart. Patient walks the distance, turns around, and comes back, and the activity is timed. Note if the gait was achieved with or without device; serial examinations should be done with the same device as in the first examination.)

(Stance and gait tests may be done barefoot if patient does have appropriate footwear; however, it should be done the same way for serial measurement.)

Circle which: Barefoot   Footwear

Also, indicate if ankle-foot   Yes   No
   orthoses are used:

1. Sitting posture (patient seated in chair with thighs together, arms folded, back unsupported; observe for 30 seconds)

   0—Normal.

   1—Mild oscillations of head/trunk without touching chair back or side.

   2—Moderate oscillations of head/trunk; needs contact with chair back or side for stability.

   3—Severe oscillations of head/trunk; needs contact with chair back or side for stability.

   4—Support on all four sides for stability.

2. Stance—feet apart (inside of feet 20 cm apart marked on floor; use stopwatch; three attempts; time in seconds)

   Trial 1 [ ]   Trial 2 [ ]   Trial 3 [ ]   Average [ ]

   0—1 min or longer.

   1—<1 min, >45 sec.

   2—<45 sec, >30 sec.

   3—<30 sec, >15 sec.

   4—<15 sec or needs hands held by assistant/device.

3. Stance—feet together (use stopwatch; three attempts; time in seconds)

   Trial 1 [ ]   Trial 2 [ ]   Trial 3 [ ]   Average [ ]

   0—1 min or longer.

   1—<1 min, >45 sec.

   2—<45 sec, >30 sec.

   3—<30 sec, >15 sec.

   4—<15 sec.

Table 12-2. *(continued)*

4. Tandem stance (use stopwatch; three attempts, dominant foot in front; time in seconds)

   Trial 1 ☐   Trial 2 ☐   Trial 3 ☐   Average ☐

   0—1 min or longer.

   1—<1 min, >45 sec.

   2—<45 sec, >30 sec.

   3—<30 sec, >15 sec.

   4—<15 sec.

5. Stance on dominant foot (use stopwatch; three attempts; time in seconds)

   Trial 1 ☐   Trial 2 ☐   Trial 3 ☐   Average ☐

   0—1 min or longer.

   1—<1 min, >45 sec.

   2—<45 sec, >30 sec.

   3—<30 sec, >15 sec.

   4—<15 sec.

6. Tandem walk (tandem walk 10 steps in straight line; performed in hallway with no furniture within reach of 1 m/3 ft and no loose carpet)

   0—Normal (able to tandem walk more than eight sequential steps).   ☐

   1—Able to tandem walk in less than perfect manner; can tandem walk more than four sequential steps but fewer than eight.

   2—Can tandem walk but fewer than four steps before losing balance.

   3—Too poorly coordinated to attempt task.

7. Gait (use stopwatch; walk 8 m/25 ft at normal pace, turn around using single step pivot and return to start; performed in hallway with no furniture within reach of 1 m/3 ft and no loose carpet)

   Device, if any: _____   ☐

   Time in seconds: _____

   0—Normal.

   1—Mild ataxia/veering/difficulty in turning; no cane/other support needed to be safe.

   2—Walks with definite ataxia; may need intermittent support/or examiner needs to walk with patient for safety's sake.

   3—Moderate ataxia/veering/difficulty in turning; walking requires cane/holding onto examiner with one hand to be safe.

   4—Severe ataxia/veering; walker or both hands of examiner needed.

   5—Cannot walk even with assistance (wheelchair bound).

Total upright stability score: ☐

Total neurologic examination score: ☐

(continued)

Table 12-2. *(continued)*

IV. Instrumental testing

    1. PaTa rate (Use a tape recorder that can play at slow and fast speeds [1.2 and 2.4 cm/sec]. Record at normal [2.4] speed. Use a digital stopwatch. Patient is seated comfortably and instructed to repeat the syllable "PaTa" as quickly and distinctly as possible for 10 sec until told to stop. Start recorder and record patient's name and date. Preset stopwatch for 10 sec. Say "go," and as soon as patient starts speaking, start timer. Say "stop" when timer beeps at end of 10 sec. Perform test twice and count number of "PaTas" for each 10 sec, using playback at slower speed. Record number for each trial and also the average score.)

        Trial 1 [   ]   Trial 2 [   ]   Average [   ]

    2. Nine hole pegboard (Make sure the stopwatch is set to 0. Introduce this section by saying, "Now, we're going to be measuring your arm and hand function." If this is the first visit, ask, "Are you right- or left-handed?" Make a note of the dominant hand for subsequent instructions. Place the Nine Hole Peg Test apparatus on the table directly in front of the patient. Arrange the apparatus so that the side with the pegs is in front of the hand being tested and the side with the empty pegboard is in front of the hand not being tested. Secure with Dycem. Read the following instructions to the patient: "On this test, I want you to pick up the pegs one at a time, using one hand only, and put them into the holes as quickly as you can in any order until all the holes are filled. Then, without pausing, remove the pegs one at a time, and return them to the container as quickly as you can. We'll have you do this two [2] times with each hand. We'll start with your [*dominant*] hand. You can hold the pegboard steady with your [*nondominant*] hand. If a peg falls onto the table, you retrieve it and continue with the task. If a peg falls on the floor, keep working on the task, and I will retrieve it for you. See how fast you can put all the pegs in and take them out again. Are you ready? Begin."

    Start timing as soon as the patient touches the first peg, and stop timing when the last peg hits the container. If a peg drops on the floor, the examiner will retrieve it and put it back in the peg box. However, if a peg drops onto the table, the patient is to retrieve it unless it is beyond his or her arm reach, in which case you can retrieve it for the patient. It is possible that a peg may fall beyond the reach of the examiner; therefore, it is recommended that you keep a few extra pegs in hand so that testing is not interrupted. Do not put extra pegs in the testing apparatus, as this may confuse the subject. Record the patient's time under "Dominant hand—trial 1." If the subject stops after having put all the pegs into the holes, prompt the subject to remove them as well by saying, "And now remove them all." If the subject begins to remove more than one peg at a time, correct him or her by saying, "Pick up one peg at a time."

    The total time to complete the task is recorded in seconds, including one decimal place rounded as needed. Round up to the next tenth if hundredths place is ≥0.05, round down if hundredths place is <0.5.)

                   Right   Left

    Trial 1 [   ]   Trial 1 [   ]

    Trial 2 [   ]   Trial 2 [   ]

    Average [   ]   Average [   ]

Validation

The scale was tested by a group of seven neurologists testing 14 patients in various stages of the disease. Inter-rater reliability was excellent for disease stage, activities of daily living, upper limb coordination, lower limb coordination, upright stability/gait, total neurologic examination, PATA rate, pegboard, and gait times. Bulbar and peripheral nerve scores were somewhat less reliable.

Administration

Testing is done by a neurologist and requires approximately 30 minutes.

Advantages

This is a new scale specifically designed for clinical trials in Friedreich's ataxia. It appears to have good reliability.

Disadvantages

It has had very limited use thus far, and further information is required to assess its overall usefulness. No information on sensitivity to change in Friedreich's has been reported. Its adaptability to other forms of progressive ataxia such as spinocerebellar ataxia has not been reported.

Summary

Friedreich's Ataxia Rating Scale is a first effort at developing a scale for scoring ataxia. Whether the scale or portions of it will be suitable for broader application in degenerative ataxias remains unknown.

The development of rating scales for the ataxias is in its infancy. There is much work to be done to establish the responsiveness and generalizability of these scales, but the Ataxia Neuropharmacology Committee of the World Federation of Neurology and the Cooperative Ataxia Group have made a good start in this area. Further development and validation of these scales is essential for the development of therapeutic trials for these diseases.

References

Filla A, De Michele G, Coppola G, et al. Accuracy of clinical diagnostic criteria for Friedreich's ataxia. *Mov Disord* 2000;15:1255–58.

Storey E, Tuck K, Hester R, et al. Inter-rater reliability of the International Cooperative Ataxia Rating Scale (ICARS) *Mov Disord* 2004;19:190–92.

Subramony SH, May W, Lynch D, et al. Measuring Friedreich ataxia: Interrater reliability of a neurologic rating scale. *Neurology* 2005;64:1261–62.

Trouillas P, Takayanagi T, Hallett M, et al. International Cooperative Ataxia Rating Scale for pharmacological assessment of the cerebellar syndrome. *J Neurol Sci* 1997; 145:205–11.

13 Assessment of Traumatic Brain Injury

Risa Nakase-Richardson, Ph.D., Frances Spinosa, R.N., Charles F. Swearingen, B.S., and Domenic Esposito, M.D.

Individuals with traumatic brain injury (TBI) manifest with a variety of symptom complexes. Initial evaluation determines severity level and need for certain types of interventions. Patients are evaluated with protocols that depend on level of neurologic responsiveness on presentation to an emergency department. Neurologic classification by Glasgow Coma Scale (GCS) and abnormalities on computed tomography scan commonly determine initial severity levels and need for subsequent intervention. During subsequent monitoring of recovery from TBI, components of the neurologic examination (e.g., command following, motor localization) have been used to indicate emergence from minimally responsive states (Giacino et al., 2002; Levin, 1995; Whyte et al., 2001).

Once an individual has returned to a responsive state, the duration of posttraumatic amnesia (PTA) has been considered one of the best indicators of TBI severity and eventual outcome (Ellenberg et al., 1996; Jennett & MacMillan, 1981; Teasdale & Jennett, 1974). PTA is considered the period of recovery after TBI during which the patient has not returned to full consciousness. Once a TBI patient returns to a responsive state

(following commands or communicates), the patient remains in an altered state of consciousness. Labels for the period of impaired consciousness after head injury have included *acute traumatic psychosis, aftereffects of concussion, traumatic confusion, delirium,* and more commonly *posttraumatic amnesia* (Russell, 1932; Russell & Nathan, 1946; Symonds, 1937). Impaired consciousness after head injury includes cognitive, behavioral, and emotional changes. Symptoms commonly cited across reports include disturbances in arousal, memory, orientation, attention, language, behavior, mood, and perception.

Characteristics of Impaired Consciousness

Cognitive Impairments—Memory

Memory impairment has consistently been reported as the defining characteristic of impaired consciousness after TBI (Russell, 1932; Russell & Nathan, 1946; Symonds, 1937). Early authors described memory impairments, including both retrograde and anterograde amnesia (Russell, 1932; Russell & Nathan, 1946;

363

Symonds, 1937). Anterograde amnesia, loss of continuous memory for ongoing events, varied in duration across individuals (Russell, 1932; Russell & Nathan, 1946; Symonds, 1937). The ability to recall specific events that occurred during the interval of impaired consciousness were reported by many and referred to as *islands of memory* (Symonds, 1937). Early authors reported that the return of memory consolidation for ongoing events and not memory for a single event after the injury signaled the conclusion of impaired consciousness or PTA (Russell, 1935; Russell & Nathan, 1946; Symonds & Russell, 1943). After resolution of impaired consciousness, individuals were left with a loss of memory for events occurring before injury and during impaired consciousness (Russell, 1935; Russell & Nathan, 1946; Symonds & Russell, 1943).

Levin, High, and Eisenberg examined the nature of memory loss during impaired consciousness and revealed that patients with TBI demonstrate impaired learning curves relative to non-TBI controls and rapid decay of new memories over time. The same memory paradigm used with patients after resolution of impaired consciousness revealed performance similar to non-TBI controls (Levin et al., 1988).

With Russell's (1932) initial conceptualization of impaired consciousness as inability to form continuous memories, establishment of methodologies to measure duration of impaired consciousness have commonly included memory tasks. In addition to information such as demographics and events surrounding the injury, Artiola et al. (1980) used a memory task of presenting examiner information as well as three pictures and evaluated spontaneous and recognition recall the following day. This paradigm demonstrated good agreement with estimates of duration of impaired consciousness by neurosurgical colleagues. A similar paradigm was implemented by Geffen et al. (1991) and Stuss and colleagues (1999, 2000), who used word lists to evaluate return of continuous memory postinjury. Schwartz et al. (1998) used both pictures and word lists and found similar time intervals for return of recall of information encoded the day before. The authors concluded that ability to recall pictures could be substituted if individuals were unable to engage in verbal memory tasks. Historically and currently, assessment paradigms of anterograde amnesia have become an integral part of neuropsychological evaluation during impaired consciousness after head injury.

Disorientation and Confusion

The inability to recall ongoing events was thought to contribute to prolonged disorientation and confab-

ulation (Russell & Nathan, 1946; Symonds, 1937). Early studies reported individuals' tendency to make sense of their environment in terms of past experiences (Russell & Nathan, 1946; Symonds, 1937). For example, Russell and Nathan (1946) described a case where an individual recalled he was in a hospital but attributed the reason to an injury he sustained 2 years earlier; thus, he was reported to be disoriented and confused regarding his current situation.

Current measures of impaired consciousness after TBI include assessment of orientation to evaluate individuals' ability to retain current information that is constantly changing (e.g., date, day of week) in addition to information regarding current circumstance (e.g., reason for hospitalization). Levin, O'Donnell, and Grossman (1979) developed a measure of orientation and amnesia to prospectively evaluate duration of impaired consciousness after TBI. Studies examining cognitive sequelae during impaired consciousness after TBI have commonly included indices of orientation (Artiola, 1980; Geffen et al., 1991; High et al., 1990; Stuss et al., 1999). High et al. (1990) prospectively evaluated TBI patients during the course of impaired consciousness and found that orientation returns in the following sequence for a majority of patients: person, place, and then time. Current measures of impaired consciousness after head injury typically include orientation evaluation.

Cognitive Impairments—Attention

Levin (1993) described difficulties focusing attention on the examiner, sustaining attention, processing information, and excessive distractibility as common impairments during early recovery. The presence of these attentional impairments contributes to the duration of anterograde amnesia during early recovery. Although disturbed attention was initially described as pervasive in PTA, few studies have systematically studied disturbed attention during PTA (Ahmed et al., 2000). Stuss et al. (1999) described that individuals regain ability to perform simple attentional tasks earlier than performance on other cognitive tasks. Performance on attentional tasks improved before obtaining a Galveston Orientation and Amnesia Test (GOAT) score (see Galveston Orientation and Amnesia Test) in target range or ability to recall three words at a 24-hour delay (Stuss et al., 1999). Work by Stuss and colleagues (1999) has documented more clearly the nature and course of attentional impairments during early recovery from TBI.

Motor Restlessness

Cerebral irritation was initially used to describe the state of motor restlessness and resistiveness occurring as consciousness remained impaired after head injury, with the consequence of elevating intracranial pressure (Russell, 1971). Initially, motor restlessness was thought to be related to the degree of cerebral pressure (Russell, 1932). After the stage of "flaccid coma," Symonds (1937) described a stage of deep stupor with "restless bodily movements such as turning over in the bed" that typically persisted for brief intervals. Levin and Grossman (1978) described one-third of patients on their neurosurgery service transitioned through a period of recovery after TBI that was marked by disinhibition of motor movements, restlessness, thrashing, and aggressiveness. In 1989, Corrigan published a measure of restlessness after TBI. Corrigan and Mysiw (1988) reported a correlation between restlessness and cognitive abilities. They reported that as cognition improved, agitation diminished. None of the high-cognitive-functioning cases concurrently demonstrated high levels of restlessness; however, low levels of cognitive functioning did not always correlate with high levels of restlessness. With the exception of the Levin and Grossman (1978) study, subsequent studies with small sample sizes examining agitation after TBI make it difficult to draw definitive conclusions regarding the prevalence and impact of restlessness after TBI (Corrigan, 1989; Corrigan & Mysiw, 1988).

Cognitive Impairments—Language

Speech and language impairments after TBI were described in the early case studies of TBI impairments (Russell, 1932; Symonds, 1937). Difficulties with production of speech, articulation, and intelligibility, paucity of speech, jargon aphasia, and automatic phrases characterized individuals in PTA (Russell, 1932). Symonds (1937) described aphasia during PTA as a dynamic process that improved as PTA resolved. The phases of improvement included return of automatic speech that could be pressured with jargon content. Case illustrations highlight perseveration of speech during examination. Abnormalities of speech are reported in studies of consecutive admissions (Gil et al., 1996; Levin et al., 1976). Anomia was reported present in 40% of 50 consecutive admissions after absence or marked reduction of confusion (Levin et al., 1976). Residual difficulties with word finding, naming, writing to dictation, and comprehension of complex, multistage commands are common after severe closed-head injury (Levin et al., 1976; Sarno, 1980; Thomsen, 1975). Gil and colleagues (1996) reported that 11% of 351 consecutive TBI admissions who were 3–18 months postinjury suffered from an aphasic syndrome. Payne-Johnson (1986) compared 20 closed-head injury patients with 15 non–closed-head injury patients and found significant differences on several tests of language between the two groups. Despite these studies, language assessment is not always emphasized during PTA due to difficulty distinguishing confusion from persistent language impairment.

Disturbed Mood and Personality Change

Altered mood or personality is not uncommon during impaired consciousness (Russell, 1932). Russell initially reported that altered personality was thought to be due to damage to higher cerebral functions that control more primitive and vulnerable emotions and behavior. His case descriptions of altered personality during impaired consciousness included being talkative, docile, aggressive, impudent, irritable, boastful, tearful, affectionate, or less reserved (Russell, 1932). After resolution of impaired consciousness, a more "civilized interaction" occurs, suggesting higher cerebral functions of control and inhibition have returned (Russell, 1932). Current authors also include descriptions of patients screaming, being combative, and emotionally labile during the early neurobehavioral manifestations after TBI (Levin, 1993; Nakase-Thompson et al., 2004). For more severely impaired patients, these behavioral changes may persist beyond impaired consciousness and are more likely to contribute to long-term disability (Greve et al., 2001; Hanks et al., 1999; Jennett & MacMillan, 1981).

Delirium

More recent research has focused on the application of delirium/confusion assessment instruments with exclusively TBI samples (Kennedy et al., 2003; Nakase-Thompson et al., 2004). Delirium is defined as a disorder with rapid onset of fluctuating disturbed consciousness and cognitive impairment due to a general medical condition (American Psychiatric Association, 1994). Delirium may comprise many symptoms, including attentional abnormalities, sleep–wake cycle disturbance, cognitive impairments, psychomotor alterations (i.e., hypoactive, hyperactive, or mixed), perceptual abnormalities, and mood lability (Trzepacz, 2002). The temporal course of delirium includes acute onset and fluctuating symptom severity that is usually reversible and may last for days or weeks (Trzepacz, 2002). Recent investigations have examined the usefulness of delirium instruments with TBI populations and found that they contribute additional information to understanding the early neurobehavioral recovery course after TBI (Kennedy et al., 2003; Nakase-Thompson et al., 2004).

Summary

The tests reviewed in this chapter include scales used during the initial evaluation of persons with TBI and subsequent monitoring through stages of impaired consciousness (coma, minimally conscious state, PTA, delirium). Bedside assessment instruments of sports-related concussions are also included. Formal evaluation (lengthier assessment batteries) are briefly described.

Scales

Glasgow Coma Scale

The GCS (Teasdale & Jennett, 1974) is a three-item measure designed to measure depth and duration of impaired consciousness or coma (Table 13-1). Scores are assigned for the severity of impairment of consciousness, with specific focus on motor responses, verbal responses, and eye opening.

Table 13-1. Glasgow Coma Scale

Response	Score
Eyes open	
Spontaneous	4
To speech	3
To pain	2
Absent	1
Verbal	
Converses/oriented	5
Converses/disoriented	4
Inappropriate	3
Incomprehensible	2
Absent	1
Motor	
Obeys	6
Localizes pain	5
Withdraws (flexion)	4
Decorticate rigidity (flexion)	3
Decerebrate rigidity (extension)	2
Absent	1

Scoring

Best responses elicited from the three subscales are scored and summed. Scores range from 3 to 15.

- Mild (GCS = 13–15)
- Moderate (GCS = 9–12)
- Severe (GCS = 3–8)

Advantages and Disadvantages

The GCS is a brief, practical instrument that can be used in various settings. It can be useful for tracking neurologic status over time. It can be rated by various health care professionals. Limitations include ceiling effects for monitoring impairment associated with more mild injuries.

Glasgow Coma Scale—Extended

The GCS—Extended (Nell et al., 2000) is the combination of the GCS and a seven-level numeric amnesia scale (Table 13-2). The extended scale gives a value for differing durations of amnesia; higher scores indicate better outcomes. It was developed to identify mild cases of concussion that may sustain lasting cognitive/behavioral deficits. This would ensure a continuity of care for patients with TBI who may otherwise be dropped from the treatment plan or prematurely discharged. Trained raters, for whom a manual is available, administer it. The amnesia scale has been shown to be easily learned and applied by emergency staff without affecting the GCS scoring itself.

Advantages and Disadvantages

The GSC—Extended allows mild cases of TBI patients, who experience differing levels of amnesia, to be maintained in the treatment loop for appropriate intervention, if needed. This also gives these patients options for compensatory rights. It also provides additional information regarding degree of confusion after TBI for which the GCS is not sensitive.

Abbreviated Injury Scale

Developed by the Association for the Advancement of Automotive Medicine (AAAM) in 1969, the Abbreviated Injury Scale (AIS) is an anatomic method of classifying traumatic injuries, not consequences of injuries (Table

Table 13-2. Amnesia Scale

Score	
7	No amnesia: client can remember impact, can remember falling and striking a solid surface, etc.
6	Amnesia for 30 min or less: client regained consciousness while still in vehicle, in street at scene of incident, etc.
5	Amnesia of 30 min to 3 hr: client remembers being loaded into ambulance, in ambulance on way to hospital, arriving at emergency room, admission to ward, etc.
4	Amnesia of 3–24 hr: determine duration by content of the first memory, which is for an event in the ward or other hospital procedure
3	Amnesia of 1–7 days
2	Amnesia of 8–30 days
1	Amnesia of 31–90 days
0	Amnesia longer than 3 mo
X	Cannot be scored—e.g., client can speak, but responses are inappropriate or unintelligible, cannot speak because unconscious, intubated, facial fractures, etc.

13-3). Injuries are assessed and categorized on a scale from 1 to 6 as follows: 1, minor; 2, moderate; 3, serious; 4, severe; 5, critical; and 6, unsurvivable (Copes et al., 1990). A score of 0 is reserved for a "no injury" classification. The anatomic regions include head/neck, face, thorax, abdomen and visceral pelvis, bony pelvis, and extremities and external regions (Copes et al., 1990). The AIS can be used singularly but is most effective when coupled with other scoring systems, such as the Injury Severity Scale (ISS), as the AIS alone does not account for multiple traumatic injuries (Baker et al., 1974).

Administration

Any trained evaluator who is proficient in the use of this scale can perform the AIS; however, the AAAM identifies the importance for the AIS to be taught by qualified trainers and that the scoring methodology be strictly followed.

Scoring

Injuries are rated per anatomic region on a scale of 1–6, correlating with a specific injury. AIS scores are

predetermined by the AAAM per specific injury (Copes et al., 1990). Therefore, to use the AIS as its authors intended, a practitioner would evaluate the patient and then assign an AIS to each of the six anatomic regions based on the specific injuries. See Table 13-3 for rating severity of injuries on the 1–6 scale.

Scale (Reprint) Availability

The AIS is available in the public domain, but the copyright and the right for development belong to the AAAM.

Advantages and Disadvantages

Although the AIS is a simple numerical method for ranking injuries for researchers, its primary disadvantage is its inability to account for the polytraumatized patient. In addition, the AIS accounts only for injuries and not for the consequences of those injuries. Copes et al. (1990) described a growing worldwide consensus in favor for the use of the AIS in conjunction with the ISS.

Injury Severity Score

The ISS (Baker et al., 1974) was developed to describe the multitrauma patient (Table 13-4). The ISS is an anatomic scoring system based on abbreviated injury descriptors. The ISS describes the overall severity of individuals with multiple traumas. The ISS range is from 1 to 75. A higher score represents a more severely injured the patient. The ISS is the most widely accepted anatomic scoring system and has proved to correlate with length of hospitalization, morbidity, and mortality.

Administration

The ISS can be administered by any trained individual proficient in its use.

Table 13-3. Abbreviated Injury Scale

Abbreviated Injury Scale Score	Injury
1	Minor
2	Moderate
3	Serious
4	Severe
5	Critical
6	Unsurvivable

Table 13-4. Injury Severity Score

Region	Injury Description	Abbreviated Injury Scale	Square Top Three
Head and neck	Cerebral contusion	3	9
Face	No injury	0	
Chest	Flail chest	4	16
Abdomen	Minor contusion of liver	2	
	Complex rupture of spleen	5	25
Extremity	Fractured femur	3	
External	No injury	0	
		Injury severity score	50

Scoring

The ISS uses the descriptors from the AIS. Only the three most severe injuries are used to calculate the ISS. Each of the three AIS descriptors are squared and then added together. An individual injury with AIS of 6 automatically receives an ISS of 75. An ISS of 15 or greater is universally accepted as a definition for a major trauma patient.

Scale (Reprint) Availability

The ISS is available in the public domain.

Advantages and Disadvantages

The ISS is virtually the only anatomic scoring system. It correlates in a linear fashion with length of stay, morbidity, and mortality. Any error in the AIS increases ISS error. Many different injury patterns can yield the same score. Injuries to different body areas are not weighted.

Revised Trauma Score

The Revised Trauma Score (RTS) is a measure of the severity of injury based on the GCS, systolic blood pressure (SBP), and respiratory rate (RR) (Table 13-5) (Champion et al., 1989). Originally, the Trauma Score was based on GCS, SBP, RR, capillary refill, and respiratory expansion calculated for both the purposes of patient triage and statistical analysis of patient outcome. However, previous studies indicate that the assessment of capillary refill and respiratory expansion is difficult to accurately assess in the field environment

(Champion et al., 1989; Hedges et al., 1987; Morris et al., 1987). For example, it is difficult to assess for capillary refill of nail beds in an environment with insufficient illumination, such as on the scene of an accident at night. There is also an inherent difficulty in qualitative assessment of respiratory expansion, independent of environment, which prevents the original TS from being executed simply and accurately (Champion et al., 1989; Kane et al., 1985). Two versions of the RTS were developed, one for practical patient triage (T-RTS) and one for statistical analysis, where the three components are weighted to provide better sensitivity and specificity of outcome (RTS), specifically with respect to head injury patients (Champion et al., 1989). Prehospital and emergency medical services personnel use the T-RTS as a method of communicating physiologic response of injury to the trauma and emergency department staff. Quality assessment personnel and researchers use the RTS as a method of patient outcome.

Administration

Any trained personnel proficient with the scoring system can perform the RTS.

Scoring

The T-RTS version is scored using the integers 0–12 (see Table 13-5). The score is computed as the sum of the coded values assigned to each of the differing physiologic parameters: GCS, SBP, and RR.

For example, an individual with a GCS of 15, SBP of 120 mm Hg, and RR of 12 per minute yields a T-RTS of 12 (4 + 4 + 4, respectively). Alternatively, an individual with a GCS of 7, SBP of 60 mm Hg, and RR of 32

Table 13-5. Revised Trauma Score

Area of Measurement	Coded Value
Systolic blood pressure (mm Hg)	
>89	4
76–89	3
50–75	2
1–49	1
0	0
Respiratory rate (spontaneous inspirations/min)*	
10–29	4
>29	3
6–9	2
1–5	1
0	0
Glasgow Coma Scale score	
13–15	4
9–12	3
6–8	2
4–5	1
3	0
Total possible points	**0–12**

*Patient-initiated, not artificial ventilations.

per minute yields a T-RTS of 7 (2 + 2 + 3, respectively). Patients triaged with a T-RTS of 11 or less should be entered into the trauma system (Champion et al., 1989). When the goal is to account for patient outcome, these three physiologic parameters are weighted and summed to provide a more sensitive and specific representation for outcome evaluation. In this case, Champion et al. (1989) defined RTS as follows:

$$RTS = (0.9368)(GCS) + (0.7326)(SBP) + (0.2908)(RR)$$

Regression analysis was used to derive these weighted values and applied as a multiplier to the raw scores of GCS, SBP, and RR, respectively (Champion et al., 1989).

Scale (Reprint) Availability

The RTS is available in the public domain.

Advantages and Disadvantages

There is good concurrence between prehospital and in-hospital providers, and, thus, RTS provides accurate transfer of information between those providers with respect to the RTS (Champion et al., 1989). The RTS correlates closely with the probability of survival (Champion et al., 1989).

Coma Recovery Scale

The Coma Recovery Scale (CRS) is a 35-item instrument designed to assess various levels of neurologic responsiveness (Giacino et al., 1991). The subscales of the CRS assess responsiveness in the areas of arousal, attention, auditory perception, visual perception, motor function, oromotor ability, communication, and initiative. The lowest item on each scale represents a reflexive response, whereas the highest item response reflects cortically based abilities (Giaciono et al., 1991).

Validation

The CRS was determined to have acceptable reliability (kappa = .83) across raters, and concurrent validity with the Disability Rating Scale (–.93) and GCS (Giacino et al., 1991).

Administration

The CRS can be administered by a trained rater.

Scale (Reprint) Availability

Contact Joe Giacino, Ph.D., of the JFK Johnson Rehabilitation Institute, Center for Head Injuries, at 2048 Oak Tree Road, Edison, NJ.

Advantages and Disadvantages

Although the CRS takes longer to administer than a GCS rating, it provides additional information important in determining level of responsiveness that has implications for rehabilitation and treatment planning. Individuals who are aphasic may not respond to items, as with comprehension demands on the GCS; thus, the CRS provides other modalities by which to determine levels of responsiveness (Ng et al., 2001).

Galveston Orientation and Amnesia Test

The GOAT is a 10-item measure that assesses orientation as well as memory for events preceding and after

Table 13-6. Galveston Orientation and Amnesia Test

Error/Points	
_____/10	1. What is your name? (2) _____ When were you born? (4) _____ Where do you live? (4) _____
_____/10	2. Where are you now? City (5) _____ Hospital (unnecessary to state name of hospital) (5) _____
_____/10	3. On what date were you admitted to the hospital (or injured)? (5) _____ How did you get to the hospital? (5) _____
_____/10	4. What is the first event you can remember *after* the injury? (5) _____ _____ Can you describe in detail (e.g., date, time, companions) the first event you recall *after* the injury? (5) _____ _____
_____/10	5. What is the last event you can remember *before* the injury? (5) _____ _____ Can you describe in detail (e.g., date, time, companions) the last event you recall *before* the injury? (5) _____ _____
_____/5	6. What time is it now? _____:_____ a.m./p.m. (–1 for each 0.5 hr off, maximum of –5)
_____/3	7. What day of the week is it? Su M T W Th F Sa (–1 for each day removed from correct one in reverse direction, maximum of –3)
_____/5	8. What day of the month is it? _____ (–1 for each day removed from correct date, maximum of –5)
_____/15	9. What is the month? J F M A M J J A S O N D (–5 for each month removed from correct one, maximum of –15)
_____/30	10. What is the year? _____ (–10 for each year removed from correct one, maximum of –30)
_____	**Total error points**
_____	**Galveston Orientation and Amnesia Test score (100 minus error points)**

TBI (Table 13-6) (Levin et al., 1979). Areas of orientation include biographic information, place, time, and current circumstances. Two items ask respondents to recall events before and after the injury. The GOAT has been used to determine the duration of PTA in numerous studies of TBI.

Validation

Inter-rater reliability has been found to be excellent (correlation coefficient = .99). Individuals with impaired scores on initial GCS were found to be in PTA longer (via GOAT assessment) than individuals with higher-level responses (Levin et al., 1979).

Scoring

Error points are assigned for incorrect response to items. Amnesia items are scored based on the coherence and potential accuracy of a respondent's answer. Total error scores can range from 0 to 108, with higher error scores indicating poorer orientation. Error scores are subtracted from 100 to determine a GOAT score (range –8 to 100).

Administration

The GOAT can be administered by trained raters.

Scale (Reprint) Availability

The GOAT is available in the public domain.

Advantages and Disadvantages

The GOAT can be incorporated into a brief bedside assessment or as part of a formal cognitive evaluation. Duration of PTA as determined by the GOAT scores has been shown to be a reliable predictor of outcome after TBI (Sherer et al., 2002). The GOAT can be difficult to administer to patients who cannot give verbal responses (e.g., secondary to intubation, aphonia, aphasia). A modified version of the GOAT that allows the respondent an opportunity to answer by pointing to the answer among four options presented in visual format has undergone recent investigation. A study of this modified version of the GOAT (scores ranging from 0 to 80) correlated poorly with the full form among acute TBI inpatients (Telmet et al., 2003). A modified version for patients with aphasia was found to have high specificity but poor sensitivity in aphasic patients (Jain et al., 1999).

Standardized Assessment of Concussion

The Standardized Assessment of Concussion (SAC) is intended to be a brief sideline examination that evaluates areas of cognition recommended by the guidelines published by the American Academy of Neurology (Table 13-7) (Kelly & Rosenberg, 1997; McCrea et al., 1997).

It is a 30-point scale with items assessing orientation (month, date, year, day of week, and time of day), immediate memory (five-word list learning task), concentration (digits backward, months in reverse order), and delayed recall (for five-word list). The maximum score on the examination is 30 points and takes approximately 5 minutes to administer. Three versions of the form were developed to minimize practice effects.

Validation

The SAC was administered to 141 football players with no history of concussion. Follow-up SAC administrations were given to six individuals immediately after sustaining a concussion. Significant differences were observed between normal controls and the concussed group on the immediate memory, delayed recall, and total score of the SAC, suggesting preliminarily that the SAC can discriminate individuals who have sustained a concussion from individuals who have not. The normative control group used in the development of the SAC had an average total score of 25.6 and 2.2 standard deviations, whereas the concussed group had an average score of 21.5, with 3.5 standard deviations. Authors recommend baseline data be collected for players during the off season to compare future administrations.

Scoring

The orientation subscale has five items worth 1 point each. The immediate memory subscale has three learning trials of a five-word list worth up to 15 points. The concentration and delayed recall subtests sum to 5 points each. The SAC total score can range from 0 to 30.

Advantages and Disadvantages

The authors of the SAC acknowledge that it was administered only to high school athletes from a specific geographical region with a relatively small clinical comparison group. Data regarding normative values are from a small sample and regarded as preliminary in nature.

Agitated Behavior Scale

The Agitated Behavior Scale is a 14-item measure of agitation, motor restlessness, and distractibility for brain injury individuals (Table 13-8) (Corrigan, 1989). The Agitated Behavior Scale was developed to allow objective assessment of abnormal behavior after neurologic disease and could be used for serial assessments to document the course of symptoms for treatment purposes. Raters indicate the frequency of various behaviors on a scale from 1 to 4. Scores range from 14 to 56, with higher scores indicating higher levels of motor restlessness (impaired behavior) and attention and lower ratings indicating lower frequency of motor restlessness.

Validation

The 14 items were originally selected from a pool of 39 items that were rated by registered nurses on a

Table 13-7.   Standardized Assessment of Concussion

Name:

Age: Sex: Examiner:

Nature of injury:

Date of exam: Time: No.:

Orientation (1 point each)

  Month:

  Date:

  Day of week:

  Year:

  Time (within 1 hr):

  Orientation score _____ (5):

Immediate memory (1 point for each correct, total over three trials)

	Trial 1	Trial 2	Trial 3
Word 1 _____	___	___	___
Word 2 _____	___	___	___
Word 3 _____	___	___	___
Word 4 _____	___	___	___
Word 5 _____	___	___	___

Immediate memory score _____ (15)

Concentration reverse digits (go to next string length if correct on first trial; stop if incorrect on both trials; 1 point each
  for each string length)

3 8 2	5 1 8	___
2 7 9 3	2 1 6 8	___
5 1 8 6 9	9 1 4 7 5	___
6 9 7 3 5 1	4 2 8 9 3 7	___

Months of the year in reverse order (1 point for entire sequence correct)

Dec.   Nov.   Oct.   Sept.   Aug.   July   June   May   April   March   Feb.   Jan.

  Concentration score _____ (5)

Delayed recall (approximately 5 min after immediate memory; 1 point each)

  Word 1

  Word 2

  Word 3

  Word 4

  Word 5

  Delayed recall score _____ (5)

Table 13-7.   *(continued)*

Summary of total scores

Orientation	_____	(5)
Immediate memory	_____	(15)
Concentration	_____	(5)
Delayed recall	_____	(5)
Total score	_____	(30)

The following may be performed between the immediate memory and delayed recall portions of this assessment when appropriate:

Neurologic screening

Recollection of the injury:

Strength:

Sensation:

Coordination:

Exertional maneuvers

1	40-yd sprint
5	Sit-ups
5	Pushups
5	Knee bends

traumatic head injury unit. The 14-item scale was subsequently validated on a new sample and found to have acceptable inter-rater reliability, internal consistency (alpha >.80), and concurrent validity with other indices of agitation.

Scoring

The total score is calculated by adding the ratings (from 1 to 4) on each of the 14 items. Raters are instructed to leave no blanks, but if a blank is left, the average rating for the other 14 items should be inserted such that the total score reflects the appropriate possible range of values. The total score is the best overall measure of the course of agitation (Corrigan & Bogner, 1994). Subscale scores are calculated by adding ratings from the component items:

- Disinhibition is the sum of items 1, 2, 3, 6, 7, 8, 9, and 10.
- Aggression is the sum of items 3, 4, 5, and 14. (It is not an error that Item #3 is in both scores.)
- Lability is the sum of items 11, 12, and 13.

To allow subscale scores to be compared to each other and to the total score, it is recommended that an average item score for each factor be calculated and multiplied by 14. This procedure provides subscale scores with the same range as each other and the total score, which is useful for graphic presentation.

Scale (Reprint) Availability

The Agitated Behavior Scale is available in the public domain.

Advantages and Disadvantages

The Agitated Behavior Scale is a brief instrument that can be used by trained medical personnel, including nursing, therapy staff, neuropsychology, and physicians.

Confusion Assessment Method

The Confusion Assessment Method (CAM) is a nine-item questionnaire and four-item algorithm for the detection and diagnosis of delirium (Tables 13-9 and

Table 13-8.   Agitated Behavior Scale

Patient: _____   Period of observation

Observation environment: _____   From: _____ a.m./p.m. __/__/__

Rater: _____   To: _____ a.m./p.m. __/__/__

At the end of the observation period, indicate whether the behavior described in each item was present and, if so, to what degree: slight, moderate, or extreme. Use the following numerical values and criteria for your ratings.

1 = Absent: The behavior is not present.

2 = Present to a slight degree: The behavior is present but does not prevent the conduct of other, contextually appropriate behavior. (The individual may redirect spontaneously, or the continuation of the agitated behavior does not disrupt appropriate behavior.)

3 = Present to a moderate degree: The individual needs to be redirected from an agitated to an appropriate behavior but benefits from such cueing.

4 = Present to an extreme degree: The individual is not able to engage in appropriate behavior due to the interference of the agitated behavior, even when external cueing or redirection is provided.

_____ 1. Short attention span, easy distractibility, inability to concentrate

_____ 2. Impulsive, impatient, low tolerance for pain or frustration

_____ 3. Uncooperative, resistant to care, demanding

_____ 4. Violent and/or threatening violence toward people or property

_____ 5. Explosive and/or unpredictable anger

_____ 6. Rocking, rubbing, moaning, or other self-stimulating behavior

_____ 7. Pulling at tubes, restraints, etc.

_____ 8. Wandering from treatment areas

_____ 9. Restlessness, pacing, excessive movement

_____ 10. Repetitive behaviors, motor and/or verbal

_____ 11. Rapid, loud, or excessive talking

_____ 12. Sudden changes of mood

_____ 13. Easily initiated or excessive crying and/or laughter

_____ 14. Self-abusiveness, physical and/or verbal

_____ **Total score**

13-10) (Inouye et al., 1990). The questionnaire involves items considered to be of diagnostic importance and adapted from the *Diagnostic and Statistical Manual of Mental Disorders III—Revised.* Item content assesses acute onset of disturbance, fluctuating course, inattention, disorganized thinking, altered level of consciousness, disorientation, memory impairment, perceptual disturbances, increased or decreased psychomotor activity, and disturbance of the sleep–wake cycle. The diagnostic algorithm was developed a priori and included four features: (1) fluctuating course, (2) inattention, (3) disorganized thinking, and (4) altered level of con-

sciousness. Individuals must demonstrate fluctuating course of symptoms, inattention, and either disorganized thinking or altered level of consciousness.

Validation

The initial validation studies indicated that the CAM demonstrated excellent sensitivity (94–100%) and specificity (90–95%) for detection of delirium when compared with a formal diagnostic psychiatric interview. Excellent convergent validity was found between the CAM and other cognitive or confusion

Table 13-9.   Confusion Assessment Method Instrument

1. Acute onset

   Is there evidence of an acute change in mental status from the patient's baseline?

2. Inattention

   A. Did the patient have difficulty focusing attention—e.g., being easily distractible or having difficulty keeping track of what was being said?

   Not present at any time during the interview

   Present at some time during interview but in mild form

   Present at some time during interview in marked form

   Uncertain

   B. (If present or abnormal) Did this behavior fluctuate during the interview—i.e., tend to come and go or increase and decrease in severity?

   Yes

   No

   Uncertain

   Not applicable

   C. (If present or abnormal) Please describe this behavior.

3. Disorganized thinking

   Was the patient's thinking disorganized or incoherent—e.g., rambling or irrelevant conversation, unclear or illogical flow of ideas, or unpredictable switching from subject to subject?

4. Altered level of consciousness

   Overall, how would you rate this patient's level of consciousness?

   Alert (normal)

   Vigilant (hyperalert, overly sensitive to environmental stimuli, startled very easily)

   Lethargic (drowsy, easily aroused)

   Stupor (difficult to arouse)

   Coma (unarousable)

   Uncertain

5. Disorientation

   Was the patient disoriented at any time during the interview—i.e., thinking that he or she was somewhere other than the hospital, using the wrong bed, or misjudging the time of day?

6. Memory impairment

   Did the patient demonstrate any memory problems during the interview—e.g., inability to remember events in the hospital or difficulty remembering instructions?

7. Perceptual disturbances

   Did the patient have any evidence of perceptual disturbances—i.e., hallucinations, illusions, or misinterpretations (e.g., thinking something was moving when it was not)?

8. Psychomotor agitation/retardation

   Part 1. At any time during the interview, did the patient have an unusually increased level of motor activity—e.g., restlessness, picking at bedclothes, tapping fingers, or making frequent sudden changes of position?

   Part 2. At any time during the interview, did the patient have an unusually decreased level of motor activity—e.g., sluggishness, staring into space, staying in one position for a long time, or moving very slowly?

9. Altered sleep–wake cycle

   Did the patient have evidence of disturbance of sleep–wake cycle—e.g., excessive daytime sleepiness with insomnia at night?

Table 13-10. Confusion Assessment Method Four-Item Diagnostic Algorithm

---

Feature 1. Acute onset and fluctuating course

This feature is usually obtained from a family member or nurse and is shown by positive responses to the following questions. Is there evidence of an acute change in mental status from the patient's baseline? Did the (abnormal) behavior fluctuate during the day—i.e., tend to come and go or increase and decrease in severity?

Feature 2. Inattention

This feature is shown by a positive response to the following question: Did the patient have difficulty focusing attention—e.g., being easily distractible or having difficulty keeping track of what was being said?

Feature 3. Disorganized thinking

This feature is shown by a positive response to the following question: Was the patient's thinking disorganized or incoherent, such as rambling or irrelevant conversation, unclear or illogical flow of ideas, or unpredictable switching from subject to subject?

Feature 4. Altered level of consciousness

This feature is shown by any answer other than "alert" to the following question: Overall, how would you rate this patient's level of consciousness? (alert [normal], vigilant [hyperalert], lethargic [drowsy, easily aroused], stupor [difficult to arouse], or coma [unarousable])?

---

indices. Excellent agreement across samples was found among independent ratings of subjects for the nine-item questionnaire (88%) and the four CAM diagnostic items (93%).

Scoring

Individuals must demonstrate fluctuating course of symptoms (feature 1), inattention (feature 2), and either disorganized thinking (feature 3) or altered level of consciousness (feature 4).

Scale (Reprint) Availability

The CAM is available in the public domain.

Advantages and Disadvantages

The CAM instrument is probably the most widely used in general hospitals and intensive care unites and can be completed in 5 minutes after clinical examina-

tion of a patient. It can be administered by physicians, nurses, and trained lay interviewers. Limitations include its difficulty in distinguishing delirium from dementia, depression, or other psychiatric conditions.

Delirium Rating Scale/Delirium Rating Scale–Revised

The Delirium Rating Scale (DRS) is a 10-item rating scale that assesses the presence and severity of various symptoms of delirium. Individual items assess temporal onset of symptoms, perceptual disturbance, hallucination type, delusions, psychomotor behavior, cognitive status, physical disorder, sleep–wake cycle, lability of mood, and variability of symptoms. Trzepacz and colleagues (1988) found that the DRS successfully discriminated patients with delirium with psychosis and dementia.

Scoring

Item scores are summed to obtain a total score that may range from 0 to 32. Scores between 8 and 12 suggest subclinical delirium; scores above 13 are consistent with delirium.

Advantages and Disadvantages

The DRS is a widely used delirium-rating instrument that has shown good psychometric properties for measuring delirium and is available in multiple languages (French, Italian, Spanish, Dutch, Mandarin Chinese, Korean, Swedish, Japanese, German, and Indian language translations). However, the DRS does have limitations in measuring aspects of a single episode of delirium (e.g., items assessing sudden onset, fluctuation of symptoms, and physical etiology). In addition, multiple domains are included in the same item (motor impairment and cognitive impairment). The DRS–Revised-98 was developed to address these limitations of the original instrument.

Delirium Rating Scale–Revised-98

The DRS–Revised-98 (Trzepacz et al., 2001) is a 16-item rating scale with two subtests. The initial subtest comprises the first 13 items that indicate severity of delirium symptoms. Items include text descriptions for scores ranging from 0 to 3. The last three items are used for diagnostic purposes and can range from 0 to 2 or 3. Items are rated based on best source information (e.g., patient examination, family interview, medical records). Some items are based on examination and history; others are based on cognitive tasks. Individual items assess temporal onset of symptoms, perceptual disturbance, delusions, psychomotor behavior, aspects of cognition (attention, language, visuospatial disturbance, short-term memory, and long-term memory), presence of a physical disorder accounting for symptoms, sleep–wake cycle disturbance, thought process abnormalities, lability of mood, and fluctuation of symptoms. Item scores are summed to obtain a total score that may range from 0 to 46 (severity and diagnostic items summed) or 0 to 39 for the severity items only. The DRS–Revised-98 has excellent reliability, with a Cronbach's coefficient alpha of .90. Inter-rater reliability is excellent, with intra-class correlation coefficients ranging from 0.98 to 0.99 Trzepacz and colleagues (2001) found that the DRS–Revised-98 successfully discriminated patients with delirium from patients with dementia, schizophrenia, depression, and other mixed groups. Severity scores of more than 15 have demonstrated excellent specificity (93%) and sensitivity (92%) in these samples.

Scale (Reprint) Availability

DRS–Revised-98 is in the public domain.

Advantages and Disadvantages

The DRS–Revised-98 was developed to address limitations of the DRS. The DRS–Revised-98 has three items that are used for initial diagnostic purposes only (temporal onset, fluctuation of symptoms, and presence of physical disorder). Thirteen additional items are included for repeated measurement within a single episode of delirium. Items are broken into multiple cognitive areas, including language, memory, orientation, visual perception, attention, and other thought process abnormalities. Motor retardation and motor restlessness are rated separately. Trained clinicians are able to rate the presence of these symptoms over time. Sources of information can vary to rate items, and some type of standardized protocol for assessing cognitive domains is needed, as they are not provided as part of the scale. Authors suggest using measures such as the Cognitive Test for Delirium (CTD) in addition to the DRS–Revised-98.

Cognitive Test for Delirium

The CTD (Hart et al., 1996, 1997) was developed to assess cognitive symptoms of delirium in acutely ill patients. The test is appropriate for patients who may not be able to give verbal responses, as items may be responded to by pointing, nodding the head, or raising the hand. The CTD consists of five subtests that assess orientation, attention span, memory, comprehension/ conceptual reasoning, and vigilance. In a study of intensive care unit patients with delirium, outpatients with dementia, and general psychiatric inpatients with depression or schizophrenia, Hart and colleagues (1996) found that the CTD successfully discriminated patients with delirium from patients with other conditions. Receiver operating characteristic analysis showed that total scores of less than 19 indicated probable delirium. At this level, sensitivity was 100% and specificity 95.1%. Kennedy and colleagues (2003) compared the CTD in a homogeneous sample of TBI patients meeting *Diagnostic and Statistical Manual of Mental Disorders IV* criteria for delirium. The CTD demonstrated acceptable sensitivity and specificity for diagnosis of delirium in the TBI population. Receiver operating characteristic analysis showed an optimal cutoff value of less than 22, yielded sensitivity of 71% and specificity of 72% compared with *Diagnostic and Statistical Manual of Mental Disorders IV* diagnosis.

Scoring

The raw scores from each subtest are converted to a common metric of 0–6. These converted scores are summed to give overall scores that range from 0 to 30.

Scale (Reprint) Availability

The CTD is available in the public domain. Contact Robert Hart, M.D.: Department of Psychiatry, P.O. Box 980268, Medical College of Virginia, Richmond, VA 23298-0268.

Advantages and Disadvantages

The CTD can be administered in 10–20 minutes. The CTD can be administered to individuals who cannot verbalize. All responses can be given gesturally so that individuals who cannot verbalize can be administered the test. Individuals with motor limitations may have difficulty responding to some test items.

Full Neuropsychological Batteries

Formal neuropsychological examinations involve quantitative assessment of cognitive functions measured through standard administration of a battery of tests. Test batteries may include a uniform series of tests that are given regardless of the patient's condition (fixed battery approach) or tailored to the individual's areas of cognitive difficulty (flexible battery approach). Formal assessment may include tests of memory, attention, visual-spatial abilities, language, executive functions, motor skills, intelligence, academic achievement, and psychosocial adjustment. The results of formal neuropsychological assessment are used to assist with treatment planning, identifying appropriate rehabilitation goals, and predicting eventual outcome (American Academy of Neurology, 1996; Boake et al., 2001; Levin, 1994; Sherer et al., 2002). Advantages over bedside mental status examinations are that neuropsychological evaluations are standardized in scoring and administration, and most of the tests have been determined to be reliable and valid (Heilman & Valenstein, 1993; Lezak, 1995). In addition, normative values are available for widely used tests, and test scores can be meaningfully compared over time and among different patients (American Academy of Neurology, 1996). Several publications describe tests, administration procedures, scoring, and interpretation (Lezak, 1995; Spreen & Strauss, 1998).

References

Ahmed S, Bierley R, Sheikh JI, et al. Post-traumatic amnesia after closed head injury: a review of the literature and some suggestions for further research. *Brain Inj* 2000; 14:765–80.

American Academy of Neurology. Report of the Therapeutics and Technology Subcommittee. Assessment: neuropsychological testing of adults. *Neurology* 1996;47: 592–99.

American Psychiatric Association. *Diagnostic and statistical manual of mental disorders* (4th ed.). Washington: American Psychiatric Association, 1994:124–29.

Artiola L, Fortuny I, Briggs M, et al. Measuring the duration of post traumatic amnesia. *J Neurol Neurosurg Psychiatry* 1980;43:377–79.

Baker SP, O'Niel B, Haddon W Jr. The Injury Severity Score: a method for describing patients with multiple injuries and evaluating emergency care. *J Trauma* 1974;14:187–96.

Boake C, Millis S, High WM Jr., et al. Using early neuropsychological testing to predict long term productivity outcome from traumatic brain injury. *Arch Phys Med Rehabil* 2002;82:761–68.

Champion HR, Sacco WJ, Copes WS, et al. A revision of the Trauma Score. *J Trauma* 1989;29:623–29.

Copes WS, Sacco WJ, Champion HR, et al. Progress in characterizing anatomic injury. Association for the Advancement of Automotive Medicine. Proceedings of the 33rd Annual Meeting. Des Plaines, IL: AAAM, 1990.

Corrigan JD. Development of a scale for assessment of agitation following traumatic brain injury. *J Clin Exp Neuropsychol* 1989;11:261–77.

Corrigan JD, Bogner JA. Factor structure of the Agitated Behavior Scale. *J Clin Exp Neuropsychol* 1994;16:386–92.

Corrigan JD, Mysiw WJ. Agitation following traumatic head injury: equivocal evidence for a discrete stage of cognitive recovery. *Arch Phys Med Rehabil* 1988;69:487–92.

Ellenberg JH, Levin HS, Saydjari C. Posttraumatic amnesia as a predictor of outcome after severe closed head injury. *Arch Neurol* 1996;53:782–91.

Geffen GM, Encel JS, Forrester GM. Stages of recovery during post-traumatic amnesia and subsequent everyday memory deficits. *Neuroreport* 1991;2:105–8.

Gil M, Cohen M, Korn C, et al. Vocational outcome of aphasic patients following severe traumatic brain injury. *Brain Inj* 1996;10:39–45.

Giacino JT, Shwall S, Childs N, et al. The minimally conscious state: definition and diagnostic criteria. *Neurology* 2002;58:349–53.

Giacino JT, Kezmarsky MA, DeLuca J, et al. Monitoring rate of recovery to predict outcome in minimally responsive patients. *Arch Phys Med Rehabil* 1991;72:897–901.

Greve KW, Sherwin E, Stanford MS, et al. Personality and neurocognitive correlates of impulsive aggression in long-term survivors of severe traumatic brain injury. *Brain Inj* 2001;15:255–62.

Hanks RA, Temkin N, Machamer J, et al. Emotional and behavioral adjustment after traumatic brain injury. *Arch Phys Med Rehabil* 1999;80:991–97.

Hart RP, Best AL, Sessler CN, et al. Abbreviated cognitive test for delirium. *J Psychosom Res* 1997;43:417–23.

Hart RP, Levenson JL, Sessler CN, et al. Validation of the Cognitive Test for Delirium in medical ICU patients. *Psychosomatics* 1996;37:533–46.

Heilman KM, Valenstein E (eds.). *Clinical neuropsychology* (3rd ed.). New York: Oxford University Press, 1993.

Hedges JR, Feero S, Moore B, et al. Comparison of prehospital trauma triage instruments in a semi-rural population. *J Emerg Med* 1987;5:197–208.

High WM, Levin HS, Gary HE. Recovery of orientation following closed-head injury. *J Clin Exp Neuropsychol* 1990;12:703–14.

Inouye SK, van Dyck CH, Alessi CA, et al. Clarifying confusion: the confusion assessment method. *Ann Intern Med* 1990;113:941–48.

Jain N, Layton BS, Murray PK. Are aphasic patients who fail the GOAT in PTA? A modified Galveston Orientation and Amnesia Test for persons with aphasia. *Clinical Neuropsychol* 1999;14:13–17.

Jennett B, MacMillan R. Epidemiology of head injury. *BMJ* 1981;282:101–4.

Kane G, Engelhardt R, Celentano J, et al. Empirical development and evaluation of prehospital triage instruments. *J Trauma* 1985;25:482–89.

Kelly JP, Rosenberg J. Practice parameter: the management of concussion in sport. Report of the quality standards committee. *Neurology* 1997;48:581–85.

Kennedy RE, Nakase-Thompson R, Sherer M, et al. Use of the cognitive test for delirium in patients with traumatic brain injury. *Psychosomatics* 2003;44:283–89.

Levin HS. A guide to clinical neuropsychological testing. *Arch Neurol* 1994;51:854–59.

Levin HS. Neurobehavioral sequelae of closed head injury. In: PR Cooper (ed.). *Head injury*. Baltimore: Williams & Wilkins, 1993:525–51.

Levin HS. Prediction of recovery from traumatic brain injury. *J Neurotrauma* 1995;12:913–22.

Levin HS, Grossman RG. Behavioral sequelae of closed head injury: a quantitative study. *Arch Neurol* 1978;35:720–27.

Levin HS, High WM, Eisenberg HM. Learning and forgetting during posttraumatic amnesia in head injured patients. *J Neurol Neurosurg Psychiatry* 1988;51:14–20.

Levin HS, O'Donnell VM, Grossman RG. The Galveston Orientation and Amnesia Test. *J Nerv Ment Dis* 1979;167:675–84.

Levin HS, Grossman RG, Kelly PJ. Aphasic disorder in patients with closed head injury. *J Neurol Neurosurg Psychiatry* 1976;39:1062–70.

Lezak MD. *Neuropsychological assessment* (3rd ed.). New York: Oxford University Press, 1995.

McCrea M, Kelly JP, Kluge J, et al. Standardized assessment of concussion in football players. *Neurology* 1997; 48:586–88.

Morris JA Jr., Auerbach PS, Marshall GA, et al. The Trauma Score as a triage tool in the prehospital setting. *JAMA* 1987;256:1319–25.

Nakase-Thompson R, Sherer M, Yablon SA, et al. Acute confusion following traumatic brain injury. *Brain Inj* 2004;18:131–42.

Ng WK, Thompson RN, Yablon SA, et al. Conceptual dilemmas in evaluating individuals with severely impaired consciousness: a case report. *Brain Inj* 2001;15:639–43.

Nell V, Yates DW, Kruger J. An extended Glasgow Coma Scale (GCS-E) with enhanced sensitivity to mild brain injury. *Arch Phys Med Rehabil* 2000;81:614–17.

Payne-Johnson JC. Evaluation of communication competence in patients with closed head injury. *J Commun Disord* 1986;19:237–49.

Russell WR. Cerebral involvement in head injury. *Brain* 1932;55:549–603.

Russell WR. Amnesia following head injuries. *Lancet* 1935;2:762–63.

Russell WR. *The traumatic amnesias*. London: Oxford Press, 1971.

Russell WR, Nathan PW. Traumatic amnesia. *Brain* 1946; 69:280–300.

Sarno MT. The nature of verbal impairment after closed head injury. *J Nerv Ment Dis* 1980;168:685–92.

Schwartz ML, Carruth F, Binns MA, et al. The course of posttraumatic amnesia: three little words. *Can J Neurol Sci* 1998;25:108–16.

Sherer M, Sander AM, Nick TG, et al. Early cognitive status and productivity outcome following traumatic brain injury: findings from the TBI model systems. *Arch Phys Med Rehabil* 2002;83:183–92.

Spreen O, Strauss E. *A compendium of neuropsychological tests: administration, norms, and commentary* (2nd ed.). New York: Oxford University Press, 1998.

Stuss DT, Binns MA, Carruth FG, et al. Prediction of recovery of continuous memory after traumatic brain injury. *Neurology* 2000;54:1337–44.

Stuss DT, Binns MA, Carruth FG, et al. The acute period of recovery from traumatic brain injury: posttraumatic amnesia or posttraumatic confusional state? *J Neurosurg* 1999;90:635–43.

Symonds CP. Mental disorder following head injury. *Proc R Soc Med* 1937;30:33–46.

Symonds CP, Russell WR. Accidental head injuries. *Lancet* 1943;1:7–10.

Teasdale G, Jennett B. Assessment of coma and impaired consciousness. A practical scale. *Lancet* 1974;2:81–84.

Telmet KL, Hanks R, Rapport LJ, et al. Reliability and validity of a modified Galveston Orientation and Amnesia Test. *J Intl Neuropsychol Soc* 2003;9:233.

Thomsen IV. Evaluation and outcome of aphasia patients with severe closed head trauma. *J Neurol Neurosurg Psychiatry* 1975;38:713–18.

Trzepacz PT, Meagher DJ, Wise MG. Neuropsychiatric aspects of delirium. In: Yudofsky SC, Hales RE (eds.). *The American Psychiatric Publishing textbook of neuropsychiatry and clinical sciences*. Washington: American Psychiatric Press, 2002:525–64.

Trzepacz PT, Baker RW, Greenhouse J. A symptom rating scale for delirium. *Psychiatry Res* 1988;23:89–97.

Trzepacz PT, Mittal D, Torres R, et al. Validation of the Delirium Rating Scale-Revised-98: comparison with the delirium rating scale and the cognitive test for delirium. *J Neuropsychiatry Clin Neurosci* 2001;13:229–42.

Whyte J, Cifu D, Dikmen S, et al. Prediction of functional outcomes after traumatic brain injury: a comparison of 2 measures of duration of unconsciousness. *Arch Phys Med Rehabil* 2001;82:1355–59.

14 Health-Related Quality-of-Life Scales for Epilepsy

James J. Cereghino, M.D.

Without warning, a person lets out a cry, falls rigidly to the ground, jerks arms and legs uncontrollably, bites the tongue, froths at the mouth, and then gradually regains consciousness (generalized tonic-clonic seizure). Another person, again without warning, stops conversation suddenly, blinks eyelids and smacks lips for only a few seconds, and then resumes conversation (absence seizure). Another person begins to stare, starts fumbling at clothes, walks around aimlessly, does not respond to other people, and then gradually returns to normal (complex partial/focal motor seizure). All of these people have epilepsy, and yet it is obvious from these brief descriptions that they are all different.

Although epilepsy has been described since before the beginning of written history, it was not until 1857 that an effective treatment was found. It was not until 1946 that it was found that generalized seizures responded to some antiepileptic drugs and partial seizures to other antiepileptic drugs. With the recognition that certain seizure types could benefit from specific treatments and with the availability of new neurophysiologic information, the International League Against Epilepsy (ILAE) attempted to standardize terminology in the 1960s. This has not proved to be an easy task and, as new information is obtained, it must be integrated into current concepts. An epileptic seizure is a discrete event characterized by a sudden, excessive discharge of neurons within the brain. Epilepsy is a chronic neurologic condition characterized by recurrent epileptic seizures. A person may have more than one type of seizure (e.g., absence plus generalized tonic-clonic) or may have only one type of seizure. The ILAE has approved an International Classification of Epileptic Seizures (Commission on Classification and Terminology, 1981) and an International Classification of Epilepsies and Epileptic Syndromes (Commission on Classification and Terminology, 1989). Under consideration is a proposed change in this terminology (Engel, 2001).

Quality of life (QOL) has proved equally difficult to define for epilepsy. It would appear that the majority of studies use the term to represent the functional effect of epilepsy and its treatment(s) upon a person, as perceived by the person. For epilepsy, this is a huge undertaking. Throughout the centuries, a person with epilepsy has sometimes been viewed as sacred and venerated and sometimes as possessed and shunned (for a history, see Temkin, 1945). As recently as the late nineteenth and early twentieth centuries, persons with epilepsy were sent to reside in colonies. It was not until the 1940s that persons were permitted to rejoin the community. Today in the twenty-first century, stigma about epilepsy persists and even exorcism may be used to treat epilepsy, but stigma in this century is usually subtle and relates to issues with independence and self-esteem.

For purposes of this chapter, health-related QOL (HRQOL) will use the three principal dimensions outlined by Devinsky (2000, p. 89): "(1) physical health (e.g., daily function, general health, severity of physical symptoms, medication side effects, pain, strength, endurance); (2) mental health (e.g., emotional well-being, self-esteem, perceived stigma, anxiety, depression, cognition); and (3) social health (e.g., social activities, relationships with family and friends)."

History of Development

The first epilepsy-specific psychosocial measure—the Washington Psychosocial Seizure Inventory (WPSI) developed by Carl Dodrill and colleagues at the University of Washington Epilepsy Center—was published in 1980 (Dodrill et al., 1980). In 1978, Dodrill had published a neuropsychological battery for epilepsy. In a brief historical review in the initial paper, Dodrill acknowledged that mental status examination in persons with epilepsy had been studied since the late nineteenth century, but that no formal battery of tests had been developed (Dodrill, 1978). By the mid-twentieth century both single tests and batteries of tests began to be used in epilepsy, although they may have been developed and standardized on other populations. In developing the neuropsychological battery, Dodrill recognized that the Halstead-Reitan Battery (Halstead, 1947; Reitan, 1966), which had been developed by his mentors, was the only comprehensive battery being used in persons with epilepsy. Dodrill correctly recognized that the Halstead-Reitan battery needed to be updated to include side effects of new antiepileptic drugs, the effects of electroencephalographic findings, gender differences, degree and type of brain damage, age at onset, and the influence of seizures on abilities such as memory, sustained attention, and verbal problem solving. The new battery would be in need of standardization, too. Although it documented intellectual functioning, emotional status, and lateral dominance, the 1978 neuropsychological battery did not meet the need to objectively measure psychosocial problems of persons with epilepsy. So, concurrently with the neuropsychological battery, the WPSI was developed.

Another approach involved the development of specific scales to measure concerns of persons with epilepsy, such as social stigma (Ryan et al., 1980) and fear of seizures (Lund & Mittan, 1982). Many of these scales were partially funded by the National Institute of Neurological Disorders and Stroke through the Comprehensive Epilepsy Programs, which were specifically formulated to stimulate clinical research in all aspects of epilepsy (Cereghino et al., 1980; Cereghino, 1982).

This was followed by the current generation of HRQOL scales developed mainly in Europe and North America. Some of these tests are quantitative, multidimensional approaches using single scales or batteries. Others are qualitative. This chapter briefly reviews the older psychosocial quantitative and qualitative unidimensional approaches. The current adult QOL measures will be reviewed. Finally assessment scales specific for children, adolescents, and families will be reviewed.

In the early 1990s, the ILAE and the International Bureau for Epilepsy (IBE), in collaboration with the World Health Organization (WHO), focused global attention on increasing public awareness and QOL of persons with epilepsy. This activity was formalized in 1997 as the ILAE/IBE/WHO Global Campaign Against Epilepsy. The ILAE Commission on Outcome Measurement in Epilepsy has published two pertinent reports. In 1998, the Commission inventoried all outcome measurements of epilepsy and its consequences, including the composite effect of epilepsy and treatment expressed as QOL (Baker et al., 1998a). In 2002, the Commission published a review of the principles of HRQOL assessment in clinical trials (Cramer, 2002). In the new proposed 5-axis ILAE Diagnostic Scheme of Epilepsy and Seizures, axis 5 is impairment. This classification will be derived from the WHO International Classification of Functioning and Disability, which is currently in preparation and will undoubtedly involve many HRQOL issues (Engel, 2001).

Recognizing the proliferation of QOL instruments, the Medical Outcomes Trust was incorporated in 1992 with "the mission of promoting the science and application of outcomes assessment, with a particular emphasis on expanding the availability and use of self- or interviewer-administered questionnaires designed to assess health and the outcome of health care from the patient's point of view" (Scientific Advisory Committee of the Medical Outcomes Trust, 2002, p. 194). The Trust created a Scientific Advisory Committee that has defined eight attributes with specific review criteria with which to evaluate QOL instruments. These are

"1. Conceptual and Measurement Model
2. Reliability
3. Validity
4. Responsiveness
5. Interpretability
6. Respondent and Administrative Burden
7. Alternative Forms
8. Cultural and Language Adaptations or Translations" (Scientific Advisory Committee of the Medical Outcomes Trust, 2002, p. 194).

Psychosocial Outcome Measures

See Table 14-1.

Washington Psychosocial Inventory

The first version of WPSI (Dodrill et al., 1980) consisted of 132 items printed on both sides of a single sheet of paper. Items were answered yes or no "*according to the self-perceived usual feeling and actions of the respondent*" (Dodrill et al., 1980, p. 124). Reliability and validation results were presented in the first paper. Currently, the WPSI contains 125 items in eight subscales. WPSI takes approximately 40 minutes to complete. A WPSI QOL subscale based on correlations with the Quality of Life in Epilepsy Scale-31 has been published (Dodrill & Batzel, 1995).

Adolescent Washington Psychosocial Inventory

The Adolescent Washington Psychological Inventory, developed by the University of Washington Epi-

Table 14-1. Psychosocial Assessments

Washington Psychosocial Inventory
Adolescent Washington Psychosocial Inventory
Sepulveda Epilepsy Battery
Epilepsy Psycho-Social Effects Scale
Stigma of Epilepsy As a Self-Concept

lepsy Center group (Batzel et al., 1991) is a 38-item, yes or no response designed to evaluate concerns of teenagers (ages 12–19). The nine scales are: family background, emotional adjustment, interpersonal adjustment, school adjustment, vocational outlook, adjustment to seizures, medical management, antisocial activity, and overall functioning. There are two validity scales—lie and rare items. Overall and subscale scores are used, and validation studies were published in the first article. The inventory takes approximately 15 minutes to complete.

Sepulveda Epilepsy Battery

Developed at the Sepulveda Veterans Administration Hospital (Lund & Mittan, 1982; Mittan, 1986; Helgeson et al., 1990), this 18-item, self-completed questionnaire assesses patient's fears related to seizures. Items have multiple responses, and an overall score is obtained. Validation studies were published (Mittan, 1986). The battery takes approximately 6 minutes to complete.

Epilepsy Psycho-Social Effects Scale

This scale assesses patient adjustment to having seizures. The 42 items in the self-completed questionnaire fall into 14 categories and use a 5-point Likert scale. Validation studies were published (Chaplin et al., 1990). The scale takes approximately 15 minutes to complete. Cross-cultural use between Sweden and the United Kingdom has been published (Chaplin & Malmgren, 1999).

Stigma of Epilepsy As a Self-Concept

A sample of 445 people with epilepsy was studied for the extent to which stigma was felt (Ryan et al., 1980). Perceived stigma was used as a measure of the extent to which people with epilepsy felt they were victims of prejudice. The final model included six independent variables: perceived limitations, seizure severity, perceived discrimination, age, sex, and years of school. The underlying theme of perceived limitations was a sense of vulnerability to the physical consequences of seizures. A single score is created for each subject by summing responses of scale items. Validation was published (Ryan et al., 1980).

Adult Quality-of-Life Assessments

See Table 14-2.

Table 14-2. Adult Quality-of-Life Measures

Epilepsy Surgery Inventory 55 (ESI-55)

Quality of Life in Epilepsy Scales (QOLIE-89, QOLIE-31, QOLIE-10)

Subjective Handling of Epilepsy Scale

Liverpool Quality-of-Life Battery

Health-Related Quality of Life Questionnaire for People with Epilepsy

RAND 36-Item Health Survey (SF-36)

Quality of Life Assessment Schedule

Well-Being and Epilepsy

Life Fulfillment Scale

Impact of Epilepsy Scale

Epilepsy Foundation of America Concerns Index

Quality of Life in Newly Diagnosed Epilepsy Instrument

Glasgow Epilepsy Outcome Scales (GEOS-66 and GEOS-35)

Side Effect and Life Satisfaction (SEALS) Inventory

Epilepsy Surgery Inventory

The Epilepsy Surgery Inventory 55 was originally used with 224 medically refractory seizure surgery patients to assess HRQOL. The generic core was the 36-item RAND Health Survey (SF-36) with 19 epilepsy-specific items added. The scales include health perception (9 items); energy/fatigue (4 items); overall QOL (2 items); social functioning (2 items); emotional well-being (5 items); cognitive functioning (5 items); physical functioning (10 items); pain (2 items); role limitation consisting of emotional (5 items), physical (5 items), and memory (5 items); and change in health over the preceding year (1 item). A total score and three composite scores are obtained by weighting and summing individual scale scores (Vickrey et al., 1992, 1994, 1995). Langfitt (1995) has reported a reliability and validity comparison study of the Epilepsy Surgery Inventory 55, the WPSI, and a generic Sickness Impact Profile in a group of people with intractable seizures. Although it has been suggested that the Epilepsy Surgery Inventory 55 may detect change with a sample size of about 20, the minimal important difference to discriminate between treatment groups has yet to be identified. For persons of normal intelligence and

reading skill, the questionnaire should take approximately 20 minutes to complete. The copyright holder is the RAND Corporation, 1700 Main Street, PO Box 2138, Santa Monica, CA, USA 90407-2138.

Quality of Life in Epilepsy Scales

See Table 14-3 where the Quality of Life in Epilepsy Scale versions are tabulated using the Medical Outcomes Trust Scientific Advisory Committee Criteria.

Subjective Handling of Epilepsy Scale

The Subjective Handling of Epilepsy Scale, based on the WHO concept of handicap, has 32 items in six subscales: work and activities (8 items), social and personal (4 items), self-perception (5 items), physical (4 items), life satisfaction (4 items), and a change scale (7 items). Scoring is on a Likert scale (1–5 for each item), and item scores are summed. The subscale score is linearly transformed onto a 0 (worst handicap) to 100 (least handicap or most satisfaction) scale. Validation and reliability data have been published (O'Donoghue et al., 1998). Populations included neurology clinic patients and post-epilepsy surgery patients at a UK university. The scale takes approximately 10 minutes to complete. The Subjective Handling of Epilepsy Scale and scoring instructions have been published (O'Donoghue et al., 1998).

Liverpool Quality-of-Life Battery

In an effort to develop a comprehensive assessment of treatment effects in medically refractory epilepsy, the Liverpool group developed the Liverpool Seizure Severity Scale (Baker et al., 1991; Smith et al., 1991; Baker et al., 1998b). The group also developed a patient-based HRQOL model for epilepsy that included physical, social, and psychological domains designed to be used as an outcome measure for longitudinal study and to measure disability in cross-sectional studies. The approach of the group is to develop batteries tailored to assist in answering specific clinical questions. The initial battery (Baker et al., 1993) included the Liverpool Seizure Severity Scale divided into the Perception and Control subscale (8 items), and Ictal and Post-Ictal subscale (11 items), seizure frequency, the Nottingham Health Profile, the Side Effect and Life Satisfaction Inventory (SEALS), Activities of Daily Living, the Social Problems Questionnaire, the Hospital Anxiety and Depression Scale, the Affect Balance Scale, the Rosenberg Self-Esteem Scale, the Profile of Mood States, and the Liverpool

Table 14-3. Quality of Life in Epilepsy Scale-89 (QOLIE-89), QOLIE-31, QOLIE-10

Concept

17 multiscales to measure health concepts of

Overall quality of life (2 items)[1]

Emotional well-being (5 items)[1]

Role limitation—emotional (5 items)

Social support (4 items)

Social isolation (2 items)

Energy/fatigue (4 items)[1]

Seizure worry (5 items)[1]

Medication effects (3 items)[1]

Health discouragement (2 items)

Work/driving/social function (11 items)[1]

Attention/concentration (9 items)[1]

Language (5 items)

Memory (6 items)

Physical function (10 items)

Pain (2 items)

Role limitation—physical (5 items)

Health perceptions (6 items)

Change in 1-yr health (1 item)

Sexual satisfaction (1 item)[2]

Overall health (1 item)[1,2]

Conceptual and empirical bases

Generic core of QOLIE-89 is RAND 36-item Health Survey 1.0 (SF-36), which was adapted from MOS instruments. QOLIE-89 contains other items from longer MOS instruments, the ESI-55, the Dartmouth COOP Chart, the Faces Scale and visual analog scale. Thirty-two items were developed de novo.

Target population

304 adult males and females having simple partial, complex partial, generalized tonic-clonic, absence, and/or myoclonic seizures of mild to moderate severity were tested in 25 U.S. sites.

Final content

An initial 98-item battery was completed and then re-administered in 3 wk. A brief neuropsychological test battery, selected neurologic examination features, a proxy's assessment of the subject's quality of life, seizure occurrence, medication(s), demographics, and health care use were also obtained. From this, the QOLIE-89 was developed. From the QOLIE-89, items were empirically selected to develop the QOLIE-31 and QOLIE-10.

Scoring

Raw, precoded, numeric values are converted via tables. T-scores can be determined for an overall score and each of the 17-scale final scores. A higher T-score reflects a more favorable quality of life. The QOLIE-10 is not scored.

Reliability

Internal consistency reliabilities (Cronbach's alpha) range from $r = 0.78$ to $r = 0.92$. All scales exceeded 0.70, and 13 scales exceeded 0.80 (see Steinbuchel et al., 2000, for discussion).

Test-retest reliabilities (Pearson product-moment correlation) ranged from $r = 0.58$ to $r = 0.86$. All scales exceeded $r = 0.70$ except for pain and medication effects. Intra-class correlation coefficients ranged from 0.58 to 0.85.

Validity

Content validity was based on patient and clinician input and literature review. An open-ended question about concerns not covered identified finances, athletic participation, pregnancy, birth defects, stigma, insomnia, and bothering with taking medication.

Construct validity was explored by factor analysis identifying four factors (epilepsy-targeted [4 scales], cognitive [3 scales], mental health [6 scales], and physical health [4 scales]). These four factors were intercorrelated, justifying the use of the overall score.

Product-moment correlations between patient self-reports and corresponding proxy reports ranged from 0.29 (role limitations, emotional) to 0.57 (work/social function). All correlations were significant at $p < .0001$.

(continued)

Table 14-3. *(continued)*

Responsiveness

Although sensitivity to group differences has been demonstrated, the ability to demonstrate small differences in outcomes (responsiveness) is still debated, and the reader should go to on-line searches for results of ongoing studies.

Interpretability

Multiple publications have reported these scales to show differences with intervention (surgery, drug treatment), but the minimal important difference to discriminate between treatment groups has yet to be identified.

Burden

For persons of normal intelligence and reading skills at a rate of 3 items per minute, the QOLIE-89 takes approximately 30 min to complete, the QOLIE-31 approximately 10 min, and the QOLIE-10 approximately 3–5 min.

Alternative modes of administration

Information on alternative modes of administration (interviewer-administered, proxy, etc.) is not available.

Cultural and language adaptations

Cross-cultural translation in more than 10 languages is now available.

Source

Scoring manual and patient inventory and permission to use the QOLIE-89 or QOLIE-31 are available from: RAND Corporation, 1700 Main Street, PO Box 2138, Santa Monica, CA, USA 90407-2138; and for the QOLIE-10: Professional Postgraduate Services, 400 Plaza Drive, Secaucus, NJ, USA 07094.

ESI-55 = Epilepsy Surgery Inventory 55; MOS = Medical Outcomes Study.
[1] QOLIE-31 and QOLIE-10 include items from these scales.
[2] Added after field testing.
Note: It is impossible to list all of the citations for the QOLIE instruments, and the reader should perform a computerized literature search such as OVID. References listed here are the first references. QOLIE-89—description: Vickrey et al., 1993a; Devinsky et al., 1995. Validation: Devinsky et al., 1995; Perrine, 1993; Perrine at al., 1995. QOLIE-31—description: Vickrey et al., 1993b; Cramer et al., 1998. Validation: Cramer et al., 1998. QOLIE-10—description and reliability: Cramer et al., 1996.

Mastery Scale (7 items). The patient population consisted of 81 medically refractory seizure patients. Validity and reliability results were published. Scores are derived for each scale with no overall score. The questionnaire took approximately 45 minutes to complete.

The Social Problems Questionnaire was recognized early on to be of limited value and was replaced with a 13-item Life Fulfillment Scale (Baker et al., 1994b) and an 8-item Impact on Epilepsy Scale (Jacoby et al., 1993) with reliability and validity tested on 75 epilepsy clinic patients (Baker et al., 1994b, see Life Fulfillment Scale and Impact of Epilepsy Scale for further discussion of these two scales). Subsequently deleted were the Nottingham Health Profile, the SEALS, Activities of Daily Living, and the Profile of Mood States. Added have been a Stigma Scale and Adverse Effects Profile. The Liverpool experience has been documented by Baker (1998).

Subsequently, a composite seizure severity scale has been developed that is based on three existing scales: the Liverpool Seizure Severity Instrument, the National Hospital Seizure Severity Scale, and the VA Seizure Frequency and Severity Rating (Cramer et al., 2002).

The Liverpool Battery is flexible. An investigator can choose measures tailored to answer specific questions. Medline search reveals multiple publications using the Liverpool Battery. Comparison across studies may be difficult if different measures have been used.

The Epilepsy and Learning Disability Questionnaire was developed for completion by parents and caregivers for learning disability persons with epilepsy. The 66-item instrument has subscales for seizure severity (14 items), drug-related side effects (18 items), mood (14 items), behavior (9 items), and single items relating to seizure-related injuries, health, and overall QOL (Baker et al., 1994a, 2000; Jacoby et al., 1996). Construct validity and reliability have been reported (Baker et al., 1994a).

The Liverpool group subsequently developed the Quality of Life in Newly Diagnosed Epilepsy Instrument (NEWQOL), which is discussed later.

Permission to use the copyrighted instruments may be obtained from Department of Neurosciences, Walton Hospital, Rice Lane, Liverpool L9 1AE, UK.

Health-Related Quality of Life Questionnaire for People with Epilepsy

The Health-Related Quality of Life Questionnaire for People with Epilepsy is a 171-item, 31-subscale, self-administered questionnaire that includes the UK version of the RAND 36-item Health Survey, a symptom check list and other generic health measures. The complete listing of scales, subscales, number of items, and source of items is in Table 14-4 (Devinsky & Cramer, 1997). Validation was with 136 epilepsy patients (Wagner et al., 1995, 1997). For persons with normal intelligence and reading ability, the questionnaire takes about 45 minutes to complete. The copyright holder is Schering-Plough Inc., Kenilworth, NJ, USA.

RAND 36-Item Health Survey and Other Generic Instruments

SF-36 refers to version 1.0 of the RAND (Hays et al., 1993) and the almost identical Medical Outcomes Study Short Form 36 Health Survey (Ware & Sherbourne, 1992). These scales were developed for broad use among various populations and are referred to as *generic*. They are usually used to assess common issues across disease groups or general issues within a population. Studies with epilepsy have used the SF-36. The questions being studied determine whether a generic or epilepsy-specific QOL measure best.

Other generic QOL instruments include the Nottingham Health Profile (Hunt et al., 1980, 1985), the Sickness Impact Profile (Bergner, 1988), the Dartmouth COOP Function Charts (Nelson et al., 1990), and the EUROQOL (EuroQol Group, 1990).

Quality of Life Assessment Schedule

This repertory grid technique allows people to construct a picture of their current QOL relative to past experiences, those of other people, and future expectations. The technique dates to 1977 (Fransella & Bannister, 1977) and uses a Construct Importance Scale in which patients identify 10 items affecting their QOL and rate the items on a subscale ranging from 1 (no problem) to 5 (could not be worse). Aggregate and profile scores are calculated. The profile score shows dif-

ferences between actual (NOW) and desired (LIKE) status. Kendrick and Trimble (1994) used the technique in persons with epilepsy and subsequently simplified and revised the QOLAS (Selai & Trimble, 1995).

In the revised version, a semi-structured interview is used. In the interview, people are invited to discuss what is important in their QOL and the ways in which their current health situation affect their QOL. Ten constructs are elicited from among the five domains of physical functioning, psychological/emotional status, social functioning, work/economic status, or cognitive abilities (two constructs from each domain). People rate their constructs with a 5-point Likert scale on how much of a problem each item is for them at the moment. Then the constructs are rated on how much of a problem they would like the construct to be. They are also asked to rate other situations and people in their lives. The current view of their life situation (NOW) is measured in relation to how far they must progress to achieve their desired state (LIKE). The shorter the distance (NOW-LIKE) may indicate a greater QOL. A global level (composite score) and individual level (profile) are obtained (Selai et al., 1994). The interviews tend to be lengthy.

Well-Being and Epilepsy

This is an assessment between current self-perception and how life would be without epilepsy. A total score is obtained from the self-administered 105-item questionnaire. There are six subscales: self-image, life fulfillment, social/interpersonal difficulties, general physical health, worries, and affect balance. Validation data have been published (Collings, 1990a, 1990b).

Life Fulfillment Scale

This scale is an adjunct to the Liverpool QOL Battery developed based on the concept of Krupinsky (1980). In the two-phase, self-administered questionnaire, the person was first asked to use a 4-point Likert scale to rate the importance of 13 aspects of daily life: (1) a good family life, (2) having close friends in whom you can confide, (3) a happy marriage (or similar relationship), (4) being happy with the area where you live, (5) having housing that meets your needs, (6) being able to do things you enjoy in your spare time, (7) enjoying a good social life, (8) being in good health, (9) being happy with yourself as a person, (10) having a job that you consider satisfying, (11) having a secure and stable job, (12) having an adequate standard of living, and (13) having enough money to do most of the things you wish.

Table 14-4.   Scales, Subscales, Number of Items, and Source of Items in the Health-Related Quality of Life Questionnaire for People with Epilepsy[a]

HQL Scales and Subscales	No. of Items[b]	Source
General HQL—SF-36 Scales		
Physical functioning	**10**	SF-36 UK version
Role functioning—physical	**4**	SF-36 UK version plus one new item
Augmented role functioning—physical	5	
Bodily pain	**2**	SF-36 UK version
General health perceptions	**5**	SF-36 UK version plus one item from the MOS
Current health	4	
Health outlook	1	
Resistance to illness	1	
Vitality	**4**	SF-36 UK version
Social functioning	**2**	SF-36 UK version
Role functioning—emotional	**3**	SF-36 UK version plus one new item
Augmented role functioning—emotional	**4**	
Mental health	**5**	SF-36 UK version
Change in health	**1**	SF-36 UK version
General HQL—additional scales		
Mental health	**18**	MH-18 (included MH-5) plus
Anxiety	4	
Depression	4	
Behavior/emotional control	5	One item from MHI-38
Positive well-being	5	
Emotional ties	4	Three items from UCLA Loneliness Scale
Overall quality of life	**1**	MOS
Cognition	**13**	Six-item MOS cognition scale plus one item from SIP
Confusion	2	
Thinking	2	One item from PERI
Concentration	2	Two items from PERI
Attention	2	One item from SIP
Memory	1	
Reasoning	1	
Psychomotor functioning	3	Two items from SIP
Epilepsy-specific HQL scales		
Mastery	**6**	Pearlin/Schooler Master Scale
Impact	**8**	Liverpool Impact Scale
Experience	**13**	New items
Worry	**9**	New items
Agitation	**2**	Health Insurance Study
Distress	**2**	MOS

Table 14-4. *(continued)*

HQL Scales and Subscales	No. of Items[b]	Source
Seizure severity scales		
Ictal	**12**	Liverpool Seizure Severity Scale
Percept	**8**	Liverpool Seizure Severity Scale
Symptoms	**16**	New items
Open-ended questions	**2**	New items

HQL = health-related quality of life; MHI = Mental Health Inventory; MOS = Medical Outcomes Study; PERI = Psychiatric Epidemiology Research Interview; SIP = Sickness Impact Profile.
[a]Development of the Health-Related Quality of Life Questionnaire for People with Epilepsy was supported by Schering-Plough International.
[b]Bold numbers indicate the overall number of items for each major domain. Nonbold numbers indicate numbers of items for each subscale.

In the second phase, the person was asked to rate his or her satisfaction with the current actual situation. Factor component analysis yielded a two-factor solution called Personal Fulfillment (accounting for 29% of variance) and Material Fulfillment (accounting for 13% of variance). Personal Fulfillment consisted of items 1–3 and 6–10 and Material Fulfillment consisted of items 4, 5, 12, and 13. Item 11 was excluded because it did not load onto either scale, so the current version rates 12 aspects of daily life. The discrepancy between the two ratings is calculated as fulfillment. Reliability and validity were published (Baker et al., 1994b). The scale takes approximately 10 minutes to complete.

Impact of Epilepsy Scale

This scale is an adjunct to the Liverpool QOL Battery used to describe the perceived impact of epilepsy on QOL. Scale items are: (1) relationship with spouse/partner, (2) relationship with other close family members, (3) social life/social activities, (4) work, (5) health, (6) relationship with friends, (7) feelings about self, and (8) plans and ambitions for the future. People were asked to rate, using a 4-point Likert scale ranging from 1 (not at all) to 4 (a lot), how much they thought that item was affected by their epilepsy and its treatment. Total impact score was obtained by summing the items, with the higher the score, the greater the perceived impact of epilepsy and treatment. Construct validity and correlation coefficients to other psychological measures have been published. Reliability in the initial study was reduced by inclusion of the work item, so the scale was revised to accommodate both employed and unem-

ployed persons, and the wording of the item has been changed (Jacoby et al., 1993). The scale takes approximately 5 minutes to complete.

Epilepsy Foundation of America Concerns Index

Originally published as the Patient-Validated Content of Epilepsy-Specific Quality-of-Life Measurement, the Epilepsy Foundation of America Concerns Index was renamed to acknowledge the research support from the Epilepsy Foundation of America to one of the developers (Dr. Gilliam) early in his career. The developers asked 81 patients with chronic epilepsy to list, in order of importance, concerns about living with epilepsy. These concerns were tabulated into 24 domains: driving, independence, employment, social embarrassment, medication dependence, mood/stress, safety/injury, medication side effects, recreation, social life, seizure unpredictability, cognitive effects of epilepsy, worry about family, seizure aversion, MD/hospital dependence, enigma of epilepsy, family worry, medical costs, future, discrimination, pregnancy/birth defects, personal hygiene, education, and self-worth. The tabulated concerns were then transposed to questions and were reviewed with the same patients in small group-structured interviews (Gilliam et al., 1997).

The current Epilepsy Foundation of America Concerns Index is composed of 20 questions that are rated on a 5-point scale which is summed into a Concerns Index score with a range from 20 to 100. Internal consistency and reproducibility data have been published (Gilliam et al., 1999). The Epilepsy Foundation of America Concerns Index takes approximately 10 minutes to complete.

Quality of Life in Newly Diagnosed Epilepsy Instrument

The Liverpool group recognized that concerns for the person newly diagnosed with epilepsy may be different than those for the person with chronic epilepsy. The developers conducted qualitative interviews with 18 people with seizure onset within 6 months and identified key themes from the interviews that were used as the basis for the structured questionnaire (Abetz et al., 2000).

NEWQOL is a self-completed battery of 93 previously validated and novel multi-item scales and single items. Of the 93 items, 81 are used to score eight multi-item scales (total of 13 subscales) that measure: anxiety/depression, social activities, symptoms, locus of control/mastery, neuropsychological problems (fatigue, memory, concentration, motor skills, and reading), social stigma, worry, and work limitations. Single-item measures are used to measure general health, number of seizures, social limitations, social support, self-concept, ambition limitations, health transition, and general limitations. An additional five items were used to examine the extent of support networks available to the patient. The NEWQOL is described in detail, with validity and reliability data, in the publication by Abetz et al. (2000). NEWQOL takes approximately 30 minutes to complete and is intended for people age 16 and older.

Glasgow Epilepsy Outcome Scale

The Glasgow scale is for use with adults with epilepsy and mental retardation. The scale was preceded by a pilot scale (Espie et al., 1998). A total of 1,007 items were generated by 48 caregivers and 46 health practitioners, and 90 items were selected to comprise four subscales: seizures, treatment, caring, and social impact. The scale can be completed by clinicians, caregivers, or family members. A 90-item Glasgow Epilepsy Outcome Scale 90 and 35-item Glasgow Epilepsy Outcome Scale 35 are available and validity and reliability data have been published (Espie et al., 2001).

Side Effect and Life Satisfaction Inventory

The original SEALS (Brown & Tomlinson, 1982) was a 50-item self-report questionnaire to identify subtle subjective side effects of antiepileptic drugs analyzed by five derived factors: mood and irritability,

general cognitive difficulties, satisfaction, fatigue, and interpersonal skills. Gillham et al. (1996) refined the five factors and reduced the number of questions to 38. The 38-item questionnaire takes approximately 15 minutes to complete, has been validated in a UK population, is available in nine cross-cultural translations, and purportedly is able to distinguish between antiepileptic drugs (Gillham et al., 2000).

Assessment Scales for Children, Adolescents, and Families

During the past decade, a proliferation of scales putatively measuring QOL in children and adolescents has been published (Table 14-5). Discussion has arisen whether these scales actually measure the people's QOL in relation to their personal expectations. The argument is made that the QOL scale must be derived from direct descriptions and definitions from the person. Are these scales measuring the person's QOL or a proxy's expectations of the QOL for the person? Although parent or proxy impressions are valid in themselves, they cannot be considered as valid substitutes for the person's perspective (McEwan et al., 2004).

The paper by McEwan et al. (2004) used criteria rating sheets defined by the Critical Appraisal Skills Programme guidelines for qualitative research (CASP, 2000) to evaluate 17 publications investigating QOL in children or adolescents (age 5–18 years). The five study quality criteria were:

Table 14-5. Child, Adolescent, and Family Quality-of-Life Measures

Health-Related Quality of Life in Epilepsy

Child Attitude Toward Illness Scale

Quality of Life in Epilepsy Inventory for Adolescents (QOLIE-AD-48)

Adolescent Stigma Scale

Impact of Childhood Illness Scale

Hague Restrictions in Childhood Epilepsy Scale

Quality of Life in Childhood Epilepsy Questionnaire

Impact of Pediatric Epilepsy Scale

Impact of Childhood Neurologic Disability Scale

Bipolar Visual Analogue Scale

Quality of Life in Pediatric Epilepsy Scale

"1. An appropriate sampling strategy (e.g., details regarding how and where participants were selected; details provided on nonparticipants; and consideration of saturation of data in relation to sampling size, i.e., ensuring theoretical saturation is obtained, where no additional data are gained by further collection, to increase reliability of findings);

2. Rigorous data analysis (e.g., explanation of how analysis was carried out; attempts to ensure the reliability of data by methods, such as feeding back results to participants, repetition of analysis by more than one researcher, and use of triangulation methods, i.e., the combination of methods to take into account as many aspects of a problem as possible);

3. Accurate interpretation of data (provision of adequate quotes to support findings);

4. A clear statement of the aims of the research with consideration of qualitative methodology as the most appropriate approach; and

5. Transferability of results (i.e., relevance of study to the wider population beyond the study sample, which is increased by use of methods to increase validity and reliability of results and provision of details of participants and non-participants)" (McEwan et al., 2004, p. 5).

Although an extensive literature search was performed, it is not clear in this author's opinion whether or not all pertinent papers were identified or whether some papers were excluded from the review for other reasons. The only QOL measure that they identified as meeting quality criteria was that of Ronen et al. (1999, 2001).

Health-Related Quality of Life in Childhood Epilepsy

Separate groups of children ages 6–12 years who function in a regular school situation and their parents were recruited from a regional Canadian epilepsy database. Nine child and 17 parent small focus groups met to analyze HRQOL components. Five components were identified: the experience of epilepsy, life fulfillment and time use, social issues, impact of epilepsy, and attribution (Ronen et al., 1999, 2001).

From this background, the group has gone on to develop two related 25-item HRQOL instruments for children with epilepsy. A 67-item questionnaire was completed independently by children ages 6–15 years with epilepsy and their parents. Results from 6- to 7-

year-olds did not have sufficient reliability and were dropped from analysis. From this, five items were chosen for each subscale. The child and parent questionnaires share four subscales and each has an additional distinct subscale. Validity and reliability were published. As expected, discrepancies were found between child and parent perspectives of QOL (Ronen et al., 2003).

Child Attitude Toward Illness Scale

The Child Attitude Toward Illness Scale consists of 13 self-administered items with a five-point response. Originally developed and validated with children ages 8–12 (Austin & Huberty, 1993), it was later extended to adolescents ages 11–17 (Heimlich et al., 2000). It takes about 5 minutes to complete. It is a generic scale and has been used to compare QOL with other diseases (Austin et al., 1992, 1994).

The Child Attitude Toward Illness Scale is one of several scales this group has included in scales measuring perceived stigma in children with epilepsy and their parents (Austin et al., 2004). Related scales developed by this group include a scale to measure psychosocial care needs of children with seizures and their parents (Austin et al., 1998) and a Seizure Self-Efficacy Scale for Children that measures degree of self-efficacy related to management of their seizures (Caplin et al., 2002).

Quality of Life in Epilepsy Inventory for Adolescents

The Quality of Life in Epilepsy Inventory for Adolescents was developed by a panel of seven experts who selected items from a variety of sources including adolescent focus groups and experiences from health professionals who work with this population. The self-administered 48 items are in eight subscales: epilepsy impact (12 items), memory/concentration (10 items), attitudes toward epilepsy (4 items), physical functioning (5 items), stigma (6 items), social support (4 items), school behavior (4 items), and health perceptions (3 items). A total summary score is obtained. Validity and reliability results have been published. The inventory takes approximately 25 minutes to complete (Cramer et al., 1999; Devinsky et al., 1999).

Adolescent Stigma Scale

The Adolescent Stigma Scale includes four questions pertaining to perceived stigma and four questions pertaining to disclosure of the diagnosis of epilepsy to others. The scale was developed and validated with 64 adolescents (ages 12–20 years) with idiopathic epilepsy. It takes about 5 minutes to complete (Westbrook et al., 1992).

Impact of Childhood Illness Scale

The Impact of Childhood Illness Scale is completed by parents. Initially, the 30-item scale pilot study involved 21 parents of children with chronic epilepsy attending a UK seizure clinic. Four aspects were considered: epilepsy and its treatment, impact on the child, impact on the parent, and impact on the family. Each question was considered in terms of frequency of the problem and degree of concern it causes (Hoare & Russsell, 1995). The scale was then administered to parents of 108 school children with chronic epilepsy (Hoare, 1993). A newer 30-item questionnaire was designed for use with children with epilepsy or diabetes and has been published (Hoare et al., 2000).

Hague Restrictions in Childhood Epilepsy Scale

The 10-item Hague Restrictions in Childhood Epilepsy Scale with 4-point Likert-type questions is to be completed by parents of children with epilepsy ages 4 to 12 or older. Validation has been published (Carpay et al., 1997). A U.S. version has been published (O'Dell et al., 1998).

Quality of Life in Childhood Epilepsy Questionnaire

The Quality of Life in Childhood Epilepsy Questionnaire, developed in Australia, is completed by guardians of children (5 years and older) and consists of an epilepsy-specific parent HRQOL scale and two generic parent scales. Five domains are covered: physical function, emotional well-being, cognitive function, social function, and behavior. Validation results have been published (Sabaz et al., 2000). The Quality of Life in Childhood Epilepsy Questionnaire has also been validated in American epilepsy patients (Sabaz et al., 2003). A self-report, epilepsy-specific scale of HRQOL for children older than 10 years is planned (Sabaz et al., 2000).

Impact of Pediatric Epilepsy Scale and Childhood Neurologic Disability Scale

The Impact of Pediatric Epilepsy Scale is an 11-item scale completed by the parent to evaluate the influence of epilepsy on the major aspects of their family and child's life. External validation from several sources and internal validation have been published. Areas covered include overall health, family relationships, social life and family activities, school, self-esteem, and loss of original hope for the child. The scale takes less than 5 minutes to complete (Camfield et al., 2001).

The Impact of Childhood Neurologic Disability Scale evaluates the impact of three additional areas: behavior, cognition, and physical/neurologic disability in children with epilepsy. Parents of children ages 2–18 years completed the 44-item scale. External validation and internal consistency were reported. Parents are asked to rate on a 4-point scale how much impact each of four conditions has had on various aspects of the child's and the family's life. The conditions are: (1) inattentiveness, impulsivity, or mood; (2) ability to think and remember; (3) neurologic or physical limitations; and (4) epilepsy (overall problem of having epilepsy—its social consequences, degree of control and types of seizures, treatment, and side effects) (Camfield et al., 2003).

A cross-validation study utilizing the Impact of Childhood Illness Scale, Impact of Childhood Neurologic Disability Scale, and the Hague Restrictions in Childhood Epilepsy Scale showed high intercorrelation, but differences between the instruments emerged and suggest that care must be taken in choosing an instrument (Sherman et al., 2002).

Bipolar Visual Analogue Scale

The Bipolar Visual Analogue Scale contains 39 bipolar adjectives denoting extreme opposites, and the child is asked to mark on a visual analogue scale 100 mm in length. Only 31 children between 9 and 13 years were studied, and 18 children were seizure-free without medication. Validity data were presented (Norby et al., 1999).

Quality of Life in Pediatric Epilepsy Scale

The Quality of Life in Pediatric Epilepsy Scale contains child and parent forms that each contain 20 questions. Eighty consecutive patients age 3 months to 18 years were asked to list in order of importance their concerns, with 80 parents and 48 children completing the forms. Twenty-one concerns were common to both parents and children; five were listed only by parents, and five listed only by children. Twenty-six domains were identified and, from this, a 20-item form generated. Validation has not yet been published (Arunkumar et al., 2000).

Conclusions

During the past decade, there has been an exponential increase in the number of QOL tests and publications. The author apologizes for any that have been missed. There are a number of review articles that also cannot be cited in this text. I do recommend a book edited by Baker and Jacoby entitled *Quality of Life in Epilepsy* (2000). The chapter in that book by Steinbuchel et al. (2000) is recommended for a summary of the psychometric properties of many of the instruments.

Evaluation criteria are being developed to evaluate instruments, which will lead to stronger instruments. Terminology is still a problem. What is the overlap between HRQOL and QOL? Are patient-reported outcome instruments truly QOL instruments? Although parent/caregiver evaluations appear to be different from the affected individual's evaluation, there appears to be a role for both, and knowing these differences may lead to useful therapy. How is QOL best measured in the learning disabled, particularly those severely affected?

Use of QOL measures is expanding. Baker (2000) has an excellent review of QOL measures in randomized, clinical, antiepileptic drug trials. The question of whether small differences in short-term outcome are truly valid appears to need more work. Many publications continue to look at surgical outcomes, vagal nerve stimulation outcomes, ketogenic diet outcomes, and other alternative therapy outcomes. A comprehensive interpretation strategy that gives results that are meaningful to a variety of audiences, including patients, clinicians, and decision makers, has been proposed (Marquis et al., 2004). How to choose the appropriate measure for the question being asked is not easy, but the good news is that there are now many choices. The instruments can presumably be used to evaluate efficacy of health care delivery systems. Evidence-based medicine, although not yet uniformly espoused, is making increasing use of QOL instruments.

The role of QOL instruments in routine clinical practice is unclear. Are they of any practical value? The reader is referred to the article by Cramer (1999) for the pros and to the article by Betts (2000) for the cons.

The interplay with increases in scientific knowledge about epilepsy and seizures cannot be overlooked. Is there a difference in QOL based on seizure type or on epilepsy syndrome? Our classification of both seizures and epilepsy is bound to change based on new genetic findings and will affect how we view QOL.

Despite our lack of knowledge on many aspects of QOL instruments, the bottom line is clear. Information gained from QOL instruments can empower patients to achieve their best possible outcome, and that is, after all, what medicine and health care are about.

References

Abetz L, Jacoby A, Baker GA, et al. Patient-based assessments of quality of life in newly diagnosed epilepsy patients: validation of the NEWQOL. *Epilepsia* 2000; 41:1119–28.

Arunkumar G, Wyllie E, Kotagal P, et al. Parent- and patient-validated content for pediatric epilepsy quality-of-life assessment. *Epilepsia* 2000;41:1474–84.

Austin JK, Dunn D, Huster G, et al. Development of scales to measure psychosocial care needs of children with seizures and their parents. *J Neurosci Nurs* 1998;30:155–60.

Austin JK, Huberty TJ. Development of the Child Attitude Toward Illness Scale. *J Pediatr Psychol* 1993;18:467–80.

Austin JK, MacLeod J, Dunn DW, et al. Measuring stigma in children with epilepsy and their parents: instrument development and testing. *Epilepsy Behav* 2004;5:472-82.

Austin JK, Risinger MW, Beckett LA. Correlates of behavior problems in children with epilepsy. *Epilepsia* 1992; 33:1115–22.

Austin JK, Smith MS, Risinger M, et al. Childhood epilepsy and asthma: comparison of quality of life. *Epilepsia* 1994;35:608–15.

Baker GA. Quality of life and epilepsy: the Liverpool experience. *Clin Ther* 1998;20(Suppl A):A2–12.

Baker GA. Use of quality of life assessment as an outcome measure in clinical research. In: Baker GA, Jacoby A (eds.). *Quality of life in epilepsy: beyond seizure counts in assessment and treatment.* Reading, UK: Harwood Academic Publishers, 2000:181–95.

Baker GA, Camfield C, Camfield P, et al. Commission On Outcome Measurement in Epilepsy, 1994–1997; Final report. *Epilepsia* 1998a;39:213–31.

Baker GA, Jacoby A (eds.). *Quality of life in epilepsy: beyond seizure counts in assessment and treatment.* Reading, UK: Harwood Academic, 2000.

Baker GA, Hesdon B, Marson AG. Quality-of-life and behavioral outcome measures in randomized controlled trials of antiepileptic drugs: a systematic review of methodology and reporting standards. *Epilepsia* 2000;41:1357–63.

Baker GA, Jacoby A, Berney T, et al. Development of an instrument to assess quality of life in children with epilepsy and learning disability. *Epilepsia* 1994a;35(Suppl 7):47(abst).

Baker GA, Jacoby A, Smith DF, et al. Development of a novel scale to assess life fulfillment as part of the further refinement of a quality-of-life model for epilepsy. *Epilepsia* 1994b;35:591–96.

Baker GA, Smith DF, Dewey M, et al. The development of a seizure severity scale as an outcome measure in epilepsy. *Epilepsy Res* 1991;8:245–51.

Baker GA, Smith DF, Dewey M, et al. The initial development of a health-related quality of life model as an outcome measure in epilepsy. *Epilepsy Res* 1993;16:65–81.

Baker GA, Smith DF, Jacoby A, et al. Liverpool seizure severity scale revisited. *Seizure* 1998b;7:201–05.

Batzel LW, Dodrill CB, Dubinsky BL. An objective method for the assessment of psychosocial problems in adolescents with epilepsy. *Epilepsia* 1991;32:202–11.

Bergner M. Development, testing, and use of the Sickness Impact Profile. In: Walker SR, Rosser MR (eds.). *Quality of life: assessment and application*. Lancaster, UK: MTP Press, 1988:79–84.

Betts T. Non est vivere, sed valere vita est* A physician reflects on quality of life. In: Baker GA, Jacoby A (eds.). *Quality of life in epilepsy: beyond seizure counts in assessment and treatment*. Reading, UK: Harwood Academic, 2000:161–70.

Brown SW, Tomlinson LL. Anticonvulsant side-effects: a self-report questionnaire for use in community surveys. *Br J Clin Pract* 1982;Suppl 18:147–49.

Camfield C, Breau L, Camfield P. Assessing the impact of pediatric epilepsy and concomitant behavioral, cognitive, and physical/neurologic disability: impact of Childhood Neurologic Disability Scale. *Develop Med Child Neurol* 2003;45:152–59.

Camfield C, Breau L, Camfield P. Impact of pediatric epilepsy on the family: a new scale for clinical and research use. *Epilepsia* 2001;42:104–12.

Caplin D, Austin JK, Dunn DW, et al. Development of a self-efficacy scale for children and adolescents with epilepsy. *Child Health Care* 2002;31:295–309.

Carpay JA, Vermeulen J, Stroink H, et al. Disability due to restrictions in childhood epilepsy. *Develop Med Child Neurol* 1997;39:521–26.

CASP. *The critical appraisal skills programme: 10 questions to help you make sense of qualitative research*. Oxford: The CASP Office, 2000.

Cereghino JJ. Comprehensive epilepsy programs in the United States—an update. In: Akimoto H, Kazamatsuri H, Seino M, et al. (eds.). *Advances in epileptology: XIIIth Epilepsy International Symposium*. New York: Raven Press, 1982:453–54.

Cereghino JJ, Penry JK, Smith LD. Comprehensive epilepsy programs in the United States. In: Canger R, Angeleri F, Penry JK (eds.). *Advances in epileptology: XIth epilepsy international symposium*. New York: Raven Press, 1980: 257–60.

Chaplin JE, Malmgren K. Cross-cultural adaptation and use of the epilepsy psycho-social effects scale: comparison between the psychosocial effects of chronic epilepsy in Sweden and the UK. *Epilepsia* 1999;40:93–96.

Chaplin JE, Yepez R, Shorvon S, et al. A quantitative approach to measuring the social effects of epilepsy. *Neuroepidemiology* 1990;9:151–58.

Collings JA. Correlates of well-being in a New Zealand epilepsy sample. *N Z Med J* 1990a;103:301–3.

Collings JA. Psychosocial well-being and epilepsy: an empirical study. *Epilepsia* 1990b;31:418–26.

Commission on Classification and Terminology of the International League Against Epilepsy. Proposal for revised clinical and electroencephalographic classification of epileptic seizures. *Epilepsia* 1981;22:489–501.

Commission on Classification and Terminology of the International League Against Epilepsy. Proposal for revised clinical and electroencephalographic classification of epilepsies and epileptic syndromes. *Epilepsia* 1989;30: 389–99.

Cramer JA. Quality of life assessment in clinical practice. *Neurology* 1999;53(Suppl 2):S49–52.

Cramer JA. ILAE Subcommission on Outcome Measurement in Epilepsy. Principles of health-related quality of life: assessment in clinical trials. *Epilepsia* 2002;43: 1084–95.

Cramer JA, Baker GA, Jacoby A. Development of a new seizure severity questionnaire: initial reliability and validity testing. *Epilepsy Res* 2002;48:187–97.

Cramer JA, Perrine K, Devinsky O, et al. A brief questionnaire to screen for quality of life in epilepsy: the QOLIE-10. *Epilepsia* 1996;37:577–82.

Cramer JA, Perrine K, Devinsky O, et al. Development and cross-cultural translations of a 31-item quality of life in epilepsy inventory. *Epilepsia* 1998;39:81–88.

Cramer JA, Westbrook LE, Devinsky O, et al. Development of the quality of life in epilepsy inventory for adolescents: the QOLIE-AD-48. *Epilepsia* 1999;40:1114–21.

Devinsky O. Quality of life in epilepsy: time to practice what we preach. *Epilepsy Behav* 2000;1:89–90.

Devinsky O, Cramer J. Health-related quality of life scales for epilepsy. In: Herndon RM (ed.). *Handbook of neurologic rating scales*. New York: Demos Vermande, 1997:209–23.

Devinsky O, Vickrey BG, Cramer JA, et al. Development of the quality of life inventory. *Epilepsia* 1995;36:1089–104.

Devinsky O, Westbrook LE, Cramer JA, et al. Risk factors for poor health-related quality of life in adolescents with epilepsy. *Epilepsia* 1999;40:1715–20.

Dodrill CB. A neuropsychological battery for epilepsy. *Epilepsia* 1978;19:611–23.

Dodrill CB, Batzel LW. The Washington Psychosocial Seizure Inventory: new developments in the light of the quality of life concept. *Epilepsia* 1995;36(Suppl 3): S220 (abst).

Dodrill CB, Batzel LW, Queisser HR, et al. An objective method for the assessment of psychological and social problems among epileptics. *Epilepsia* 1980;21:123–35.

Engel J Jr. ILAE Commission Report. A proposed diagnostic scheme for people with epileptic seizures and with epilepsy: report of the ILAE Task Force on classification and terminology. *Epilepsia* 2001;42:796–803.

Espie CA, Paul A, Graham M, et al. The Epilepsy Outcome Scale: the development of a measure for use with carers of people with epilepsy and intellectual disabilities. *J Intellect Disabil Res* 1998;42:90–96.

Espie CA, Watkins J, Duncan R, et al. Development and validation of the Glasgow Epilepsy Outcome Scale (GEOS): a new instrument for measuring concerns about epilepsy in people with mental retardation. *Epilepsia* 2001; 42:1043–51.

EuroQol Group. EuroQol—a new facility for the measurement of health-related quality of life. *Health Policy* 1990;16:199–208.

Fransella F, Bannister D. *A manual for repertory grid technique.* London: Academic Press, 1977.

Gilham R, Baker G, Thompson P, et al. Standardisation of a self-report questionnaire for use in evaluating cognitive, affective, and behavioural side-effects of antiepileptic drug treatments. *Epilepsy Res* 1996;24:47–55.

Gilham R, Bryant-Comstock L, Kane K. Validation of the side effect and life satisfaction (SEALS) inventory. *Seizure* 2000;9:458–63.

Gilliam F, Kuzniecky R, Faught E, et al. Patient-validated content of epilepsy-specific quality-of-life measurement. *Epilepsia* 1997;38:233–36.

Gilliam F, Kuzniecky R, Meador K, et al. Patient-oriented outcome assessment after temporal lobectomy for refractory epilepsy. *Neurology* 1999;53:687–94.

Halstead WC. *Brain and intelligence: a quantitative study of the frontal lobes.* Chicago: University of Chicago Press, 1947.

Hays RD, Sherbourne C, Mazel E. The RAND 36-item health survey 1.0 *Health Econ* 1993;2:217–27.

Heimlich TE, Westbrook LE, Austin JK, et al. Brief report: adolescents' attitudes toward epilepsy: further validation of the Child Attitude Toward Illness Scale (CATIS). *J Pediatr Psychol* 2000;25:339–45.

Helgeson DC, Mittan R, Tan SY, et al. Sepulveda Epilepsy Education: the efficacy of a psychoeducational treatment program in treating medical and psychosocial aspects of epilepsy. *Epilepsia* 1990;31:75–82.

Hoare P. The quality of life of children with chronic epilepsy and their families. *Seizure* 1993;2:269–75.

Hoare P, Mann H, Dunn S. Parental perception of the quality of life among children with epilepsy or diabetes with a new assessment questionnaire. *Qual Life Research* 2000;9:637–44.

Hoare P, Russell M. The quality of life of children with chronic epilepsy and their families: preliminary findings with a new assessment measure. *Dev Med Child Neurol* 1995;37:689–96.

Hunt SM, McKenna SP, McEwen J, et al. A quantitative approach to perceived health status: a validation study. *J Epidemiol Community Health* 1980;34:281–86.

Hunt SM, McEwan J, McKenna SP. Measuring health status: a new tool for clinicians and epidemiologists. *J R Coll Gen Pract* 1985;35:185–88.

Jacoby A, Baker G, Bryant-Comstock L, et al. Lamotrigine add-on therapy is associated with improvement in mood in patients with severe epilepsy. *Epilepsia* 1996; 37(Suppl 5):202(abst).

Jacoby A, Baker G, Smith D, et al. Measuring the impact of epilepsy: the development of a novel scale. *Epilepsy Research* 1993;16:83–88.

Kendrick AM, Trimble MR. Repertory grid technique in the assessment of quality of life in patients with epilepsy: the quality of life assessment schedule. In: Trimble MR, Dodson WE (eds.). *Epilepsy and quality of life.* New York: Raven Press, 1994:151–64.

Krupinsky J. Health and quality of life. *Soc Sci Med* 1980; 14A:203–11.

Langfitt JT. Comparison of the psychometric characteristics of three quality of life measures in intractable epilepsy. *Qua Life Res* 1995;4:101–14.

Lund GF, Mittan RJ. The urban epilepsy program at the King/Drew Medical Center. *Urban Health* 1982;11:30–32.

Marquis P, Chassany O, Abetz L. A comprehensive strategy for the interpretation of quality-of-life data based on existing methods. *Value in Health* 2004;7:93–104.

McEwan MJ, Espie CA, Metcalfe J. A systematic review of the contribution of qualitative research to the study of quality of life in children and adolescents with epilepsy. *Seizure* 2004;13:3–14.

Mittan RJ. Fear of seizures. In: Whitman S, Hermann B (eds.). *Psychopathology in epilepsy: social dimensions.* New York: Oxford University Press, 1986:90–121.

Nelson EC, Landgraf JM, Hays RD, et al. The functional status of patients: how can it be measured in physicians' offices? *Med Care* 1990;28:1111–26.

Norby U, Carlsson J, Beckung E, et al. Self-assessment of well-being in a group of children with epilepsy. *Seizure* 1999;8:228–34.

O'Dell C, Lightstone L, Shinnar S, et al. Impact of childhood seizures on quality of life: perceptions of parents and children. *Epilepsia* 1998;39(Suppl 6):223–24 (abst).

O'Donoghue MF, Duncan JS, Sander JW. The subjective handicap of epilepsy. A new approach to measuring treatment outcome. *Brain* 1998;121:317–43.

Perrine KR. A new quality-of-life inventory for epilepsy patients: interim results. *Epilepsia* 1993;34(Suppl 4):S28–33.

Perrine KR, Devinsky O, Meador KJ, et al. The relationship of neuropsychological functioning to quality of life in epilepsy. *Arch Neurol* 1995;52:997–1003.

Reitan RM. A research program on the psychological effects of brain lesions in human beings. In: NR Ellis (ed.). *International review of research in mental retardation* (Vol. 1). New York: Academic Press, 1966:153–218.

Ronen GM, Rosenbaum P, Law M, et al. Health-related quality of life in childhood disorders: a modified focus group technique to involve children. *Qual Life Res* 2001; 10:71–79.

Ronen GM, Rosenbaum P, Law M, et al. Health-related quality of life in childhood epilepsy: the results of children's participation in identifying the components. *Dev Med Child Neurol* 1999;41:554–59.

Ronen GM, Streiner DL, Rosenbaum P, et al. Health-related quality of life in children with epilepsy: development and validation of self-report and parent proxy measures. *Epilepsia* 2003;44:598–612.

Ryan R, Kempner K, Emlen AC. The stigma of epilepsy as a self-concept. *Epilepsia* 1980;21:433–44.

Sabaz M, Cairns DR, Lawson JA, et al. Validation of a new quality of life measure for children with epilepsy. *Epilepsia* 2000;41:765–74.

Sabaz M, Lawson JA, Cairns DR, et al. Validation of the quality of life in childhood epilepsy questionnaire in American epilepsy patients. *Epilepsy Behav* 2003;4:680–91.

Scientific Advisory Committee of the Medical Outcomes Trust. Assessing health status and quality-of-life instruments: attributes and review criteria. *Qual Life Res* 2002;11:193–205.

Selai CE, Kendrick A, Trimble MR. New method for measuring quality of life based on repertory grid technique. *Epilepsia* 1994;35(Suppl 7):47(abst).

Selai CE, Trimble MR. Quality of life based on repertory grid technique. *Epilepsia* 1995;36(Suppl 3):S220(abst).

Sherman EM, Slick DJ, Connolly MB, et al. Validity of three measures of health-related quality of life in children with intractable epilepsy. *Epilepsia* 2002;43: 1230–38.

Smith DF, Baker GA, Dewey M, et al. Seizure frequency, patient-perceived seizure severity and the psychosocial consequences of intractable epilepsy. *Epilepsy Res* 1991;9:231–41.

Steinbuchel NV, Heel S, Bullinger M. A review of currently available quality of life measures. In: Baker GA, Jacoby A (eds.). *Quality of life in epilepsy: beyond seizure counts in assessment and treatment.* Reading, UK: Harwood Academic, 2000:65–101.

Temkin O. *The falling sickness: a history of epilepsy from the Greeks to the beginning of modern neurology.* Baltimore: The Johns Hopkins Press, 1945.

Vickrey BG, Hays RD, Engel J, et al. Outcome assessment for epilepsy surgery: the impact of measuring health-related quality of life. *Ann Neurol* 1995;37:158–66.

Vickrey BG, Hays RD, Graber J, et al. A health-related quality of life instrument for patients evaluated for epilepsy surgery. *Med Care* 1992;30:299–319.

Vickrey BG, Hays RD, Rausch R, et al. Quality of life in epilepsy surgery patients as compared to outpatients with hypertension, diabetes, heart disease, and/or depressive symptoms. *Epilepsia* 1994;35:597–607.

Vickrey BG, Perrine KR, Hays RD, et al. *Scoring manual and patient inventory. Quality of Life in Epilepsy QOLIE-89* (Version 1.0). Santa Monica, CA, 1993a.

Vickrey BG, Perrine KR, Hays RD, et al. *Scoring manual for the QOLIE-31* (Version 1.0). Santa Monica, CA, 1993b.

Wagner AK, Ehrenberg BL, Tran TA, et al. Patient-based health status measurement in clinical practice: a study of its impact on epilepsy patients' care. *Qual Life Res* 1997;6:329–41.

Wagner AK, Keller SD, Kosinski M, et al. Advances in methods for assessing the impact of epilepsy and antiepileptic drug therapy on patients' health-related quality of life. *Qual Life Res* 1995;4:115–34.

Ware JE, Sherbourne CD. A 36-item short form health survey (SF-36). I. Conceptual framework and item selection. *Med Care* 1992;30:473–83.

Westbrook LE, Bauman LJ, Shinar S. Applying stigma theory to epilepsy: a test of a conceptual model. *J Pediatr Psychol* 1992;17:633–49.

15 Rehabilitation Outcome Measures

Samuel T. Gontkovsky, Psy.D., and Risa Nakase-Richardson, Ph.D.

Rehabilitation, both as a science and a form of intervention, is concerned with the facilitation of functional recovery for persons with disabling and chronic health conditions. Multidisciplinary in nature, the field of rehabilitation encompasses professionals practicing within various disciplines including physiatry, neurology, urology, surgery, psychiatry, psychology, biomedical engineering, nursing, physical therapy, occupational therapy, speech-language pathology, respiratory therapy, social work, and vocational rehabilitation. Offering unique contributions to patient care while working toward a common goal, professionals within the field of rehabilitation function in a dynamic fashion to prepare individuals physically, cognitively, emotionally, socially, and vocationally for the fullest possible life compatible within the confines of particular existing strengths and limitations (Campbell, 1996).

The process of rehabilitation may be conceptualized along three dimensions (Jarvis & Barth, 1994). Initially, *treatment is restorative*, aimed at directly restoring the structure and function of injured tissues.

When restoration is not possible, intervention is targeted toward the *development of alternative strategies* to compensate for lost or damaged function. The rehabilitation process then shifts to the *provision of external aids and equipment* to facilitate independence in circumstances where restoration of functioning and use of compensatory techniques fail to do so.

In light of this three-stage model, formal assessment within the rehabilitation milieu establishes the initial level of functioning following onset of a medical illness or injury and, consequently, provides the requisite data for development of an appropriate program of intervention. Measures then are used to track progress and/or evaluate outcomes over time. The comprehensive, multidisciplinary, and evolving nature of rehabilitation, in conjunction with increasing pressure from policy makers to formally document individual response to intervention, has resulted in the development of numerous instruments specifically for rehabilitation. Moreover, the recently developed standard for classification of functioning, disability, and health by the World Health Organization (WHO), has resulted in the incorporation of an assortment of rehabilitation measures that initially were developed for use in various other treatment settings.

International Classification of Functioning, Disability, and Health

The International Classification of Functioning, Disability, and Health (ICF; WHO, 2001) is a revision of the International Classification of Impairments, Disabilities, and Handicaps (ICIDH; WHO, 1980). It serves as the present standard for multipurpose classification in rehabilitation by providing a unified, consistent language and framework for the description of, as well as a scientific basis for, the understanding and investigation of health and health-related states, outcomes, and determinants. In contrast to the ICIDH, which served as a consequences-of-disease classification, the ICF functions as a components-of-health model, identifying the constituents of health and taking a neutral stand with respect to etiological mechanisms. Intended to be used in a complementary fashion with the WHO International Classification of Diseases—Tenth Revision, the ICF provides a standard method for demonstrating that varying levels of function may be seen within the same disease classification.

The ICF is organized along two primary dimensions, with each having two corresponding components of classification. Part 1—functioning and disability—considers health and health-related states according to (1) body functions and structures and (2) activities and participation. Part 2—contextual factors—examines health and health-related states based on (1) environmental factors and (2) personal factors. Each of these four components is comprised of various domains and may be expressed both in positive and in negative terms.

Body functions and structures are the physiologic and anatomic aspects of health and health-related states, respectively, which may sustain impairments involving an anomaly, defect, or loss that represents a deviation from certain generally accepted population standards. The term *body* refers to the human organism as a whole, encompassing all anatomic structures and functions including the brain and its corresponding psychological processes, both cognitive and emotional. Impairments, as delineated by the ICF, are not contingent on etiology and represent not the underlying pathology of the body but rather the manifestations of that pathology. Impairments may be conceptualized further as temporary

or permanent; progressive, regressive, or static; and intermittent or continuous.

The activities and participation component of functioning and disability embodies a plethora of domains, including but not limited to communication, mobility, self-care, interpersonal interactions, and community involvement. *Activities* are defined by the ICF as the executions of various tasks or actions, which may be limited by health or health-related states. *Participation* represents involvement in life situations that may be restricted by health and health-related states. Activities and participation may be moderated both by performance and capacity. The performance qualifier of ICF offers a formal standard for considering the impact of various environmental factors on activities and participation. Performance difficulties may exist in the absence of impairment, arising directly from aspects of the social environment. The capacity qualifier of ICF provides a method to reflect the environmentally adjusted ability of the individual. The gap between performance and capacity denotes the differential impact of current and uniform environments, thereby providing a framework for environmental modification in order to improve performance.

Contextual factors represent the complete and subjective life experiences that, individually or collectively, may influence health and health-related states. Contextual factors may be classified either as environmental or as personal. *Environmental factors* comprise the physical, social, and attitudinal milieu in which individuals function on a daily basis. Such factors, which are external to the individual, may exert either a positive or a negative influence on performance within the confines of society, capacity to execute actions or tasks, and/or structure and function of the body. Indeed, environmental factors, by definition, interact with the components of body functions and structures as well as activities and participation. Environmental factors may be conceptualized on an individual level, encompassing the physical and material features of the home and workplace settings as well as direct contacts with family, peers, and strangers. They also may be viewed on a societal level, involving both formal and informal societal structures, services, and institutions such as governmental agencies, legal regulations, and generally held ideologies.

Personal factors reflect the unique background of the individual, as acquired through life experiences, which are not part of the present health condition, *per se*, but may act to influence disability. Personal factors include various demographic characteristics of an individual, such as age, educational level, race, ethnicity, gender, socioeconomic status, and occupation, as well as broad psychosocial influences, including general patterns of behavior and character style, past and present familial and social relationships, patterns of coping, and psychological strengths. Although not formally classified by the ICF, personal factors are included in the model, given their probable effect on the outcomes of various interventions.

In contrast to the ICIDH model, which viewed impairment, disability, and handicap in a linear paradigm, conceptualization of disability within the framework of the ICF is biopsychosocial in nature, providing a coherent view of varying perspectives of health from biological, individual, and social standpoints. Interactions among the aforementioned components of the ICF model are dynamic and complex, often occurring in unpredictable ways to influence disability. This movement away from the consequences-of-disease model to a components-of-health model has important implications with respect to assessment within the context of rehabilitation. Formal evaluation in light of the ICF necessarily posits a more global, or holistic, view of the individual, with an increased emphasis on health-related quality of life. Although not provided for explicitly within the framework of the ICF, systematic examination of personal factors and their impact upon outcome inevitably will assume a more prominent position in the process of rehabilitation.

Outcome Measures

Barthel Index

The Barthel Index (Mahoney & Barthel, 1965) is a 10-item measure developed to assess functional independence in personal care and mobility in persons with neuromuscular or musculoskeletal disorders. Items emphasize various activities of daily living, including feeding, transferring, personal hygiene, toileting, bathing, mobility, dressing, and controlling bowel and bladder functions (Table 15-1). Each item is assigned a score of 0, 5, 10, or 15, with differential weighting reflecting the relative importance of each disability with respect to level of assistance required for performance. Items are summed to obtain a total score ranging from 0 to 100, with a score of 100 representing the highest degree of independence. Excellent internal consistency reliability has been demonstrated in persons with stroke undergoing rehabilitation, with Cron-

bach's coefficient alphas of 0.87 at time of admission and 0.92 at time of discharge (Shah et al., 1989). Adequate inter-rater and test-retest reliabilities also have been shown, with kappa scores of 0.70–0.88 (Loewen & Anderson, 1988) and 0.98 (Wolfe et al., 1991), respectively. Barthel Index scores have been found to be predictive of living arrangements, productivity, and overall independent living in individuals with stroke (DeJong & Branch, 1982). Higher Barthel Index scores also have been associated with decreased mortality rates at 6 months following hospital admission (Wylie, 1967) and shorter lengths of hospital stay (Granger et al., 1979b). Significant correlations have been reported between the Barthel Index and the Motricity Index ($r = 0.73$–0.77; Wade & Hewer, 1987), Katz Index of Activities of Daily Living ($r = 0.77$; Gresham et al., 1980), Kennedy Self-Care Evaluation ($r = 0.42$; Gresham et al., 1980) and PULSES profile ($r = -0.74$ to -0.90; Granger et al., 1979a). Adapted versions of the Barthel Index, which propose to increase the utility of the scale, have been proposed by Collin et al. (1988), Granger et al. (1979a), and Shah et al. (1989). The Barthel Index and relevant guidelines for administration may be obtained from the Web site: http://www.neuro. mcg.edu/mcgstrok/Indices/Barthel_Ind.htm.

Berg Balance Scale

The Berg Balance Scale (BBS; Berg et al., 1989, 1992) is a 14-item rating measure originally developed to assess risk for falls in persons following stroke by examining ability to maintain positions or movements of increasing difficulty with diminishing base of support from sitting and standing to single leg stance (Table 15-2). Items are rated according to a five-point ordinal scale and are summed for a total score ranging from 0–56, with higher scores indicating a greater degree of independence and safety. Point deductions are implemented in cases where the examinee fails to meet time or distance specifications, requires supervision, touches an external support, or obtains assistance from the examiner. A cutoff point of more than 45 has been reported as highly specific for identifying persons at low risk for falls (Thorbahn & Newton, 1996). The BBS maintains excellent internal consistency, with Cronbach's coefficient alpha of 0.96 for the total score and ranging from 0.72 to 0.90 for individual items. Inter-rater reliability of 0.99 for the total score and ranging from 0.71 to 0.99 for individual items also has been reported. Construct validity has been established through the demonstration of signifi-

Table 15-1.   Barthel Index (BI)

	With Help	Independent
1. Feeding (if food needs to be cut up = help)	5	10
2. Moving from wheelchair to bed and return (includes sitting up in bed)	5–10	15
3. Personal toilet (wash face, comb hair, shave, clean teeth)	0	5
4. Getting on and off toilet (handling clothes, wipe, flush)	5	10
5. Bathing self	0	5
6. Walking on level surface (or if unable to walk, propel wheelchair)	10	15
*Score only if unable to walk	*0	*5
7. Ascend and descend stairs	5	10
8. Dressing (includes tying shoes, fastening fasteners)	5	10
9. Controlling bowels	5	10
10. Controlling bladder	5	10

A patient scoring 100 BI is continent, feeds self, dresses self, can get up out of a bed and chair, bathes self, walks at least a block, and can ascend and descend stairs. This does not mean that the patient is able to live alone: The patient may not be able to cook, keep house, and meet the public, but is able to get along without attendant care.

Definition and discussion of scoring

1. Feeding

   10 Independent. The patient can feed self a meal from a tray or table when someone puts the food within reach. The patient must put on an assistive device if this is needed, cut up the food, use salt and pepper, spread butter, etc. The patient must accomplish this in a reasonable time.

   5 Some help is necessary (with cutting up food, etc., as listed above).

2. Moving from wheelchair to bed and return

   15 Independent in all phases of this activity. Patient can safely approach the bed in wheelchair, lock brakes, lift footrests, move safely to bed, lie down, come to a sitting position on the side of the bed, change the position of the wheelchair, if necessary, to transfer back into it safely, and return to the wheelchair.

   10 Either some minimal help is needed in some step of this activity or the patient needs to be reminded or supervised for safety of one or more parts of this activity.

   5 Patient can come to a sitting position without the help of a second person but needs to be lifted out of bed, or if patient transfers with a great deal of help.

3. Doing personal toilet

   5 Patient can wash hands and face, comb hair, clean teeth, and shave. Patient may use any kind of razor but must put in blade or plug in razor without help as well as get it from drawer or cabinet. Female patients must put on own makeup, if used, but need not braid or style hair.

4. Getting on and off toilet

   10 Patient is able to get on and off toilet, fasten and unfasten clothes, prevent soiling of clothes, and use toilet paper without help. Patient may use a wall bar or other stable object for support, if needed. If it is necessary to use a bedpan instead of a toilet; patient must be able to place it on a chair, empty it, and clean it.

   5 Patient needs help because of imbalance or in handling clothes or in using toilet paper.

5. Bathing self

   5 Patient may use a bathtub, a shower, or take a complete sponge bath. Patient must be able to do all the steps involved in whichever method is used without another person being present.

Table 15-1.   *(continued)*

6. Walking on a level surface

   15   Patient can walk at least 50 yd without help or supervision. Patient may wear braces or prostheses and use crutches, canes, or a walkerette but not a rolling walker. Patient must be able to lock and unlock braces, if used, assume the standing position and sit down, get the necessary mechanical aides into position for use, and dispose of them when they sit. (Putting on and taking off braces is scored under dressing.)

   10   Patient needs help or supervision in any of the above but can walk at least 50 yd with a little help.

   Propelling a wheelchair

   5   Patient cannot ambulate but can propel a wheelchair independently. Patient must be able to go around corners, turn around, maneuver the chair to a table, bed, toilet, etc. Patient must be able to push a chair at least 50 yd. Do not score this item if the patient gets score for walking.

7. Ascending and descending stairs

   10   Patient is able to go up and down a flight of stairs safely without help or supervision. Patient may and should use handrails, canes, or crutches, when needed. Patient must be able to carry canes or crutches as they ascend or descend stairs.

   5   Patient needs help with or supervision of any one of the above items.

8. Dressing and undressing

   10   Patient is able to put on and remove and fasten all clothing, and tie shoelaces (unless it is necessary to use adaptations for this). The activity includes putting on and removing and fastening corset or braces when these are prescribed. Such special clothing as suspenders, loafer shoes, or dresses that open down the front, may be used when necessary.

   5   Patient needs help in putting on and removing or fastening any clothing. Patient must do at least half the work. Patient must accomplish this in a reasonable time.

   Women need not be scored on use of a brassiere or girdle unless these are prescribed garments.

9. Continence of bowels

   10   Patient is able to control bowels and has no accidents. Patient can use a suppository or take an enema when necessary (as for spinal cord injury patients who have had bowel training).

   5   Patient needs help in using a suppository or taking an enema or has occasional accidents.

10. Controlling bladder

   10   Patient is able to control bladder day and night. Spinal cord injury patients who wear an external device and leg bag must put them on independently, clean and empty bag, and stay dry day and night.

   5   Patient has occasional accidents or cannot wait for the bedpan or get to the toilet in time or needs help with an external device.

A score of 0 is given in all of the above activities when the patient cannot meet the criteria as defined above.

The advantage of the BI is its simplicity. It is useful in evaluating a patient's state of independence before treatment, progress as the patient undergoes treatment, and status when the patient reaches maximum benefit. It can easily be understood by all who work with a patient and can accurately and quickly be scored by anyone who adheres to the definitions of items listed above. The total score is not as significant or meaningful as the breakdown into individual items, because these indicate where the deficiencies are.

Any applicant to a chronic hospital who scores 100 BI should be evaluated carefully before admission to see whether such hospitalization is indicated. Discharged patients with 100 BI should not require further physical therapy but may benefit from a home visit to see whether any environmental adjustments are indicated. Encouragement by family and others may be necessary for a patient to maintain his or her degree of independence.

From Mahoney FI, Barthel DW. Functional evaluation: the Barthel Index. *MD State Med J* 1965;14:61–5, with permission.

Table 15-2. Berg Balance Scale

Balance Item	0	1	2	3	4
Sitting unsupported					
Change of position: sit to stand					
Change of position: stand to sit					
Transfers					
Standing unsupported					
Standing with eyes closed					
Standing with feet together					
Tandem standing					
Standing on one leg					
Turning trunk (feet fixed)					
Retrieving object from floor					
Turning 360 degrees					
Stool stepping					
Reaching forward while standing					

These tasks are graded from 0 to 4. Normal performance is scored 4, which means the task was completed independently in a normal period of time. Progressively fewer points are scored as the time required to complete the task is increased or as greater assistance is needed with 0 for complete inability to perform the task.

Adapted from Berg K, Wood-Dauphinee S, Williams JI, et al. Measuring balance in the elderly: preliminary development of an instrument. *Physiotherapy Canada* 1989;41:304–11; and Berg K, Wood-Dauphinee S, Williams JI, et al. Measuring balance in the elderly: validation of an instrument. *Can J Public Health* 1992;2:S7–11.

cant positive correlations between the BBS and both the Barthel Index and Fugl-Meyer Assessment of Sensorimotor Recovery after Stroke (FM). BBS scores have been found to discriminate between persons according to their use of mobility aids and have been shown to be predictive of inpatient rehabilitation length of stay and discharge destination (Wee et al., 2003). The BBS and relevant instructions for administration may be obtained from the Web site: http://www.chcr.brown.edu/Balscale.doc.

Chedoke-McMaster Stroke Assessment

The Chedoke-McMaster Stroke Assessment (Gowland et al., 1993) is a two-part measure developed to evaluate physical impairments and disabilities affecting individuals with stroke. The impairment inventory portion of the assessment provides a basis for determining the presence and severity of common physical impairments following stroke, to classify or stratify patients for treatment planning and monitoring of status over time. This section of the measure consists of six dimensions (shoulder pain, postural control, arm, hand, leg, and foot), each rated based on a 7-point scale corresponding to a revision of the seven stages of motor recovery as delineated by Brunnstrom (1970). Ratings are summed to provide a total score ranging from 7 to 42, with higher scores indicating a lesser degree of motor impairment. An additional scale in this portion of the measure is designed specifically to evaluate severity of shoulder pain. The disability inventory portion of the assessment (Table 15-3) serves to measure change in physical disability, apart from the arm, and is designed to be used in conjunction with the Uniform Data System for Medical Rehabilitation, which includes the Functional Independence Measure (FIM). Comprised

Table 15-3. Chedoke-McMaster Stroke Assessment: Disability Inventory

Gross Motor Function Index

   1. Supine to side lying on strong side

   2. Supine to side lying on weak side

   3. Side lying to long sitting through strong side

   4. Side lying to sitting on side of the bed through strong side

   5. Side lying to sitting on side of the bed through weak side

   6. Standing

   7. Transfer to and from bed toward strong side

   8. Transfer to and from bed toward weak side

   9. Transfer up and down from floor and chair

   10. Transfer up and down from floor and standing

Walking Index

   11. Walking indoors

   12. Walking outdoors, over rough ground, ramps, and curbs

   13. Walking outdoors several blocks

   14. Stairs

   15. Age- and sex-appropriate walking distance (in meters) for 2 min (2-point bonus)

Item scoring based on the Functional Independence Measure 7-point ordinal scale.

From Gowland C, Stratford P, Ward M, et al. Measuring physical impairment and disability with the Chedoke-McMaster Stroke Assessment. *Stroke* 1993;24:58–63, with permission.

of a 10-item, 70-point gross motor function index and a 5-item, 30-point walking index, the disability inventory provides important information for evaluation of both outcome and effectiveness of therapeutic interventions. Strong reliability of the Chedoke-McMaster Stroke Assessment was reported by Gowland et al. (1993), with intra-class correlation coefficients ranging from 0.85 to 0.98 for the dimensions and indexes and from 0.97 to 0.99 for the total score. Construct and concurrent validity of the measure also was established through significant correlations with the FM and FIM. Additionally, the disability inventory of the Chedoke-McMaster Stroke Assessment was found to be considerably more responsive to change in status relative to the FIM. The disability inventory portion of the Chedoke-McMaster Stroke Assessment was published by Gowland et al. (1993). The impairment inventory portion of the measure as well as relevant guidelines for administration and scoring may be obtained from the Institute of Applied Science at McMaster University in Hamilton, Ontario, Canada.

Community Integration Questionnaire

The Community Integration Questionnaire (CIQ; Willer et al., 1993) is a 15-item scale originally designed to measure return to family and community life following traumatic brain injury. Subscales for the CIQ include Home Integration (degree to which persons are involved in household affairs), Social Integration (level of persons' participation in activities outside of the home), and Productive Activities (degree to which persons are out of the house during the day engaging in work, school, or volunteer-related activities). Subtotals for each of these domains are generated based on the frequency of engaging in roles and activities, and responses are weighted according to level of independence in performing roles and activities. Subscales are summed to yield a total score for community integration ranging from 0 to 29. Test-retest reliability for the CIQ was reported to be 0.93 for home integration, 0.86 for social integration, and 0.83 for productive activities (Willer et al., 1993). Correspondence between patients with traumatic brain injury and proxy reports on the individual items of the CIQ were found to be adequate, with kappas ranging from 0.42 to 0.94 (Sander et al., 1997). CIQ total score as well as all three subscale scores have been found to differentiate persons with traumatic brain injury from persons without traumatic brain injury, and CIQ total score has been reported to differentiate among individuals with traumatic brain injury residing in different settings (Willer et al., 1994). Scores on the CIQ have been demonstrated to correlate significantly with scores on the Craig Handicap Assessment and Reporting Technique (CHART) in persons with traumatic brain injury, and the CIQ has been indicated to be the most appropriate instrument for characterizing community participation in this population (Zhang et al., 2002). Scores on the CIQ also have been shown to correlate significantly with life satisfaction in persons with traumatic brain injury (Burleigh et al., 1998; Heinemann & Whiteneck, 1995). The CIQ and relevant information concerning administration, scoring, and interpretation may be obtained from the Center for Outcome Measurement in Brain Injury Web site, http://www.tbims.org/combi/index.html, which is sponsored by the National Institute of Disability and Rehabilitation Research through its Traumatic Brain Injury Model Systems Program. Permission for use of the scale may be procured from Barry Willer at the Centre for Research on Community Integration at the Ontario Brain Injury Association, Thorold, Ontario, Canada.

Coping with Health Injuries and Problems

Coping with Health Injuries and Problems (CHIP; Endler & Parker, 1992) is a 32-item scale assessing potential strategies for coping with the occurrence of a health condition. The CHIP is comprised of four subscales (distraction, palliative, instrumental, and emotional preoccupation), each consisting of eight items, with subscale items distributed strategically to control for order effects. The distraction subscale assesses the extent to which actions and cognitions aimed at avoiding preoccupation with the health problem are used in coping. The palliative subscale examines the degree to which coping involves use of various self-help responses to alleviate the unpleasantness of the situation, such as resting or modifying the surroundings. The instrumental subscale focuses on task-oriented strategies that may be used to cope with the health problem, including active problem solving or acquisition of information about the particular illness or injury. The emotional preoccupation subscale assesses the extent to which coping involves focusing on the emotional consequences of the health problem, such as fantasizing. Examinees are asked to rate each of the 32 items according to a 5-point scale ranging from 1 (not at all) to 5 (very much) based on the extent to which engagement in each behavior has occurred since onset of the particular health problem. Reliability of the CHIP has been demonstrated with internal consistency estimates for its subscales ranging from 0.65 to 0.84 (Endler & Parker, 1992) and test-retest reliabilities ranging from 0.64 to 0.85 (Endler et al., 1998a). Exploratory factor analysis has revealed all 32 items of the CHIP to load at least moderately on their respective matching factors and low or very low on remaining factors (Endler & Parker, 1992). Furthermore, the construct validity of the CHIP has been demonstrated in studies examining the relationship between this measure and other tests of coping (Amirkhan, 1990; Gontkovsky & Parker, 2004; Endler et al., 1998b). The

CHIP manual and protocol forms may be obtained from Multi-Health Systems, Inc., North Tonawanda, New York.

Craig Handicap Assessment and Reporting Technique

The CHART (Whiteneck et al., 1992) is a 27-item measure originally developed to evaluate degree of community integration following rehabilitation for individuals with spinal cord injury. Test items, which focus on observable criteria, yield scores across five subscales (physical independence, mobility, occupation, social integration, and economic self-sufficiency). To expand the applicability of the instrument to a wider range of disability groups (i.e., individuals with cognitive and/or behavioral disturbances secondary to brain injury), the CHART was revised with the addition of five new items to assess a sixth domain of handicap (Table 15-4), entitled Cognitive Independence (Mellick et al., 1999). Scores across each of the six subscales of the revised 32-item CHART range from 0 to 100, resulting in a total score for the measure of 0–600, with higher scores indicating a lesser degree of handicap or greater degree of social and community participation. Rasch analysis was used to verify the scaling and scoring procedures of the original CHART (Whiteneck et al., 1992). Test-retest reliability for the original version was found to be 0.93 for the total score and between 0.80 and 0.95 for the five subscales. Participant-proxy correlations of 0.83 and 0.81 for the CHART total score also have been reported for the original (Dijkers, 1991) and revised versions (Mellick et al., 1999), respectively. Validity of the CHART was established through demonstration by independent classification of significant differences between low and high handicap groups on the total score as well as the physical independence, mobility, occupation, and social integration subscales (Whiteneck et al., 1992). Scores on the revised CHART also have been shown to discriminate among impairment categories (e.g., multiple sclerosis, spinal cord injury, stroke, traumatic brain injury) in a direction that parallels increasing disability (Walker et al., 2003) and have been demonstrated to correlate significantly with scores on the FIM in stroke survivors (Segal & Schall, 1995). A short form of the CHART, consisting of 19 items that generate scores for the same six subscales of the full revised version, also has been developed and has been demonstrated to possess adequate reliability and validity. The CHART and relevant information

Table 15-4.   Craig Handicap Assessment and Reporting Technique—Revised

1. How many hours in a typical 24-hr day do you have someone with you to provide physical assistance for personal care activities, such as eating, bathing, dressing, toileting, and mobility?

    _____ hours of paid assistance

    _____ hours unpaid (family, others)

2. Not including any regular care, as reported above, how any hours in a typical month do you occasionally have assistance with such things as grocery shopping, laundry, housekeeping, or infrequent medical needs because of disability?

    _____ hours per month

3. Who takes responsibility for instructing and directing your attendants and/or caregivers?

    _____ Self

    _____ Someone else

    _____ Not applicable, do not use attendant care

4. How much time is someone with you in your home to assist you with activities that require remembering, decision making, or judgment?

    _____ Someone else is always with me to observe or supervise.

    _____ Someone else is always around, but they only check on me now and then.

    _____ Sometimes I am left alone for an hour or two.

    _____ Sometimes I am left alone for most of the day.

    _____ I have been left alone all day and all night, but someone checks in on me.

    _____ I am left alone without anyone checking on me.

5. How much of the time is someone with you to help you with remembering, decision making, or judgment when you go away from your home?

    _____ I am restricted from leaving, even with someone else.

    _____ Someone is always with me to help with remembering, decision making, or judgment when I go anywhere.

    _____ I go to places on my own as long as they are familiar.

    _____ I do not need help going anywhere.

6. How often do you have difficulty communicating with other people?

    _____ I almost always have difficulty.

    _____ I sometimes have difficulty.

    _____ I almost never have difficulty.

7. How often do you have difficulty remembering important things that you must do?

    _____ I almost always have difficulty.

    _____ Sometimes I have difficulty.

8. How much of your money do you control?

    _____ None, someone makes all money decisions for me.

    _____ A small amount of spending money is given to me periodically.

    _____ Most of my money, but someone does help me make major decisions.

    _____ I make all my own money decisions (or if married, in joint participation with my partner).

9. On a typical day, how many hours are you out of bed?

    _____ hours

(continued)

Table 15-4. *(continued)*

10. In a typical week, how many days do you get out of your house and go somewhere?

    _____ days

11. In the last year, how many nights have you spent away from your home (excluding hospitalization)?

    _____ None

    _____ 1–2

    _____ 3–4

    _____ 5 or more

12. Can you enter and exit your home without any assistance from someone?

    _____ Yes

    _____ No

13. In your home, do you have independent access to your sleeping area, kitchen, bathroom, telephone, and TV (or radio)?

    _____ Yes

    _____ No

14. Can you use your transportation independently?

    _____ Yes

    _____ No

15. Does your transportation allow you to get to all the places you would like to go?

    _____ Yes

    _____ No

16. Does your transportation let you get out whenever you want?

    _____ Yes

    _____ No

17. Can you use your transportation with little or no advance notice?

    _____ Yes

    _____ No

18. How many hours per week do you spend working in a job for which you get paid?

    _____ hours (occupation: _____)

19. How many hours per week do you spend in school working toward a degree or in an accredited technical training program (including hours in class and studying)?

    _____ hours

20. How many hours per week do you spend in active homemaking including parenting, housekeeping, and food preparation?

    _____ hours

21. How many hours per week do you spend in home maintenance activities such as gardening, house repairs, or home improvement?

    _____ hours

22. How many hours per week do you spend in ongoing volunteer work for an organization?

    _____ hours

Table 15-4. *(continued)*

23. How many hours per week do you spend in recreational activities such as sports, exercise, playing cards, or going to the movies? Please do not include time spent watching TV or listening to the radio.

    _____ hours

24. How many hours per week do you spend in other self-improvement activities such as hobbies or leisure reading? Please do not include time spent watching TV or listening to the radio.

    _____ hours

25. Do you live alone? (If yes, skip to question 26.)

    _____ Yes

    _____ No

    25a. (If you don't live alone) do you live with a spouse or significant other?

    _____ Yes

    _____ No

    25b. How many children do you live with? _____

    25c. How many other relatives do you live with? _____

    25d. How many roommates do you live with? _____

    25e. How many attendants do you live with? _____

26. (If you don't live with a spouse or significant other) are you involved in a romantic relationship?

    _____ Yes

    _____ No

27. How many relatives (not in your household) do you visit, phone, or write to at least once a month?

    _____ Number of relatives

28. How many business or organizational associates do you visit, phone, or write to at least once a month?

    _____ Number of associates

29. How many friends (non-relatives contacted outside business or organization settings) do you visit, phone, or write to at least once a month?

    _____ Number of friends

30. With how many strangers have you initiated conversation in the last month (e.g., to ask information or place an order)?

    _____ Number of strangers

31. Approximately what was the combined annual income, in the last year, of all family members in your household? (Consider all sources including wages and earnings, disability benefits, pensions and retirement income, income from court settlements, investments and trust funds, child support and alimony, contributions from relatives, and any other source.)

    $_____

32. Approximately how much did you pay last year for medical care expenses? (Consider any amounts paid by yourself or the family members in your household and not reimbursed by insurance or benefits.)

    $_____

From Mellick D, Walker N, Brooks CA, et al. Incorporating the cognitive independence domain into CHART. *J Rehabil Outcomes Meas* 1999;3:12–21, with permission.

concerning administration, scoring, and interpretation may be obtained from Craig Hospital, Englewood, Colorado, or from the Center for Outcome Measurement in Brain Injury Web site, http://www.tbims.org/combi/index.html.

Davidson Trauma Scale

The Davidson Trauma Scale (DTS; Davidson, 1996) is a 17-item self-report measure, which examines symptoms of post-traumatic stress disorder along the dimensions of frequency and severity using five-point scales. Specifically, examinees are asked to respond to individual test items according to frequency of symptom occurrence during the past week, from 0 (not at all) to 4 (every day) and distress level associated with each occurring symptom, from 0 (not at all distressing) to 4 (extremely distressing). Test items were developed based on diagnostic criteria as specified by the Fourth Edition of the *Diagnostic and Statistical Manual of Mental Disorders* (American Psychiatric Association, 1994). A DTS total score ranging from 0 to 136 is generated based upon subscores from three symptom clusters, namely intrusion, avoidance/numbing, and hyperarousal. Reliability of the DTS has been demonstrated with a test-retest coefficient of 0.86 and internal consistency coefficients (i.e., split-half reliability and coefficient alpha) of >0.90. A cutoff point of 40 on the DTS total score, which has been demonstrated to yield a positive predictive value of 0.92 and negative predictive value of 0.79, has been proposed as most clinically precise for diagnostic accuracy (Davidson, 1996). The DTS also has been shown to be sensitive to change in post-traumatic stress disorder symptomatology over time (Davidson, 1996; Gontkovsky et al., 2004) as well as improvement in posttraumatic stress disorder symptomatology following treatment (Davidson, 1996). The DTS manual and protocol forms may be obtained from Multi-Health Systems, Inc., North Tonawanda, New York.

Disability Rating Scale

The Disability Rating Scale (DRS; Rappaport et al., 1982) is a 30-point measure consisting of eight items corresponding to the following areas of functioning: eye opening; verbalization; motor response; level of cognitive ability for feeding, toileting, and grooming; overall level of independence; and employability (paid employment, academic enrollment, or home-making). Each area of functioning is rated on a scale of 0 to either 3, 4, or 5, with higher scores representing greater impairment, or lower level of functioning (Table 15-5). Ratings are summed to yield a total score ranging from 0 to 29, with 29 representing the lowest level of functioning, consistent with a vegetative state. Individuals without any disability would be assigned a score of 0. The DRS was developed on an inpatient rehabilitation unit with individuals with moderate to severe traumatic brain injury. It has been found to be a reliable and valid instrument that can be self-administered or scored through interview with the patient and/or a family member (Gouvier et al., 1987; Hall et al., 1985; Rappaport et al., 1982). The DRS also can be administered via telephone interview. Concurrent validity has been established with significant correlations between the first three items of the DRS and auditory, visual, and somatosensory brain evoked potentials ($r = 0.38$–0.78; Rappaport et al., 1982). Hall et al. (1985) reported the DRS was significantly correlated with the Glasgow Outcome Scale at two time intervals post injury ($r = 0.57$ at rehabilitation admission, $r = 0.67$ at rehabilitation discharge). The DRS also has been found to correlate with the Stover Zeiger Scale at time of hospital admission and discharge ($r = 0.92$ at hospital admission, $r = 0.80$ at hospital discharge; Gouvier et al., 1987). Excellent inter-rater reliability has been reported with coefficients ranging from 0.97 to 0.98 (Gouvier et al., 1987; Rappaport et al., 1982). The DRS has been used in a wide variety of investigations examining outcome for individuals after brain injury (Bowers & Kofroth, 1989; Eliason & Topp, 1984; Hall et al., 1985; Hall et al., 1993). The primary disadvantage of the measure is its insensitivity to mild brain injuries (Hall et al., 1996). The DRS and relevant information concerning administration, scoring, and interpretation may be obtained from the Center for Outcome Measurement in Brain Injury Web site: http://www.tbims.org/combi/index.html.

Fugl-Meyer Assessment of Sensorimotor Recovery after Stroke

The FM (Fugl-Meyer et al., 1975) is a performance-based measure that provides quantitative assessment of voluntary movement, balance, sensation, passive

Table 15-5. Disability Rating Scale

1. Eye Opening	2. Communication Ability	3. Motor Response
_____0 Spontaneous	_____0 Oriented	_____0 Obeying
_____1 To speech	_____1 Confused	_____1 Localizing
_____2 To pain	_____2 Inappropriate	_____2 Withdrawing
_____3 None	_____3 Incomprehensible	_____3 Flexing
	_____4 None	_____4 Extending
		_____5 None

4. Feeding*	5. Toileting*	6. Grooming*
_____0 Complete	_____0 Complete	_____0 Complete
_____1 Partial	_____1 Partial	_____1 Partial
_____2 Minimal	_____2 Minimal	_____2 Minimal
_____3 None	_____3 None	_____3 None

7. Level of Functioning (Physical and Cognitive Disability)	8. Employability (As Full-Time Worker, Homemaker, or Student)
_____0 Completely independent	_____0 Not restricted
_____1 Independent in special environment	_____1 Selected jobs, competitive
_____2 Mildly dependent—limited assist (nonresident helper)	_____2 Sheltered workshop, noncompetitive
_____3 Moderately dependent—moderate assist (person in home)	_____3 Not employable
_____4 Markedly dependent (assist all major activities, all times)	
_____5 Totally dependent (24-hr nursing care)	

*Knows how and when to feed, toilet, or groom self.
From Rappaport M, Hall KM, Hopkins K, et al. Disability Rating Scale for severe head trauma: coma to community. *Arch Phys Med Rehabil* 1982;63:118–23, with permission.

range of motion, and pain. The FM is based on the patterns of motor recovery delineated by Twitchel (1951). Items in the motor section were developed from the seven stages of motor recovery following stroke described by Brunnstrom (1970), and items in the passive range of motion section were derived based on the standards of the American Academy of Orthopaedic Surgeons. Test items are rated according to a 3-point ordinal scale from 0 (no function) to 2 (full function), secondary to direct observation of patient functioning. Scores across the five sections are summed for a maximum total score of 226 (Fugl-Meyer et al., 1975). The measure has been found to possess adequate inter-rater and test-retest reliabilities, particularly for the total scale (Beckerman et al., 1996; Duncan et al., 1983). A multitude of investigations have examined the validity of the FM, with results generally being favorable (Feys et al., 2000; Lin & Sabbahi, 1999; Malouin et al., 1994; Wood-Dauphinee et al., 1990). The total motor score is the most commonly used subscale of the FM, and various investigators have proposed numerical ranges for categorization of stroke severity (Duncan et al., 1994; Fugl-Meyer, 1980; Fugl-Meyer et al., 1975), which may be used for clinical and/or research purposes.

Functional Independence Measure

The FIM (Keith et al., 1987) is an 18-item instrument developed for use as part of the Uniform Data System for Medical Rehabilitation to assess disability and estimate burden of care (Granger, 1998) in persons undergoing inpatient rehabilitation. FIM items, which evaluate various aspects of motor functioning (e.g., eating, grooming, bathing, dressing, toileting, transferring, ambulating, bowel and bladder control) and cognition (e.g., communication, social interaction, problem solving, memory), are rated according to a seven-level ordinal scale from complete dependence to complete independence. Total scores range from 18 to 126, with higher scores reflecting a greater degree of independence. Excellent internal consistency reliability for the FIM has been reported, with Cronbach's coefficient alphas >0.90 (Dodds et al., 1993). The measure also has been demonstrated to possess excellent inter-rater and test-retest reliabilities, with reported interclass correlations for both >0.90 (Chau et al., 1994; Ottenbacher et al., 1994; Segal & Schall, 1994). FIM scores have been demonstrated to be predictive of amount of assistance required by persons with multiple sclerosis (Granger et al., 1990) and to correlate significantly with total nursing contact time in patients with traumatic brain injury and spinal cord injury (Heinemann et al., 1997). The FIM also has been found to be sensitive to change in patient status over time (Dodds et al., 1993; Sharrack et al., 1999; van der Putten et al., 1999). The FIM has become proprietary; however, relevant information concerning administration, scoring, and interpretation may be obtained from the Uniform Data System for Medical Rehabilitation Web site: http://www.udsmr.org.

Glenrose Ambulation Rating

The Glenrose Ambulation Rating (GAR; McIntosh et al., 1999) is a five-item ordinal measure designed to provide a descriptive indication of ambulation in persons with brain injury and stroke. The scale assesses ambulation ability according to velocity, distance, and level of assistance required by the

patient and considers potential environmental barriers through rating of ambulation on both indoor surfaces and outdoor terrain. An additional scale, which is not scored as part of the formal measure, evaluates ability to ascend and descend stairs (Table 15-6). Initial inter-relater reliability was examined by determining point-to-point agreement between therapists' scoring. Results revealed 95% agreement between raters for the GAR total score and 93% agreement between raters for the stair item (McIntosh et al., 1999). The GAR has been found to correlate significantly with the BBS ($p = .86$) and the Physiotherapy Clinical Outcomes Variables Scale ($p = .88$). In addition, the GAR has been demonstrated to better differentiate patients with higher functional abilities relative to the BBS and the Clinical Outcomes Variables Scale, and both the total score and stair scale of the GAR have been shown to be responsive to change in patient ambulation ability from admission to discharge (McIntosh et al., 1999).

Head Injury Semantic Differential Scale

The Head Injury Semantic Differential Scale (HISDS; Tyerman & Humphrey, 1984) is a 20-item measure designed to assess self-concept according to the semantic differential paradigm, as developed by Osgood and colleagues (1957) and described further by Snider and Osgood (1969). Examinees are required to rate 20 bipolar adjective pairs (Table 15-7), selected by the authors for their adjudged relevance to head injury, based on a 7-point scale (1 at the negative pole and 7 at the positive pole). Ratings are summed for a total score ranging from 20 to 140, with higher scores indicating a more positive view of self. Investigations examining ratings on the HISDS of persons with head injury have revealed all aspects of self-concept to be more negative postinjury (Tyerman & Humphrey, 1984; Wright & Telford, 1996). Strong internal reliability of the HISDS has been demonstrated by Tyerman with a Cronbach's coefficient alpha of 0.88 and a split half Guttman's coefficient of 0.87 (see Ellis-Hill & Horn, 2000). Construct validity of the HISDS has been supported by research demonstrating a significant positive association between the total score on this measure and that of the Tennessee Self-Concept Scale—Second Edition (TSCS-2; Fitts & Warren, 1996) in a sample of patients with acquired brain injury (Vickery et al., 2005). HISDS self-scores have been shown to be significantly and negatively corre-

Table 15-6. Glenrose Ambulation Rating

0 Non-functional ambulator

__ Unable to walk or required more than one (1) person to assist to walk on any surface

__ Uses wheelchair full-time

1 Dependent ambulator

__ Requires assistance/supervision of one (1) person on all surfaces

__ Able to walk ≤10 m

__ Walks for some functional activity outside of therapy

2 Independent indoor ambulator

__ Independent on all indoor surfaces including carpets, hardwood, and linoleum floors

__ Able to walk ≥50 m

__ Requires assistance/supervision of one (1) person to walk on all outdoor surfaces

3 Limited outdoor ambulator

__ Independent on outdoor surfaces but requires assistance/supervision on ice/snow

__ Velocity less than 0.9 meters per second (<0.9 m/sec)

__ May need to use a wheelchair for distances ≥500 m and/or in crowds

4 Unlimited ambulator

__ Independent on all indoor surfaces and outdoor surfaces, including ice and snow

__ Able to walk >500 m

__ Velocity greater than or equal to 0.9 meters per second (≥0.9 m/sec)

__ Does not use a wheelchair

Stairs

__ 0 Unable to do stairs

__ 1 Requires assistance/supervision of __ person(s)

__ 2 Independent on stairs with a railing, number of stairs __

__ 3 Independent on stairs without a railing, number of stairs __

From McIntosh L, Woronuk J, May L, et al. Development of the Glenrose Ambulation Rating (GAR): validity and inter-rater reliability. *J Rehabil Outcomes Measurement* 1999;3:1–11, with permission.

Table 15-7. Head Injury Semantic Differential Scale Adjective Pairs

Original Version

Bored—Interested	Forgetful—Mindful
Unhappy—Happy	Irritable—Calm
Helpless—In control	Unfeeling—Caring
Worried—Relaxed	Clumsy—Agile
Dissatisfied—Satisfied	Dependent—Independent
Unattractive—Attractive	Inactive—Active
Unhopeful—Hopeful	Difficult—Cooperative
Lack confidence—Self-confident	Withdrawn—Talkative
Emotional—Stable	Unfriendly—Friendly
Worthless—Valuable	Stupid—Clever

Updated Version

Bored—Interested	Aggressive—Unaggressive
Unhappy—Happy	Irritable—Calm
Helpless—In Control	Unfeeling—Caring
Worried—Relaxed	Incapable—Capable
Dissatisfied—Satisfied	Dependent—Independent
Unattractive—Attractive	Inactive—Active
Despondent—Hopeful	Uncooperative—Cooperative
Lack confidence—Self-confident	Withdrawn—Talkative
Unstable—Stable	Unfriendly—Friendly
Worthless—Of value	Impatient—Patient

Adapted from Ellis-Hill CS, Horn S. Change in identity and self-concept: a new theoretical approach to recovery following a stroke. *Clin Rehabil* 2000;14:279–87; and Tyerman A, Humphrey M. Changes in self-concept following severe head injury. *Int J Rehabil Res* 1984;7:11–23.

lated with scores on the Leeds Scale for emotional distress (see Ellis-Hill & Horn, 2000). Furthermore, a significant negative relationship has been reported between scores on the HISDS and scores on the Beck Depression Inventory—Second Edition (Beck et al., 1996), suggesting a poorer view of self is associated with higher levels of reported depressive symptomatology (Vickery et al., 2005). Ellis-Hill and Horn (2000) used an updated version of the HISDS, comprised of many of the same adjective pairs but with half reversed, to examine change in self-concept following stroke. Reliability of this updated version has been demonstrated with a Cronbach's coefficient alpha of 0.93 and a split half Guttman's coefficient of 0.93 (Ellis-Hill & Horn, 2000).

Mayo-Portland Adaptability Inventory

The Mayo-Portland Adaptability Inventory, presently in its fourth revision (MPAI-4; Malec & Lezak, 2003), is a 35-item measure developed to evaluate the physical, cognitive, emotional, behavioral, and social sequelae of acquired brain injury during the postacute phase of recovery. The first 29 items of the MPAI-4 yield three subscales (Ability Index, Adjustment Index, and Participation Index) that consider the major obstacles to community integration and provide important information for planning programs of rehabilitation. Items comprising the Ability Index focus primarily on aspects of patient sensory, motor, and cognitive functioning. Items comprising the Adjustment Index emphasize mood and social interactions. Items comprising the Participation Index consider social contacts, initiation, and money management. The remaining six items allow for recording of additional pre- and postinjury information that may not represent direct or typical sequelae of acquired brain injury, including alcohol and drug use, psychotic symptoms, law violations, and the presence of other conditions that may influence physical and/or cognitive functioning but that should be considered nonetheless in clinical planning. Item reliability for the MPAI-4 has been found to be excellent, with coefficients ≥0.94 for the full scale and ≥0.89 for the three subscales. Scores on the MPAI scales have been shown to correlate significantly with scores on the DRS, Rancho Level of Cognitive Functioning Scale, and various measures of neuropsychological status and have been found to be predictive of job placement after participation in vocational rehabilitation (Bohac et al., 1997; Malec et al., 2000; Malec & Thompson, 1994). The authors of the MPAI-4 maintain copyright to the measure; however, the scale and relevant information concerning administration, scoring, and interpretation may be obtained from the Center for Outcome Measurement in Brain Injury Web site, http://www.tbims.org/combi/index.html and may be used without fee or other charge.

Medical Outcomes Study 36-Item Short-Form Health Survey

The Medical Outcomes Study 36-Item Short-Form Health Survey (SF-36; Ware & Sherbourne, 1992; Ware et al., 1993) was developed to serve as an indicator of perceived health status. This multidimensional survey is comprised of eight subscales, which assess physical functioning, role limitations related to physical health problems, bodily pain, general health perceptions, vitality, social functioning, role limitations related to emotional problems, and mental health. One additional item, which is scored separately from the remainder of the test, evaluates perceived change in health status. Item response choices range from dichotomous classifications to six-level Likert-type ordinal classifications (Table 15-8). Total scores across the eight subscales range from 0 to 100, with higher scores indicating better health status. Physical and mental health subcomponents, which have a mean of 50 and standard deviation of 10, also may be derived (Ware et al., 1994). Good internal consistency reliability has been demonstrated in multiple and diverse clinical samples, with Cronbach's coefficient alphas of 0.80–0.96 in patients with chronic stroke (Dorman et al., 1998) and 0.77–0.94 in patients with multiple sclerosis (Freeman et al., 2000). Adequate inter-rater and test-retest reliabilities also have been shown, with intra-class correlations ranging from 0.15 to 0.67 (Segal & Schall, 1994) and 0.30 to 0.93 (Dorman et al., 1998; Ruta et al., 1998), respectively. Convergent/discriminant validity of the SF-36 subscales has been well established (Brazier et al., 1992; Dorman et al., 1999; Freeman et al., 2000; Ruta et al., 1998), and subscale scores have been found to be predictive of patient hospitalization and mortality (McHorney, 1996). An updated version of the SF-36 includes expanded item response choices to allow for more comprehensive evaluation across selected subscales, and an acute version of the survey has been developed for use in circumstances when effects of treatment are expected to occur rapidly (Finch et al., 2002). The SF-36 and relevant guidelines for administration, scoring, and interpretation may be obtained from the Web site: http://www.sf-36.com.

Multidimensional Health Locus of Control Scales

The Multidimensional Health Locus of Control Scales (MHLC; Wallston et al., 1978, 1994) are 18-item

Table 15-8.   SF-36 Health Status Questions and Response Categories

1. In general would you say your health is:

   Excellent _____   Very good _____   Good _____   Fair _____   Poor _____

2. *Compared to 1 year ago,* how would you rate your health in general *now?*

   Much better now than 1 year ago _____

   Somewhat better now than 1 year ago _____

   About the same _____

   Somewhat worse now than 1 year ago _____

   Much worse now than 1 year ago _____

3. The following items are about activities you might do during a typical day. Does *your health now limit you in these activities?* If so, how much?

   a. *Vigorous activities,* such as running, lifting heavy objects, participating in strenuous sports

   b. *Moderate activities,* such as moving a table, pushing a vacuum cleaner, bowling, or playing golf

   c. Lifting or carrying groceries

   d. Climbing *several* flights of stairs

   e. Climbing *one* flight of stairs

   f. Bending, kneeling, or stooping

   g. Walking *more than a mile*

   h. Walking *several blocks*

   i. Walking *one block*

   j. Bathing or dressing yourself

   Response categories: Yes, limited a lot; Yes, limited a little; No, not limited at all.

4. During the *past 4 weeks,* have you had any of the following problems with your work or other regular daily activities *as a result of your physical health?*

   a. Cut down the *amount of time* you spent on work or other activities

   b. *Accomplished less* than you would like

   c. Were limited in the *kind* of work or other activities

   d. Had difficulty performing the work or other activities (e.g., it took extra effort)

   Response categories: Yes; No.

5. During the *past 4 weeks,* have you had any of the following problems with your work or other regular daily activities *as a result of any emotional problems* (e.g., feeling depressed or anxious)?

   a. Cut down the *amount of time* you spent on work or other activities

   b. *Accomplished less* than you would like

   c. Didn't do work or other activities as *carefully* as usual

   Response categories: Yes; No.

6. During the *past 4 weeks,* to what extent has your *physical health or emotional problems* interfered with your normal social activities with family, friends, neighbors, or groups?

   Response categories: Not at all; Slightly; Moderately; Quite a bit; Extremely.

7. How much *bodily* pain have you had during the *past 4 weeks?*

   Response categories: None; Very mild; Mild; Moderate; Severe; Very severe.

(continued)

Table 15-8.   *(continued)*

8. During the *past 4 weeks*, how much did *pain* interfere with your normal work (including both work outside the home and housework)?

Response categories: Not at all; A little bit; Moderately; Quite a bit; Extremely.

9. These questions are about how you feel and how things have been with you *during the past 4 weeks*. For each question, please give the one answer that comes closest to the way you have been feeling. How much of the time during the past 4 weeks:

a. Did you feel full of pep?

b. Have you been a very nervous person?

c. Have you felt so down in the dumps that nothing could cheer you up?

d. Have you felt calm and peaceful?

e. Did you have a lot of energy?

f. Have you felt downhearted and blue?

g. Did you feel worn out?

h. Have you been a happy person?

i. Did you feel tired?

Response categories: All of the time; Most of the time; A good bit of the time; Some of the time; A little of the time; None of the time.

10. During the *past 4 weeks*, how much of the time has your *physical health or emotional problems* interfered with your social activities (like visiting with friends, relatives, etc.)?

Response categories: All of the time; Most of the time; Some of the time; A little of the time; None of the time.

11. How *true or false* is *each* of the following statements for you?

a. I seem to get sick a little easier than other people.

b. I am as healthy as anybody I know.

c. I expect my health to get worse.

d. My health is excellent.

Response categories: Definitely true; Mostly true; Don't know; Mostly false; Definitely false.

From Ware JE, Sherbourne CD. The MOS 36-item short-form health survey (SF-36) I. Conceptual framework and item selection. *Medical Care* 1992;30:473–83. Modified to include response categories. Copied with permission of the Medical Outcomes Trust.

measures assessing subjective beliefs regarding the degree of perceived control over personal health status. MHLC items reflect health beliefs along multiple dimensions, which are rated according to a 6-point scale ranging from 1 (strongly disagree) to 6 (strongly agree). Parallel forms of the measure (A and B) originally were published by Wallston et al. (1978) to assess general health beliefs in the absence of a specified health condition. Both forms examine health beliefs along two primary dimensions. Internal locus of control describes the extent to which health status is judged to be contingent on personal behavior, whereas external locus of control describes the extent to which health status is believed to be a consequence of the behavior of others (Powerful Others subscale) or the result of fate or luck (Chance subscale). Form C of the MHLC (Wallston et al., 1994) was developed as a general-purpose, condition-specific locus of control scale, which could be adapted for use with any medical or health-related condition (Table 15-9). Form C also is comprised of internal and external locus of control subscales. Consistent with forms A and B, form C includes the external dimension of Chance. However, the Powerful

Table 15-9. Multidimensional Health Locus of Control Scale: Form C

Instructions: Each item below is a belief statement about your medical condition with which you may agree or disagree. Beside each statement is a scale that ranges from strongly disagree (1) to strongly agree (6). For each item, we would like you to circle the number that represents the extent to which you agree or disagree with that statement. The more you agree with a statement, the higher will be the number you circle. The more you disagree with a statement, the lower will be the number you circle. Please make sure that you answer *every item* and that you circle *only one* number per item. This is a measure of your personal beliefs; obviously, there are no right or wrong answers.

	SD	MD	D	A	MA	SA
1. If my condition worsens, it is my own behavior that determines how soon I will feel better again.	1	2	3	4	5	6
2. As to my condition, what will be will be.	1	2	3	4	5	6
3. If I see my doctor regularly, I am less likely to have problems with my condition.	1	2	3	4	5	6
4. Most things that affect my condition happen to me by chance.	1	2	3	4	5	6
5. Whenever my condition worsens, I should consult a medically trained professional.	1	2	3	4	5	6
6. I am directly responsible for my condition getting better or worse.	1	2	3	4	5	6
7. Other people play a big role in whether my condition improves, stays the same, or gets worse.	1	2	3	4	5	6
8. Whatever goes wrong with my condition is my own fault.	1	2	3	4	5	6
9. Luck plays a big part in determining how my condition improves.	1	2	3	4	5	6
10. In order for my condition to improve, it is up to other people to see that the right things happen.	1	2	3	4	5	6
11. Whatever improvement occurs with my condition is largely a matter of good fortune.	1	2	3	4	5	6
12. The main thing that affects my condition is what I myself do.	1	2	3	4	5	6
13. I deserve the credit when my condition improves and the blame when it gets worse.	1	2	3	4	5	6
14. Following doctor's orders to the letter is the best way to keep my condition from getting any worse.	1	2	3	4	5	6
15. If my condition worsens, it's a matter of fate.	1	2	3	4	5	6
16. If I am lucky, my condition will get better.	1	2	3	4	5	6
17. If my condition takes a turn for the worse, it is because I have not been taking proper care of myself.	1	2	3	4	5	6
18. The type of help I receive from other people determines how soon my condition improves.	1	2	3	4	5	6

SD = strongly disagree; MD = moderately disagree; D = slightly disagree; A = slightly agree; MA = moderately agree; SA = strongly agree.

Adapted from Wallston KA, Stein MJ, Smith CA. Form C of the MHLC scales: a condition-specific measure of locus of control. *J Pers Assess* 1994;63:534–53; and Wallston KA, Wallston BS, DeVillis R. Development of the multidimensional health locus of control (MHLC) scales. *Health Educ Monogr* 1978;6:160–70.

Others subscale is replaced with two independent subscales labeled Doctors and Other People. The reliability and validity of forms A and B have been demonstrated across a number of investigations (Marshall et al., 1990; Robinson-Whelen & Storant, 1992; Wallston et al., 1978). Most appropriate for use within the rehabilitation milieu given its condition-specific basis, form C of the MHLC has been found to possess strong psychometric properties, with subscale internal consistency estimates ranging from 0.70 to 0.85 and test-retest reliabilities ranging from 0.35 to 0.80 in clinical samples. Convergent, discriminant, and concurrent validities of form C have been demonstrated, in that scores across the majority of its subscales have been found to be significantly correlated in expected directions with theoretically related constructs of pain, helplessness, and depression as well as significantly and positively correlated with respective subscales of form B (Wallston et al., 1994). The MHLC scales and relevant guidelines for administration, scoring, and interpretation may be obtained from the Web site: http://www.vanderbilt.edu/nursing/kwallston/mhlcscales.htm.

Rancho Level of Cognitive Functioning Scale

The Rancho Level of Cognitive Functioning Scale (LCFS; Hagen et al., 1972) originally was developed for use in patients post-coma as a means for evaluating and monitoring cognitive status, planning treatment interventions, and classifying level of outcome. Patient evaluation with this measure results in classification into one of eight levels of functioning ranging from I, no response, during which the patient is unresponsive to external stimuli, to VIII, purposeful—appropriate, during which the patient is alert, oriented, and functional (Table 15-10). Excellent inter-rater and test-retest reliabilities of the LCFS have been reported, with Spearman rho coefficients of 0.89 and 0.82 (Gouvier et al., 1987), respectively. The LCFS also has been shown to possess adequate validity, with demonstrated positive associations with the Stover Zeiger Scale and Glasgow Outcome Scale (Gouvier et al., 1987). Additionally, the LCFS has been found to be useful in determining the potential of patients with brain injury to return to work and/or school (Cifu et al., 1997; Rao & Kilgore, 1992). The LCFS and relevant information concerning administration, scoring, and interpretation may be obtained from the Center for Outcome Measure-

ment in Brain Injury Web site: http://www.tbims.org/combi/index.html.

Satisfaction with Life Scale

The Satisfaction with Life Scale (SWLS; Diener et al., 1985) is a five-item measure of global life satisfaction. Conceptualized as the cognitive component of subjective well-being (Andrews & Withey, 1976), life satisfaction involves a judgmental process by which a comparison of perceived life circumstances with a unique, self-imposed set of standards is made (Pavot & Diener, 1993; Shin & Johnson, 1978). Items are rated based on a 7-point scale ranging from 1 (strongly disagree) to 7 (strongly agree) and are summed for a total score ranging from 5 to 35, with higher scores indicating a greater degree of life satisfaction (Table 15-11). Psychometric properties of the SWLS have been examined in a number of investigations, with results demonstrating internal consistency estimates ranging from 0.79 to 0.89 and test-retest reliability ranging from 0.54 to 0.84 (see Pavot & Diener, 1993, for a review). Factor analyses also consistently have supported that the SWLS measures a single dimension of global life satisfaction. Considerable evidence exists demonstrating the convergence of the SWLS with various other ratings of subjective well-being and life satisfaction. Construct validity of the SWLS is further supported by significant correlations in the expected directions between scores on this measure and scores on measures of anxiety (Arrindell et al., 1991), depression (Arrindell et al., 1991; Blais et al., 1989), negative affect (Larsen et al., 1985), extraversion (Pavot & Diener, 1993), and self-concept (Gontkovsky & Parker, 2004). Additionally, SWLS scores have been found to be associated with multiple demographic, social, functional, and clinical characteristics in individuals with spinal cord injury (Dijkers, 1999). The SWLS and relevant information concerning administration, scoring, and interpretation may be obtained from the Center for Outcome Measurement in Brain Injury Web site: http://www.tbims.org/combi/index.html.

Service Obstacles Scale

The Service Obstacles Scale (SOS; Marwitz & Kreutzer, 1996) is a six-item measure developed to assess the perceptions of patients with traumatic brain injury and

Table 15-10. Rancho Level of Cognitive Functioning Scale

1. No response. Patient appears to be in a deep sleep and is completely unresponsive to any stimuli presented to him/her.

2. Generalized response. Patient reacts inconsistently and nonpurposefully to stimuli in a nonspecific manner. Responses are limited in nature and are often the same regardless of stimulus presented. Responses may be physiologic changes, gross body movements, and vocalization. Responses are likely to be delayed. The earliest response is to deep pain.

3. Localized response. Patient reacts specifically, but inconsistently, to stimuli. Responses are directly related to the type of stimulus presented, as in turning head toward a sound or focusing on an object presented. The patient may withdraw an extremity and vocalize when presented with a painful stimulus. May follow simple commands in an inconsistent, delayed manner, such as closing the eyes, hand squeezing, or extending an extremity. Once external stimuli are removed, the patient may lie quietly. He/she may also show a vague awareness of self and body by responding to discomfort by pulling at nasogastric tube, catheter, or resisting restraints. May show a bias toward responding to some persons, especially family and friends, but not to others.

4. Confused—agitated. Patient is in a heightened state of activity with severely decreased ability to process information. He/she is detached from the present and responds primarily to his/her own internal confusion. Behavior is frequently bizarre and nonpurposeful relative to immediate environment. May cry out or scream out of proportion to stimuli even after removal, may show aggressive behavior, attempt to remove restraints or tube, or crawl out of bed in a purposeful manner. Patient does not discriminate among persons or objects and is unable to cooperate directly with treatment efforts. Verbalization is frequently incoherent or inappropriate to the environment. Confabulation may be present; he/she may be hostile. Gross attention to environment is very brief, and selective attention often nonexistent. Being unaware of present events, patient lacks short-term recall and may be reacting to past events. Unable to perform self-care activities, such as sitting, reaching, and ambulating, as part of his/her agitated state but not as a purposeful act or on request, necessarily.

5. Confused—inappropriate. Patient appears alert and is able to respond to simple commands fairly consistently. However, with increased complexity of commands or lack of any external structure, responses are nonpurposeful, random, or, at best, fragmented toward any desired goal. May show agitated behavior, but not on stimulus. Has gross attention to the environment, is highly distractible, and lacks ability to focus attention to a specific task without frequent redirection. With structure, may be able to converse on a very simple level for short periods of time. Verbalization is often inappropriate; confabulation may be triggered by present events. Memory is severely impaired, with confusion of past and present in reaction to ongoing activity. Patient does not initiate functional tasks and often shows inappropriate use of objects with external direction. May be able to perform previously learned tasks when structured for him/her, but is unable to learn new information. Responds best to self, body, comfort, and, often, family members. The patient can usually perform self-care activities with assistance and may accomplish feeding with supervision. Management on the unit is often a problem if the patient is physically mobile, as he/she may wander off, either randomly or with vague intention of "going home."

6. Confused—appropriate. Patient shows goal-directed behavior, but is dependent on external input for direction. Response to discomfort is appropriate, and patient is able to tolerate unpleasant stimuli (e.g., nasogastric tube when needed is explained). Follows simple directions consistently, and shows carryover for tasks he/she has learned (e.g., self-care). Responses may be incorrect due to memory problems, but are appropriate to the situation. The patient shows increased ability to process information with little or no anticipation or prediction of events. Past memories show more depth and detail than recent memory. The patient may show some awareness of situation by realizing he/she does not know an answer. The patient no longer wanders and is inconsistently oriented to time and place. Selective attention to tasks may be impaired, especially with difficult tasks, and in unstructured settings, but is functional for common daily activities (30 min with structure). May show a vague recognition of some staff, has increased awareness of self, family, and basic needs (as food), again in an appropriate manner, in contrast to level 5.

7. Automatic—appropriate. Patient appears appropriate and oriented within hospital and home settings, goes through daily routine automatically, but frequently robot-like, with minimal-to-absent confusion, but has shallow recall of what he/she has been doing. Shows increased awareness of self, body, family, foods, people, and interaction in the environment. Has superficial awareness of, but lacks insight into, his/her condition; decreased judgment and problem-solving and lacks realistic planning for the future. Shows carryover for new learning but at a decreased rate. Requires minimal supervision for learning and for safety purposes. With structure, is able to initiate tasks or social and recreational activities in which he/she now has interest. Judgment remains impaired, such that he/she is unable to drive a car.

8. Purposeful—appropriate. Patient is alert and oriented, is able to recall and integrate past and recent events and is aware of and responsive to his/her culture. Shows carryover for new learning, if acceptable to him/her and his/her life role, and needs no supervision once activities are learned. Within physical capabilities, the patient is independent in home and community skills, including driving. Vocational rehabilitation to determine ability to return as a contributor to society (perhaps in a new capacity) is indicated. May continue to show decreases relative to premorbid abilities in quality and rate of processing, abstract reasoning, tolerance for stress, and judgment in emergencies or unusual circumstances. Social, emotional, and intellectual capacities may continue to be at a decreased level, but patient is functional in society.

From Hagen C, Malkmus D, Durham P. *Levels of cognitive functioning.* Downey, CA: Rancho Los Amigos Hospital, 1972, with permission.

Table 15-11. Satisfaction with Life Scale

Below are five statements with which you may agree or disagree. Using the 1–7 scale below, indicate your agreement with each item by placing the appropriate number on the line preceding that item. Please be open and honest in your responding. The 7-point scale is as follows:

1 = Strongly disagree

2 = Disagree

3 = Slightly disagree

4 = Neither agree or disagree

5 = Slightly agree

6 = Agree

7 = Strongly agree

___ 1. In most ways my life is close to my ideal.

___ 2. The conditions of my life are excellent.

___ 3. I am satisfied with my life.

___ 4. So far I have gotten the important things I want in life.

___ 5. If I could live my life over, I would change almost nothing.

From Diener E, Emmons RA, Larsen RJ, et al. The Satisfaction with Life Scale. *J Pers Assess* 1985;49:71–75, with permission.

---

their caregivers with regard to quality and accessibility of brain injury services provided within the community. Scale items (Table 15-12), which solicit information concerning obstacles to receiving brain injury services, knowledge and availability of resources, and satisfaction with quality of care, are rated according to a 7-point scale ranging from 1 (strongly disagree) to 7 (strongly agree). The SOS has been shown to have good internal consistency, with estimates ranging from 0.56 to 0.77 for the items evaluating satisfaction with amount of professional help, quality of brain injury treatment, and adequacy of resources and from 0.29 to 0.48 for the remaining items, which include evaluation of transportation and financial issues (Kolakowsky-Hayner et al., 2000). SOS scores have been found to be associated with scores on the Family Needs Questionnaire, with individuals who report a greater number of unmet needs being likely to report more obstacles to services and greater dissatisfaction with community

resources. Lower quality of life ratings also have been associated with reports of increased obstacles and decreased satisfaction with community resources (Kolakowsky-Hayner et al., 2000). Primary components of the SOS, revealed by correlational analyses, include satisfaction with treatment resources, finances as an obstacle to receipt of services, and transportation as an obstacle to receipt of services. The SOS and relevant information concerning administration, scoring, and interpretation may be obtained from the Center for Outcome Measurement in Brain Injury Web site: http://www.tbims.org/combi/index.html.

Supervision Rating Scale

The Supervision Rating Scale (SRS; Boake, 1996) is a measure developed to assess the degree of supervision that a patient receives from caregivers. Level of supervision is rated according to a 13-point ordinal scale (Table 15-13), which can optionally be grouped into five ranked categories (independent, overnight supervision, part-time supervision, full-time indirect supervision, and full-time direct supervision). Ratings are derived from information acquired through interviews with the patient and an informant who has directly observed the level of supervision received by the patient. Inter-rater reliability of the SRS has been found to be adequate, with intra-class correlation of 0.86 and weighted kappa of 0.64. SRS ratings have been associated with type of living arrangement and with independence in self-care and instrumental activities of daily living. SRS ratings also were found to be strongly associated with ratings on the DRS and Glasgow Outcome Scale (Boake, 1996). The SRS and relevant information concerning administration, scoring, and interpretation may be obtained from the Institute for Rehabilitation Research, Houston, Texas, or from the Center for Outcome Measurement in Brain Injury Web site: http://www.tbims.org/combi/index.html.

Tennessee Self-Concept Scale

The TSCS-2 (Fitts & Warren, 1996) is an 82-item revision of the original Tennessee Self-Concept Scale (Fitts, 1965) developed to evaluate self-concept along physical, moral, personal, family, social, and academic/work dimensions. The TSCS-2 provides sum-

Table 15-12.   Services Obstacle Scale

1. I am dissatisfied with the amount of professional help and services being provided.

_____ 1. Strongly disagree

_____ 2. Disagree

_____ 3. Slightly disagree

_____ 4. Neither agree nor disagree

_____ 5. Slightly agree

_____ 6. Agree

_____ 7. Strongly agree

2. Transportation is a major obstacle toward getting enough help.

_____ 1. Strongly disagree

_____ 2. Disagree

_____ 3. Slightly disagree

_____ 4. Neither agree nor disagree

_____ 5. Slightly agree

_____ 6. Agree

_____ 7. Strongly agree

3. Lack of money to pay for medical, rehabilitation, and injury-related services is a major problem.

_____ 1. Strongly disagree

_____ 2. Disagree

_____ 3. Slightly disagree

_____ 4. Neither agree nor disagree

_____ 5. Slightly agree

_____ 6. Agree

_____ 7. Strongly agree

4. I don't know if there are good brain-injury treatment resources in the community.

_____ 1. Strongly disagree

_____ 2. Disagree

_____ 3. Slightly disagree

_____ 4. Neither agree nor disagree

_____ 5. Slightly agree

_____ 6. Agree

_____ 7. Strongly agree

5. For brain injury–related problems, there are very few resources in the community.

_____ 1. Strongly disagree

_____ 2. Disagree

_____ 3. Slightly disagree

_____ 4. Neither agree nor disagree

_____ 5. Slightly agree

_____ 6. Agree

_____ 7. Strongly agree

6. I have little confidence in the quality of care now being provided.

_____ 1. Strongly disagree

_____ 2. Disagree

_____ 3. Slightly disagree

_____ 4. Neither agree nor disagree

_____ 5. Slightly agree

_____ 6. Agree

_____ 7. Strongly agree

From Marwitz JH, Kreutzer JS. *The Service Obstacles Scale (SOS)*. Richmond, VA: Medical College of Virginia, Virginia Commonwealth University, 1996, with permission.

mary scores for those previously listed aspects of self-concept as well as for total self-concept and conflict (the degree to which self-concept is differentiated by assertion through agreement with positive items or by negation through disagreement with negative items). Supplementary scores, delineated on a theoretical basis only, examine a presumed subjective internal frame of reference across the domains of identity, satisfaction, and behavior. The measure also yields multiple validity scores designed to identify defensive, guarded, socially desirable, or other unusual or dis-torted patterns of responding. Items are rated according to a 5-point scale ranging from 1 (always false) to 5 (always true). Reliability of the TSCS-2 has been sufficiently demonstrated, with internal consistency estimates ranging from 0.81 to 0.95 (median, 0.80) and test-retest reliability estimates from 0.47 to 0.82 (median, 0.76). The validity of the TSCS-2 has been established through principal components analysis as well as correlational analyses illustrating significant associations between scores on this measure and scores on other tests of self-concept and personality. A

Table 15-13. Supervision Rating Scale

Level 1: Independent

1   The patient lives alone or independently. Other persons can live with the patient, but they cannot take responsibility for supervision (e.g., a child or elderly person).

2   The patient is unsupervised overnight. The patient lives with one or more persons who *could* be responsible for supervision (e.g., a spouse or roommate), but they are *all* sometimes absent overnight.

Level 2: Overnight supervision

3   The patient is only supervised overnight. One or more supervising persons are always present overnight, but they are *all* sometimes absent for the rest of the day.

Level 3: Part-time supervision

4   The patient is supervised overnight and part-time during waking hours, but is allowed on independent outings. One or more supervising persons are always present overnight and are also present during part of waking hours every day. However, the patient is sometimes allowed to leave the residence without being accompanied by someone who is responsible for supervision.

5   The patient is supervised overnight and part-time during waking hours, but is unsupervised during working hours. Supervising persons are *all* sometimes absent for enough time for them to work full-time outside the home.

6   The patient is supervised overnight and during most waking hours. Supervising persons are *all* sometimes absent for periods longer than 1 hr, but less than the time needed to hold a full-time job away from home.

7   The patient is supervised overnight and during almost all waking hours. Supervising persons are *all* sometimes absent for periods shorter than 1 hr.

Level 4: Full-time indirect supervision

8   The patient is under full-time indirect supervision. At least one supervising person is *always* present, but the supervising person does not check on the patient more than once every 30 min.

9   Same as No. 8 plus requires overnight safety precautions (e.g., a deadbolt on outside door).

Level 5: Full-time direct supervision

10   The patient is under full-time direct supervision. At least one supervising person is always present, and the supervising person checks on the patient more than once every 30 min.

11   The patient lives in a setting in which the exits are physically controlled by others (e.g., a locked ward).

12   Same as No. 11 plus a supervising person is designated to provide full-time, line-of-sight supervision (e.g., an escape watch or suicide watch).

13   The patient is in physical restraints.

From Boake C. Supervision Rating Scale: a measure of functional outcome. *Arch Phys Med Rehabil* 1996;77:765–72, with permission.

20-item short form of the TSCS-2, comprised of scale items found to correlate most highly with full measure Total Self-Concept and representative of the various self-concept dimensions listed previously, may be administered in circumstances precluding use of the full instrument. This short form has been reported to be sound from a psychometric perspective, with an internal consistency reliability of 0.84 and a correlation of 0.94 with the total self-concept score of the full measure (Fitts & Warren, 1996). The TSCS-2 manual and protocol forms may be obtained from Western Psychological Services, Los Angeles, California.

Conclusion

Consistent with the predictions of Coulthard-Morris et al. (1997) at the time of the publication of the first edition of this text, assessment of treatment outcomes in rehabilitation has shifted dramatically over the past decade to include an increased emphasis on issues such as health-related quality of life and psychological well-being. Broadening evaluations, which consider a more holistic view of the individual, parallel the standards set forth in the recently developed ICF and should function not only to facilitate the establishment of more effective and efficient programs of intervention but also to form the foundation on which to better monitor individual progress over time. The completion of more comprehensive assessments, despite their importance, may pose pragmatic challenges for rehabilitation professionals secondary to public policy provisions limiting the length of inpatient rehabilitation stays as a means for reducing direct health care costs.

This chapter reviews several formal outcome measures, which may be used in the rehabilitation setting to systematically evaluate health and health-related states according to the ICF model. Although selected instruments highlighted in this discussion are suitable, either with or without modification, for use with individuals under the age of 18 years or include alternate forms for assessment of adolescents and children, the focus has been on the presentation of measures appropriate for use by rehabilitation professionals in the examination of adults. Existing instruments that might be used for evaluation in the context of rehabilitation are far too numerous to review in a single chapter. Indeed, every measure described in this text, arguably, could be used as an outcome measure in the rehabilitation milieu, given the assertion that the ICF is universal in its application. The responsibility for choosing the most relevant outcome measures for use in a particular case rests with the rehabilitation professional and should be guided by the various components of the ICF model.

References

American Psychiatric Association. *Diagnostic and statistical manual of mental disorders* (4th ed.). Washington: American Psychiatric Association, 1994.

Amirkhan JH. A factor analytically derived measure of coping: the Coping Strategy Indicator. *J Pers Soc Psychol* 1990;59:1066–74.

Andrews FM, Withey SB. *Social indicators of well-being: America's perception of life quality.* New York: Plenum Press, 1976.

Arrindell WA, Meeuwesen L, Huyse FJ. The Satisfaction with Life Scale (SWLS): psychometric properties in a non-psychiatric medical outpatients sample. *Pers Individ Dif* 1991;12:117–23.

Beck AT, Steer RA, Brown GK. *Beck Depression Inventory—second edition manual.* San Antonio: Psychological Corporation, 1996.

Beckerman H, Vogelaar TW, Lankhorst GJ, et al. A criterion for stability of the function of the lower extremity in stroke patients using the Fugl-Meyer Assessment scale. *Scand J Rehabil Med* 1996;28:3–7.

Berg K, Wood-Dauphinee S, Williams JI, et al. Measuring balance in the elderly: Preliminary development of an instrument. *Physiotherapy Canada* 1989;41:304–11.

Berg K, Wood-Dauphinee S, Williams JI, et al. Measuring balance in the elderly: validation of an instrument. *Can J Public Health* 1992;2:S7–11.

Blais MR, Vallerand RJ, Pelletier LG, et al. L'Echelle de satisfaction de vie: validation Canadienne-Francaise du "Satisfaction with Life Scale." *Can J Behav Sci* 1989;21:210–23.

Boake C. Supervision Rating Scale: a measure of functional outcome. *Arch Phys Med Rehabil* 1996;77:765–72.

Bohac DL, Malec JF, Moessner AM. Factor analysis of the Mayo-Portland Adaptability Inventory: structure and validity. *Brain Inj* 1997;11:469–82.

Bowers D, Kofroth L. Comparison: Disability Rating Scale and Functional Independence Measure during recovery from traumatic brain injury. *Arch Phys Med Rehabil* 1989;70:A58.

Brazier JE, Harper R, Jones NM, et al. Validating the SF-36 Health Survey questionnaire: new outcome measure for primary care. *BMJ* 1992;305:160–4.

Brunnstrom S. *Movement therapy in hemiplegia: a neurophysiological approach.* New York: Harper and Row, 1970.

Burleigh SA, Farber RS, Gillard M. Community integration and life satisfaction after traumatic brain injury: long-term findings. *Am J Occup Ther* 1998;52:45–52.

Campbell RJ. *Psychiatric dictionary* (7th ed.). New York: Oxford University Press, 1996.

Chau N, Daler S, Andre JM, et al. Inter-rater agreement of two functional independence scales: the Functional Independence Measure (FIM) and a subjective uniform continuous scale. *Disabil Rehabil* 1994;16:63–71.

Cifu DX, Keyser-Marcus L, Lopez E, et al. Acute predictors of successful return to work 1 year after traumatic brain injury: a multicenter analysis. *Arch Phys Med Rehabil* 1997;78:125–31.

Collin C, Wade DT, Davies S, et al. The Barthel ADL Index: a reliability study. *Int Disabil Stud* 1988;10:61–3.

Coulthard-Morris L, Burks JS, Herndon RM. Rehabilitation outcome measures. In: Herndon RM (ed.). *Handbook of neurologic rating scales.* New York: Demos Vermande, 1997:225–64.

Davidson J. *Davidson Trauma Scale.* North Tonawanda, NY: Multi-Health Systems, 1996.

DeJong G, Branch LG. Predicting the stroke patient's ability to live independently. *Stroke* 1982;13:648–55.

Diener E, Emmons RA, Larsen RJ, et al. The Satisfaction with Life Scale. *J Pers Assess* 1985;49:71–5.

Dijkers M. Scoring CHART: survey and sensitivity analysis. *J Am Paraplegia Soc* 1991;14:85–6.

Dijkers MP. Correlates of life satisfaction among persons with spinal cord injury. *Arch Phys Med Rehabil* 1999; 80:867–76.

Dodds TA, Martin TP, Stolov WC, et al. A validation of the functional independence measurement and its performance among rehabilitation inpatients. *Arch Phys Med Rehabil* 1993;74:531–36.

Dorman PJ, Dennis M, Sandercock P. How do scores on the EuroQol relate to scores on the SF-36 after stroke? *Stroke* 1999;30:2146–51.

Dorman P, Slattery J, Farrell B, et al. Qualitative comparison of the reliability of health status assessments with the EuroQol and SF-36 questionnaires after stroke. *Stroke* 1998;29:63–8.

Duncan PW, Goldstein LB, Horner RD, et al. Similar motor recovery of upper and lower extremities after stroke. *Stroke* 1994;25:1181–88.

Duncan PW, Propst M, Nelson SG. Reliability of the Fugl-Meyer Assessment of Sensorimotor Recovery following cerebrovascular accident. *Phys Ther* 1983;63:1606–10.

Eliason M, Topp B. Predictive validity of Rappaport's Disability Rating Scale in subjects with acute brain dysfunction. *Phys Ther* 1984;64:1357.

Ellis-Hill CS, Horn S. Change in identity and self-concept: a new theoretical approach to recovery following a stroke. *Clin Rehabil* 2000;14:279–87.

Endler NS, Courbasson CMA, Fillion L. Coping with cancer: the evidence for the temporal stability of the French-Canadian version of the Coping with Health Injuries and Problems (CHIP). *Pers Individ Dif* 1998a;25:711–17.

Endler NS, Parker JDA. *Coping with Health Injuries and Problems (CHIP) manual.* North Tonawanda, NY: Multi-Health Systems, 1992.

Endler NS, Parker JDA, Summerfeldt LJ. Coping with health problems: developing a reliable and valid multidimensional measure. *Psychol Assess* 1998b;10:195–205.

Feys H, Van Hees J, Bruyninck F, et al. Value of somatosensory and motor evoked potentials in predicting arm recovery after stroke. *J Neurol Neurosurg Psychiatry* 2000;68:323–31.

Finch E, Brooks D, Stratford PW, et al. *Physical rehabilitation outcome measures: a guide to enhanced clinical decision making* (2nd ed.). Toronto: Canadian Physiotherapy Association, 2002.

Fitts WH. *Tennessee Self-Concept Scale (TSCS) manual.* Los Angeles: Western Psychological Services, 1965.

Fitts WH, Warren WL. *Tennessee Self-Concept Scale—Second Edition (TSCS:2) manual.* Los Angeles: Western Psychological Services, 1996.

Freeman JA, Hobart JC, Langdon DW, et al. Clinical appropriateness: a key factor in outcome measure selection: the 36-Item Short Form Health Survey in multiple sclerosis. *J Neurol Neurosurg Psychiatry* 2000;68:150–56.

Fugl-Meyer AR. Post-stroke hemiplegia assessment of physical properties. *Scand J Rehabil Med* 1980;7(Suppl): 85–93.

Fugl-Meyer AR, Jaasko L, Leyman I, et al. The post-stroke hemiplegic patient 1. A method for evaluation of physical performance. *Scand J Rehabil Med* 1975;7:13–31.

Gontkovsky ST, Parker R. *Relationship between coping, self-esteem, self-concept, and life satisfaction after spinal cord injury.* Poster session presented at the annual meeting of the American Psychological Society, Chicago, IL, 2004.

Gontkovsky ST, Vickery CD, Parker R, et al. *Early evolution of posttraumatic stress disorder symptomatology following traumatic spinal cord injury.* Poster session presented at the annual meeting of the American Association of Spinal Cord Injury Psychologists and Social Workers, Las Vegas, NV, 2004.

Gouvier WD, Blanton PD, LaPorte KK, et al. Reliability and validity of the Disability Rating Scale and the Levels of Cognitive Functioning Scale in monitoring recovery from severe head injury. *Arch Phys Med Rehabil* 1987; 68:94–7.

Gowland C, Stratford P, Ward M, et al. Measuring physical impairment and disability with the Chedoke-McMaster Stroke Assessment. *Stroke* 1993;24:58–63.

Granger CV. The emerging science of functional assessment: our tool for outcomes analysis. *Arch Phys Med Rehabil* 1998;79:235–40.

Granger CV, Albrecht GL, Hamilton BB. Outcome of comprehensive medical rehabilitation: measurement by PULSES profile and the Barthel Index. *Arch Phys Med Rehabil* 1979a;60:145–54.

Granger CV, Cotter AC, Hamilton BB, et al. Functional assessment scales: a study of persons with multiple sclerosis. *Arch Phys Med Rehabil* 1990;71:870–75.

Granger CV, Dewis LS, Peters NC, et al. Stroke rehabilitation: analysis of repeated Barthel Index measures. *Arch Phys Med Rehabil* 1979b;60:14–7.

Gresham GE, Phillips TF, Labi ML. ADL status in stroke: relative merits of three standard indexes. *Arch Phys Med Rehabil* 1980;61:355–58.

Hagen C, Malkmus D, Durham P. *Levels of cognitive functioning.* Downey, CA: Rancho Los Amigos Hospital, 1972.

Hall KM, Cope N, Rappaport M. Glasgow Outcome Scale and Disability Rating Scale: comparative usefulness in following recovery in traumatic head injury. *Arch Phys Med Rehabil* 1985;66:35–7.

Hall KM, Hamilton B, Gordon WA, et al. Characteristics and comparisons of functional assessment indices: Disability Rating Scale, Functional Independence Measure and Functional Assessment Measure. *J Head Trauma Rehabil* 1993;8:60–74.

Hall KM, Mann N, High W, et al. Functional measures after traumatic brain injury: ceiling effects of FIM, FIM+FAM, DRS and CIQ. *J Head Trauma Rehabil* 1996; 11:27–39.

Heinemann AW, Kirk P, Hastie BA, et al. Relationship between disability measures and nursing effort during medical rehabilitation for patients with traumatic brain and spinal cord injury. *Arch Phys Med Rehabil* 1997; 78:143–49.

Heinemann AW, Whiteneck GG. Relationships among impairment, disability, handicap and life satisfaction in persons with traumatic brain injury. *J Head Trauma Rehabil* 1995;10:54–63.

Jarvis PE, Barth JT. *The Halstead-Reitan Neuropsychology Battery: a guide to interpretation and clinical applications.* Odessa, FL: Psychological Assessment Resources, 1994.

Keith RA, Granger CV, Hamilton BB, et al. The Functional Independence Measure: a new tool for rehabilitation. In: Eisenberg MG, Grzesiak RC (eds.). *Advances in clinical rehabilitation.* New York: Springer, 1987:6–18.

Kolakowsky-Hayner SA, Kreutzer JS, Miner D. Validation of the Service Obstacle Scale for the traumatic brain injury population. *Neurorehabilitation* 2000;14:151–58.

Larsen RJ, Diener E, Emmons RA. An evaluation of subjective well-being measures. *Soc Indic Res* 1985;17:1–18.

Lin FM, Sabbahi M. Correlation of spasticity with hyperactive stretch reflexes and motor dysfunction in hemiplegia. *Arch Phys Med Rehabil* 1999;80:526–30.

Loewen SC, Anderson BA. Reliability of the Modified Motor Assessment Scale and Barthel Index. *Phys Ther* 1988; 68:1077–81.

Mahoney FI, Barthel DW. Functional evaluation: the Barthel Index. *MD State Med J* 1965;14:61–5.

Malouin F, Pichard L, Bonneau C, et al. Evaluating motor recovery early after stroke: comparison of the Fugl-Meyer and the Motor Assessment Scale. *Arch Phys Med Rehabil* 1994;75:1206–12.

Malec JF, Buffington ALH, Moessner AM, et al. A medical/vocational case coordination system for persons with brain injury: an evaluation of employment outcomes. *Arch Phys Med Rehabil* 2000;81:1007–15.

Malec JF, Lezak MD. *Manual for the Mayo-Portland Adaptability Inventory (MPAI-4).* Center for Outcome Measurement in Brain Injury Web site, 2003.

Malec JF, Thompson JM. Relationship of the Mayo-Portland Adaptability Inventory to functional outcome and cognitive performance measures. *J Head Trauma Rehabil* 1994;9:1–15.

Marshall GN, Collins BE, Crooks VC. A comparison of two multidimensional health locus of control instruments. *J Pers Assess* 1990;54:181–90.

Marwitz JH, Kreutzer JS. *The Service Obstacles Scale (SOS).* Richmond, VA: Medical College of Virginia, Virginia Commonwealth University, 1996.

McHorney CA. Measuring and monitoring general health status in elderly persons: practical and methodological issues in using the SF-36 Health Survey. *Gerontologist* 1996;36:571–83.

McIntosh L, Woronuk J, May L, et al. Development of the Glenrose Ambulation Rating (GAR): validity and inter-rater reliability. *J Rehabil Outcomes Meas* 1999; 3:1–11.

Mellick D, Walker N, Brooks CA, et al. Incorporating the cognitive independence domain into CHART. *J Rehabil Outcomes Meas* 1999;3:12–21.

Osgood C, Suci G, Tannenbaum P. *The measurement of meaning.* Urbana, IL: University of Illinois Press, 1957.

Ottenbacher KJ, Mann WC, Granger CV, et al. Inter-rater agreement and stability of functional assessment in the community-based elderly. *Arch Phys Med Rehabil* 1994; 75:1297–301.

Pavot W, Diener E. Review of the Satisfaction with Life Scale. *Psychol Assess* 1993;5:164–72.

Rao N, Kilgore KM. Predicting return to work in traumatic brain injury using assessment scales. *Arch Phys Med Rehabil* 1992;73:911–16.

Rappaport M, Hall KM, Hopkins K, et al. Disability Rating Scale for severe head trauma: coma to community. *Arch Phys Med Rehabil* 1982;63:118–23.

Robinson-Whelen S, Storant M. Factorial structure of two health belief measures among older adults. *Psychol Aging* 1992;7:209–13.

Ruta DA, Hurst NP, Kind P, et al. Measuring health status in British patients with rheumatoid arthritis: reliability, validity and responsiveness of the Short-Form 36-Item Health Survey (SF-36). *Br J Rheumatol* 1998; 37:425–36.

Sander AM, Seel RT, Kreutzer JS, et al. Agreement between persons with traumatic brain injury and their relatives regarding psychosocial outcome using the Community Integration Questionnaire. *Arch Phys Med Rehabil* 1997;78:353–57.

Segal ME, Schall RR. Determining functional/health status and its relation to disability in stroke survivors. *Stroke* 1994;25:2391–97.

Segal ME, Schall RR. Assessing handicap of stroke survivors. A validation study of the Craig Handicap Assessment and Reporting Technique. *Am J Phys Med Rehabil* 1995;74:276–86.

Shah S, Vanclay F, Cooper B. Improving the sensitivity of the Barthel Index for stroke rehabilitation. *J Clin Epidemiol* 1989;42:703–9.

Sharrack B, Hughes RA, Soudain S, et al. The psychometric properties of clinical rating scales used in multiple sclerosis. *Brain* 1999;122(Pt 1):141–59.

Shin DC, Johnson DM. Avowed happiness as an overall assessment of the quality of life. *Social Indicators Research* 1978;5:475–92.

Snider JG, Osgood CE. *Semantic differential technique: a source book.* Chicago: Aldine, 1969.

Thorbahn LDB, Newton RA. Use of the Berg Balance Test to predict falls in elderly persons. *Phys Ther* 1996;76:576–82.

Twitchel TE. The restoration of motor function following hemiplegia in man. *Brain* 1951;74:443–80.

Tyerman A, Humphrey M. Changes in self-concept following severe head injury. *Int J Rehabil Res* 1984;7:11–23.

van der Putten JJ, Hobart JC, Freeman JA, et al. Measuring change in disability after inpatient rehabilitation: comparison of the responsiveness of the Barthel Index and the Functional Independence Measure. *J Neurol Neurosurg Psychiatry* 1999;66:480–84.

Vickery CD, Gontkovsky ST, Caroselli JS. Self-concept and quality of life following acquired brain injury: a pilot investigation. *Brain Inj* 2005;19:657–65.

Wade DT, Hewer RL. Functional abilities after stroke: measurement, natural history and prognosis. *J Neurol Neurosurg Psychiatry* 1987;50:177–82.

Walker N, Mellick D, Brooks CA, et al. Measuring participation across impairments groups using the Craig Handicap Assessment and Reporting Technique. *Am J Phys Med Rehabil* 2003;82:936–41.

Wallston KA, Wallston BS, DeVellis R. Development of the multidimensional health locus of control (MHLC) scales. *Health Education Monographs* 1978;6:160–70.

Wallston KA, Stein MJ, Smith CA. Form C of the MHLC scales: a condition-specific measure of locus of control. *J Pers Assess* 1994;63:534–53.

Ware JE, Kosinski M, Keller SD. *SF-36 physical and mental summary scales: a user's manual.* Boston: The Health Institute, New England Medical Center, 1994.

Ware JE, Sherbourne CD. The MOS 36-Item Short-Form Health Survey (SF-36): I. Conceptual framework and item selection. *Med Care* 1992;30:473–81.

Ware JE, Snow KK, Kosinski M, et al. *SF-36 Health Survey: manual and interpretation guide.* Boston: The Health Institute, New England Medical Center, 1993.

Wee JY, Wong H, Palepu A. Validation of the Berg Balance Scale as a predictor of length of stay and discharge destination in stroke rehabilitation. *Arch Phys Med Rehabil* 2003;84:731–35.

Whiteneck GG, Charlifue SW, Gerhart KA, et al. Quantifying handicap: a new measure of long-term rehabilitation outcomes. *Arch Phys Med Rehabil* 1992;73:519–26.

Willer B, Ottenbacher KJ, Coad ML. The Community Integration Questionnaire: a comparative examination. *Am J Phys Med Rehabil* 1994;73:103–11.

Willer B, Rosenthal M, Kreutzer JS, et al. Assessment of community integration following rehabilitation for traumatic brain injury. *J Head Trauma Rehabil* 1993; 8:75–87.

Wolfe CD, Taub NA, Woodrow EJ, et al. Assessment of scales of disability and handicap for stroke patients. *Stroke* 1991;22:1242–44.

Wood-Dauphinee SW, Williams JI, Shapiro SH. Examining outcome measures in a clinical study of stroke. *Stroke* 1990;21:731–39.

World Health Organization. *International Classification of Impairments, Disabilities, and Handicaps.* Geneva: World Health Organization, 1980.

World Health Organization. *International Classification of Functioning, Disability, and Health.* Geneva: World Health Organization, 2001.

Wright J, Telford, R. Psychological problems following minor head injury: a prospective study. *Br J Clin Psychol* 1996; 35:399–412.

Wylie, CM. Measuring end results of rehabilitation of patients with stroke. *Public Health Rep* 1967;82:893–98.

Zhang L, Abreu BC, Gonzales V, et al. Comparison of the Community Integration Questionnaire, the Craig Handicap Assessment and Reporting Technique, and the Disability Rating Scale in traumatic brain injury. *J Head Trauma Rehabil* 2002;17:497–509.

16 Human Immunodeficiency Virus–Associated Cognitive Impairment

Giovanni Schifitto, M.D., and Michelle D. Gaugh, M.A.

Cognitive impairment is one of the most common neurological complications of human immunodeficiency virus (HIV) infection. Before the introduction of highly active antiretroviral therapy in 1996, it was projected that 15–20% of acquired immunodeficiency syndrome (AIDS) patients would develop dementia. The course of dementia in the early 1980s was rapid, with a median survival of 6 months. In this context, Price and Brew (1988) proposed the AIDS dementia complex (ADC) staging intended to favor the follow-up of patients and research initiatives. To facilitate the consensus on terminology and criteria for HIV-associated neurologic disorders, the American Academy of Neurology (AAN) AIDS Task Force convened a multispecialty working group, and a report from this meeting was published in 1991 (Janssen et al., 1991).

More recently, operationalization of Price and Brew ADC staging and of the AAN recommendations for ADC and minor cognitive/motor disorder have been published (Marder et al., 1996, 2003). An additional HIV dementia scale was proposed by Power et al. (1995) but has not been widely used.

Acquired Immunodeficiency Syndrome Dementia Complex Clinical Staging

The ADC is divided into six stages, from normal mental and motor function (stage 0) to a nearly vegetative state (stage 4) (Table 16-1). The stages increase by one unit from 0–4 except for the subclinical stage that is scored 0.5. The scale is based primarily on functional disability with supporting neurological and neuropsychological evaluation. In addition, functional deficits at these stages may or may not be due to neurologic disease.

To overcome some of this limitation, investigators from the Northeast AIDS Dementia Consortium have standardized the use of neurologic, neuropsychological, and functional performance to derive ADC staging (see Table 16-1). The standard neurologic exam includes the motor subscale (part III) of the Unified Parkinson Disease Rating Scale (Goetz et al., 1995). The battery of neuropsychological tests used is shown in Table 16-2; however, equivalent neuropsychological tests to assess similar cognitive domains can be used (Janssen et al., 1991; Butters et

Table 16-1. Acquired Immunodeficiency Syndrome (AIDS) Dementia Complex Staging

ADC Stage	Characteristics	New Criteria: NEAD Modification
Stage 0 (normal)	Normal mental and motor function.	NP impression is 0, *even if* cognitive complaints are present.
Stage 0.5 (subclinical or equivocal)	Absent, minimal, or equivocal symptoms *without impairment of work or capacity to perform ADL*. Mild signs (snout response, slowed ocular or extremity movements) may be present. Gait and strength are normal.	1. NP impression is 0 *and* any CNS neuro findings, *or* any IADL functional impairment. 2. NP impression is 1 *and* no IADL functional impairment.
Stage 1 (mild)	Able to perform all but the more *demanding aspects of work* or ADL but with unequivocal evidence (signs or symptoms that may include performance on neuropsychological testing) of functional intellectual or motor impairment. Can walk without assistance.	1. NP impression is 1 *and* abnormalities in both CNS neurologic examination *and* IADL function. 2. NP impression is 2 *but* no abnormalities in *either* CNS neurologic examination *or* IADL function.
Stage 2 (moderate)	Able to perform *basic activities of self-care* but cannot work or maintain the more demanding aspects of daily life. Ambulatory but may require a single prop.	1. NP impression is 2 *and* any abnormality in one of the two domains (CNS neurologic examination *or* IADL function). 2. NP impression is 2 *and* mild to moderate abnormalities in both CNS neurologic examination *and* IADL function; however, neither severe.
Stage 3 (severe)	*Major intellectual incapacity* (cannot follow news or personal events, cannot sustain complex conversation, considerable slowing of all output) *or motor* disability (cannot walk unassisted, requiring walker or personal support, usually with slowing and clumsiness of arms as well).	1. NP impression is 2 *and* severe abnormalities in both CNS neurologic examination *and* IADL function. 2. NP impression is 2 *and* mild to moderate abnormalities in CNS neurologic examination *and* severe IADL functional impairment *and* severe gait impairment. 3. NP impression is 3 *and* gait is mild to moderately impaired.
Stage 4 (end stage)	*Nearly vegetative.* Intellectual and social comprehension and output are at a rudimentary level. Nearly or absolutely mute. Paraparetic or paraplegic with urinary and fecal incontinence.	1. Unable to perform NP testing because of cognitive-motor impairments. 2. Unable to walk on CNS basis.

ADC = AIDS dementia complex; ADL = activities of daily living; CNS = central nervous system; IADL = instrumental activities of daily living; NEAD = Northeast AIDS Dementia Consortium; NP impression = this may be the global cognitive impression or the quantitative global neuropsychological impression.

Table 16-2. Algorithm for Determining Quantitative Global Impression of Cognitive Function

Neuropsychological Domain	Test	Subtest
Verbal memory	Rey Auditory Verbal Learning Test	Trial 5
		Delayed recall
		Delayed recognition
Visual memory	Rey Complex Figure	Delayed recall
Visuoconstruction	Rey Complex Figure	Copy
Frontal/executive	Odd Man Out	(total score)
	Verbal Fluency	(total score)
Psychomotor	Digit Symbol	(total score)
	California Computerized Assessment Package	Choice
		Sequential
Motor speed	Grooved Pegboard	Dominant
		Non-dominant

Note: A score of ≥1 SD below the appropriate norm earns 1 point. A score ≥2 SD below the appropriate norm earns 2 points. Thus, the range of the summary impairment score is 0–24. A summary impairment score of (0–1) = quantitative global impression of 0 (normal); a summary impairment score of (2–6) = quantitative global impression of 1 (mild); a summary impairment score of (7–14) = quantitative global impression of 2 (moderate); a summary impairment score of (15–24) = a quantitative global impression of 3 (severe).

al., 1990). The global neuropsychological impression used in this modified ADC staging requires the availability of a neuropsychologist. The kappa statistics for pairwise agreement among the four Northeast AIDS Dementia Consortium sites for ADC staging ranged from 0.70 to 0.91. Reasonable results were also obtained when the neuropsychological impression was computer generated (0.62–0.79), adopting the schema shown in Table 16-2. In this regard, a computerized ADC algorithm can be generated, facilitating the use of ADC staging in multicenter studies.

American Academy of Neurology Criteria for Human Immunodeficiency Virus–Associated Acquired Immunodeficiency Syndrome Dementia Complex and Minor Cognitive-Motor Disorder

The AAN criteria for ADC introduce more detailed requirements for the presence of cognitive, neurologic and behavioral abnormalities (Table 16-3). The staging of mild, moderate, and severe is based on func-

tional disability with self-independence lost in the moderate and severe stages of ADC. A milder form of cognitive impairment, minor cognitive-motor disorder, was also introduced (Table 16-4), and it may be compared to Price and Brew stage 0.5.

Marder et al. (2003) have proposed an operationalization of the AAN criteria for ADC and minor cognitive-motor disorder (Tables 16-5 and 16-6). As for the ADC operationalization, a computer-generated algorithm can be derived, providing a tool that can simplify the use of ADC or minor cognitive-motor disorder outcomes in multicenter studies.

Human Immunodeficiency Virus Dementia Scale

The HIV Dementia Scale has a structure similar to the Mini-Mental State Examination but the use of timing tests stresses psychomotor speed, a known abnormality in subcortical dementias. The usefulness of the HIV Dementia Scale is that it can be easily administered and requires only a few minutes to complete. The scale was validated in a relatively small sample that included 29

Table 16-3.   American Academy of Neurology Criteria for HIV-1–Associated Dementia Complex[a]

Probable (must have each of the following):

1. Acquired abnormality in at least two of the following cognitive abilities (present for at least 1 mo): attention/concentration, speed of processing of information, abstraction/reasoning, visuospatial skills, memory/learning, and speech/language. The decline should be verified by reliable history and mental status examination. In all cases, when possible, history should be supplemented by neuropsychological testing.

Cognitive dysfunction causing impairing of work or activities of daily living[b] (objectively verifiable or by report of a key informant). This impairment should not be attributable solely to severe system illness.

2. At least one of the following:

   a. Acquired abnormality in motor function or performance verified by clinical examination (e.g., slowed rapid movements, abnormal gait, limb incoordination, hyperreflexia, hypertonia, or weakness), neuropsychological tests (e.g., fine motor speed, manual dexterity, perceptual motor skills), or both.

   b. Decline in motivation or emotional control or change in social behavior. This may be characterized by any of the following: change in personality with apathy, inertia, irritability, emotional liability, or new onset of impaired judgment characterized by socially inappropriate behavior or disinhibition.

3. Absence or clouding of consciousness during a period long enough to establish the presence of No. 1.

4. Evidence of another etiology, including active CNS opportunistic infection or malignancy, psychiatric disorders (e.g., depressive disorder), active alcohol or substance use, or acute or chronic substance withdrawal, must be sought from history, physical and psychiatric examination, and appropriate laboratory and radiologic investigation (e.g., lumbar puncture, neuroimaging). If another potential etiology (e.g., major depression) is present, it is not the cause of the above cognitive, motor, or behavioral symptoms and signs.

Possible (must have one of the following):

1. Other potential etiology present (must have each of the following):

   a. As above (see Probable) Nos. 1, 2, and 3.

   b. Other potential etiology is present but the cause of No. 1 above is uncertain.

2. Incomplete clinical evaluation (must have each of the following):

   a. As above (see Probable) Nos. 1, 2, and 3.

   b. Etiology cannot be determined (appropriate laboratory or radiologic investigations not performed).

CNS = central nervous system; HIV = human immunodeficiency virus.

[a]For research purposes, HIV-1–associated dementia complex can be coded to describe the major features: HIV-1–associated dementia complex requires criteria 1, 2a, 2b, 3, and 4; HIV-1–associated dementia complex (motor) requires criteria 1, 2a, 3, and 4; HIV-1–associated dementia complex (behavior) requires criteria 1, 2b, 3, and 4.

[b]The level of impairment due to cognitive dysfunction should be assessed as follows:

Mild: Decline in performance at work, including work in the home, that is conspicuous to others. Unable to work at usual job, although may be able to work at a much less demanding job. Activities of daily living or social activities are impaired but not to a degree making the person completely dependent on others. More complicated daily tasks or recreational activities cannot be undertaken. Capable of basic self-care such as feeding, dressing, and maintaining personal hygiene, but activities such as handling money, shopping, using public transportation, driving a car, or keeping track of appointments or medications are impaired.

Moderate: Unable to work, including work in the home. Unable to function without some assistance of another in daily living, including dressing, maintaining personal hygiene, eating, shopping, handling money, and walking, but able to communicate basic needs.

Severe: Unable to perform any activities of daily living without assistance. Requires continual supervision. Unable to maintain personal hygiene; nearly or absolutely mute.

Table 16-4. American Academy of Neurology Criteria for HIV-1–Associated Minor Cognitive/Motor Disorder

Probable (must have each of the following):

1. Cognitive/motor/behavioral abnormalities (must have each of the following):

   a. At least two of the following acquired cognitive, motor, or behavior symptoms (present for at least 1 mo) verified by reliable history (when possible, from an informant):

      1. Impaired attention or concentration

      2. Mental slowing

      3. Impaired memory

      4. Slowed movements

      5. Incoordination

      6. Personality change, or irritability or emotional lability

   b. Acquired cognitive/motor abnormality verified by clinical neurologic examination or neuropsychological testing (e.g., fine motor speed, manual dexterity, perceptual motor skills, attention/concentration, speed of processing of information, abstraction/reasoning, visuospatial skills, memory/learning, or speech/language).

2. Disturbance from cognitive/motor/behavioral abnormalities (see No. 1) causes mild impairment of work or activities of daily living* (objectively verifiable or by report of a key informant).

3. Does not meet criteria for HIV-1–associated dementia complex or HIV-1–associated myelopathy.

4. No evidence of another etiology, including active CNS opportunistic infection or malignancy, or severe systemic illness determined by appropriate history, physical examination, and laboratory and radiologic investigation (e.g., lumbar puncture, neuroimaging). The above features should not be attributable solely to the effects of active alcohol or substance use, acute or chronic substance withdrawal, adjustment disorder, or other psychiatric disorders.

Possible (must have one of the following):

1. Other potential etiology present (must have each of the following):

   a. As above (see Probable) Nos. 1, 2, and 3.

   b. Other potential etiology is present and the cause of the cognitive/motor/behavioral abnormalities is uncertain.

2. Incomplete clinical evaluation (must have each of the following):

   a. As above (see Probable) Nos. 1, 2, and 3.

   b. Etiology cannot be determined (appropriate laboratory or radiologic investigations not performed).

CNS = central nervous system; HIV = human immunodeficiency virus.

*Able to perform all but the most demanding aspects of work or activities of daily living. Performance at work is mildly impaired but able to maintain usual job; social activities may be mildly impaired, but person is not dependent on others. Can feed self, dress, and maintain personal hygiene; handle money; shop; use public transportation; or drive a car, but complex daily tasks such as keeping track of appointments or medications may be occasionally impaired.

Table 16-5. Modification of American Academy of Neurology Criteria for Human Immunodeficiency Virus-1–Associated Dementia Complex

Criteria for 1 and 2 must be met:

1. Scores 1 SD below age- and education-adjusted norms on two of eight neuropsychological tests or 2 SDs below the norms on one of eight tests.

2. Requires assistance or has difficulty (due to either physical or cognitive deficit) in one of the following IADL:

    Using the telephone

    Handling money

    Taking medication

    Performing light housekeeping

    Doing laundry

    Preparing meals

    Shopping for groceries

    Getting to places out of walking distance

and must meet either 1 or 2 of the following:

1. Any impairment in the following: lower extremity strength, coordination, finger tapping, alternating hand movements, leg agility, or performance on grooved pegboard 2 SDs below mean (dominant hand).

2. Self-reported frequent depression that interferes with function, loss of interest in usual activities or emotional lability, or irritability.

Staging of ADC

   Mild: must attribute IADL to a cognitive source

   Moderate: satisfies neurologic and psychiatric criteria for mild ADC plus functional impairment in either telephone use, medication taking, or money handling plus two or three other IADLs or ADLs (indoor mobility, eating, dressing, grooming, toileting, getting in and out of bed, bathing) attributed to a cognitive source

   Severe: satisfies neurologic and psychiatric criteria for moderate ADC and has in addition to impairment in telephone use, medication taking, or money handling at least four IADLs or ADLs attributed to a cognitive source

ADC = AIDS dementia complex; ADL = activities of daily living; AIDS = acquired immunodeficiency syndrome; IADL = instrumental activities of daily living.

Table 16-6. Modification of American Academy of Neurology Criteria for Human Immunodeficiency Virus-1 (HIV-1)–Associated Minor Cognitive/Motor Disorder

Does not meet criteria for HIV-1–associated cognitive/motor disorder and meets 1 and 2 of the following:

1. Deficit in at least two of the following:

    Mental slowing: digit symbol at least 1 SD below age- and education-adjusted norms

    Memory: Rey Auditory Verbal Learning Test (total) at least 1 SD below norms

    Motor dysfunction: any impairment in finger tapping or pronation/supination

    Incoordination: mild impairment in gait or clumsiness

    Emotional lability or apathy/withdrawal

2. Deficit in at least one of the role function measures attributed in part to cognitive function:

    Need for frequent rests

    Cut down on amount of time in activities

    Accomplish less than desired

    Cannot perform activities as carefully as one would like

    Limited in work or activities

    Difficulty performing activities

    Requires special assistance to perform activities

HIV-negative individuals, 29 HIV-positive asymptomatic patients, 35 nondemented AIDS patients, 30 ADC stage 1 and 2, and 7 ADC stage 3 and 4 subjects.

The scale consists of four subtests: (a) timed written alphabet (uppercase letters) or numbers from 1 to 26 if the patient is unable to use the alphabet, (b) recall of four items at 5 minutes, (c) timed copy of a recognizable cube, and (d) antisaccadic errors. For the antisaccadic errors task, the patient is looking at the examiner's nose. The examiner holds both index fingers level with the patient's shoulders and asks the patient to look at the moving finger (practicing with both index fingers). Then the patient is asked to look only from nose to nonmoving finger in 20 trials. An error is recorded when the patient looks at the moving finger.

The maximum score of the scale is 16 (a = 6; b = 4; c = 2; d = 4), details of the scoring are listed in Table 16-7. In the validation study, AIDS patients scored 12.7 ± 3.17, ADC 1 and 2 scored 8.04 ± 3.81, and ADC stages 3 and 4 scored 3.5 ± 2.28.

Table 16-7. Human Immunodeficiency Virus Dementia Scale

---

1. Memory—registration

   Give four words to recall (dog, hat, green, peach)—1 sec to say each. Then ask the patient all 4 after you have said them.

2. Attention

   Anti-saccadic eye movements: 20 commands _____errors in 20 trials

   ≤3 errors = 4

   4 errors = 3

   5 errors = 2

   6 errors = 1

   >6 errors = 0

3. Psychomotor speed

   Ask patient to write the alphabet in uppercase letters horizontally across the page and record time: ____ sec

   ≤21 sec = 6

   21.1–24.0 sec = 5

   24.1–27.0 sec = 4

   27.1–30.0 sec = 3

   30.1–33.0 sec = 2

   33.1–36.0 sec = 1

   >36 sec = 0

4. Memory—recall

   Ask for four words from registration, above. Give 1 point for each correct. For words not recalled, prompt with "semantic " clue as follows: animal (dog), piece of clothing (hat), color (green), fruit (peach). Give 0.5 point for each correct answer after prompting.

5. Construction

   Copy the cube below; record time; _____ sec

   <25 sec = 2; 25–35 sec = 1; >35 sec = 0

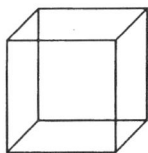

Score _____/16

References

Butters N, Grant I, Haxby J, et al. Assessment of AIDS-related cognitive change: recommendations of the NIMH workshop on neuropsychological assessment approaches. *J Clin Exp Neuropsychol* 1990;12:963–78.

Goetz GC, Stebbins GT, Chmura TA, et al. Teaching tape for the motor section of the Unified Parkinson's Disease Rating Scale. *Mov Dis* 1995;10:263–66.

Janssen RS, Cornblath DR, Epstein LG, et al. Nomenclature and research case definitions for neurological manifestations of Human Immunodeficiency Virus type-1 (HIV-1) infection, report from the American Academy of Neurology AIDS Task Force. *Neurology* 1991;41:778–85.

Marder K, Albert S, Dooneief G, et al. Clinical confirmation of the American Academy of Neurology algorithm for HIV-1 associated cognitive/motor disorder. *Neurology* 1996;47:1247–53.

Marder K, Albert SM, McDermott MP, et al. Inter-rater reliability of a clinical staging of HIV-associated cognitive impairment. *Neurology* 2003;60:1467–73.

Power C, Selnes OA, Grim JA, et al. HIV Dementia Scale: a rapid screening test. *J Acq Imm Def Syn Hum Retrovirol* 1995;8:273–78.

Price RW, Brew BJ. The AIDS dementia complex. *J Infect Dis* 1988;158:1079–83.

17 Summary and Conclusions

Robert M. Herndon, M.D.

Advances in therapy for neurologic disease are dependent on high-quality clinical trials. The quality of clinical trials, in turn, depends on the validity, precision, reliability, and sensitivity of the measures used to validate therapeutic efficacy. Substantial progress has been made in the development of new and better neurological scales since 1997, yet much remains to be done. Many existing scales need improvement, whereas others need further validation. Given the large number of available scales, scale selection plays an important role in the planning of clinical trials. A scale with the appropriate properties is essential. Some of the factors that need to be considered that were discussed in Chapter 1 include:

Validity
  Face validity
  Construct validity
  Content validity
  Criterion-related validity
  Ecological validity
  Predictive validity

Reliability (accuracy)
Reproducibility (precision)
Sensitivity within the disease range to be tested (responsiveness to change in the underlying condition but not to day-to-day fluctuation in symptoms)
Efficiency—in terms of examiner and patient burden

The primary consideration in scale selection remains how well the scale will accomplish the task at hand. Reliability, reproducibility, and sensitivity largely determine the numbers needed in clinical trials. Use of accepted valid scales is important if trial results are to be widely accepted. Scale efficiency also affects costs and patient acceptance. It is difficult to recruit and retain subjects in a trial if the testing is long and arduous and patient dropout affects the number needed and validity of the result.

The number of scales and measures available for some disorders is quite large whereas, for others, few or no scales are available. Ataxia scales are a recent development, and further validation and refinement of these new scales can be expected. Surrogate measures such as magnetic resonance imaging in multiple sclerosis (MS) or positron emission tomography in Parkinson's disease still have limited acceptance but are gradually becoming established. On the other hand, older scales often need to be included in trials, despite their limitations, so that current trial results can be compared with results of previous trials. Thus, while the Multiple Sclerosis Functional Composite Scale has greater sensitivity and reliability, MS trials still need to include the Kurtzke Expanded Disability Status Scale, which has been used in almost all of the clinical trials in MS, has the advantage of familiarity, and allows comparison of current trials with previous trial results.

Generic *Quality of Life Scales* have become increasingly important in recent years and are now required by the Food and Drug Administration for trials of new medications. They add a great deal to our ability to assess the value of new therapies. They cover the total effect of the treatment, providing an overall appreciation of both positive and negative effects. They are covered only to a very limited extent in this volume, mainly with regard to specific diseases where they form the base for a disease-specific, quality-of-life scale. Those interested in exploring generic quality-of-life scales are referred to specific texts on the subject such as McDowell and Newell's *Measuring Health* (McDowell & Newell, 1996).

Over the next decade, we can expect to see development of more tools for measurement of neurologic disease. We are also likely to see rating scales used increasingly for monitoring disease progression and for staging neurologic disease and planning treatment. Already, payers are insisting that patients meet certain criteria to receive medications. We have seen this in MS for the use of interferons and glatiramer acetate and for the use of cholinomimetics and memantine for dementia in the Veterans Affairs medical centers. We can expect to see more requirements for measurement of disease progression and requirements for staging of disease as new and more expensive medications are added to our armamentarium.

Reference

McDowell I, Newell C. *Measuring health* (2nd ed.). New York: Oxford University Press, 1996.

Index